# MEDICAL ABBREVIATIONS:

## 24,000 Conveniences at the Expense of Communications and Safety

### *11th Edition*

Neil M Davis, MS, PharmD, FASHP

Professor Emeritus, Temple University
  School of Pharmacy, Philadelphia, PA,
Editor Emeritus, Hospital Pharmacy
President, Safe Medication Practices
  Consulting, Inc.

published by

**Neil M Davis Associates**
**1143 Wright Drive**
**Huntingdon Valley, PA 19006-2721**

Phone (215) 947-1752 (9 AM-4:30 PM EST, Mon-Fri)
FAX (215) 938-1937
Website www.medabbrev.com
E-mail med@neilmdavis.com

# Contents

# Dedication

This book is dedicated to Julie, my wife, for her support, patience, assistance, and love.

# Acknowledgments

The assistance of Evelyn Canizares, Vicki Bell, Ann Sandt Kishbaugh, Kelly Hogate, Matthew Davis, Robin Miller, Ben Miller, Danial Baker, and Suzette Knight is gratefully acknowledged.

I would like to express my deep appreciation to the many contributions received from readers for their suggested additions and corrections. Please continue to send these to—

Dr. Neil M Davis
1143 Wright Drive
Huntingdon Valley PA 19006-2721
FAX (215) 938 1937
Website www.medabbrev.com
E-mail    med@neilmdavis.com

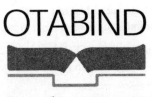

# OTABIND

**Bound to stay open**

The pages in this book open easily and lie flat, a result of the Otabind bookbinding process. Otabind combines advanced adhesive technology and a free-floating cover to achieve books that last longer and are bound to stay open.

# Preface

## Website-Version Access Information

Along with the purchase of each book, the book owner, at no extra cost, is entitled to a single-user license for access to the Internet version of this 11th edition. This license is valid for 24 months from the date of the initial log-in. Internet Explorer 4.0, Netscape 4.0, or AOL 5.0 can meet the minimum browser requirement.

### Features of the Web-Version
- Updated monthly (suggestions from users are welcomed and will be incorporated).
- Can instantaneously search for the meanings of abbreviations and acronyms.
- Has a reverse-search feature, for example, looking for all the abbreviations that contain the word "laparoscopic."
- Can search for cross-referenced generic and brand names of drugs.
- Can search through the listings of symbols, lists, and normal laboratory values.
- Quick access to a list of dangerous abbreviations, an explanation as to why they are dangerous, and suggested alternatives to be used.
- Can read the full-text of the introductory chapters of the book.

### Initial One-time Log-in
- Access the Website at *www.medabbrev.com*
- Click the **Register** button (on the top-left of the screen)
- You will be asked for the 8-letter access code that appears on the front inside cover of the book. This will be the only time you are asked for this code.
- At this point just follow the directions.
- You must agree to the Single-User License Agreement which is presented.
- Note your sign-in name and your self-assigned password. This name/password will only permit one access at a time, so keep this information confidential to ensure your ready access to the site.

A copy of the Multi-User Site License agreement and its price list is available by clicking the "Submit Suggestions" button on *www.medabbrev.com* where you can type a request to receive it.

## Searching for the Meaning of an Abbreviation on the Web-version

- Use upper OR lower case letters as the search engine is NOT case sensitive.
- Use normal upper OR lower case letters as the search engine is NOT sensitive to whether the letters are **bold-face** or *italicized.*
- Superscripts and subscripts are to be entered as regular text.
- For other details, just follow the simple instructions shown on the Website. The Web-version of the book is the same as the print version except for the fact that it is searchable and is updated monthly.

# Chapter 1
# Introduction

**L**isted are current acronyms, symbols, and other abbreviations and 24,000 of their possible meanings. This list has been compiled to assist individuals in reading and transcribing medical records, medically-related communications, and prescriptions. The list, although current and comprehensive, represents a portion of abbreviations in use and their many possible meanings as new ones are being coined every day.

## WARNING

Abbreviations are a convenience, a time saver, a space saver, and a way of avoiding the possibility of misspelling words. However, a price can be paid for their use. Abbreviations are sometimes not understood, misread, or are interpreted incorrectly. Their use lengthens the time needed to train individuals in the health fields, wastes the time of healthcare workers in tracking down their meaning, at times delays the patient's care, and occasionally results in patient harm.

The publication of this list of abbreviations is not an endorsement of their legitimacy. It is not a guarantee that the intended meaning has been correctly captured, or an indication that they are in common use. Where uncertainty exists, the one who wrote the abbreviation must be contacted for clarification.

There are many variations in how an abbreviation can be expressed. Anterior-posterior has been written as AP, A.P., ap, and A/P. Since there are few standards and those who use abbreviations do not necessarily follow these standards, this book only shows anterior-posterior as AP. This is done to make it easier to find the meaning of an abbreviation as all the meanings of AP are listed together. This elimination of unnecessary duplication also keeps the book at a convenient size, thus enabling it to be sold at a reasonable price.

When an abbreviation is made up of a series of abbreviations, it may not be listed as such. In such instances, the meaning may be determined by looking up each set of abbreviations, as in the example of DTP$_a$-HIB-PNU-MEN, which means, diphtheria, tetanus toxoids, acellular pertussis; *Haemophilus influenzae* type b conjugate; pneumococcal (*Streptococcus pneumoniae*) conjugate; meningococcal (*Neisseria meningitidis*) conjugate (serogroups unspecified) vaccine.

Lower case letters are used when firm custom dictates as in Ag, Na, mCi, etc. The first letter of brand names are capitalized, whereas nonproprietary names appear in lower case.

The abbreviation AP is listed as meaning doxorubicin and cisplatin. The reason for this apparent disparity is that the official generic names (United States Adopted Names) are shown rather than the brand names Adriamycin® and Platinol AQ®. In the case of LSD, the official name, lysergide, is given, rather than the chemical name, lysergic acid diethylamide. The Latin derivations for older medical and pharmaceutical abbreviations (t.i.d., *ter in die,* three times daily) may be found in *Remington.*[1]

Some abbreviations which have been encountered or that have been suggested for addition to the book have not been added. Some were obscene or completely insensitive.

Abbreviations for medical facility names create problems as they are usually not recognized by the readers in other geographic areas. A clue to the fact that one is dealing with such an abbreviation is when it ends with MC, for Medical Center; HS, for Health System; MH, for Memorial Hospital; CH, for Community Hospital; UH, for University Hospital; and H, for Hospital.

When an abbreviation which ends with "s" can not be found it might be a plural form of a listed abbreviation.

When an abbreviation cannot be found in this book or when the listed meaning(s) do not make sense, there is a possibility that the abbreviation has been misread. As an example, a reader could not find the meaning of HHTS. On closer examination it really was +HTS, not HHTS. Also EWT could not be identified because it was really ENT.

Some common French and Spanish abbreviations are listed in the book. Because of language structure differences, abbreviations are often reversed, as in the case of HIV, which in Spanish and French is abbreviated as VIH.

Chapter 7 contains a cross-referenced list of 3,400 generic and brand drug names. The list contains names of commonly prescribed and new drugs. Brand names have their first letter capitalized whereas generic names are in lower case. This list will enable readers to obtain the generic name for brand name products or brand names for generic names. It will also serve as a spelling check.

Coded drug names and abbreviations for drug names are found in the chapter on abbreviations (Chapter 4).

Chapter 8 is a table of normal laboratory values. Both the conventional and international values are listed. Each laboratory publishes a list of its normal values. These local lists should be reviewed to see if there are significant differences.

The Council of Biology Editors (CBE), in their 1983 edition of the *CBE Style Manual* listed about 600 abbreviations gathered from 15 internationally recognized authorities and organizations.[2] The majority of these symbols and abbreviations tend to be more scientifically oriented than those which would appear in medical records. In the few situations where the CBE abbreviations differ from what is presented in this book, the CBE abbreviation has been placed in parentheses after the meaning. As is the practice in the United States, mL has been used rather than ml and the spelling of liter, meter, etc. is used rather than litre and metre, even though ml, litre, and metre are listed in the *CBE Style Manual*. A new edition of the *CBE Style Manual* was published in 1995.[3] Again, in this edition, emphasis is placed on scientific abbreviations.

An examination of the abbreviations, acronyms, symbols, and their 24,000 meanings is a testimonial to the problems and dangers associated with most undefined abbreviations.

### References

1. Gennaro AR, ed. Remington's Pharmaceutical Sciences, 20th ed. Phila., PA: Lippincott Williams and Wilkins, 2000.

2. CBE Style Manual, 5th ed. Bethesda, MD: Council of Biology Editors; 1983.

3. Scientific Style and Format: The CBE Manual for Authors, Editors, and Publishers, 6th Ed. Council of Biological Editors-Cambridge University Press. Cambridge UK, New York, Victoria Australia: 1995.

If you encounter abbreviations which are not in this book or on the web-version, please send them to—

Neil M Davis
1143 Wright Drive
Huntingdon Valley, PA 19006

or E-mail them to med@neilmdavis.com
or fax them to 215 938 1937

---

Have you investigated the web-version of this book?
See the Preface for access instructions.

- It is instantaneously searchable for the meanings of abbreviations
- It is reverse searchable (search for all abbreviations containing the word "cardiac")
- Each month, about 100 new entries are added

# Chapter 2

# Dangerous, Contradictory, and/or Ambiguous Abbreviations

Healthcare organizations are advised by the Joint Commission on Accreditation of Healthcare Organizations to formulate a list of dangerous abbreviations which should NOT be used. An example of such a list, which has been adopted from the Institute of Safe Medication Practice Inc. list, is shown as Table 1.

Many inherent problems associated with abbreviations contribute to or cause errors. Reports of such errors have been published routinely.[1–5]

**Abbreviations and symbols can easily be misread or interpreted in an unintended manner. For example:**

(1) "HCT250 mg" was intended to mean hydrocortisone 250 mg but was interpreted as hydrochlorothiazide 50 mg (HCTZ50 mg).

(2) Flucytosine was improperly abbreviated as 5 FU, causing it to be read as fluorouracil. Flucytosine is abbreviated 5 FC and fluorouracil is 5 FU.

(3) Floxuridine was improperly abbreviated as 5 FU, causing it to be read as fluorouracil. Floxuridine is abbreviated FUDR and fluorouracil is 5 FU.

(4) MTX was thought to be mechlorethamine. MTX is methotrexate and mechlorethamine is abbreviated HN2.

(5) **The abbreviation "U" for unit is the most dangerous one in the book, having caused numerous tenfold insulin and heparin overdoses. The word unit should never be abbreviated.** The handwritten U for unit has been mistaken for a zero, causing tenfold errors. The handwritten U has also been read as the number four, six, and as "cc."

**Table 1. Dangerous abbreviations and dosage designations**

| Problem term | Reason | Suggested term |
|---|---|---|
| O.D. for once daily | Interpreted as right eye | Write "once daily" |
| q.o.d. for every other day | Interpreted as meaning "every once a day" or read as q.i.d. | Write "every other day" |
| q.d. for once daily | Read or interpreted as q.i.d. | Write "once daily" |
| q.n. for every night | Read as every hour | Write "every night," "HS," or nightly |
| q hs for every night | Read as every hour | Use "HS" or "at bedtime" |
| TIW for three times a week | Interpeted as T/W (Tuesday & Wednesday); as twice a week; as TID (three times daily) | Write "three times a week" |
| U for Unit | Read as 0, 4, 6, or cc | Write "unit" |
| O.J. for orange juice | Read as OD or OS | Write "orange juice" |
| μg (microgram) | When handwritten, misread as mg | Write "mcg" |
| sq or sub q for subcutaneous | The q is read as every | Use "subcut" |
| IU for international unit | Misread as IV (intravenous) | Use "units" |
| AU for each ear | Read as OU (each eye) | Spell out "each ear" |
| ss for sliding scale or half in the Apothecary system | Read as the number 55 | Spell out "sliding scale" or "1/2" |
| Chemical symbols | Not understood or misunderstood | Write full name |

6

**Table 1. Dangerous abbreviations and dosage designations (continued)**

| Problem term | Reason | Suggested term |
|---|---|---|
| Lettered abbreviations for drug names or drug protocols | Not understood or misunderstood | Use generic or brand name(s) |
| Apothecary symbols or terms per os for by mouth D/C for discharge | Not understood or misunderstood OS read as left eye Interpreted as discontinue (orders for discharge medications result in premature discontinuance of current medication) | Use metric system Use "by mouth," "orally," or "PO" Write "discharge" |
| T/d for one per day / (a slash mark) for with, and, or per | Read as t.i.d. Read as a one | Use "once daily" Use, "and," "with," or "per" |
| Roman numerals | Not understood or misinterpreted (iv read as intravenous rather than 4; iii, X, L, and M, not understood) | Use Arabic numerals (4, 3, 10, 50, 100, etc.) |
| > and < | Not understood or the meaning is reversed | Use "greater than" or "less than" |
| Drug name and dosage not separated by space | Inderal40 mg misread as Inderal 140 mg | Always leave a space between a drug name, dose, and unit of measure |
| Trailing zeros; 1.0 mg Naked decimal point; .5 mL | Decimal point not seen causing tenfold overdose Decimal point not seen causing tenfold overdose | Omit zero; 1 mg Add zero; 0.5 mL |

7

(6) OD, meant to signify once daily, has caused Lugol's solution to be given in the right eye.

(7) OJ meant to signify orange juice, looked like OS and caused saturated solution of potassium iodide to be given in the left eye.

(8) IVP, meant to signify intravenous push (Lasix 20 mg IVP), caused a patient to be given an intravenous pyelogram which is the usual meaning of this abbreviation.

(9) Na Warfarin (sodium warfarin) was read as "No Warfarin."

(10) The abbreviation "s" for "without" has been thought to mean "with" (c).

(11) The order for PT, intended to signify a laboratory test order for prothrombin time, resulted in the ordering of a physical therapy consultation.

(12) The abbreviation "TAB," meant to signify Triple Antibiotic (a coined name for a hospital sterile topical antibiotic mixture), caused patients to have their wounds irrigated with a diet soda. At another facility, with the same set of circumstances, they did not have TAB®, so they used Diet Shasta.®

(13) A slash mark (/) has been mistaken for a one, causing a patient to receive a 100 unit overdose of NPH insulin when the slash was used to separate an order for two insulin doses:

6 units regular insulin/20 units NPH insulin

(14) Vidarabine, an antiviral agent, was ordered as ara-A; however, ara-C, which is cytarabine, an antineoplastic agent, was given.

(15) On several occasions, pediatric strength diphtheria-tetanus toxoids (DT) have been confused with adult strength tetanus-diphtheria toxoids (Td).

(16) DTP is commonly understood to refer to diphtheria-tetanus-pertussis vaccine, but in some hospitals it is also used as shorthand for a sedative cocktail of Demerol, Thorazine, and Phenergan. Several cases have occurred where a child was vaccinated rather than given the sedative mixture.

(17) What does the abbreviation MR mean? Some will guess measles-rubella vaccine (M-R-Vax II, Merck), while others will assume mumps-rubella vaccine (Biavax II, Merck).

(18) The abbreviation TIW (three times a week) was thought to mean Tuesday and Wednesday when the I was read as a slash mark. Due to confirmation bias (you see what you know), this uncommon abbreviation is seen as the more commonly used TID (three times a day).

(19) PCA, meant to be procainamide, was interpreted as patient-controlled analgesia.

(20) $PGE_1$ (alprostadil, Caverject) was read as P6 E1 (Alcon's ophthalmic 6% pilocarpine and 1% epinephrine solution).

(21) A nurse transcribed an oral order for the antibiotic aztreonam as AZT, which was subsequently thought to be the antiviral drug zidovudine.

(22) An order for TAC 0.1%, intended to mean triamcinolone cream, was interpreted as tetracaine, Adrenalin, and cocaine solution.

(23) An order for SPA (salt poor albumin) was overlooked because it was not recognized as a drug order.

(24) Therapy was delayed and considerable professional time was wasted when an order for "Bactrim SS q 12 h on S/S" had to be clarified (Bactrim Single Strength every 12 hours on Saturday and Sunday).

(25) A physician wrote an order stating "may take own supply of EPO". The physician meant evening primrose oil, not Epogen (epoetin alfa).

(26) 4-MP was recommended to treat ethylene glycol poisoning. The medical resident mistakenly interpreted this as 6-MP (6-mercaptopurine). 4-MP is fomepizole (4 methylpyrazole) and 6-MP is mercaptopurine (6-mercaptopurine).

(27) An order for lomustine stated it was to be given at "hs". This was misinterpreted as to mean every night. After continuous administration, toxicity resulted in the patient's death. The drug is normally given once every 6 weeks. State complete orders such as "HS × 1 dose today," "HS nightly," or "HS nightly PRN for sleep."

(28) The directions for an order for Cortisporin Otic Solution indicated "Three drops in ® ear TID." The patient was given the drops in the rear rather than the right ear.

(29) There have been mix-ups between IL-2 and IL-11 when IL-2 is expressed as IL-II (Roman numeral 2). The II has been read as "IL eleven," and vice versa.

IL-2 (interleukin 2) is aldesleukin (Proleukin) and IL-11 is oprelvekin (Neumega).

(30) A drug was ordered "Q 10 h." It was read as QID (four times daily). Drugs should not be ordered at unusual hourly intervals such as every 10, 18, or 36 hours, as this has resulted in a host of errors. Standard times are every 2, 3, 4, 6, 8, or 12 hours; once, twice, three, or four times daily; every other day, or Monday, Wednesday, and Friday and once weekly.

The author would appreciate receiving other examples of abbreviations that have been misinterpreted causing error or delays so that this section can be expanded.

A prescription could be written with directions as follows: "OD OD OD," to mean one drop in the right eye once daily!

Abbreviations should not be used for drug names as they are particularly dangerous. As previously illustrated, there is the possibility that the writer may, through mental error, confuse two abbreviations and use the wrong one. Similarly, the reader may attribute the wrong meaning to an abbreviation. To further confound the problem, some drug name abbreviations have multiple meanings (see ATR, CPM, CPZ, GEM, NITRO, and PBZ in Table 2). The abbreviation AC has been used for three different cancer chemotherapy combinations to mean Adriamycin and either cyclophosphamide, carmustine, or cisplatin.

Beside causing medication errors and incorrect interpretation of medical records, abbreviations can create problems because treatment is delayed while a health professional seeks clarification for the meaning of the abbreviation used. Abbreviations should not be used to designate drugs or combinations of drugs.

Certain meanings of abbreviations in the book are followed by a warning, "this is a dangerous abbreviation." This warning could be placed after many abbreviations, but was reserved for situations where errors have been published because these abbreviations were used or where the meaning is critical and not likely to be known. If no alternative abbreviation is suggested, then the term should be spelled out rather than abbreviated. Such warning statements should also appear after every abbreviation for a drug or drug combination.

## Table 2. Examples of abbreviations that have contradictory or ambiguous meanings

| | |
|---|---|
| ABP | = ambulatory blood pressure |
| | arterial blood pressure |
| | |
| ACU | = acute receiving unit |
| | ambulatory care unit |
| | |
| AMI | = amifostine |
| | amitriptyline |
| | |
| APC | = advanced pancreatic cancer |
| | advanced prostate cancer |
| | |
| ATR | = atropine |
| | atracurium |
| | |
| AZT | = zidovudine |
| | azathioprine |
| | |
| BO | = bowel open |
| | bowel obstruction |
| | |
| CAS | = carotid artery stenosis |
| | cerebral arteriosclerosis |
| | coronary artery stenosis |
| | |
| CF | = cystic fibrosis |
| | Caucasian female |
| | calcium leucovorin (citrovorum factor) |
| | complement fixation |
| | cancer-free |
| | cardiac failure |
| | coronary flow |
| | contractile force |
| | Christmas factor |
| | count fingers |
| | cisplatin and fluorouracil |
| | |
| CLD | = chronic liver disease |
| | chronic lung disease |
| | |
| CPM | = cyclophosphamide |
| | chlorpheniramine maleate |
| | |
| CPZ | = chlorpromazine |
| | Compazine |

| | |
|---|---|
| DW | = dextrose in water |
| | distilled water |
| | deionized water |
| | |
| DXM | = dexamethasone |
| | dextromethorphan |
| | |
| ESLD | = end-stage liver disease |
| | end-stage lung disease |
| | |
| FEC | = fluorouracil, epirubicin, and cyclophosphamide |
| | fluorouracil, etoposide, and cisplatin |
| | |
| GD | = Graves disease |
| | Gaucher disease |
| | |
| GEM | = gemfibrozil |
| | gemicitabine |
| | |
| HD | = Hansen disease |
| | Hodgkin disease |
| | Huntington disease |
| | |
| ICA | = internal carotid artery |
| | intracranial abscess |
| | intracranial aneurysm |
| | |
| IAI | = intra-abdominal infection |
| | intra-abdominal injury |
| | intra-amniotic infection |
| | |
| IT | = intrathecal |
| | intratracheal |
| | intratumoral |
| | |
| LFD | = lactose-free diet |
| | low fat diet |
| | low fiber diet |
| | |
| MP | = melphalan; prednisone |
| | mitoxantrone; prednisone |
| | |
| MPM | = malignant peritoneal mesothelioma |
| | malignant pleural mesothelioma |

| | |
|---|---|
| MS | = morphine sulfate |
| | multiple sclerosis |
| | mitral stenosis |
| | musculoskeletal |
| | medical student |
| | minimal support |
| | muscle strength |
| MS | = mental status |
| | milk shake |
| | mitral sound |
| | morning stiffness |
| MTD | = maximum tolerated dose |
| | minimum toxic dose |
| MTZ | = mirtazapine |
| | mitoxantrone |
| MV | = mechanical ventilation |
| | manual ventilation |
| NBM | = no bowel movement |
| | normal bowel movement |
| | nothing by mouth |
| NE | = no effect |
| | no enlargement |
| | not evaluated |
| NITRO | = nitroglycerin |
| | sodium nitroprusside |
| OLB | = open-liver biopsy |
| | open-lung biopsy |
| PBL | = primary breast lymphoma |
| | primary brain lymphoma |
| PBZ | = phenylbutazone |
| | pyribenzamine |
| | phenoxybenzamine |
| PORT | = postoperative radiotherapy |
| | postoperative respiratory therapy |

| | |
|---|---|
| PVO | = peripheral vascular occlusion |
| | portal vein occlusion |
| | pulmonary venous occlusion |
| | |
| RS | = Reiter syndrome |
| | Reye syndrome |
| | Raynaud disease (syndrome) |
| | rumination syndrome |
| | |
| S & S | = swish and spit |
| | swish and swallow |
| | |
| SAD | = social anxiety disorder |
| | seasonal affective disorder |
| | |
| SDBP | = seated, standing, or supine diastolic blood pressure |
| | |
| SJS | = Schwartz-Jampel syndrome |
| | Stevens-Johnson syndrome |
| | Swyer-James syndrome |
| | |
| SSE | = saline solution enema |
| | soapsuds enema |
| | |
| STF | = special tube feeding |
| | standard tube feeding |
| | |
| TICU | = thoracic intensive care unit |
| | transplant intensive care unit |
| | trauma intensive care unit |
| | |
| TMZ | = temazepam |
| | temozolomide |
| | |
| TS | = Tay-Sachs (disease) |
| | Tourette syndrome |
| | Turner syndrome |
| | |
| VAD | = vincristine, doxorubicin, (Adriamycin) and dexamethasone |
| | vincristine, doxorubicin (Adriamycin) and dactinomycin |

14

## Table 2. Examples of abbreviations that have contradictory or ambiguous meanings (*continued*)

| VAP | = vincristine, Adriamycin, and prednisone |
| | vincristine, Adriamycin, and procarbazine |
| | vincristine, actinomycin D, and Platinol AQ |
| | vincristine, asparaginase, and prednisone |

## References

1. Davis NM, Cohen MR. Medication errors: causes and prevention. Huntingdon Valley, PA: Neil M Davis Associates; 1983.

2. Cohen MR. Medication error reports. Hosp Pharm (appears monthly from 1975 to the present).

3. Cohen MR. Medication errors. Nursing 2001 (appears monthly, starting in Nursing 77, to the present).

4. Davis NM. Med Errors. Am J Nursing (appears monthly from 1994 to 1995).

5. Cohen MR. Medication Errors. American Pharmaceutical Assoc. Wash. DC, 1999.

# Chapter 3

# A Healthcare Controlled Vocabulary

Presently there are no standards for abbreviations used in prescribers' orders, consultations, written prescriptions, standing orders, computer order sets, nurse's medication administration records, pharmacy profiles, hospital formularies, etc. Because in the healthcare field everyone does their own thing, there are many variations. These variations in the way abbreviations are expressed are not always understood and at times are misinterpreted. They cause delays in initiating therapy, cause accidents, waste time for everyone in clarifying these documents, lengthen the time it takes to train those working in the healthcare field, lengthen hospital stays, and waste money.

A controlled vocabulary similar to what is used in the aviation industry is needed. Everyone in the aviation industry "follows the book," and uses a controlled vocabulary. All pilots and air traffic controllers say, "alfa", "bravo", "charlie." See Table 1, the phonetic alphabet. They do not go off on their own and say "adam", "beef", "candy!" They say "one three," not thirteen, because thirteen sounds like thirty. Radio transmission in the aviation industry is not easy to decipher, yet because precision is critical everything possible is done to eliminate error. To prevent errors all radio transmissions are given only in English, every transmission is given in the same order and must be immediately repeated by the receiver to make sure it was heard correctly. Written and oral communication in the medical professions are just as critical and are also not easy to decipher, so establishing a controlled vocabulary is also necessary in this industry.

Listed below are six organizations that have ongoing projects related to standardizing medical terminology:

Computer-Based Patient Record Institute, Inc.
1000 East Woodfield Rd. Suite 102
Schuamburg, IL 60173

The United States Pharmacopeial Convention, Inc.
12601 Twinbrook Parkway
Rockville, MD, 20852

National Library of Medicine
Unified Medical Language Systems
8600 Rockville Pike
Bethesda, MD, 20894

Council of Biological Editors, through their Scientific Style and Format: The CBE Manual for Authors, Editors, and Publishers, 6th Ed. Council of Biological Editors; Cambridge University Press, Cambridge UK, New York, Victoria Australia: 1995

American Medical Association, through their American Medical Assoc. Manual of Style, 9th Edition. AMA, Chicago, 1998

American Association of Medical Transcriptionists through their AAMT Book of Style for Medical Transcriptions, 2nd Edition. American Assoc. for Medical Transcriptions, Modesta CA, 2002

Listed below (Table 2) is the start of a Healthcare Controlled Vocabulary. The basis for this controlled vocabulary is established standard terminology and the result of 37 years of studying medical errors by this author.

It is anticipated that a Healthcare Controlled Vocabulary, with professional organizations' input and backing, will grow and someday evolve into an "official standard." Your suggestions and comments are vital to this growth and eventual recognition. It is always safest to avoid the use of abbreviations unless they are well known in your work environment.

## Table 1. Phonetic Alphabet

The International Civil Aviation Organization phonetic alphabet is used by the aviation industry when communications conditions are such that the information cannot be readily received without their use. Health professionals also should use it when it is necessary to orally spell critical information.

| Character | Telephony | Phonic |
|-----------|-----------|--------|
| A | Alfa | (AL-FAH) |
| B | Bravo | (BRAH-VOH) |
| C | Charlie | (CHAR-LEE) or (SHAR-LEE) |
| D | Delta | (DELL-TA) |
| E | Echo | (ECK-OH) |
| F | Foxtrot | (FOKS-TROT) |
| G | Golf | (GOLF) |
| H | Hotel | (HOH-TEL) |
| I | India | (IN-DEE-AH) |
| J | Juliett | (JEW-LEE-ETT) |
| K | Kilo | (KEY-LOH) |
| L | Lima | (LEE-MAH) |
| M | Mike | (MIKE) |
| N | November | (NO-VEM-BER) |
| O | Oscar | (OSS-CAH) |
| P | Papa | (PAH-PAH) |
| Q | Quebec | (KEH-BECK) |
| R | Romeo | (ROW-ME-OH) |
| S | Sierra | (SEE-AIR-RAH) |
| T | Tango | (TANG-GO) |
| U | Uniform | (YOU-NEE-FORM) or (OO-NEE-FORM) |
| V | Victor | (VIK-TAH) |
| W | Whiskey | (WIS-KEY) |
| X | X-ray | (ECKS-RAY) |
| Y | Yankee | (YANG-KEY) |
| Z | Zulu | (ZOO-LOO) |
| 1 | One | (WUN) |
| 2 | Two | (TOO) |
| 3 | Three | (TREE) |
| 4 | Four | (FOW-ER) |
| 5 | Five | (FIFE) |
| 6 | Six | (SIX) |
| 7 | Seven | (SEV-EN) |
| 8 | Eight | (AIT) |
| 9 | Nine | (NIN-ER) |
| 0 | Zero | (ZEE-RO) |

**Table 2. Examples of a Controlled Vocabulary**

| Standard | What **not** to use or do | Comments |
|---|---|---|
| 100 mg (100 space mg) | 100mg (100 no space mg) | The USP* standard way of expressing a strength is to leave a space between the number and its units. Leaving this space makes it easier to read the number as can be seen below.<br><br>1mg    1 mg<br>10mg   10 mg<br>100mg  100 mg |
| 1 mg | 1.0 mg | This is a USP standard. When a trailing zero is used, the decimal point is sometimes not seen thus causing a tenfold overdose. These overdoses have caused injury and death. |
| 0.1 mL | .1 mL | When the decimal point is not seen, this is read as 1 mL, causing a ten fold overdose. |
| once daily (Do not abbreviate.) | The abbreviation OD<br><br>The abbreviation QD | The classic meaning for OD is right eye. Liquids intended to be given once daily are mistakenly given in the right eye.<br><br>When the Q is dotted too aggressively it looks like Q.I.D. and the medication is given four times daily. When a lower case q is used, the tail of the q has come up between the q and the d to make it look like qid.<br><br>In the United Kingdom, Q.D. means four times daily |
| unit (Do not abbreviate. Write "unit" using a lower-case u) | The abbreviation U | The handwritten U is mistaken for a zero when poorly written causing a 10 fold overdose (i.e. 6 U regular insulin is read as 60). The poorly written U has also been read as a 4, 6, and cc. Write "unit," leaving a space between the number and the word unit. |

20

**Table 2. (cont.)**

| Standard | What **not** to use or do | Comments |
|---|---|---|
| mg (lower case mg with no period) | mg., Mg, Mg, MG, mgm, mgs | The USP standard expression is the mg |
| mL (lower case m with a capital L, no period) | mL., ml, ml, mls, mLs, cc | The USP standard expression is the mL |
| Use generic names or brand names | Do not abbreviate drug names or combinations of drugs, such as CPZ, PBZ, NTG, MS, 5FC, MTX, 6MP, MOPP, ASA, HCTZ, etc.<br><br>Do not use shortened names or chemical names | Abbreviated drug names and acronyms are not always known to the reader; at times they have more than one possible meaning, or are thought to be another drug.<br><br>When the chemical name "6 mercaptopurine" has been used, six doses of mercaptopurine have been mistakenly administered. The generic name, mercaptopurine, should be used.<br><br>When an unofficial shortened version of the name norfloxacin, norflox was used, Norflex was mistakenly given.<br><br>An order for Aredia was read as Adriamycin, as some professionals abbreviated the name Adriamycin as "Adria" which looks like Aredia. |
| The metric system | The apothecary system (grains, drams, minims, ounces, etc.) | The Apothecary system is so rarely used it is not recognized or understood. The symbol for minim (♏) is read as mL; the symbol for one dram (3 T) is read as 3 tablespoons, and gr (grain) is read as gram. |
| Use properly placed commas for numbers above 999, as in 10,000, or 5,000,000 | 5000000 | Many people have difficulty in reading large numbers such as 5000000. The use of commas helps the reader to read these numbers correctly. |

*(continued)*

21

**Table 2. (cont.)**

| Standard | What **not** to use or do | Comments |
|---|---|---|
| 600 mg<br>When possible, do not use decimal expressions.<br>25 mcg | 0.6 g<br><br>0.025 mg | A USP standard. The elimination of decimals lessens the chance for error.<br><br>Mistakes are made when reading numbers less than 1 with decimals. |
| Use specific concentrations and the time in which intravenous potassium chloride should be administered. | Do not use the term "bolus" in conjunction with the administration of potassium chloride injection. | Some physicians will erroneously indicate that potassium chloride injection should be "bolused" or be given "IV push," vaguely meaning that it should not be dripped in slowly. Many deaths have been reported when prescribers have been taken literally and the potassium chloride was given by bolus or IV push for fluid-restricted patients, orders should be specific such as, "20 mEq of potassium chloride in 50 mL of 5% dextrose to run over 30 minutes." |
| use "and" | Do not use a slash (/) mark or the symbol "&" | A slash mark looks like a one. An order written "6 units regular insulin/20 units NPH insulin," was read as 120 units of NPH insulin.<br><br>The symbol "&" has been read as a 4. |
| Orally transmitted medical orders should be read back as heard for verification. | Do not assume that one has spoken or heard correctly. | During oral communications, speakers misspeak and/or transcribers mishear. To minimize these errors, the transmitter must speak clearly and slowly, the transcriber must repeat what was transcribed, and the transmitter must listen attentively when this is being done. Errors are less likely to occur when the prescription is complete. When spelling out words, use the phonetic alphabet shown in Table 1. |

**Table 2. (cont.)**

| Standard | What **not** to use or do | Comments |
|---|---|---|
| When prescriptions are written or orally transmitted they must be complete.<br>• dosage form must be specified<br>• strength must be specified<br>• directions must be specified<br>• included in the directions must be the purpose or indication. | Incomplete orders | Prescribers on occasion think of one drug and mistakenly order another. Nurses and pharmacists on occasion misread prescriptions because of error, poor handwriting or poor oral communications, or look-alike or sound-alike drugs.[1]<br><br>When the prescription is complete and the purpose or indication is included, these errors are less likely to occur. Listing the purpose or indication on the prescription label will assist in increasing patient adherence. |
| Written communications must be legible. | Illegible handwriting | Those who cannot or will not write legibly must print (if this would be legible), type, use a computer, or have an employee write for them and then immediately verify and sign the document. |
| Prescribe specific doses. | Do not prescribe 2 ampuls or 2 vials | There is often more than one size or concentration of drug available. Failing to be specific will lead to unintended doses being administered. |
| Establish a list of dangerous abbreviations which should not be used | Use dangerous abbreviations. | See Chapter 2 of this book "Dangerous, Contradictory, and/or Ambiguous Abbreviations." |
| Use h or hr for hour | ° | An order written as q 4° has been read as q 40 or the symbol ° has not been understood. |
| Specify amount of drug to be given in a single dose.[2] | Specify total amount of drug to be administered over a period of time. | Orders such as ....1,600 mg over 4 days have caused death when mistakenly given as a single dose. Order should state ....400 mg once daily for four days (2-1-03 to 2-4-03) |

*USP = United States Pharmacopeia
1. Davis NM. Look-alike and sound alike drug names. Hosp Pharm 2001, 36, No. 11, Supplement Wall-chart (Call 1-800-223-0554).
2. Kohler D. Standardizing the expression & nomenclature of cancer treatment regimens. Am J Health-System Pharm. 1998;55;137–44

If you encounter abbreviations which are not in this book or on the web-version, please send them to—

Neil M Davis
1143 Wright Drive
Huntingdon Valley, PA 19006

or E-mail them to med@neilmdavis.com
or fax them to 215 938 1937

---

Have you investigated the web-version of this book? See the Preface for access instructions.

- It is instantaneously searchable for the meanings of abbreviations
- It is reverse searchable (search for all abbreviations containing the word "cardiac")
- Each month, about 100 new entries are added

# Chapter 4

# Lettered Abbreviations and Acronyms

Where an abbreviation contains numbers, symbols, punctuation, spaces, etc., they are *not* considered during alphabetizing (6 MP is listed under MP). Entries beginning with a *Greek letter* are alphabetized where the name of the letter would be found alphabetically.

The letter-by-letter (dictionary) system of alphabetizing is used ("*ad lib*" is listed under ADL).

Brand names (proprietary names) have their first letter capitalized, whereas nonproprietary (generic) names are in lower-case letters.

The listing of symbols, numbers, and Greek letters can be found in Chapter 5.

See WARNING in chapter 1.

## A

| | |
|---|---|
| A | accommodation |
| | *Acinetobacter* |
| | adenine |
| | age |
| | alive |
| | ambulatory |
| | angioplasty |
| | anterior |
| | anxiety |
| | apical |
| | arterial |
| | artery |
| | Asian |
| | assessment |
| | auscultation |

| | |
|---|---|
| A+ | blood type A positive (A positive is preferred) |
| A− | blood type A negative (A negative is preferred) |
| A′ | ankle |
| @ | at |
| (a) | axillary temperature |
| $\overline{a}$ | before |
| $A_1$ | aortic first heart sound |
| $A_2$ | aortic second sound |
| A250 | 5% albumin 250 mL |
| A1000 | 5% albumin 1000 mL |
| A II | angiotensin II |
| AA | acetic acid |
| | achievement age |
| | active assistive |
| | acute asthma |
| | affected area |
| | affirmative action |
| | African American |

| | | | |
|---|---|---|---|
| | Alcoholics Anonymous | AACG | acute-angle closure glaucoma |
| | alcohol abuse | | |
| | alopecia areata | AACLR | arthroscopic anterior cruciate ligament reconstruction |
| | alveolar-arterial gradient | | |
| | amino acid | | |
| | anaplastic astrocytoma | AAD | acid-ash diet |
| | anti-aerobic | | antibiotic-associated diarrhea |
| | antiarrhythmic agent | | |
| | aortic aneurysm | $A_1AD$ | alpha$_1$-antitrypsin deficiency |
| | aplastic anemia | | |
| | arm ankle (pulse ratio) | AADA | Abbreviated Antibiotic Drug Application |
| | ascending aorta | | |
| | audiologic assessment | $[A\text{-}a]Do_2$ | alveolar-arterial oxygen tension gradient |
| | Australia antigen | | |
| | authorized absence | AAE | active assistance exercise |
| | automobile accident | | acute allergic encephalitis |
| | cytarabine (ara-C) and doxorubicin (Adriamycin) | AAECS | amino acid enriched cardioplegic solution |
| *aa* | of each | A/AEX | active assistive exercise |
| A&A | aid and attendance | AAF | African-American female |
| | arthroscopy and arthrotomy | AAFB | alcohol acid-fast bacilli |
| | awake and aware | AAG | alpha-1-acid glycoprotein |
| A-a | alveolar arterial (gradient) | AAH | acute alcoholic hepatitis |
| a/A | arterial-alveolar (gradient) | | atypical adenomatous hyperplasia |
| AIIA | Angiotensin II antagonist | AAI | acute alcohol intoxication |
| AAA | abdominal aortic aneurysmectomy (aneurysm) | | arm-ankle index |
| | | | atlantoaxial instability |
| | | | atrial demand-inhibited (pacemaker) |
| | acute anxiety attack | | |
| | Area Agencies on Aging | AAK | atlantoaxial kyphosis |
| | aromatic amino acids | AAL | anterior axillary line |
| A&AA | active and active assistive | AAM | African-American male |
| AAAASF | American Association for Accreditation of Ambulatory Surgery Facilities | | amino acid mixture |
| | | AAMI | age-associated memory impairment |
| | | AAMS | acute aseptic meningitis syndrome |
| AAAE | amino acid activating enzyme | AAN | AIDS-associated neutropenia |
| AAAHC | Accreditation Association of Ambulatory Health Care | | analgesic abuse nephropathy |
| | | | analgesic-associated nephropathy |
| AAC | Adrenalin, atropine, and cocaine | | attending's admission notes |
| | advanced adrenocortical cancer | AANA | American Association of Nurse Anesthetists |
| | antimicrobial agent-associated colitis | AAO | alert, awake, & oriented |
| | augmentative and alternative communication | AAO × 3 | awake and oriented to time, place, and person |
| | | AAOC | antacid of choice |
| AACD | aging-associated cognitive decline | AAP | acute anterior poliomyelitis |

| | | | |
|---|---|---|---|
| | American Academy of Pediatrics (guidelines) | $A_1AT$ | alpha$_1$-antitrypsin |
| | assessment adjustment pass | $A_1AT\text{-}P_i$ | alpha$_1$-antitrypsin (phenotyping) |
| AAPC | antibiotic-associated pseudomembranous colitis | AAU | acute anterior uveitis |
| | | AAV | adeno-associated vector |
| | | | adeno-associated virus |
| AAPMC | antibiotic-associated pseudomembranous colitis | AAVV | accumulated alveolar ventilatory volume |
| | | AAWD | antiandrogen withdrawal |
| a/ApO$_2$ | arterial-alveolar oxygen tension ratio | AB | abortion |
| | | | Ace® bandage |
| AAPSA | age-adjusted prostate-specific antigen | | antibiotic |
| | | | antibody |
| AAR | antigen-antiglobulin reaction | | Aphasia Battery |
| | | | apical beat |
| | automated anesthesia record | | armboard |
| | | | products meeting bioequivalence requirements for generic pharmaceuticals |
| AARF | atlantoaxial rotatory fixation (subluxation; dislocation) | | |
| AAROM | active-assistive range of motion | $A\beta$ | beta-amyloid peptide |
| | | A/B | acid-base ratio |
| AAS | acute abdominal series | | apnea/bradycardia |
| | allergic Aspergillus sinusitis | $A > B$ | air greater than bone (conduction) |
| | androgenic-anabolic steroid | A & B | apnea and bradycardia |
| | | | assault and battery |
| | Ann Arbor stage (Hodgkin disease staging system) | AB+ | AB positive blood type (AB positive preferred) |
| | | AB− | AB negative blood type (AB negative preferred) |
| | aortic arch syndrome | | |
| | atlantoaxis subluxation | ABBI | Advanced Breast Biopsy Instrumentation |
| | atypical absence seizure | | |
| AASCRN | amino acid screen | ABC | abacavir (Ziagen) |
| AASH | adrenal androgen-stimulating hormone | | abbreviated blood count |
| | | | absolute band counts |
| AAST | American Association for the Surgery of Trauma (trauma grading) | | absolute basophil count |
| | | | advanced breast cancer |
| | | | airway, breathing, and circulation |
| AAST-OIS | American Association for the Surgery of Trauma—Organ Injury Scale | | all but code (resuscitation order) |
| | | | aneurysmal bone cyst |
| AAT | activity as tolerated | | antigen-binding capacity |
| | alpha-antitrypsin | | apnea, bradycardia, and cyanosis |
| | androgen ablation therapy | | |
| | at all times | | applesauce, bananas, and cereal (diet) |
| | atrial demand-triggered (pacemaker) | | argon-beam coagulator |
| | atypical antibody titer | | aspiration, biopsy and cytology |
| | automatic atrial tachycardia | | artificial beta cells |

27

automated blood count
(no differential)

avidin-biotin complex

**ABCD** amphotericin B
cholesteryl sulfate
complex (Amphotec;
amphotericin B colloid
dispersion)

**a**symmetry, **b**order
irregularity, **c**olor
variation, and **d**iameter
more than 6 mm
(melanoma warning
signs in a mole)

automated blood count
(differential done
manually)

**ABCDE** botulism toxoid
pentavalent

**ABCS** automated blood count,
STKR (differential done
by machine)

**ABD** after bronchodilator

automated border
detection

type of plain gauze
dressing

**Abd** abdomen

abdominal

abductor

**ABDCT** atrial bolus dynamic
computer tomography

**ABD GR** abdominal girth

**ABD PB** abductor pollicis brevis

**ABD PL** abductor pollicis longus

**ABE** acute bacterial
endocarditis

adult basic education

botulism equine trivalent
antitoxin

**ABECB** acute bacterial
exacerbations of
chronic bronchitis

**ABEP** auditory brain stem-
evoked potentials

**ABF** aortobifemoral
(bypass)

**ABG** air/bone gap

aortoiliac bypass graft

arterial blood gases

axiobuccogingival

**ABH** Ativan, Benadryl, and
Haldol

**ABI** ankle brachial index
(ankle-to-arm systolic
blood pressure ratio)

atherothrombotic brain
infarction

auditory brainstem
implant

**ABID** antibody identification

**A Big** atrial bigeminy

**ABK** aphakic bullous
keratopathy

**ABL** abetalipoproteinemia

allograft bound
lymphocytes

axiobuccolingual

**ABLB** alternate binaural loudness
balance

**ABLC** amphotericin B lipid
complex (Abelcet)

**A/B Mods** apnea/bradycardia
moderate stimulation

**ABMS** autologous bone marrow
support

**A/B MS** apnea/bradycardia mild
stimulation

**ABMT** autologous bone marrow
transplantation

**ABN** abnormality(ies)

advance beneficiary
notice

**abnl bld** abnormal bleeding

**ABNM** American Board of
Nuclear Medicine

**abnor.** abnormal

**ABO** absent bed occupant

blood group system (A,
AB, B, and O)

**ABP** ambulatory blood pressure

androgen-binding protein

arterial blood pressure

**ABPA** allergic bronchopulmo-
nary aspergillosis

**ABPM** allergic bronchopulmo-
nary mycosis

ambulatory blood pressure
monitoring

**ABQAURP** American Board of
Quality Assurance and
Utilization Review
Physicians

**ABR** absolute bed rest

auditory brain-stem
response

| | | | |
|---|---|---|---|
| ABRS | acute bacterial rhinosinusitis | | acyclovir |
| | | | adenocarcinoma |
| ABS | absent | | against clinical advice |
| | absorbed | | aminocaproic acid |
| | absorption | | (Amicar) |
| | Accuchek® blood sugar | | anterior cerebral artery |
| | acute brain syndrome | | anterior communicating |
| | admitting blood sugar | | artery |
| | Alterman-Bishop stent | | anticanalicular antibodies |
| | antibody screen | AC/A | accommodation |
| | at bedside | | convergence– |
| ABSS | Anderson Behavioral | | accommodation (ratio) |
| | State Scale | ACABS | acute community-acquired |
| A/B SS | apnea/bradycardia self- | | bacterial sinusitis |
| | stimulation | ACAD | anterior circulation arterial |
| ABT | aminopyrine breath test | | dissection |
| | antibiotic therapy | ACAS | acute community-acquired |
| ABVD | Adriamycin®, bleomycin, | | sinusitis |
| | vinblastine, and | | asymptomatic carotid |
| | dacarbazine (DTIC) | | artery study |
| ABW | actual body weight | ACAT | acyl coenzyme A: |
| ABx | antibiotics | | cholesterol |
| AC | abdominal circumference | | acyltransferase |
| | acetate | ACB | alveolar-capillary block |
| | acromioclavicular | | antibody-coated bacteria |
| | activated charcoal | | aortocoronary bypass |
| | acute | | before breakfast |
| | African Caribbean | AcB | assist with bath |
| | air conditioned | AC & BC | air and bone conduction |
| | air conduction | ACBE | air contrast barium enema |
| | anchored catheter | ACBG | aortocoronary bypass |
| | antecubital | | graft |
| | anticoagulant | ACBT | active cycle of breathing |
| | arm circumference | | techniques |
| | assist control | ACC | acalculous cholecystitis |
| | autologous cell | | accident |
| | before meals | | accommodation |
| | (*a.c.* preferred) | | adenoid cystic carcinomas |
| | doxorubicin (Adriamycin) | | administrative control |
| | and cyclophosphamide | | center |
| *a.c.* | before meals | | advanced colorectal |
| A-C | Astler-Coller (stages of | | cancer |
| | colorectal cancer | | ambulatory care center |
| A/C | anterior chamber of the eye | | amylase creatinine |
| | assist/control | | clearance |
| A & C | alert and cooperative | | anterior cingulate cortex |
| A₁C | glycosylated hemoglobin | | automated cell count |
| | A₁C | ACCE | Academic Clinical |
| 5-AC | azacitidine | | Coordinator Educator |
| 9AC | rubitecan (9-aminocamp- | AcCoA | acetyl-coenzyme A |
| | tothecin) | ACCR | amylase creatinine |
| ACA | acrodermatitis chronica | | clearance ratio |
| | atrophicans | ACCU | acute coronary care unit |

| ACCU✔ | Accucheck® (blood glucose monitoring) | | arm girth, chest depth, and hip width |
| ACD | absolute cardiac dullness | ACh | acetylcholine |
| | absorbent cover dressing | ACHA | air-conduction hearing aid |
| | acid-citrate-dextrose | AChE | acetylcholinesterase |
| | allergic contact dermatitis | AChEIs | acetylcholinesterase inhibitors |
| | anemia of chronic disease | | |
| | anterior cervical diskectomy | ACHES | abdominal pain, chest pain, headache, eye problems, and severe leg pains (early danger signs of oral contra-ceptive adverse effects) |
| | anterior chamber depth | | |
| | anterior chamber diameter | | |
| | anterior chest diameter | | |
| | before dinner | | |
| | dactinomycin (actinomycin D) | AC & HS | before meals and at bedtime |
| ACDC | antibody complement-dependent cytolysis | ACI | acceleration index |
| | | | adrenal cortical insufficiency |
| AC-DC | bisexual (homo- and heterosexual) | | aftercare instructions |
| | | | anabolic-catabolic index |
| ACDDS | Alcoholism/Chemical Dependency Detoxification Service | | anemia of chronic illness |
| | | | autologous chondrocyte implantation |
| ACDF | anterior cervical diskectomy and fusion | ACIOL | anterior chamber intraocular lens |
| ACDFs | adult children from dysfunctional families | ACIP | Advisory Committee on Immunization Practices (of the Centers for Disease Control and Prevention) |
| ACDK | acquired cystic disease of the kidney | | |
| ACDs | anticonvulsant drugs | | |
| ACE | adrenocortical extract | ACIS | automated cellular imaging system |
| | adverse clinical event | | |
| | aerosol-cloud enhancer | ACJ | acromioclavicular joint |
| | angiotensin-converting enzyme | A/CK | Accuchek® |
| | | ACL | accessory collateral ligament (hand) |
| | antegrade colonic enema | | |
| | doxorubicin (Adriamycin), cyclophosphamide, and etoposide | | anterior cruciate ligament (knee) |
| | | aCL | anticardiolipin (antibody) |
| ACEI | angiotensin-converting enzyme inhibitor | ACLA | aclarubicin |
| | | ACLF | adult congregate living facility |
| ACF | aberrant crypt focus | | |
| | accessory clinical findings | ACLR | anterior cruciate ligament repair |
| | acute care facility | ACLS | advanced cardiac (cardio-pulmonary) life support |
| | anterior cervical fusion | | |
| ACG | accelerography | | Allen Cognitive Level Screen |
| | angiocardiography | | |
| ACGME | Accreditation Council for Graduate Medical Education | ACM | alternative/complementary medicine |
| ACH | adrenal cortical hormone | | Arnold-Chiari malformation |
| | aftercoming head | | |

| | |
|---|---|
| ACME | aphakic cystoid macular edema |
| | Automated Classification of Medical Entities |
| ACMT | advanced combined modality therapy |
| ACMV | assist-controlled mechanical ventilation |
| ACN | acute conditioned neurosis |
| ACNP | Acute Care Nurse Practitioner |
| ACNU | nidran |
| ACOA | Adult Children of Alcoholics |
| ACOG | American College of Obstetricians and Gynecologists |
| A COMM A | anterior communicating artery |
| ACOS-OG | American College of Surgeons Oncology Group |
| ACP | accessory conduction pathway |
| | acid phosphatase |
| | adamantinomatous craniopharyngioma |
| | adenocarcinoma of the prostate |
| | ambulatory care program |
| | anesthesia-care provider |
| | antrochoanal polyp |
| ACPA | anticytoplasmic antibodies |
| AC-PC line | anterior commissure-posterior commissure line |
| AC-PH | acid phosphatase |
| ACPO | acute colonic pseudo-obstruction |
| ACPP | adrenocorticopolypeptide |
| ACPPD | average cost per patient day |
| ACPP PF | acid phosphatase prostatic fluid |
| ACPS | anterior cervical plate stabilization |
| ACQ | acquired |
| | Areas of Change Questionnaire |
| ACR | adenomatosis of the colon and rectum |
| | albumin to creatinine ratio |

| | |
|---|---|
| | anterior chamber reformation |
| | anticonstipation regimen |
| ACR20 | American College of Rheumatology rating scale (20% or more improvement) |
| ACRC | advanced colorectal cancer |
| ACS | anterior compartment syndrome |
| | acute confusional state |
| | acute coronary syndromes |
| | American Cancer Society |
| | anodal-closing sound |
| | automated corneal shaper |
| | before supper |
| ACSF | anterior cervical spine fixation |
| | artificial cerebrospinal fluid |
| ACSL | automatic computerized solvent litholysis |
| ACSVBG | aortocoronary saphenous vein bypass graft |
| ACSW | Academy of Certified Social Workers |
| ACT | activated clotting time |
| | aggressive comfort treatment |
| | allergen challenge test |
| | anticoagulant therapy |
| | assertive community treatment (program) |
| ACT-D | dactinomycin |
| Act Ex | active exercise |
| ACTG | AIDS Clinical Trial Group |
| ACTH | corticotropin (adrenocorticotropic hormone) |
| ACT-Post | activated clotting time post-filter |
| ACT-Pre | activated clotting time pre-filter |
| ACTSEB | anterior chamber tube shunt encircling band |
| ACU | ambulatory care unit |
| ACUP | adenocarcinoma of unknown primary (origin) |
| ACUV | air-contrast ultrasound venography |

A

| | | | |
|---|---|---|---|
| ACV | acyclovir (Zovirax) | ADC | Aid to Dependent Children |
| | amifostine, cisplatin, and vinblastine | | AIDS (acquired immune deficiency syndrome) dementia complex |
| | assist control ventilation | | |
| | atrial/carotid/ventricular | | anxiety disorder clinic |
| A-C-V | A wave, C wave, and V wave | | apparent diffusion coefficient (radiology) |
| ACVD | acute cardiovascular disease | | average daily census |
| ACVP | doxorubicin (Adriamycin), cyclophosphamide, vincristine, and prednisone | | average daily consumption |
| | | ADCA | autosomal dominant cerebellar ataxia |
| | | ADCC | antibody-dependent cellular cytotoxicity |
| ACW | anterior chest wall | A.D.C. VAAN DIML | mnemonic for formatting physician orders: **A**dmit, **D**iagnosis, **C**ondition, **V**itals, **A**ctivity, **A**llergies, **N**ursing procedures, **D**iet, **I**ns and outs, **M**edication, **L**abs |
| | apply to chest wall | | |
| acyl-CoA | acyl coenzyme A | | |
| AD | accident dispensary | | |
| | admitting diagnosis | | |
| | advance directive (living will) | | |
| | air dyne | | |
| | alternating days (this is a dangerous abbreviation) | ADD | adduction |
| | Alzheimer disease | | annual disability density |
| | androgen deprivation | | attention-deficit disorder |
| | antidepressant | | average daily dose |
| | assistive device | ADDH | attention-deficit disorder with hyperactivity |
| | atopic dermatitis | | |
| | axis deviation | ADDL | additional |
| | right ear | ADDM | adjustment disorder with depressed mood |
| A&D | admission and discharge | | |
| | alcohol and drug | ADDP | adductor pollicis |
| | ascending and descending | ADDs | AIDS (acquired immune deficiency syndrome)-defining diseases |
| | vitamins A and D | | |
| ADA | adenosine deaminase | | |
| | American Dental Association | ADDU | alcohol and drug dependence unit |
| | American Diabetes Association | ADE | acute disseminated encephalitis |
| | | | adverse drug event |
| | Americans with Disabilities Act | ADEM | acute disseminating encephalomyelitis |
| | anterior descending artery | ADE-NOCA | adenocarcinoma |
| ADAM | adjustment disorder with anxious mood | | |
| ADAS | Alzheimer Disease Assessment Scale | ADEPT | antibody-directed enzyme prodrug therapy |
| ADAS-COG | Alzheimer Disease Assessment Scale-Cognitive Subscale | ADFT | atrial defibrillation threshold |
| ADAT | advance diet as tolerated | ADFU | agar diffusion for fungus |
| ADAU | adolescent drug abuse unit | ADG | atrial diastolic gallop |
| ADB | amorous disinhibited behavior | | axiodistogingival |
| | | ADH | antidiuretic hormone |

32

|           | atypical ductal hyperplasia |       | anatomical dead space |
| ADHD      | attention-deficit hyperactivity disorder |  | anonymous donor's sperm |
| ADI       | acute diaphragmatic injury |  | antibody deficiency syndrome |
|           | allowable (acceptable) daily intake | ADs | advance directives (living wills) |
|           | axiodistoincisal | ADSU | ambulatory diagnostic surgery unit |
| A-DIC     | doxorubicin and dacarbazine | ADT | admission, discharge, and transfer |
| Adj Dis   | adjustment disorder |       | alternate-day therapy |
| Adj D/O   | adjustment disorder |       | androgen deprivation treatment (therapy) |
| ADL       | activities of daily living |  | |
| ADLG      | average duration of life gained |  | anticipate discharge tomorrow |
| *ad lib*  | as desired |                | any damn thing (a placebo) |
|           | at liberty |                | |
| ADM       | abductor digiti minimi (muscle) |  | Auditory Discrimination Test |
|           | administered (dose) | ADTP | Adolescent Day Treatment Program |
|           | admission |                | |
|           | adrenomedullin |            | Alcohol-Dependence Treatment Program |
|           | doxorubicin (Adriamycin) | ADTR | Academy of Dance Therapists, Registered |
| ADMA      | asymmetrical dimethyl arginine |  | |
| ADME      | absorption, distribution, metabolism, and | ADU | automated dispensing unit |
|           | excretion | ADV | adenovirus vaccine, not otherwise specified |
| ADO       | axiodisto-occlusal |        | |
| Ad-OAP    | doxorubicin, vincristine, cytarabine, and | ADV$_4$ | adenovirus vaccine, type 4, live, oral |
|           | prednisone | ADV$_7$ | adenovirus vaccine, type 7, live, oral |
| ADOL      | adolescent |               | |
| ADON      | Assistant Director of Nursing | A5D5W | alcohol 5%, dextrose 5% in water for injection |
| ADP       | arterial demand pacing | ADX | audiological diagnostic |
|           | adenosine diphosphate | AE | above elbow (amputation) |
| ADPKD     | autosomal dominant polycystic kidney disease |  | accident and emergency (department) |
|           |                           |       | acute exacerbation |
| ADPV      | anomaly of drainage of pulmonary vein |  | adaptive equipment |
|           |                           |       | adverse event |
| ADQ       | abductor digiti quinti |    | air entry |
|           | adequate |                  | anoxic encephalopathy |
| ADR       | acute dystonic reaction |   | antiembolitic |
|           | adverse drug reaction |     | arm ergometer |
|           | alternative dispute resolution |  | aryepiglottic (fold) |
|           | doxorubicin (Adriamycin) | A&E | accident and emergency (department) |
| ADRD      | Alzheimer disease and related disorders | AEA | above-elbow amputation |
|           |                           |       | anti-endomysium antibody |
| ADRIA     | doxorubicin (Adriamycin) |  | |
| ADRV      | adult diarrhea rotavirus | AEB | as evidenced by |
| ADS       | admission day surgery |     | atrial ectopic beat |

| | | | |
|---|---|---|---|
| AEC | at earliest convenience | AET | alternating esotropia |
| AECB | acute exacerbations of chronic bronchitis | | atrial ectopic tachycardia |
| | | AF | acid-fast |
| AECG | ambulatory electrocardiogram | | afebrile |
| | | | amniotic fluid |
| AECOPD | acute exacerbation of chronic obstructive pulmonary disease | | anterior fontanel |
| | | | antifibrinogen |
| | | | aortofemoral |
| AED | antiepileptic drug | | ascitic fluid |
| | automated (automatic) external defibrillator | | atrial fibrillation |
| | | AFB | acid-fast bacilli |
| AEDD | anterior extradural defects | | aorto-femoral bypass |
| AEDF | absent end-diastolic flow (umbilical-artery Doppler ultrasonography) | | aspirated foreign body |
| | | AFB$_1$ | aflatoxin B$_1$ |
| | | AFBG | aortofemoral bypass graft |
| | | AFBY | aortofemoral bypass (graft) |
| AEDP | assisted end-diastolic pressure | AFC | adult foster care |
| | | | air filled cushions |
| | automated external defibrillator pacemaker | | alveolar fluid clearance |
| | | AFDC | Aid to Family and Dependent Children |
| AEE | asthma-exacerbation episodes | | |
| | | AFE | amniotic fluid embolization |
| AEEU | admission entrance and evaluation unit | | |
| | | AFEB | afebrile |
| AEG | air encephalogram | AFEU | ante partum fetal evaluation unit |
| | Alcohol Education Group | | |
| AEIOU TIPS | mnemonic for the diagnosis of coma: Alcohol, Encephalopathy, Insulin, Opiates, Uremia, Trauma, Infection, Psychiatric, and Syncope | AF/FL | atrial fibrillation/atrial flutter |
| | | aFGF | acidic fibroblast growth factor |
| | | AFH | angiomatoid fibrous histiocytoma |
| | | | anterior facial height |
| AELBM | after each loose bowel movement | AFI | acute febrile illness |
| | | | amniotic fluid index |
| AEM | active electrode monitor | A fib | atrial fibrillation |
| | ambulatory electrogram monitor | AFIP | Armed Forces Institute of Pathology |
| | antiepileptic medication | AFKO | ankle-foot-knee orthosis |
| AEP | auditory evoked potential | AFL | air/fluid level |
| AEq | age equivalent | | atrial flutter |
| AER | acoustic evoked response | AFLP | acute fatty liver of pregnancy |
| | albumin excretion rate | | |
| | auditory evoked response | | amplified fragment length polymorphism |
| Aer. M. | aerosol mask | | |
| AERS | adverse event reporting system | A Flu | atrial flutter |
| | | AFM | acute *Plasmodium falciparum* malaria |
| AERs | adverse event reports | | |
| Aer. T. | aerosol tent | | atomic force microscopy |
| AES | adult emergency service | | doxorubicin (Adriamycin), fluorouracil, and methotrexate |
| | anti-embolic stockings | | |
| AEs | adverse events | | |

| | |
|---|---|
| AFM×2 | double-aerosol face mask |
| AFO | ankle-fixation orthotic |
| | ankle-foot orthosis |
| AFOF | anterior fontanel—open and flat |
| AFP | acute flaccid paralysis |
| | alpha-fetoprotein |
| | anterior faucial pillar |
| | ascending frontal parietal |
| AFQT | Armed Forces Qualification Test |
| AFRD | acute febrile respiratory disease |
| AFRIMS | Armed Forces Research Institute of Medical Sciences |
| AFRRI | Armed Forces Radiological Research Institute |
| AFRS | allergic fungal rhinosinusitis |
| AFS | allergic fungal sinusitis |
| Aft/Dis | aftercare/discharge |
| AFV | amniotic fluid volume |
| AFVSS | afebrile, vital signs stable |
| AFX | air-fluid exchange |
| AG | abdominal girth |
| | adrenogenital |
| | aminoglycoside |
| | Amsler grid |
| | anion gap |
| | antigen |
| | antigravity |
| | atrial gallop |
| Ag | silver |
| A/G | albumin to globulin ratio |
| AGA | accelerated growth area |
| | acute gonococcal arthritis |
| | androgenetic alopecia |
| | antigliadin antibody |
| | appropriate for gestational age |
| | average gestational age |
| AGAS | accelerated graft atherosclerosis |
| AG/BL | aminoglycoside/beta-lactam |
| AGC | absolute granulocyte count |
| | advanced gastric cancer |
| AGCUS | atypical glandular cells of undetermined significance |

| | |
|---|---|
| AGD | agar gel diffusion |
| AGE | acute gastroenteritis |
| | advanced glycation end product(s) |
| | angle of greatest extension |
| | anterior gastroenterostomy |
| AGECAT | automatic geriatric examination for computer-assisted taxonomy |
| AGF | angle of greatest flexion |
| AGG | agammaglobulinemia |
| aggl. | agglutination |
| AGI | alpha-glucosidase inhibitor |
| AGL | acute granulocytic leukemia |
| A GLAC-TO-LK | alpha galactoside leukocytes |
| AGN | acute glomerulonephritis |
| AgNO$_3$ | silver nitrate |
| AgNORs | argyrophilic nucleolar organizer regions (staining) |
| $\alpha_1$-AGP | alpha$_1$-acid glycoprotein |
| AGPT | agar-gel precipitation test |
| AGS | adrenogenital syndrome |
| AG SYND | adrenogenital syndrome |
| AGT | alanine-glyoxylate aminotransferase |
| | angiotensinogen |
| AGTT | abnormal glucose tolerance test |
| AGU | aspartylglycosaminuria |
| AGUS | atypical glandular cells of uncertain significance |
| AGVHD | acute graft-versus-host disease |
| AGVI | Ahmed glaucoma valve implantation |
| AH | abdominal hysterectomy |
| | amenorrhea and hirsutism |
| | amenorrhea-hyperprolac-tinemia |
| | antihyaluronidase |
| | auditory hallucinations |
| A&H | accident and health (insurance) |
| AHA | acetohydroxamic acid (Lithostat®) |
| | acquired hemolytic anemia |
| | American Health Association (guidelines) |

| | | | |
|---|---|---|---|
| | autoimmune hemolytic anemia | AHN | adenomatous hyperplastic nodule |
| AHAs | alpha hydroxy acids | | Assistant Head Nurse |
| AHase | antihyaluronidase | AHO | Albright hereditary osteodystrophy |
| AHB$_c$ | hepatitis B core antibody | | |
| AHC | acute hemorrhagic conjunctivitis | AHP | acute hemorrhagic pancreatitis |
| | acute hemorrhagic cystitis | | acute hepatic panel (see page 362) |
| | Adolescent Health Center | | American Herbal Pharmacopeia and Therapeutic Compendium |
| | alternating hemiplegia of childhood | | |
| | avoidable hospitalization conditions | | |
| AHCA | Agency for Healthcare Administration | AhpF | alkyl hydroperoxide reductase, F isomer |
| | American Healthcare Association | AHS | adaptive hand skills |
| | | | allopurinol hypersensitivity syndrome |
| AHCPR | Agency for Health Care Policy and Research | | |
| AHCs | academic health centers | | Alpers-Huttenlocher syndrome |
| AHD | alien-hand syndrome | | |
| | antecedent hematological disorder | | antiepileptic hypersensitivity syndrome |
| | arteriosclerotic heart disease | AHSA | Assistant Health Services Administrator |
| | autoimmune hemolytic disease | AHSCT | autologous hemopoietic stem-cell transplantation |
| AHE | acute hemorrhagic encephalomyelitis | AHST | autologous hematopoietic stem cell transplantation |
| AHEC | Area Health Education Center | | |
| AHF | antihemophilic factor | AHT | alternating hypertropia |
| | Argentine hemorrhagic fever (Junin virus) vaccine | | autoantibodies to human thyroglobulin |
| AHF-M | antihemophilic factor (human), method M, (monoclonal purified) | AHTG | antihuman thymocyte globulin |
| | | AI | accidentally incurred |
| AHFS | American Hospital Formulary Service | | apical impulse |
| | | | allergy index |
| AHG | antihemophilic globulin | | aortic insufficiency |
| AHGS | acute herpetic gingival stomatitis | | artificial insemination |
| | | | artificial intelligence |
| AHHD | arteriosclerotic hyper-tensive heart disease | A & I | Allergy and Immunology (department) |
| AHI | apnea-hypopnea index | | auscultation and inspection |
| AHJ | artificial hip joint | | |
| AHL | apparent half-life | AIA | Accommodation Independence Assessment |
| AHM | ambulatory Holter monitoring | | |
| AHMO | anterior horizontal mandibular osteotomy | | allergen-induced asthma |
| | | | allyl isopropyl acetamide |
| | | | anti-insulin antibody |

|  | aspirin-induced asthma | AIM | anti-inflammatory medication |
|---|---|---|---|
| AI-Ab | anti-insulin antibody |  |  |
| AIBF | anterior interbody fusion | AIMS | Abnormal Involuntary Movement Scale |
| AICA | anterior inferior cerebellar artery |  | Arthritis Impact Measurement Scales |
|  | anterior inferior communicating artery | AIN | acute interstitial nephritis |
| AICBG | anterior interbody cervical bone graft |  | anal intraepithelial neoplasia |
| AICD | activation-induced cell death |  | anterior interosseous nerve |
|  | automatic implantable cardioverter/defibrillator | AINS | anti-inflammatory non-steroidal |
| AICM | anti-inflammatory controller medication | AIO | all-in-one (lipid emulsion, protein, carbohydrate, and electrolytes combined total parenteral nutrition) |
| AICS | acute ischemic coronary syndromes |  |  |
| AID | absolute iron deficiency |  |  |
|  | acute infectious disease | AIOD | aortoiliac occlusive disease |
|  | aortoiliac disease | AION | anterior ischemic optic neuropathy |
|  | artificial insemination donor | AIP | acute infectious polyneuritis |
|  | automatic implantable defibrillator |  | acute intermittent porphyria |
| AIDH | artificial insemination donor husband |  | asymptomatic inflammatory prostatitis |
| AIDKS | acquired immune deficiency syndrome with Kaposi sarcoma | AIPC | androgen-independent prostate cancer |
| AIDP | acute inflammatory demyelinating polyradiculoneuropathy | AIR | accelerated idioventricular rhythm |
|  |  |  | acetylcholine-induced relaxation |
| AIDS | acquired immunodeficiency syndrome | AIS | Abbreviated Injury Score |
|  |  |  | acute ischemic stroke |
| AIE | acute inclusion body encephalitis |  | adolescent idiopathic scoliosis |
| AIEOP | Italian Association of Pediatric Hematology and Oncology (cancer study group) |  | anti-insulin serum |
|  |  | AISA | acquired idiopathic sideroblastic anemia |
| AIF | aortic-iliac-femoral | AIS/ISS | Abbreviated Injury Scale/Injury Severity Score |
| AIH | artificial insemination with husband's sperm |  |  |
|  | autoimmune hepatitis | AIT | adoptive immunotherapy |
| AIHA | autoimmune hemolytic anemia |  | auditory integration therapy |
| AIHD | acquired immune hemolytic disease | AITN | acute interstitial tubular nephritis |
| AIIS | anterior inferior iliac spine | AITP | autoimmune thrombocytopenia purpura |
| AILD | angioimmunoblastic lymphadenopathy with dysproteinemia | AIU | absolute iodine uptake |
|  |  |  | adolescent inpatient unit |

| | | | |
|---|---|---|---|
| AIVC | absence of the inferior vena cava | ALBUMS | aldehyde linker-based ultrasensitive mismatch scanning |
| AIVR | accelerated idioventricular rhythm | ALC | acute lethal catatonia |
| AJ | ankle jerk | | alcohol |
| AJCC | American Joint Committee on Cancer | | alcoholic liver cirrhosis |
| | | | allogeneic lymphocyte cytotoxicity |
| AJO | apple juice only | | alternate level of care |
| AJR | abnormal jugular reflex | | Alternate Lifestyle Checklist |
| AK | above-knee (amputation) | | axiolinguocervical |
| | actinic keratosis | ALCA | anomalous left coronary artery |
| | artificial kidney | | |
| AKA | above-knee amputation | ALCL | anaplastic large-cell lymphoma |
| | alcoholic ketoacidosis | | |
| | all known allergies | ALC R | alcohol rub |
| | also known as (a.k.a. preferred) | ALD | adrenoleukodystrophy |
| | | | alcoholic liver disease |
| a.k.a. | also known as | | aldolase |
| AKP | anterior knee pain | ALDH | aldehyde dehydrogenase |
| AKS | alcoholic Korsakoff syndrome | ALDO | aldosterone |
| | | ALDOST | aldosterone |
| | arthroscopic knee surgery | ALF | acute liver failure |
| AKU | artificial kidney unit | | arterial line filter |
| AL | acute leukemia | | assisted living facility |
| | argon laser | ALFT | abnormal liver function tests |
| | arterial line | | |
| | assisted living | ALG | antilymphoblast globulin |
| | axial length | | antilymphocyte globulin |
| | left ear | ALGB | adjustable laparoscopic gastric banding |
| Al | aluminum | | |
| ALA | alpha-linolenic acid (α-linolenic acid) | ALH | atypical lobular hyperplasia |
| | | ALI | Abbott Laboratories, Inc. |
| | alpha-lipoic acid | | |
| | aminolevulinic acid (Levulan) | | acute lung injury |
| | | | argon laser iridotomy |
| | antileukotriene agent | ALIF | anterior lumbar intradiskal fusion |
| | antilymphocyte antibody | | |
| | as long as | A-line | arterial catheter |
| ALAC | antibiotic-loaded acrylic cement | ALJ | administrative law judge |
| | | ALK | alkaline |
| ALAD | abnormal left axis deviation | | automated lamellar keratoplasty |
| ALA-GLN | alanyl-glutamine | | |
| ALARA | as low as reasonably achievable | ALK Ø | alkaline phosphatase |
| | | ALK ISO | alkaline phosphatase isoenzymes |
| ALAT | alanine aminotransferase (also ALT; SGPT) | | |
| | | ALK-P | alkaline phosphatase |
| ALAX | apical long axis | ALK PHOS ISO | alkaline phosphatase isoenzyme |
| ALB | albumin | | |
| | albuterol | ALL | acute lymphoblastic leukemia |
| | anterior lenticular bevel | | |

| | acute lymphocytic leukemia | | argon laser trabeculo-plasty |
| | allergy | | autolymphocyte therapy |
| ALLD | arthroscopic lumbar laser diskectomy | 2 *alt* | every other day (this is a dangerous abbreviation) |
| ALLO | allogeneic | ALTB | acute laryngotracheobron-chitis |
| Allo-BMT | allogeneic bone marrow transplantation | ALTE | acute (aberrant, apparent) life threatening event |
| Allo-HCT | allogenic hematopoietic cell transplant | *alt hor* | every other hour (this is a dangerous abbreviation) |
| ALM | acral lentiginous melanoma | ALTP | argon laser trabeculo-plasty |
| | alveolar lining material | ALUP | Alupent |
| | autoclave-killed *Leishmania major* | ALv | attachment level (dental) |
| ALMI | anterolateral myocardial infarction | ALVAD | abdominal left ventricular assist device |
| ALN | anterior lower neck | ALWMI | anterolateral wall myocardial infarct |
| | anterior lymph node | | |
| | axillary lymph nodes | ALZ | Alzheimer disease |
| ALND | axillary lymph node dissection | AM | adult male |
| | | | aerosol mask |
| ALNM | axillary lymph node metastasis | | amalgam |
| | | | anovulatory menstruation |
| ALO | apraxia of eyelid opening | | anterior midpapillary |
| | axiolinguo-occlusal | | morning (a.m.) |
| ALOC | altered level of consciousness | | myopic astigmatism |
| Al(OH)₃ | aluminum hydroxide | AMA | advanced maternal age |
| ALOS | average length of stay | | against medical advice |
| ALP | alkaline phosphatase | | American Medical Association |
| | argon laser photocoagulation | | antimitochondrial antibody |
| | Alupent | AMAC | adults molested as children |
| ALPS | autoimmune lymphoproliferative syndrome | AMBI | acute multiple brain infarcts |
| ALPZ | alprazolam (Xanax) | AM Care | brushing teeth, washing face and hands |
| ALR | adductor leg raise | AMAD | morning admission |
| ALRI | acute lower-respiratory-tract infection | AM/ADM | morning admission |
| | anterolateral rotary instability | AMAG | adrenal medullary autograft |
| ALS | acid-labile subunit | AMAL | amalgam |
| | acute lateral sclerosis | AMAN | acute motor axonal neuropathy |
| | advanced life support | AMAP | American Medical Accreditation Program |
| | amyotrophic lateral sclerosis | | as much as possible |
| | antilymphocyte serum | Amask | aerosol mask |
| ALSG | Australian Leukemia Study Group | AMAT | anti-malignant antibody test |
| ALT | alanine aminotransferase (SGPT) | | |

|  |  |
|---|---|
| | Arm Motor Ability Test |
| A-MAT | amorphous material |
| AMB | ambulate |
| | ambulatory |
| | amphotericin B |
| | as manifested by |
| AMBER | advanced multiple beam equalization radiography |
| AMC | arm muscle circumference |
| | arthrogryposis multiplex congenita |
| AM/CR | amylase to creatinine ratio |
| AMD | age-related macular degeneration |
| | arthroscopic microdiskectomy |
| | axiomesiodistal |
| | dactinomycin (actinomycin D) |
| | methyldopa (alpha methyldopa) |
| AME | agreed medical examination |
| | anthrax meningoencephalitis |
| | apparent mineralocorticoid excess (syndrome) |
| | Aviation Medical Examiner |
| AMegL | acute megakaryoblastic leukemia |
| AMES-LAN | American sign language |
| AMF | aerobic metabolism facilitator |
| | amifostine (Ethyol) |
| | autocrine motility factor |
| AMG | acoustic myography |
| | aminoglycoside |
| | axiomesiogingival |
| | Federal Republic of Germany's equivalent to United States Food, Drug, and Cosmetic Act |
| AMGA | American Medical Group Association |
| AMI | acute myocardial infarction |
| | amifostine (Ethyol) |
| | amitriptyline |
| | axiomesioincisal |
| AMKL | acute megakaryocytic leukemia |

| AML | acute myelogenous leukemia |
|---|---|
| | angiomyolipoma |
| | anterior mitral leaflet |
| AMLOS | arithmetic mean length of stay |
| AMLR | auditory midlatency response |
| | Marketing Authorization Application (French) |
| AMM | agnogenic myeloid metaplasia |
| AMML | acute myelomonocytic leukemia |
| AMMOL | acute myelomonoblastic leukemia |
| AMN | adrenomyeloneuropathy |
| amnio | amniocentesis |
| AMN SC | amniotic fluid scan |
| AMOL | acute monoblastic leukemia |
| AMOVA | analysis of molecular variance |
| AMP | adenosine monophosphate |
| | ampere |
| | ampicillin |
| | ampul |
| | amputation |
| | antipressure mattress |
| AMPLE | allergies, medications, past medical history, last meal, events leading to admission (used for history and physical examination) |
| AMPPE | acute multifocal placoid pigment epitheliopathy |
| A-M pr | Austin-Moore prosthesis |
| AMPT | metyrosine (alphamethylpara tyrosine) |
| AMR | acoustic muscle reflex |
| | alternating motion rates |
| AMRI | anterior medial rotary instability |
| AMS | acute maxillary sinusitis |
| | acute mountain sickness |
| | aggravated in military service |
| | altered mental status |
| | amylase |
| | aseptic meningitis syndrome |
| | atypical mole syndrome |

auditory memory span

m-AMSA amsacrine (acridinyl anisidide)

AMSAN acute motor sensory axonal neuropathy

AMSIT portion of the mental status examination:
A—appearance,
M—mood,
S—sensorium,
I—intelligence,
T—thought process

AMT abbreviated mental test
Adolph's Meat Tenderizer
allogeneic (bone) marrow transplant
aminopterin
amount

AMTS Abbreviated Mental Test Score

AMU accessory-muscle use

AMV alveolar minute ventilation
assisted mechanical ventilation

AMY amylase

AMY/CR amylase/creatinine ratio

AN acoustic neuromas
amyl nitrate
anorexia nervosa
anticipatory nausea
Associate Nurse
avascular necrosis

ANA American Nurses Association
antinuclear antibody

ANAD anorexia nervosa and associated disorders

ANADA Abbreviated New Animal Drug Application

ANAG acute narrow angle glaucoma

ANA SWAB anaerobic swab

ANC absolute neutrophil count

ANCA antineutrophil cytoplasmic antibody

anch anchored

ANCN absolute neutrophil count nadir

ANCOVA analysis of covariance

AND anterior nasal discharge
axillary node dissection

ANDA Abbreviated New Drug Application

anes anesthesia

ANF antinuclear factor
atrial natriuretic factor

ANG angiogram

ANG II angiotensin II

ANGIO angiogram

ANH acute normovolemic hemodilution
artificial nutrition and hydration

ANISO anisocytosis

ANK ankle
appointment not kept

ANLL acute nonlymphoblastic leukemia

ANM Assistant Nurse Manager

ANN artificial neural network(s)
axillary node-negative

ANNA artificial neural network analysis

ANOVA analysis of variance

ANP Adult Nurse Practitioner
atrial natriuretic peptide (anaritide acetate)
axillary node–positive

ANPR advanced notice of proposed rule making

ANS answer
autonomic nervous system

ANSER Aggregate Neurobehavioral Student Health and Education Review

ANSI American National Standards Institute

ANT anterior
anthrax vaccine, not otherwise specified
enpheptin (2-amino-5-nitrothiazol)

ANT$_a$ anthrax vaccine, absorbed

*ante* before

ANTI A:AGT anti–blood group A antiglobulin test

Anti bx antibiotic

anti-D anti-D immune globulin

anti-GAD antibodies to glutamic acid decarboxylase

anti-HBc antibody to hepatitis B core antigen (HBcAg)

41

| | | | |
|---|---|---|---|
| anti-HBe | antibody to hepatitis B e antigen (HBeAg) | | anaplastic oligodendroglioma |
| anti-HBs | antibody to hepatitis B surface antigen (HBsAg) | | arterial occlusive disease Assistant-Officer-of-the-Day |
| ant sag D | anterior sagittal diameter | AODA | alcohol and other drug abuse |
| ANTU | alpha naphthylthiourea | | |
| ANUG | acute necrotizing ulcerative gingivitis | AODM | adult-onset diabetes mellitus |
| ANV | acute nausea and vomiting | A of 1 | assistance of one |
| ANX | anxiety | A of 2 | assistance of two |
| | anxious | AOI | area of induration |
| ANZDATA | Australia and New Zealand Dialysis and Transplant Registry | ao-il | aorta-iliac |
| | | AOIVM | angiographically occult intracranial vascular malformation |
| AO | abdominal obesity | | |
| | Agent Orange | AOL | augmentation of labor |
| | anterior oblique | AOLC | acridine-orange leukocyte cytospin |
| | aorta | | |
| | aortic opening | AOLD | automated open lumbar diskectomy |
| | aortography | | |
| | axio-occlusal | AOM | acute otitis media |
| | plate, screw (orthopedics) | | alternatives of management |
| | right ear | | |
| A-O | atlanto-occipital (joint) | AONAD | alert, oriented, and no acute distress |
| A/O | alert and oriented | | |
| A & O | alert and oriented | AOO | anodal opening odor continuous arterial asynchronous pacing |
| A&O × 3 | awake and oriented to person, place, and time | | |
| | | AOP | anemia of prematurity |
| A&O × 4 | awake and oriented to person, place, time, and object | | anodal opening picture aortic pressure apnea of prematurity |
| | | AOR | adjusted odds ratio Alvarado Orthopedic Research at own risk auditory oculogyric reflex |
| AOA | anaplastic oligoastrocytoma | | |
| AOAA | aminooxoacetic acid | | |
| AOAP | as often as possible | | |
| AOB | alcohol on breath | AORT REGURG | aortic regurgitation |
| AOBS | acute organic brain syndrome | | |
| | | AORT STEN | aortic stenosis |
| AOC | abridged ocular chart | | |
| | advanced ovarian cancer | AOS | ambulatory outpatient surgery anode opening sound antibiotic order sheet aortic ostial stenoses arrived on scene |
| | amoxicillin, omeprazole, and clarithromycin | | |
| | anode opening contraction | | |
| | antacid of choice | | |
| | area of concern | | |
| AOCD | anemia of chronic disease | AOSC | acute obstructive suppurative cholangiotomy |
| AOCL | anodal opening clonus | | |
| AOD | adult-onset diabetes | | |
| | alcohol and (and/or) other drugs | AOSD | adult-onset Still disease |
| | alleged onset date | AOTB | alcohol on the breath |

42

| | | | |
|---|---|---|---|
| AOTe | anodal opening tetanus | | activated protein C |
| AP | abdominoperineal | | acute |
| | acute pancreatitis | | pharyngoconjunctiivitis |
| | aerosol pentamidine | | (fever) |
| | alkaline phosphatase | | adenoidal-pharyngeal- |
| | angina pectoris | | conjunctival |
| | antepartum | | adenomatous polyposis of |
| | anterior-posterior (x-ray) | | the colon and rectum |
| | apical pulse | | advanced pancreatic |
| | appendectomy | | cancer |
| | appendicitis | | advanced prostate cancer |
| | arterial pressure | | Ambulatory Payment |
| | arthritis panel | | Classification |
| | (see page 362) | | antigen-presenting cell |
| | atrial pacing | | aspirin, phenacetin, and |
| | attending physician | | caffeine (no longer |
| | doxorubicin (Adriamycin); | | marketed in the US) |
| | cisplatin (Platinol AQ) | | asymptomatic prostate |
| A&P | active and present | | cancer |
| | anterior and posterior | | atrial premature |
| | assessment and plans | | contraction |
| | auscultation and | | autologous packed cells |
| | percussion | APCD | adult polycystic disease |
| A/P | ascites/plasma ratio | APCE | affinity probe capillary |
| $A_2 > P_2$ | second aortic sound | | electrophoresis |
| | greater than second | APCIs | atrial peptide clearance |
| | pulmonic sound | | inhibitors |
| APA | aldosterone-producing | APCKD | adult polycystic kidney |
| | adenoma | | disease |
| | American Psychiatric | APD | acid peptic disease |
| | Association | | action potential duration |
| | anticipatory postural | | afferent pupillary defect |
| | adjustment | | anterior-posterior diameter |
| | antiphospholipid antibody | | atrial premature |
| APAA | anterior parietal artery | | depolarization |
| | aneurysm | | automated peritoneal |
| APACHE | Acute Physiology and | | dialysis |
| | Chronic Health | | pamidronate disodium |
| | Evaluation | | (aminohydroxypropylidene |
| APAD | anterior-posterior | | diphosphate) |
| | abdominal diameter | APDC | Anxiety and Panic |
| APAG | antipseudomonal | | Disorder Clinic |
| | aminoglycosidic | APDT | acellular pertussis vaccine |
| | penicillin | | with diphtheria and |
| APAP | acetaminophen (N acetyl- | | tetanus toxoids |
| | para-aminophenol) | APE | absolute prediction error |
| APB | abductor pollicis brevis | | acute psychotic episode |
| | atrial premature beat | | acute pulmonary edema |
| APBSCT | autologous peripheral | | Adriamycin, cisplatin |
| | blood stem cell | | (Platinol), and etoposide |
| | transplantation | | anterior pituitary extract |
| APC | absolute phagocyte | APER | abdominoperineal excision |
| | count | | of the rectum |

| | |
|---|---|
| APG | ambulatory patient group |
| | Apgar (score) |
| Apgar | appearance (color), pulse (heart rate), grimace (reflex irritability), activity (muscle tone), and respiration (score reflecting condition of newborn) |
| APH | adult psychiatric hospital |
| | alcohol-positive history |
| | antepartum hemorrhage |
| APhA | American Pharmacists Association |
| APHIS | Animal and Plant Health Inspection Service |
| API | active pharmaceutical ingredients |
| | Asian-Pacific Islander |
| APIS | Acute Pain Intensity Scale |
| APIVR | artificial pacemaker-induced ventricular rhythm |
| APKD | adult polycystic kidney disease |
| | adult-onset polycystic kidney disease |
| APL | abductor pollicis longus |
| | accelerated painless labor |
| | acute promyelocytic leukemia |
| | anterior pituitary-like (hormone) |
| | chorionic gonadotropin |
| AP & L | anteroposterior and lateral |
| APLA | antiphospholipid antibody |
| APLD | automated percutaneous lumbar diskectomy |
| APLS | antiphospholipid syndrome |
| APMPPE | acute posterior multifocal placoid pigment epitheliopathy |
| APMS | acute pain management service |
| APN | acquired pendular nystagmus |
| | acute panautonomic neuropathy |
| | acute pyelonephritis |
| | Advanced Practice Nurse |
| APO | adverse patient occurrence |
| | apolipoprotein A-1 |

| | |
|---|---|
| | doxorubicin (Adriamycin), prednisone, and vincristine (Oncovin) |
| APO(a) | apolipoprotein (A) |
| APOE | apolipoprotein E |
| APOE-4 | apolipoprotein-E (gene) |
| APOLT | auxiliary partial orthotopic liver transplantation |
| APOPPS | adjustable postoperative protective prosthetic socket |
| APP | alternating pressure pad |
| | amyloid precursor protein |
| | appetite |
| APPG | aqueous procaine penicillin G (dangerous terminology; since it is for intramuscular use only; write as penicillin G procaine) |
| appr. | approximate |
| appt. | appointment |
| APPY | appendectomy |
| APR | abdominoperineal resection |
| | acute radiation proctitis |
| AP & R | apical and radial (pulses) |
| APRN | Advanced Practice Registered Nurse |
| APRT | abdominopelvic radiotherapy |
| APRV | airway pressure release ventilation |
| APS | Acute Physiology Scoring (system) |
| | adult protective services |
| | Adult Psychiatric Service |
| | antiphospholipid syndrome |
| APSAC | anistreplase (anisoylated plasminogen streptokinase activator complex) |
| APSD | Alzheimer presenile dementia |
| APSP | assisted peak systolic pressure |
| APSS | Associated Professional Sleep Societies |
| aPTT | activated partial thromboplastin time |

| | | | |
|---|---|---|---|
| APU | ambulatory procedure unit | | any reliable brand |
| | antepartum unit | ARBOR | arthropod-borne virus |
| APUD | amine precursor uptake and decarboxylation | ARBOW | artificial rupture of bag of water |
| APV | amprenavir (Agenerase) | ARC | abnormal retinal correspondence |
| APVC | partial anomalous pulmonary venous connection | | AIDS-related complex |
| | | | Alcohol Rehabilitation Center |
| APVR | aortic pulmonary valve replacement | | anomalous retinal correspondence |
| APW | aortopulmonary window | | American Red Cross |
| aq | water | ARCBS | American Red Cross Blood Services |
| AQ | accomplishment quotient | | |
| aq dest | distilled water | ARD | acute respiratory disease |
| AQLQ-J | Asthma Quality of Life Questionnaire—Juniper | | adult respiratory distress |
| | | | antibiotic removal device |
| AQLQ-M | Asthma Quality of Life Questionnaire—Marks | | antibiotic retrieval device |
| A quad | atrial quadrageminy | | aphakic retinal detachment |
| AR | Achilles reflex | ARDMS | American Registry of Diagnostic Medical Sonographers |
| | acoustic reflex | | |
| | active resistance | | |
| | airway resistance | ARDS | adult respiratory distress syndrome |
| | alcohol related | | |
| | allergic rhinitis | ARE | active-resistive exercises |
| | androgen receptor | ARF | acute renal failure |
| | ankle reflex | | acute respiratory failure |
| | aortic regurgitation | | acute rheumatic fever |
| | Argyll Robertson (pupil) | | amylase-rich food (flour) |
| | assisted respiration | | |
| | at risk | ARG | alkaline reflux gastritis |
| | aural rehabilitation | | arginine |
| | autorefractor | | |
| Ar | argon | | |
| A&R | adenoidectomy with radium | ARGNB | antibiotic-resistant gram-negative bacilli |
| | advised and released | ARH | autosomal recessive hypercholesterolemia |
| A-R | apical-radial (pulses) | | |
| ARA | Action Research Arm (test) | ARHL | age-related hearing loss |
| | | ARHNC | advanced resected head and neck cancer |
| | adenosine regulating agent | ARI | acute renal insufficiency |
| ara-A | vidarabine (Vira-A) | | acute respiratory infection |
| ara-AC | fazarabine | | aldose reductase inhibitor |
| ara-C | cytarabine | | arousal index |
| ARAD | abnormal right axis deviation | ARL | acquired immunodeficiency syndrome (AIDS)-related lymphoma |
| ARAS | ascending reticular activating system | | |
| | | | average remaining lifetime |
| | atherosclerotic renal-artery stenosis | ARLD | alcohol-related liver disease |
| ARB | angiotensin II receptor blocker | ARM | anxiety reaction, mild |

artificial rupture of
  membranes

**ARMD** age-related macular
  degeneration

**ARMS** alveolar
  rhabdomyosarcoma
  amplification refractory
  mutation system

**ARN** acute retinal necrosis

**ARND** alcohol-related
  neurodevelopmental
  disorder

**ARNP** Advanced Registered
  Nurse Practitioner

**AROM** active range of motion
  artifical rupture of
  membranes

**ARP** absolute refractory
  period
  acute radiation proctitis
  alcohol rehabilitation
  program

**ARPE** amylase-rich pleural
  effusion

**ARPF** anterior release posterior
  fusion

**ARPKS** autosomal recessive
  polycystic kidney
  disease

**ARPT** acid reflux provocation
  test

**ARR** absolute risk reduction
  anterior rectal resection
  arrive

**ARROM** active resistive range of
  motion

**ARRT** American Registry of
  Radiologic
  Technologists

**ARS** antirabies serum

**ART** Accredited Record
  Technician (for newer
  title, see RHIT)
  Achilles (tendon) reflex
  test
  acoustic reflex
  threshold(s)
  antiretroviral therapy
  arterial
  assessment, review, and
  treatment
  assisted reproductive
  technology

automated reagin test (for
  syphilis)

**ARTIC** articulation

**Art T** art therapy

**ARU** acute receiving unit
  alcohol rehabilitation
  unit

**ARV** AIDS-related virus
  antiretroviral

**ARVC** arrhythmogenic right
  ventricular
  cardiomyopathy

**ARVD** arrhythmogenic right
  ventricular dysplasia
  atherosclerotic
  renovascular disease

**ARVMB** anomalous right
  ventricular muscle
  bundles

**ARW** Accredited Rehabilitation
  Worker

**ARWY** airway

**AS** activated sleep
  anabolic steroid
  anal sphincter
  androgen suppression
  Angelman syndromes
  ankylosing spondylitis
  anterior synechia
  anxiety sensitivity
  aortic stenosis
  atherosclerosis
  atropine sulfate
  AutoSuture®
  doctor called through
  answering service
  left ear

**ASA** American Society of
  Anesthesiologists
  argininosuccinate
  aspirin (acetylsalicylic
  acid)
  as soon as
  atrial septal aneurysm

**ASA I** **American Society of
  anesthesiologists'
  classification**
  Healthy patient with
  localized pathological
  process

**ASA II** A patient with mild to
  moderate systemic
  disease

| | | |
|---|---|---|
| ASA III | A patient with severe systemic disease limiting activity but not incapacitating | |
| ASA IV | A patient with incapacitating systemic disease | |
| ASA V | Moribund patient not expected to live. (These are American Society of Anesthesiologists' patient classifications. Emergency operations are designated by "E" after the classification.) | |
| 5-ASA | mesalamine (5-aminosalicylic acid) (this is a dangerous abbreviation as it is mistaken for five aspirin tablets) | |
| ASAA | acquired severe aplastic anemia | |
| ASACL | American Society of Anesthesiologists Classification | |
| ASAD | arthroscopic subacromial decompression | |
| AS/AI | aortic stenosis/aortic insufficiency | |
| A's & B's | apnea and bradycardia | |
| ASAP | Alcohol and Substance Abuse Program | |
| | as soon as possible | |
| ASAT | aspartate aminotransferase (also AST; SGOT) | |
| ASB | anesthesia standby | |
| | asymptomatic bacteriuria | |
| ASBO | adhesive small-bowel obstruction | |
| ASBS | American Society of Bariatric Surgery | |
| ASC | altered state of consciousness | |
| | ambulatory surgery center | |
| | anterior subcapsular cataract | |
| | antimony sulfur colloid | |
| | apocrine skin carcinoma | |
| | ascorbic acid | |
| ASCAD | atherosclerotic coronary artery disease | |

| | |
|---|---|
| ASCCC | advanced squamous cell cervical carcinoma |
| ASCCHN | advanced squamous cell carcinoma of the head and neck |
| ASCI | acute spinal cord injury |
| ASCO | American Society of Clinical Oncology |
| ASCR | autologous stem cell rescue |
| ASCS | autologous stem cell support |
| ASCT | autologous stem cell transplantation |
| ASCUS | atypical squamous cell of undetermined significance |
| ASCVD | arteriosclerotic cardiovascular disease |
| ASCVR | arteriosclerotic cardiovascular renal disease |
| ASD | aldosterone secretion defect |
| | androstenedione |
| | annual summary dose (ionizing radiation) |
| | atrial septal defect |
| | autism spectrum disorder(s) |
| ASD I | atrial septal defect, primum |
| ASD II | atrial septal defect, secundum |
| ASDA | American Sleep Disorders Association (criteria) |
| ASDH | acute subdural hematoma |
| ASE | abstinence symptom evaluation |
| | acute stress erosion |
| ASEX | Arizona Sexual Experiences (sexual dysfunction scale) |
| ASF | anterior spinal fusion |
| | asymmetric screen film (radiology) |
| ASFR | age-specific fertility rate |
| ASH | asymmetric septal hypertrophy |
| AsH | hypermetropic astigmatism |
| ASHD | arteriosclerotic heart disease |

| | | | |
|---|---|---|---|
| ASI | active specific immunotherapy | ASP | acute suppurative parotitis |
| | Anxiety Status Inventory | | acute symmetric polyarthritis |
| aSi | amorphous silicon | | antisocial personality |
| ASIA | **American Spinal Injury Association (Score)** | | application service provider |
| | A-Complete—No preservation of any motor and/or sensory function below the zone of injury | | asparaginase |
| | | | aspartic acid |
| | | ASPDV | anterior superior pancreaticoduodenal vein |
| | B-Incomplete—Preserved sensation | ASPVD | arteriosclerotic peripheral vascular disease |
| | C-Incomplete—Preserved motor (nonfunctional) | ASR | aldosterone secretion rate |
| | D-Incomplete—Preserved motor (functional) | | automatic speech recognition |
| | E-Complete Recovery | ASRA | Alcohol Severity Rating Scale |
| ASIH | absent, sick in hospital | ASS | anterior superior supine |
| ASIMC | absent, sick in medical center | | aspirin (some European countries) |
| ASIS | anterior superior iliac spine | | assessment |
| | | asst | assistant |
| ASK | antistreptokinase | AST | allergy skin test |
| ASKase | antistreptokinase | | Aphasia Screening Test |
| ASL | American Sign Language | | aspartate aminotransferase (SGOT) |
| | antistreptolysin (titer) | | astemizole |
| ASLO | antistreptolysin-O | | astigmatism |
| ASLV | avian sarcoma and leukosis virus (Rous virus) | AstdVe | assisted ventilation |
| | | ASTH | asthenopia |
| | | ASTI | acute soft tissue injury |
| AsM | myopic astigmatism | AS TOL | as tolerated |
| ASMA | antismooth-muscle antibody | ASTIG | astigmatism |
| | | ASTRO | astrocytoma |
| ASMI | anteroseptal myocardial infarction | ASTM | American Society for Testing and Materials |
| ASO | aldicarb sulfoxide | ASTZ | antistreptozyme test |
| | allele-specific oligodeoxynucleotide (probes) | ASU | acute stroke unit |
| | | | ambulatory surgical unit |
| | Amplatzer Septal Occluder | ASV | antisnake venom |
| | | ASVD | arteriosclerotic vessel disease |
| | antisense oligonucleotides | ASYM | asymmetric(al) |
| | antistreptolysin-O titer | ASX | asymptomatic |
| | arterial switch operation | AT | abdominothoracic |
| | arteriosclerosis obliterans | | activity therapy (therapist) |
| | automatic stop order | | Addiction Therapist |
| As₂O₃ | arsenic trioxide (Trisenox) | | anaerobic threshold |
| ASOT | antistreptolysin-O titer | | antithrombin |
| ASOTP | Affiliate Sex Offender Treatment Provider | | applanation tonometry |
| | | | ataxia-telangiectasia |

48

| | |
|---|---|
| | atraumatic |
| | atrial tachycardia |
| AT 10 | dihydrotachysterol |
| ATA | atmosphere absolute |
| ATB | antibiotic |
| | aquatic therapy bar |
| | atypical tuberculosis |
| ATC | acute toxic class |
| | aerosol treatment chamber |
| | alcoholism therapy classes |
| | all-terrain cycle |
| | antituberculous chemoprophylaxis |
| | around-the-clock |
| | Arthritis Treatment Center |
| | Athletic Trainer, Certified |
| ATCC | American Type Culture Collection |
| ATD | antithyroid drug(s) |
| | anticipated time of discharge |
| | asphyxiating thoracic dystrophy |
| | autoimmune thyroid disease |
| ATE | adipose tissue extraction |
| AT-EI | assistive technology and environmental interventions |
| ATEM | analytical transmission electron microscopy |
| ATF | Alcohol, Tobacco, and Firearms (Bureau) |
| At Fib | atrial fibrillation |
| ATFL | anterior talofibular ligament |
| AT III FUN | antithrombin III functional |
| ATG | antithymocyte globulin |
| ATHR | angina threshold heart rate |
| ATI | Abdominal Trauma Index |
| | acute traumatic ischemia |
| ATL | Achilles tendon lengthening |
| | adult T-cell leukemia |
| | anterior temporal lobectomy |
| | anterior tricuspid leaflet |
| | antitension line |
| | atypical lymphocytes |
| ATLL | adult T-cell leukemia lymphoma |
| ATLP | anterior thoracolumbar locking (implant) plate |

| | |
|---|---|
| ATLS | acute tumor lysis syndrome |
| | advanced trauma life support |
| ATM | acute transverse myelitis |
| | ataxia telangiectasia mutated (gene) |
| | atmosphere |
| At ma | atrial milliamp |
| ATN | acute tubular necrosis |
| ATNC | atraumatic normocephalic |
| aTNM | autopsy staging of cancer |
| ATNR | asymmetrical tonic neck reflex |
| ATO | arsenic trioxide (Trisenox) |
| ATOD-C | Alcohol, Tobacco and Other Drugs, Certified |
| ATP | addiction treatment program |
| | adenosine triphosphate |
| | anterior tonsillar pillar |
| | autoimmune thrombocytopenia purpura |
| ATP III | Adult Treatment Panel III |
| ATPase | adenosine triphosphatase |
| ATPS | ambient temperature & pressure, saturated with water vapor |
| ATR | Achilles tendon reflex |
| | atracurium (Tracrium) |
| | atrial |
| | atropine |
| ATRA | all-*trans* retinoic acid (tretinoin-Vesanoid®) |
| atr fib | atrial fibrillation |
| ATRO | atropine |
| ATRX | acute transfusion reaction |
| ATU | alcohol treatment unit |
| ATV | all-terrain vehicle |
| ATS | American Thoracic Society (guidelines) |
| | antimony trisulfide |
| | antitetanic serum (tetanus antitoxin) |
| | anxiety tension state |
| ATSO | admit to (the) service of |
| ATSO4 | atropine sulfate |
| ATT | alternating triple therapy |
| | antitetanus toxoid |
| | arginine tolerance test |

| | |
|---|---|
| ATTN | attention |
| ATTR | amyloid transtyretin |
| at. wt | atomic weight |
| ATZ | anal transitional zone |
| AU | allergenic (allergy) units |
| | arbitrary units |
| | both ears (this is a dangerous abbreviation, as it may be seen as OU [both eyes]) |
| Au | gold |
| A/U | at umbilicus |
| 198$_{Au}$ | radioactive gold |
| AUA score | American Urological Association—pertains to benign prostatic hypertrophy symptoms |
| AUB | abnormal uterine bleeding |
| AuBMT | autologous bone marrow transplant |
| AUC | area under the curve |
| AUC$_t$ | area under the curve to last time point |
| AUD | amplifiable units of DNA (deoxyribonucleic acid) |
| | arthritis of unknown diagnosis |
| | auditory |
| AUD COMP | auditory comprehension |
| AUDIT | Alcohol Use Disorders Identification Test |
| AUG | acute ulcerative gingivitis |
| AUGIB | acute upper gastrointestinal bleeding |
| AUIC | area under the inhibitory curve |
| AUL | acute undifferentiated leukemia |
| AUR | acute urinary retention |
| AUS | acute urethral syndrome |
| | artificial urinary sphincter |
| | auscultation |
| AUTO | autologous |
| AUTO SP | automatic speech |
| AV | anteverted |
| | anticipatory vomiting |
| | arteriovenous |
| | atrioventricular |
| | auditory visual |
| | auriculoventricular |
| A:V | arterial-venous (ratio in fundi) |

| | |
|---|---|
| AVA | anthrax vaccine, adsorbed |
| | aortic valve atresia |
| | arteriovenous anastomosis |
| AVB | atrioventricular block |
| | Aventis Behring |
| AVC | acrylic veneer crown |
| | aortic valve classification |
| | atrioventricular conduction |
| AVD | aortic valve disease |
| | apparent volume of distribution |
| | arteriosclerotic vascular disease |
| | atrioventricular delay |
| | cerebrovascular accident (French, Spanish) |
| AVDP | asparaginase, vincristine, daunorubicin, and prednisone |
| | avoirdupois |
| AVDO$_2$ | arteriovenous oxygen difference |
| AVE | aortic valve echocardiogram |
| | atrioventricular extrasystole |
| AVED | ataxia with isolated vitamin E deficiency |
| AVF | arteriovenous fistula |
| | augmented unipolar foot (left leg) |
| avg | average |
| AVGS | autologous vein graft stent |
| AVGs | ambulatory visit groups |
| AVH | acute viral hepatitis |
| AVHB | atrioventricular heart block |
| AVJA | atrioventricular junction ablation |
| AVJR | atrioventricular junctional rhythm |
| AVL | augmented unipolar left (left arm) |
| AVLT | auditory verbal learning test |
| AVM | arteriovenous malformation |
| AVN | arteriovenous nicking |
| | atrioventricular node |
| | avascular necrosis |
| AVNB | atrioventricular nodal block |

| | |
|---|---|
| AVNR | atrioventricular nodal re-entry |
| AVNRT | atrioventricular node recovery time |
| | atrioventricular nodal re-entry tachycardia |
| A-VO$_2$ | arteriovenous oxygen difference |
| AVOC | avocation |
| AVP | arginine vasopressin |
| | Aventis Pasteur |
| AVPU | alert, (responds to) verbal (stimuli), (responds to) painful (stimuli), unresponsive (mnemonic used by EMTs to judge patients' level of consciousness) |
| AVR | aortic valve replacement |
| | augmented unipolar right (right arm) |
| AVRP | atrioventricular refractory period |
| AVRT | atrioventricular reciprocating tachycardia |
| AVS | atriovenous shunt |
| AVSD | atrioventricular septal defect |
| AVSS | afebrile, vital signs stable |
| AVT | atrioventricular tachycardia |
| | atypical ventricular tachycardia |
| AvWS | acquired von Willebrand syndrome |
| AW | abdominal wall |
| | abnormal wave |
| | airway |
| A/W | able to work |
| A&W | alive and well |
| AWA | alcohol withdrawal assessment |
| | as well as |
| A waves | atrial contraction wave |
| AWB | autologous whole blood |
| AWDW | assault with a deadly weapon |
| AWE | acetowhite epithelium |
| AWI | anterior wall infarct |
| AWMI | anterior wall myocardial infarction |

| | |
|---|---|
| AWO | airway obstruction |
| AWOL | absent without leave |
| AWP | airway pressure |
| | average wholesale price |
| AWRU | active wrist rotation unit |
| AWS | alcohol withdrawal seizures (syndrome) |
| AWSA | Alcohol Withdrawal Severity Assessment (scale) |
| AWU | alcohol withdrawal unit |
| ax | axillary |
| AXB | axillary block |
| AXC | aortic cross clamp |
| ax-fem.fem. | axilla-femoral-femoral (graft) |
| AXND | axillary node dissection |
| AXR | abdomen x-ray |
| AxSYM® | immunodiagnostic testing equipment |
| AXT | alternating exotropia |
| AY | acrocyanotic (infant color) |
| AZA | azathioprine (Imuran) |
| AZA-CR | azacitidine |
| 5-AZC | azacitidine |
| AzdU | azidouridine |
| AZE | azelastine hydrochloride (Astelin) |
| AZM | acquisition zoom magnification |
| AZQ | diaziquone |
| AZT | zidovudine (azidothymidine; Retrovir) |
| A-Z test | Aschheim-Zondek test (diagnostic test for pregnancy) |

51

# B

| | | |
|---|---|---|
| B | bacillus | |
| | bands | |
| | bilateral | |
| | black | |
| | bloody | |
| | bolus | |
| | both | |
| | botulism (Vaccine B is botulism toxoid) | |
| | brother | |
| | buccal | |
| | See "Plan B" | |
| Ⓑ | both | |
| B+ | blood type B positive (B positive is preferred) | |
| B− | blood type B negative (B negative is preferred) | |
| B₁ | thiamine HCl | |
| B I | Billroth I (gastric surgery) | |
| B II | Billroth II (gastric surgery) | |
| B₂ | riboflavin | |
| B₃ | nicotinic acid | |
| b/4 | before | |
| B₅ | pantothenic acid | |
| B₆ | pyridoxine HCl | |
| B₇ | biotin | |
| B₈ | adenosine phosphate | |
| B₉ | benign | |
| B₁₂ | cyanocobalamin | |
| B19 | parvovirus B19 | |
| BA | backache | |
| | Baptist | |
| | benzyl alcohol | |
| | bile acid | |
| | biliary atresia | |
| | blood agar | |
| | blood alcohol | |
| | bone age | |
| | Bourns assist | |
| | branchial artery | |
| | broken appointment | |
| | bronchial asthma | |
| | buccoaxial | |
| | butyric acid | |
| Ba | barium | |
| B > A | bone greater than air | |
| B < A | bone less than air | |

| | |
|---|---|
| B & A | brisk and active |
| BAA | beta-adrenergic agonist |
| BAAM | Beck airway airflow monitor |
| Bab | Babinski |
| BAC | benzalkonium chloride |
| | blood-alcohol concentration |
| | bronchioloalveolar carcinoma |
| | buccoaxiocervical |
| BACE | beta-site APP (amyloid precursor protein)-cleaving enzyme |
| BACI | bovine anti-cryptosporidium immunoglobulin |
| BACM | blocking agent corticosteroid myopathy |
| BACON | bleomycin, doxorubicin, lomustine, vincristine, and mechlorethamine |
| BACOP | bleomycin, Adriamycin®, cyclophosphamide, vincristine, and prednisone |
| BACPAC | Bulk Activities Post Approval Change |
| BACs | bacterial artificial chromosomes |
| BACT | bacteria |
| | base-activated clotting time |
| BAD | bipolar affective disorder |
| | blunt aortic disruption |
| BADL | basic activities of daily living |
| BaE | barium enema |
| BAE | bronchial artery embolization |
| BAEDP | balloon aortic end diastolic pressure |
| BAEP | brain stem auditory evoked potential |
| BAERs | brain stem auditory evoked responses |
| BaEV | baboon endogenous virus |
| BAG | buccoaxiogingival |
| BAHA | bone-anchored hearing aid |
| BAI | breath-actuated inhalers |
| | Brief Assessment Interview |

| | | | |
|---|---|---|---|
| BAK cage | an interbody fusion system used to stabilize the spine | BAVP | balloon aortic valvuloplasty |
| BAL | balance | BAU | bioequivalent allergy units |
| | blood-alcohol level | BAV | bicuspid aortic valve |
| | British antilewisite (dimercaprol) | BAW | bronchoalveolar washing |
| | bronchoalveolar lavage | BB | baby boy |
| BALB | binaural alternate loudness balance | | backboard |
| | | | back to back |
| BALF | bronchoalveolar lavage fluid | | bad breath |
| | | | bed bath |
| B-ALL | B cell acute lymphoblastic leukemia | | bed board |
| | | | beta-blocker |
| BALT | bronchus-associated lymphoid tissue | | blanket bath |
| | | | blood bank |
| BaM | barium meal | | blow bottle |
| BAN | British Approved Name | | blue bloaters |
| BAND | band neutrophil (stab) | | body belts |
| BANS | back, arm, neck and scalp | | both bones |
| BAO | basal acid output | | breakthrough bleeding |
| BAP | blood agar plate | | breast biopsy |
| BAPS | balance activation proprioceptive system | | brush biopsy |
| | | | buffer base |
| | biomechanical ankle platform system | B&B | bismuth and bourbon |
| | | | bowel and bladder |
| BAPT | Baptist | B/B | backward bending |
| Barb | barbiturate | BBA | born before arrival |
| BARN | bilateral acute retinal necrosis | BBB | baseball bat beating |
| | | | blood-brain barrier |
| BAR Troche | Benadryl, Ativan, and Reglan troche | | bundle branch block |
| | | BBBB | bilateral bundle branch block |
| BAS | behavioral activation system | | |
| | | BBC | Brown-Buerger cystoscope |
| | bile acid sequestrants | BBD | baby born dead |
| | boric acid solution | | before bronchodilator |
| BaS | barium swallow | | benign breast disease |
| BASA | baby aspirin (81 mg chewable tablets of aspirin) | BBE | biofield breast examination |
| | | BBFA | both bones forearm |
| BASIS | Basic Achievement Skills Individual Screener | BBFP | blood and body fluid precautions |
| | | BBI | Bowman Birk inhibitor |
| BASK | basket cells | BBIC | Bowman Birk inhibitor concentrate |
| baso. | basophil | | |
| BASO STIP | basophilic stippling | BBL | bottle blood loss |
| | | BBM | banked breast milk |
| BAT | Behavioral Avoidance Test | BBOW | bulging bag of water |
| | blunt abdominal trauma | BBP | blood-borne pathogen |
| | borreliacidal-antibody test | | butyl benzyl phthalate |
| | brightness acuity tester | BBR | bibasilar rales |
| BATO | boronic acid adduct of technetium oxime | BBS | Berg Balance Scale |
| batt | battery | | bilateral breath sounds |

| | | | |
|---|---|---|---|
| BBSE | bilateral breath sounds equal | BC/BS | Blue Cross/Blue Shield |
| BBSI | Brigance Basic Skills Inventory | BCC | basal cell carcinoma birth control clinic |
| BBT | basal body temperature Buteyko breathing technique | BCCa BCD | basal cell carcinoma basal cell dysplasia bleomycin, cyclophosphamide, and dactinomycin borderline of cardiac dullness |
| BB to MM | belly button to medial malleolus | | |
| B Bx | breast biopsy | | |
| BC | back care | BCDCSW | Board Certified Diplomate in Clinical Social Work |
| | basket catheter | | |
| | battered child | BCDH | bilateral congenital dislocated hip |
| | bed and chair | | |
| | beta carotene | BCE | basal cell epithelioma beneficial clinical event |
| | bicycle | | |
| | birth control | B cell | B lymphocyte |
| | bladder cancer | BCETS | Board Certified Expert in Traumatic Stress |
| | blood culture | | |
| | Blue Cross | BCF | basic conditioning factor Baylor core formula |
| | bone conduction | | |
| | Bourn control | BCG | bacille Calmette-Guérin vaccine bicolor guaiac |
| | breast cancer | | |
| | buccocervical | | |
| | buffalo cap (cap for intravenous line) | BCH | benign coital headache |
| | | BCHA | bone-conduction hearing aid |
| B/C | because | | |
| | blood urea nitrogen/creatinine ratio | BChE | butyrylcholinesterase |
| | | BCI | blunt carotid injury |
| | | BCIR | Barnett continent intestinal reservoir |
| B&C | bed and chair | | |
| | biopsy and curettage | BCL | basic cycle length bio-chemoluminescence |
| | board and care | | |
| | breathed and cried | B/C/L | BUN,(blood urea nitrogen),creatinine, lytes (electrolytes) |
| BCA | balloon catheter angioplasty | | |
| | basal cell atypia | B-CLL | B-cell chronic lymphocytic leukemia |
| | bicinchoninic acid | | |
| | brachiocephalic artery | BCLP | bilateral cleft lip and palate |
| BCAA | branched-chain amino acids | | |
| | | BCLS | basic cardiac life support |
| BC < AC | bone conduction less than air conduction | BCM | below costal margin birth control medication birth control method body cell mass |
| BC > AC | bone conduction greater than air conduction | | |
| B. cat | *Branhamella catarrhalis* | BCME | bis (chloromethyl) ether |
| B-CAVe | bleomycin, lomustine (CCNU), doxorubicin (Adriamycin), and vinblastine (Velban) | BCNP | Board Certified Nuclear Pharmacist |
| | | BCNU | bacteria-controlled nursing unit carmustine |
| BCB | Brilliant cresyl blue (stain) | | |
| BCBR | bilateral carotid body resection | BCOC | bowel care of choice bowel cathartic of choice |

| | | | |
|---|---|---|---|
| BCP | biochemical profile | | 1,4-butanediol |
| | birth control pills | | United Kingdom |
| | blood cell profile | | abbreviation for twice a |
| | carmustine, cyclophos- | | day |
| | phamide, and | B-D | Becton Dickinson and |
| | prednisone | | Company |
| BCPAP | Broun continuous | BDAE | Boston Diagnostic |
| | positive airway pressure | | Aphasia Examination |
| BCQ | breast central | BDAS | balloon dilation atrial |
| | quadrantectomy | | septostomy |
| BCR | bicaudate ratio | BDBS | Bonnet-Dechaume-Blanc |
| | breakpoint cluster region | | syndrome |
| | (gene) | BDC | burn-dressing change |
| | bulbocavernosus reflex | BDCM | bromodichloromethane |
| BCRE | black cohosh root extract | BDD | body dysmorphic disorder |
| BCRS | Brief Cognitive Rate | | bronchodilator drugs |
| | Scale | BDE | bile duct exploration |
| BCRT | breast-conservation | BDF | bilateral distal femoral |
| | followed by radiation | | black divorced female |
| | therapy | BDI | Beck Depression |
| BCS | battered child syndrome | | Inventory |
| | breast-conserving surgery | | bile duct incision |
| | Budd-Chiari syndrome | | bile duct injury |
| BCSF | bone cell stimulating | BDI SF | Beck Depression |
| | factor | | Inventory-Short Form |
| BCSS | bone cell stimulating | BDL | below detectable limits |
| | substance | | bile duct ligation |
| BCT | Bag Carrying Test | B-DLCL | diffuse large B-cell |
| | breast-conserving therapy | | lymphoma |
| | broad complex | BDM | black divorced male |
| | tachycardias | BDNF | brain-derived neurotrophic |
| BCTP | bi-component triton tri-n- | | factor |
| | butyl phosphate | B-DOPA | bleomycin, dacarbazine, |
| BCU | burn care unit | | vincristine (Oncovin), |
| BCUG | bilateral cystourethrogram | | prednisone, and |
| BCVA | best corrected visual | | doxorubicin |
| | acuity | | (Adriamycin) |
| BCVI | blunt cerebrovascular | BDP | beclomethasone |
| | injury | | dipropionate |
| BD | band neutrophil | | best demonstrated |
| | base deficit | | practice |
| | base down | BDR | background diabetic |
| | behavior disorder | | retinopathy |
| | Behçet disease | BDV | Borna disease virus |
| | bile duct | BE | bacterial endocarditis |
| | bipolar disorder(s) | | barium enema |
| | birth date | | Barrett esophagus |
| | birth defect | | base excess |
| | blood donor | | below elbow |
| | brain dead | | bread equivalent |
| | bronchial drainage | | breast examination |
| | bronchodilator | B ↑ E | both upper extremities |
| | buccodistal | B ↓ E | both lower extremities |

| | | | |
|---|---|---|---|
| B & E | brisk and equal | B/F | bound-to-free ratio |
| BEA | below-elbow amputation | B & F | back and forth |
| BEAC | carmustine (BiCNU), etoposide, cytarabine (ara-C), and cyclophosphamide | %BF | percentage of body fat |
| | | BFA | baby for adoption |
| | | | basilic forearm |
| | | | bifemoral arteriogram |
| BEACOPP | bleomycin, etoposide, doxorubicin (Adriamycin), cyclophosphamide, vincristine (Oncovin), procarbazine, and prednisone | BFC | benign febrile convulsion |
| | | bFGF | basic fibroblast growth factor |
| | | BFL | breast firm and lactating |
| | | B-FLY | butterfly |
| | | BFM | Berlin-Frankfurt-Munster (cancer study group) |
| BEAM | brain electrical activity mapping | | black married female |
| | | | body fat mass |
| | | | bright field microscope |
| | carmustine BCNU), etoposide, cytarabine (ara-C), and methotrexate | BFNC | benign familial neonatal convulsions |
| | | BFP | biologic false positive |
| BEAR | Bourn electronic adult respirator | | blue fluorescent protein |
| | | BFR | blood filtration rate |
| BEC | bacterial endocarditis | | blood flow rate |
| BECs | bronchial epithelial cells | B. frag | Bacillus fragilis |
| BED | binge-eating disorder | BFT | bentonite flocculation test |
| | biochemical evidence of disease | | biofeedback training |
| | | BFU$_e$ | erythroid burst-forming unit |
| | biological effective dose | | |
| | biological equivalent dose | BG | baby girl |
| BEE | basal energy expenditure | | basal ganglia |
| BEF | bronchoesophageal fistula | | blood glucose |
| BEGA | best estimate of gestational age | | bone graft |
| | | B-G | Bender-Gestalt (test) |
| BEH | behavior | BGA | Bundesgesundheitsamt (German drug regulatory agency) |
| | benign essential hypertension | | |
| Beh Sp | behavior specialist | B-GA-LACTO | beta galactosidase |
| BEI | bioelectric impedance | | |
| | butanol-extractable iodine | BGC | basal-ganglion calcification |
| BEL | blood ethanol level | | |
| BEP | bleomycin, etoposide, and cisplatin (Platinol) | BGCT | benign glandular cell tumor |
| | | BGDC | Bartholin gland duct cyst |
| | brain stem evoked potentials | BGDR | background diabetic retinopathy |
| BE-PEG | balanced electrolyte with polyethylene glycol | BGL | blood glucose level |
| | | BGM | blood glucose monitoring |
| BEV | billion electron volts | | |
| | bleeding esophageal varices | bGS | biopsy Gleason score |
| | | BGT | Bender-Gestalt test |
| BF | black female | | blood glucose testing |
| | bone fragment | BGTT | borderline glucose tolerance test |
| | boyfriend | | |
| | breakfast fed | | |
| | breast-feed | BH | bowel habits |

| | | | |
|---|---|---|---|
| | breath holding | *b.i.d.* | twice daily |
| BHA | butylated hydroxyanisole | BIDA | amonafide |
| BHC | benzene hexachloride | BIDS | bedtime insulin, daytime |
| | Braxton Hicks | | sulfonylurea |
| | contractions | BIF | bifocal |
| bHCG | beta human chorionic | BIG | botulism immune globulin |
| | gonadotropin | | Breast International Group |
| BHD | carmustine, hydroxyurea, | BIGEM | bigeminal |
| | and dacarbazine | BIH | benign intracranial |
| B-HEXOS- | beta hexosaminidase A | | hypertension |
| A-LK | leukocytes | | bilateral inguinal hernia |
| BHI | biosynthetic human | BIL | bilateral |
| | insulin | | brother-in-law |
| | brain-heart infusion | BILAT | bilateral short leg case |
| BHMCO | behavioral health managed | SLC | |
| | care organization | BILAT | bilateral salpingo- |
| BHN | bridging hepatic necrosis | SXO | oophorectomy |
| BHR | bronchial hyperrespon- | Bili | bilirubin |
| | siveness (hyperactivity) | BILI-C | conjugated bilirubin |
| BHP | boarding home placement | BIL MRY | bilateral myringotomy |
| | British Herbal | BIMA | bilateral internal |
| | Pharmacopeia | | mammary arteries |
| BHS | Beck Hopelessness Scale | BIN | twice a night (this is a |
| | beta-hemolytic | | dangerous abbreviation) |
| | streptococci | BIND | Biological Investigational |
| | breath-holding spell | | New Drug |
| BHT | borderline hypertensive | BIO | binocular indirect |
| | breath hydrogen test | | ophthalmoscopy |
| | butylated hydroxytoluene | BIOF | biofeedback |
| BI | Barthel Index | BIP | bipolar affective disorder |
| | base in | | bleomycin, ifosfamide, |
| | Boehringer Ingelheim | | and cisplatin (Platinol) |
| | Pharmaceuticals, Inc. | | brain injury program |
| | bowel impaction | BiPAP | bilevel (biphasic) positive |
| | brain injury | | airway pressure |
| Bi | bismuth | BiPD | biparietal diameter |
| BIA | bioelectrical impedance | BIPP | bismuth iodoform paraffin |
| | analysis | | paste |
| | biospecific interaction | BIR | back internal rotation |
| | analysis | BIRB | Biomedical Institutional |
| BIB | brought in by | | Review Board |
| BIBA | brought in by ambulance | BIS | behavioral inhibition |
| BIC | brain injury center | | system |
| BICAP | bipolar electrocoagulation | | Bispectral Index |
| | therapy | Bi-SLT | bilateral, sequential single |
| Bicarb | bicarbonate | | lung transplantation |
| BiCNU® | carmustine | bisp | bispinous diameter |
| BICROS | bilateral contralateral | BIT | behavioral inattention test |
| | routing of signals | BIVAD | bilateral ventricular |
| BICU | burn intensive care unit | | (biventricular) assist |
| BID | brought in dead | | device |
| *BID* | twice daily | BIW | twice a week (this is a |
| | (b.i.d. preferred) | | dangerous abbreviation) |

| | | | |
|---|---|---|---|
| BIZ-PLT | bizarre platelets | BLEED | ongoing *b*leeding, *l*ow |
| BJ | Bence Jones (protein) | | blood pressure, *e*levated |
| | biceps jerk | | prothrombin time, |
| | body jacket | | *e*rratic mental status, |
| | bone and joint | | and unstable comorbid |
| BJE | bone and joint | | *d*isease (risk factors for |
| | examination | | continued |
| | bones, joints, and | | gastrointestinal |
| | extremities | | bleeding) |
| BJI | bone and joint infection | BLEO | bleomycin sulfate |
| BJM | bones, joints, and | BLESS | bath, laxative, enema, |
| | muscles | | shampoo, and shower |
| BJOA | basal joint osteoarthritis | BLG | bovine beta-lactoglobulin |
| BJP | Bence Jones protein | BLIC | beta-lactamase inhibitor |
| BK | below knee (amputation) | | combination |
| | bradykinin | BLIP | beta-lactamase inhibiting |
| | bullous keratopathy | | protein |
| BKA | below-knee-amputation | BLL | bilateral lower lobe |
| BKC | blepharokerato- | | blood lead level |
| | conjunctivitis | | brows, lids, and lashes |
| bkft | breakfast | BLLS | bilateral leg strength |
| Bkg | background | BLM | bleomycin sulfate |
| BKTT | below-knee to toe (cast) | BLN | bronchial lymph nodes |
| BKWC | below-knee walking cast | BLOBS | bladder obstruction |
| BKWP | below-knee walking | BLOC | brief loss of |
| | plaster (cast) | | consciousness |
| BL | baseline (fetal heart rate) | BLPB | beta-lactamase-producing |
| | bioluminescence | | bacteria |
| | bland | BLPO | beta-lactamase-producing |
| | blast cells | | organism |
| | blood level | BLQ | both lower quadrants |
| | blood loss | BLR | blood flow rate |
| | blue | BLS | basic life support |
| | bronchial lavage | | Bureau of Labor Statistics |
| | Burkitt lymphoma | BLT | blood-clot lysis time |
| B/L | brother-in-law | | brow left transverse |
| BLA | Biological License | B.L. unit | Bessey-Lowry units |
| | Application | BLV | bovine leukemia virus |
| BLB | Boothby-Lovelace- | BM | bacterial meningitis |
| | Bulbulian (oxygen | | black male |
| | mask) | | bone marrow |
| | bronchoscopic lung | | bone metastases |
| | biopsy | | bowel movement |
| BLBK | blood bank | | breast milk |
| BLBS | bilateral breath sounds | BMA | biomedical application |
| BL = BS | bilateral equal breath | | bismuth subsalicylate, |
| | sounds | | metronidazole, and |
| bl cult | blood culture | | amoxicillin |
| B-L-D | breakfast, lunch, and | | bone marrow aspirate |
| | dinner | | British Medical |
| bldg | bleeding | | Association |
| bld tm | bleeding time | BMAT | basic motor ability |
| BLE | both lower extremities | | test(s) |

| | | | |
|---|---|---|---|
| BMB | bone marrow biopsy | | bone marrow transplant |
| BMBF | German Ministry of Education and Research | BMTH | bismuth, metronidazole, tetracycline, and a histamine H$_2$-receptor antagonist |
| BMC | bone marrow cells | | |
| | bone marrow culture | BMTN | bone marrow transplant neutropenia |
| | bone mineral content | | |
| BMD | Becker muscular dystrophy | BMTT | bilateral myringotomy with tympanic tubes |
| | bone marrow depression | BMTU | bone marrow transplant unit |
| | bone mineral density | | |
| BME | basal medium Eagle (diploid cell culture) | BMU | basic multicellular unit |
| | | BMY | Bristol-Myers Squibb |
| | biomedical engineering | BN | bladder neck |
| | brief maximal effort | | bulimia nervosa |
| BMET | basic metabolic panel (see page 362) | BNBAS | Brazelton Neonatal Behavioral Assessment |
| BMF | between meal feedings | BNC | binasal cannula |
| | black married female | | bladder neck contracture |
| BMFDS | Burke-Marsden-Fahn dystonia rating scale | BNCT | boron neutron capture therapy |
| BMG | benign monoclonal gammopathy | BNE | but not exceeding |
| | | BNF | British National Formulary |
| BMI | body mass index | | |
| BMJ | bones, muscles, joints | BNI | blind nasal intubation |
| BMK | birthmark | BNL | below normal limits |
| BMM | black married male | | breast needle localization |
| | bone marrow micrometastases | Bn M | bone marrow |
| | | BNO | bladder neck obstruction |
| BMMC | bone marrow mononuclear T cells | | bowels not open |
| | | BNP | brain natriuretic peptide |
| BMMM | bone marrow micrometastases | | B-type natriuretic peptide (nesiritide [Natrecor]) |
| B-MODE | brightness modulation | BNPA | binasal pharyngeal airway |
| BMP | basic metabolic profile (panel) (see page 362) | BNR | bladder neck retraction |
| | | BNS | benign nephrosclerosis |
| | behavior management plan | BNT | back to normal |
| | | | Boston Naming Test |
| BMPC | bone marrow plasmacytosis | BO | base out |
| | | | because of |
| BMPs | bone-morphogenic proteins | | behavior objective |
| BMR | basal metabolic rate | | body odor |
| | best motor response | | bowel obstruction |
| BMRM | bilateral modified radical mastectomy | | bowel open |
| | | | bucco-occlusal |
| BMS | Bristol-Myers Squibb Company | B & O | belladonna & opium (suppositories) |
| | burning mouth syndrome | BOA | behavioral observation audiometry |
| BMT | bilateral myringotomy and tubes | | born on arrival |
| | | | born out of asepsis |
| | bismuth subsalicylate, metronidazole, and tetracycline | BOB | ball-on-back |
| | | BOC | beats of clonus |

| | | | |
|---|---|---|---|
| BOD | bilateral orbital decompression | | birthplace |
| | burden of disease | | blood pressure |
| Bod Units | Bodansky units | | body powder |
| BOE | bilateral otitis externa | | British Pharmacopeia |
| BOH | Board of Health | | bullous pemphigoid |
| | bundle of His | | bypass |
| BOLD | bleomycin, vincristine (Oncovin®), lomustine, and dacarbazine | BP-200 | Bourn Infant Pressure Ventilator |
| | | BPA | birch pollen allergy |
| | blood oxygenation level dependent | BPAD | bipolar affective disorder |
| | | BPb | whole blood lead concentration |
| BOM | benign ovarian mass | | |
| | bilateral otitis media | BPCF | bronchopleural cutaneous fistula |
| BOMA | bilateral otitis media, acute | | |
| | | BPI | bipolar disorder, Type I |
| BOME | bilateral otitis media with effusion | BPII | bipolar type II disorder |
| | | BPD | benzoporphyrin derivative |
| BOMP | bleomycin, vincristine (Oncovin), mitomycin, and cisplatin (Platinol AQ) | | biparietal diameter |
| | | | borderline personality disorder |
| | | | bronchopulmonary dysplasia |
| BOO | bladder outlet obstruction | BPd | diastolic blood pressure |
| BOOP | bronchitis obliterans-organized pneumonia | BPD/DS | biliopancreatic diversion with a duodenal switch (surgery for obesity) |
| BOP | bleeding on probing | | |
| BOR | bowels open regularly | BPF | bronchopleural fistula |
| | bronchia-oto-renal (syndrome) | BPH | benign prostatic hypertrophy |
| BORN | State Board of Registration in Nursing | BPG | bypass graft penicillin G benzathine (Bicillin L-A; Permapen) for IM use only |
| BORospA | borreliosis (Lyme disease, *Borrelia* sp.) vaccine, outer surface protein A | | |
| BOS | base of support | BPI | bactericidal/permeability increasing (protein) |
| | bronchiolitis obliterans syndrome | | Brief Pain Inventory |
| BOSS | Becker orthopedic spinal system | BPIG | bacterial polysaccharide immune globulin |
| BOT | base of tongue | BPL | benzylpenicilloylpolylysine |
| | borderline ovarian tumors | BPLA | blood pressure, left arm |
| BOU | burning on urination | BPLND | bilateral pelvic lymph node dissection |
| BOUGIE | bougienage | | |
| BOVR | Bureau of Vocational Rehabilitation | BPM | beats per minute breaths per minute |
| BOW | bag of water | BPN | bacitracin, polymyxin B, and neomycin sulfate |
| BOW-I | bag of water–intact | | |
| BOW-R | bag of water–ruptured | BPO | benzoyl peroxide |
| BP | bathroom privileges | | bilateral partial oophorectomy |
| | bed pan | | |
| | bench press | BPP | biophysical profile |
| | benzoyl peroxide | BPPP | bilateral pedal pulses present |
| | bipolar | | |

| BP,P,R,T, | blood pressure, pulse, respiration, and temperature | | blunt thoracic abdominal trauma |
| BPPV | benign paroxysmal positional vertigo | BRATT | bananas, rice (rice cereal), applesauce, tea, and toast |
| BPR | blood per rectum | BRB | blood-retinal barrier |
| | blood pressure recorder | | bright red blood |
| BPRS | Brief Psychiatric Rating Scale | BRBR | bright red blood per rectum |
| BPS | bilateral partial salpingectomy | BRBPR | bright red blood per rectum |
| | blood pump speed | BRC | bladder reconstruction |
| BPs | systolic blood pressure | BRCM | below right costal margin |
| BPSD | behavioral and psychological symptoms of dementia | BrdU | bromodeoxyuridine |
| | | BRex | breathing exercise |
| | | Br Fdg | breast-feeding |
| | bronchopulmonary segmental drainage | BRFS | biochemical relapse-free survival |
| BPT | BioPort Corporation | BRFSS | Behavioral Risk Factor Surveillance System |
| BPV | benign paroxysmal vertigo | | |
| | benign positional vertigo | BRJ | brachial radialis jerk |
| | bovine papilloma virus | BRM | biological response modifiers |
| Bq | becquerel | | |
| BQL | below quantifiable levels | BRN | brown |
| BQR | brequinar sodium | BRO | brother |
| BR | bathroom | BROM | back range of motion |
| | bedrest | BRONK | bronchoscopy |
| | Benzing retrograde | BRP | bathroom privileges |
| | birthing room | BR RAO | branch retinal artery occlusion |
| | blink reflex | | |
| | bowel rest | BR RVO | branch retinal vein occlusion |
| | brachioradialis | | |
| | breech | BRS | baroreceptor reflex sensitivity |
| | bridge | | |
| | bright red | BrS | breath sounds |
| | brown | BRSV | bovine respiratory syncytial virus |
| Br | bromide | | |
| | bromine | BRU | basic remodeling unit (osteon) |
| BRA | bananas, rice (rice cereal), and applesauce | | |
| | | | brucellosis (*Brucella melitensis*) vaccine |
| | brain | | |
| BRCA1 | breast cancer gene 1 | BRVO | branch retinal vein occlusion |
| BRCA2 | breast cancer gene 2 | | |
| BRADY | bradycardia | BS | barium swallow |
| BRANCH | branch chain amino acids | | bedside |
| BRAO | branch retinal artery occlusion | | before sleep |
| | | | Behçet syndrome |
| BRAS | bilateral renal artery stenosis | | Bennett seal |
| | | | blind spot |
| BRAT | bananas, rice (rice cereal), applesauce, and toast | | blood sugar |
| | | | Blue Shield |
| | Baylor rapid autologous transfuser | | bone scan |
| | | | bowel sounds |

breath sounds

B & S    Bartholin and Skene (glands)

bending and stooping

Brown and Sharp (suture sizes)

BS×4    bowel sounds in all four quadrants

BSA    body surface area

bowel sounds active

Brief Scale of Anxiety

BSAB    Balthazar Scales of Adaptive Behavior

BSAb    broad-spectrum antibiotics

BSAP    bone-specific alkaline phosphatase

BSB    bedside bag

body surface burned

BSC    basosquamous (cell) carcinoma

bedside care

bedside commode

best supportive care

biological safety cabinet

burn scar contracture

BSCC    bedside commode chair

Bjork-Shiley convexoconcave (valves)

BSCVA    best spectacle-corrected visual acuity

BSD    baby soft diet

bedside drainage

BSE    bovine spongiform encephalopathy

breast self-examination

BSEC    bedside easy chair

BSepF    black separated female

BSepM    black separated male

BSER    brain stem evoked responses

BSF    black single female

busulfan

BSG    Bagolini striated glasses

brain stem gliomas

BSGA    beta streptococcus group A

BSI    bloodstream infection

body substance isolation

brain stem injury

BSL    Biological Safety Level

blood sugar level

BSL-1    Biosafety Level 1

BS L base    breath sounds diminished, left base

BSM    black single male

blood safety module

BSN    Bachelor of Science in Nursing

bowel sounds normal

BSNA    bowel sounds normal and active

BSNMT    Bachelor of Science in Nuclear Medicine Technology

BSNT    breast soft and nontender

BSNUTD    baby shots not up to date

BSO    bilateral salpingo-oophorectomy

l-buthionine sulfoximine

bSOD    bovine superoxide dismutase

BSOM    bilateral serous otitis media

BSP    body substance precautions

bone sialoprotein

Bromsulphalein®

BSPA    bowel sounds present and active

BSPM    body surface potential mapping

BSR    body stereotactic radiosurgery

bowels sounds regular

BSRI    Bem Sex Role Inventory

BSRT (R)    Bachelor of Science in Radiologic Technology (Registered)

BSS    Baltimore Sepsis Scale

bedside scale

bismuth subsalicylate

black silk sutures

BSS®    balanced salt solution

BSSG    sitogluside

BSSO    bilateral sagittal split osteotomy

BSSS    benign sporadic sleep spikes

BSST    breast self-stimulation test

BST    bedside testing

bovine somatotropin

brief stimulus therapy

BSU    Bartholin, Skene, urethra (glands)

behavioral science unit

| | | | |
|---|---|---|---|
| BSu | blood sugar | | bitubal interruption |
| BSUTD | baby shots up to date | BTKA | bilateral total knee arthroplasty |
| | Base Service Unit | | |
| BSW | Bachelor of Social Work | BTL | bilateral tubal ligation |
| | bedscale weight | BTM | bilateral tympanic membranes |
| BT | bedtime | | |
| | behavioral therapy | | bismuth subcitrate, tetracycline, and metronidazole |
| | bituberous | | |
| | bladder tumor | | |
| | Blalock-Taussig (shunt) | BTMEAL | between meals |
| | bleeding time | BTO | bilateral tubal occlusion |
| | blood transfusion | BTP | bismuth tribromophenate |
| | blood type | | |
| | blunt trauma | | breakthrough pain |
| | brain tumor | BTPABA | bentiromide |
| | breast tumor | BTPS | body temperature pressure saturated |
| | bowel tones | | |
| Bt | *Bacillus thuringiensis* | BTR | bladder tumor recheck |
| B-T | Blalock-Taussig (shunt) | BTS | Blalock-Taussig shunt |
| B/T | between | BTSH | bovine thyrotropin |
| Bt# | bottle number | BTU | behavior therapy unit |
| BTA | below the ankle | BTW | back to work |
| | bladder tumor antigen | | between |
| | bladder tumor-associated analytes | BTW M | between meals |
| | | BTX | Botulinum toxin type A (Botox) |
| | botulinum toxic type A (Botox) | | |
| | | BtxA | botulinum toxin type A (Botox) |
| BTA-A | botulinum toxin type A (Botox) | | |
| | | BU | base up (prism) |
| BTB | back to bed | | below umbilicus |
| | beat-to-beat (variability) | | Bodansky units |
| | breakthrough bleeding | | burn unit |
| BTBV | beat-to-beat variability | | busulfan |
| BTC | bilateral tubal cautery | BUA | broadband ultrasound attenuation |
| | biliary tree cancer | | |
| | bladder tumor check | BUCAT | busulfan, carboplatin, and thiotepa |
| | by the clock | | |
| BTE | Baltimore Therapeutic Equipment | BuCy | busulfan and cyclophosphamide |
| | | BUD | budesonide (Rhinocort) |
| | behind-the-ear (hearing aid) | BUdR | bromodeoxyuridine |
| | | BUE | both upper extremities |
| | bisected, totally embedded | BUFA | baby up for adoption |
| BTF | blenderized tube feeding | BUN | blood urea nitrogen |
| | | | bunion |
| BTFS | breast tumor frozen section | BUO | bleeding of undetermined origin |
| | | | |
| BTG | beta thromboglobulin | BUR | back-up rate (ventilator) |
| B-Thal | beta thalassemia | Burd | Burdick suction |
| BTHOOM | beats the hell out of me (better stated as "differed diagnosis") | BUS | Bartholin, urethral, and Skene glands |
| | | | bladder ultrasound |
| BTI | biliary tract infection | | bulbourethral sling |

| BUSV | Bartholin urethral Skeins vagina |
| BUT | biopsy urease test |
| | break up time |
| BV | bacterial vaginitis |
| | biological value |
| | blood volume |
| BVAD | biventricular assist device |
| BVD | bovine viral diarrhea |
| BVDU | bromovinlydeoxyuridine (brivudin) |
| BVE | blood volume expander |
| BVF | bulboventricular foramen |
| BVH | biventricular hypertrophy |
| BVL | bilateral vas ligation |
| BVM | bag valve mask |
| BVMG | Bender Visual-Motor Gestalt (test) |
| BVO | branch vein occlusion |
| BVR | Bureau of Vocational Rehabilitation |
| BVRO | bilateral vertical ramus osteotomy |
| BVRT | Benton Visual Retention Test |
| BVT | bilateral ventilation tubes |
| BW | bandwidth (radiology) |
| | birth weight |
| | bite-wing (radiograph) |
| | body water |
| | body weight |
| B & W | Black and White (milk of magnesia & aromatic cascara fluidextract) |
| BWA | bed-wetter admission |
| BWCS | bagged white cell study |
| BWF | Blackwater fever |
| BWFI | bacteriostatic water for injection |
| BWidF | black widowed female |
| BWidM | black widowed male |
| BWS | battered woman syndrome |
| | Beckwith-Wiedemann syndrome |
| BWs | bite-wing (x-rays) |
| BWT | bowel wall thickness |
| BWX | bite-wing x-ray |
| Bx | biopsy |
| B × B | back-to-back |

| BX BS | Blue Cross and Blue Shield |
| BXM | B-cell crossmatch |
| ΦBZ | phenylbutazone |
| BZD | benzodiazepine |
| BZDZ | benzodiazepine |

# C

| | |
|---|---|
| C | ascorbic acid |
| | carbohydrate |
| | Catholic |
| | Caucasian |
| | Celsius |
| | centigrade |
| | *C*hlamydia |
| | clubbing |
| | conjunctiva |
| | constricted |
| | cyanosis |
| | cytosine |
| | hundred |
| $\bar{c}$ | with |
| C′ | cervical spine |
| C+ | with contrast |
| C− | without contrast |
| C 1 | cyclopentolate 1% ophthalmic solution (Cyclogyl) |
| $C_1$–$C_7$ | cervical vertebra 1 through 7 |
| $C_1$–$C_8$ | cervical nerves 1 through 8 |
| $C_1$–$C_9$ | precursor molecules of the complement system |
| $C_1$–$C_{12}$ | cranial nerves 1 to 12 |
| C3 | complement C3 |
| C4 | complement C4 |
| CI-CV | Drug Enforcement Agency scheduled substances class one through five |
| $C_{II}$ | second cranial nerve |
| CA | cancelled appointment |
| | *Candida albicans* |
| | carcinoma |
| | cardiac arrest |
| | carotid artery |
| | celiac artery |
| | cellulose acetate (filter) |
| | Certified Acupuncturist |
| | chronologic age |
| | Cocaine Anonymous |
| | community-acquired |
| | compressed air |
| | continuous aerosol |
| | coronary angioplasty |
| | coronary artery |

| | |
|---|---|
| Ca | calcium |
| C/A | conscious, alert |
| Ca++ | calcification |
| | calcium |
| CA 125 | cancer antigen 125 |
| C&A | Clinitest® and Acetest® |
| CAA | coloanal anastamosis |
| | crystalline amino acids |
| CAAP-1 | Certified Associate Addiction Professional Level 1 |
| CAB | catheter-associated bacteriuria |
| | cellulose acetate butyrate |
| | combined androgen blockade |
| | complete atrioventricular block |
| | coronary artery bypass |
| CAB-BAGE | coronary artery bypass graft |
| CABG | coronary artery bypass graft |
| CaBI | calcium bone index |
| CaBP | calcium-binding protein |
| CABS | coronary artery bypass surgery |
| CAC | cardioacceleratory center |
| | Certified Alcohol Counselor |
| | Community Action Center |
| | coronary artery calcification |
| CACI | computer-assisted continuous infusion |
| $CaCl_2$ | calcium chloride |
| $CaCO_3$ | calcium carbonate |
| CACP | cisplatin |
| CACS | cancer-related anorexia/cachexia |
| CAD | cadaver (kidney donor) |
| | calcium alginate dressing |
| | computer-aided diagnosis |
| | computer-aided dispatch |
| | coronary artery disease |
| CADAC | Certified Alcohol and Drug Abuse Counselor |
| CADASIL | cerebral autosomal dominant arteriopathy with subcortical infarcts and leukoencephalopathy |

| | | |
|---|---|---|
| CADD® | Computerized Ambulatory Drug Delivery (pump) | |
| CADL | communication activities of daily living (speech/cognitive test) | |
| CADP | computer-assisted design of prosthesis | |
| CADRF | coronary artery disease risk factors | |
| CADXPL | cadaver transplant | |
| CAE | cellulose acetate electrophoresis | |
| | coronary artery endarterectomy | |
| | cyclophosphamide, doxorubicin (Adriamycin), and etoposide | |
| ℭAEC | cardiac arrhythmia evaluation center | |
| CaEDTA | calcium disodium edetate | |
| CAF | chronic atrial fibrillation | |
| | controlled atrial flutter/fibrillation | |
| | cyclophosphamide, doxorubicin (Adriamycin), and fluorouracil | |
| CAFF | controlled atrial fibrillation/flutter | |
| CAFT | Clinitron® air fluidized therapy | |
| CAG | chronic atrophic gastritis | |
| | closed angle glaucoma | |
| | continuous ambulatory gamma globin (infusion) | |
| | coronary arteriography | |
| CaG | calcium gluconate | |
| CAGE | a questionnaire for alcoholism evaluation C Have you ever felt the need to cut down on your drinking? A Have you ever felt annoyed by criticism of your drinking? G Have you ever felt guilty abut your drinking? E Have you ever taken a drink (eye opener) first thing in the morning? | |
| CAH | chronic active hepatitis | |

| | | |
|---|---|---|
| | chronic aggressive hepatitis | |
| | congenital adrenal hyperplasia | |
| CAHB | chronic active hepatitis B | |
| CAI | carbonic anhydrase inhibitors | |
| | carboxyamide aminoimidazoles | |
| | carotid artery injury | |
| | computer-assisted instructions | |
| 'caid | Medicaid | |
| CAIV | cold-adapted influenza virus vaccine | |
| CAL | callus | |
| | calories (cal) | |
| | chronic airflow limitation | |
| $C_{alb}$ | albumin clearance | |
| cal ct | calorie count | |
| CALD | chronic active liver disease | |
| CALGB | Cancer and Leukemia Group B | |
| CALI | chromophore-assisted laser inactivation | |
| CALLA | common acute lympho-blastic leukemia antigen | |
| CAM | campylobacter vaccine | |
| | Caucasian adult male | |
| | cell adhesion molecules | |
| | child abuse management | |
| | complementary and alternative medicine | |
| | confusion assessment method | |
| | controlled ankle motion | |
| | cystic adenomatoid malformation | |
| CAMA | corrected-arm-muscle area | |
| CAMCOG | Cambridge Cognitive Examination | |
| CAMD | computer-aided molecular design | |
| CAMF | cyclophosphamide, Adriamycin, methotrexate, and fluorouracil | |
| CAMP | cyclophosphamide, doxorubicin (Adriamycin), methotrexate, and procarbazine | |

| | | | | |
|---|---|---|---|---|
| cAMP | cyclic adenosine monophosphate | | CAPLA | computer-assisted product license application |
| CAMs | cell adhesion molecules | | CaPPS | calcium pentosan polysulfate |
| CAN | contrast-associated nephropathy cord around neck | | CAPS | aspects of **c**ognition, **a**ffective state, **p**hysical condition, and **s**ocial factors (patient assessment; parameters) |
| CA/N | child abuse and neglect | | | |
| CANC | cancelled | | | |
| c-ANCA | antineutrophil cytoplasmic antibody | | | caffeine, alcohol, pepper, and spicy food (dietary restrictions) |
| CANDA | computer-assisted new drug application | | | |
| CAN-KLB | *Candida albicans, Klebsiella pneumoniae* vaccine | | CAPWA | computerized arterial pulse waveform analysis |
| CANP | Certified Adult Nurse Practitioner | | CAR | cardiac ambulation routine carotid artery repair coronary artery revascularization Coxsackie adenovirus receptor |
| CAO | chronic airway (airflow) obstruction | | | |
| CaO₂ | arterial oxygen concentration | | | |
| CAOS | computer-assisted orthopedic surgery | | CA-RA | common adductor-rectus abdominis |
| CaOx | calcium oxalate | | CARB | carbohydrate |
| CAP | cancer of the prostate capsule cellulose acetate phthalate Certified Addiction Professional cervical acid phosphatase chaotic atrial tachycardia chemistry admission profile chloramphenicol community-acquired pneumonia compound action potentials cyclophosphamide, doxorubicin (Adriamycin), and cisplatin | | CARBO | Carbocaine® carboplatin |
| | | | CARD | Cardiac Automatic Resuscitative Device |
| | | | CARES | Cancer Rehabilitation Evaluation System |
| | | | CARF | Commission on Accreditation of Rehabilitation Facilities |
| | | | CARM | Centre for Adverse Reactions Monitoring (New Zealand) |
| | | | C-arm | fluoroscopy image intensifier |
| | | | CARN | Certified Addiction Registered Nurse |
| CaP | cancer of the prostate | | CART | classification and regression tree |
| Ca/P | calcium to phosphorus ratio | | CARTI | community-acquired respiratory tract infection(s) |
| CAPA | Corrective and Preventive Action (related to FDA) | | CAS | carotid artery stenosis cerebral arteriosclerosis Chemical Abstracts Service Clinical Asthma Score combined androgen suppression |
| CAPB | central auditory processing battery | | | |
| CAPD | central auditory processing disorder continuous ambulatory peritoneal dialysis | | | |

|  | | |
|---|---|---|
|  | computer-assisted surgery | CAVE |
|  | coronary artery stenosis | |
| CASA | cancer-associated serum antigen | |
|  | Center on Addiction and Substance Abuse | |
|  | computer-assisted semen analysis | CAVH |
| CaSC | carcinoma of the sigmoid colon | |
| CASHD | coronary arteriosclerotic heart disease | CAVHD |
| CASP | Child Analytic Study Program | CAVM |
| CASS | computer-aided sleep system | CAV-P-VP |
| CAST® | color allergy screening test | |
| CASWCM | Certified Advanced Social Work Case Manager | |
| CAT | Cardiac Arrest Team | CAVR |
|  | carnitine acetyl transferase | |
|  | cataract | CAVS |
|  | Children's Apperception Test | CAVU |
|  | coital alignment technique | |
|  | computed axial tomography | CAW |
|  | methcatinone | |
| CATH | catheter | CAX |
|  | catheterization | Ca x P |
|  | Catholic | |
| CATS | catecholamines | CB |
| CATT | card agglutination test with stained trypanosomes | |
| CAU | Caucasian | |
| CAUTI | catheter-associated urinary tract infection | c/b |
| CAV | computer-aided ventilation | C & B |
|  | congenital absence of vagina | |
|  | cyclophosphamide, doxorubicin (Adriamycin), and vincristine | CBA |
| CAV-1 | canine adenovirus type 1 | |
| CAVB | complete atrioventricular block | CBAPF |
| CAVC | common artrioventricular canal | CBASP |

| CAVE | Content Analysis of Verbatim Explanation |
|---|---|
|  | cyclophosphamide, doxorubicin, (Adriamycin) vincristine, and etoposide |
| CAVH | continuous arteriovenous hemofiltration |
| CAVHD | continuous arteriovenous hemodialysis |
| CAVM | cerebral arteriovenous malformation |
| CAV-P-VP | cyclophosphamide, doxorubicin (Adriamycin), vincristine, cisplatin, and etoposide |
| CAVR | continuous arteriovenous rewarming |
| CAVS | calcific valve stenosis |
| CAVU | continuous arteriovenous ultrafiltration |
| CAW | carbonaceous-activated water (Willard Water) |
| CAX | central axis |
| Ca x P | calcium times phosphorus product |
| CB | cesarean birth |
|  | chronic bronchitis |
|  | code blue |
|  | conjugated bilirubin (direct) |
| c/b | complicated by |
| C & B | chair and bed |
|  | crown and bridge |
| CBA | chronic bronchitis and asthma |
|  | cost-benefit analysis |
|  | County Board of Assistance |
| CBAPF | Certified Board of Addiction Professionals |
| CBASP | Cognitive Behavioral Analysis System of Psychotherapy |
| CBAVD | congenital bilateral absence of the vas deferens |
| CBC | carbenicillin |
|  | complete blood count |
|  | contralateral breast cancer |
| CBCDA | carboplatin |

| | | | |
|---|---|---|---|
| CBCL | Child Behavior Checklist | | coarse breath sounds |
| CBCT | community based clinical trials | | Cruveilhier-Baumgarten syndrome |
| CBD | closed bladder drainage common bile duct corticobasal degeneration | CBT | cognitive behavioral therapy |
| | | CBU | cumulative breath units |
| CBDE | common bile duct exploration | CBV | central blood volume cyclophosphamide, carmustine (BiCNu), and etoposide (VePesid) |
| CBE | charting by exception child birth education | | |
| CBER | Center for Biologics Evaluation and Research (FDA) | CBZ | carbamazepine (Tegretol) |
| | | CBZE | carbamazepine epoxide |
| | | CC | cardiac catheterization |
| CBF | cerebral blood flow | | Catholic |
| CBFS | cerebral blood flow studies | | cerebral concussion chief complaint |
| CBFV | cerebral blood flow velocity | | choriocarcinoma chronic complainer |
| CBG | capillary blood glucose | | circulatory collapse |
| CBGM | capillary blood glucose monitor | | clean catch (urine) comfort care |
| CBH | collimated beam handpiece (for laser) | | complications and comorbidity |
| CBI | Caregiver Burden Index continuous bladder irrigation | | coracoclavicular cord compression corpus callosum |
| CBM | cryopreserved bone marrow | | creatinine clearance critical condition |
| CBN | chronic benign neutropenia collected by nurse | | cubic centimeter (cc), (mL) with correction (with glasses) |
| CBP | chronic benign pain copper-binding protein | $C_c$ | concentration of drug in the central compartment |
| CBPP | contagious bovine pleuropneumonia | C/C | cholecystectomy and operative cholangiogram complete upper and lower dentures |
| CBPS | congential bilateral perisylvian syndrome coronary bypass surgery | | |
| CBR | carotid bodies resected chronic bedrest clinical benefit responders complete bedrest | CCII | Clinical Clerk–2nd year |
| | | C & C | cold and clammy |
| CBRAM | controlled partial rebreathing-anesthesia method | CCA | calcium-channel antagonist Certified Coding Associate circumflex coronary artery common carotid artery concentrated care area countercurrent chromatography critical care area |
| CB RRR s M/R/G | cardiac beat, regular rhythm and rate without murmurs, rubs, or gallops | | |
| CBrS | clear breath sounds | | |
| CBS | Caregiver Burden Screen Charles Bonnet syndrome chronic brain syndrome | CCAM | congential cystic adenomatoid malformation (of the lung) |

C

69

| | | |
|---|---|---|
| CCAP | capsule cartilage articular preservation | |
| CCAT | common carotid artery thrombosis | |
| C-CATODSW | Certified Clinical Alcohol, Tobacco and Other Drugs Social Worker | |
| CCB | calcium channel blocker(s) Community Care Board corn, callus, and bunion | |
| CCBT | Certified Cognitive Behavioral Therapist | |
| CCC | Cancer Care Center central corneal clouding (Grade 0+ to 4+) Certificate of Clinical Competency child care clinic Comprehensive Cancer Center | |
| C/cc | colonies per cubic centimeter | |
| CC & C | colony count and culture | |
| CCC-A | Certificate of Clinical Competence in Audiology | |
| CCCE | Clinical Center Coordinator Educator | |
| CCC-SP | Certificate of Clinical Competence in Speech-Language Pathology | |
| CCD | charged-coupled device childhood celiac disease chin-chest distance clinical cardiovascular disease | |
| CCDC | Certified Chemical Dependency Counselor | |
| CCDC-1 | Certified Chemical Dependency Counselor, Level One | |
| CCDS | color-coded duplex sonography | |
| CCE | clubbing, cyanosis, and edema countercurrent electrophoresis | |
| CCF | cephalin cholesterol flocculation Cleveland Clinic Foundation compound comminuted fracture | |

congestive cardiac failure
crystal-induced chemotactic factor

| | |
|---|---|
| CCFE | cyclophosphamide, cisplatin, fluorouracil, and estramustine |
| CCFs | chronic-care facilities |
| CCG | Children's Cancer Group |
| CCH | community care home Cook County Hospital |
| CCHD | complex congenital heart disease cyanotic congenital heart disease |
| CCHF | Congo-Crimean hemorrhagic fever |
| CCHS | congenital central hypoventilation syndrome |
| CCI | chronic coronary insufficiency Correct Coding Initiative corrected count increment |
| CCJAP | Certified Criminal Justice Addiction Professional |
| CCJAS | Certified Criminal Justice Addiction Specialist |
| CCK | cholecystokinin |
| CCK-OP | cholecystokinin octapeptide |
| CCK-PZ | cholecystokinin pancreozymin |
| CCL | cardiac catheterization laboratory critical condition list |
| CCl$_4$ | carbon tetrachloride |
| CCLE | chronic cutaneous lupus erythematosus |
| CCM | calcium citrate malate cerebral cavernous malformation Certified Care Manager children's case management cyclophosphamide, lomustine (CCNU; CeeNU), and methotrexate |
| CCMHC | Certified Clinical Mental Health Counselor |
| CCMSU | clean catch midstream urine |

| | | | |
|---|---|---|---|
| CCMU | critical care medicine unit | | closed cranial trauma |
| CCN | continuing care nursery | | congenitally corrected |
| CCNS | cell cycle-nonspecific | | transposition (of the |
| CCNU | lomustine (CeeNu) | | great vessels) |
| CCO | continuous cardiac output | | Critical Care Technician |
| | Corporate Compliance | | crude coal tar |
| | Officer | CCTGA | congenitally corrected |
| C-collar | cervical collar | | transposition of the |
| CCP | crystalloid cardioplegia | | great arteries |
| CCPD | continuous cycling | CCT in | crude coal tar in |
| | (cyclical) peritoneal | PET | petroleum |
| | dialysis | CCTV | closed circuit television |
| CCR | California Cancer | CCU | coronary care unit |
| | Registry | | critical care unit |
| | cardiac catheterization | CCUA | clean catch urinalysis |
| | recovery | CCUP | colpocystourethropexy |
| | continuous complete | CCV | Critical Care Ventilator |
| | remission | | (Ohio) |
| | counterclockwise rotation | | critical closing volume |
| C$_{cr}$ | creatinine clearance | CCW | childcare worker |
| CCRC | Certified Clinical | | counterclockwise |
| | Research Coordinator | CCWR | counterclockwise rotation |
| | continuing care residential | CCX | complications |
| | community | CCY | cholecystectomy |
| CCRN | Certified Critical Care | CD | cadaver donor |
| | Registered Nurse | | candela |
| CCRT | combined chemo- | | Castleman disease |
| | radiotherapy | | celiac disease |
| CCRU | critical care recovery unit | | cervical dystonia |
| CCS | cell cycle-specific | | cesarean delivery |
| | certified coding specialist | | character disorder |
| | color contrast sensitivity | | chemical dependency |
| CC & S | cornea, conjunctiva, and | | childhood disease |
| | sclera | | chronic dialysis |
| CCSA | Canadian Cardiovascular | | circular dichroism |
| | Society Angina (score) | | closed drainage |
| CCSK | clear cell sarcoma of the | | clusters of differentiation |
| | kidney | | common duct |
| CCSP | Certified Chiropractic | | communication disorders |
| | Sports Physician | | complementarity- |
| | Clara cell secretory | | determining |
| | protein | | complicated delivery |
| CCS-P | Certified Coding | | conjugate diameter |
| | Specialist, Physician- | | continuous drainage |
| | Based | | conventional denture |
| CCSS | Childhood Cancer | | convulsive disorder |
| | Survivor Study | | cortical dysplasia |
| CCT | calcitriol | | Crohn disease |
| | carotid compression | | cumulative doses |
| | tomography | | cyclodextran |
| | Certified Cardiographic | | cytarabine and |
| | Technician | | daunorubicin |
| | closed cerebral trauma | Cd | cadmium |

concentration of drug
C/D cigarettes per day
cup-to-disk ratio
CD4 antigenic marker on
helper/inducer T cells
(also called OKT 4, T4,
and Leu3)
CD8 antigenic marker on
suppressor/cytotoxic T
cells (also called OKT
8, T8, and Leu 8)
C&D curettage and desiccation
cystectomy and diversion
cytoscopy and dilatation
CDA Certified Dental Assistant
chenodeoxycholic acid
(chenodiol)
congenital dyserythro-
poietic anemia
2-CDA cladribine (Leustatin;
chlorodeoxyadenosine)
CDAD *Clostridium difficile*-
associated diarrhea
CDAI Crohn Disease Activity
Index
CDAK Cordis Dow Artificial
Kidney
CDAP continuous distended
airway pressure
CDB cough and deep breath
CDC calculated day of
confinement
cancer detection center
carboplatin, doxorubicin,
and cyclophosphamide
Centers for Disease
Control and Prevention
Certified Drug Counselor
chenodeoxycholic acid
(chenodiol)
*Clostridium difficile* colitis
CDCA chenodeoxycholic acid
(chenodiol)
CDCP Centers for Disease
Control and Prevention
(CDC is official
abbreviation)
CDCR conjunctivo-
dacryocystorhinostomy
CDD Certificate of Disability
for Discharge
*Clostridium difficile*
disease

cytidine deaminase
CDDP cisplatin
CDE canine distemper
encephalitis
Certified Diabetes
Educator
common duct exploration
CDER Center for Drug
Evaluation and
Research (FDA)
CDFI color Doppler flow
imaging
CDG carbohydrate-deficient
glycoprotein
congenital disorders of
glycosylation
CDGE constant denaturant gel
electrophoresis
CDGP constitutional delay of
growth and puberty
CDH chronic daily headache
congenital diaphragmatic
hernia
congenital dislocation of
hip
congenital dysplasia of
the hip
CDHP 5-chloro-2 4-
dihydroxypyridine
CDI Children's Depression
Inventory
clean, dry, and intact
color Doppler imaging
Cotrel Duobosset
Instrumentation
CDIC *Clostridium difficile*-
induced colitis
C Dif *Clostridium difficile*
CDK climatic droplet
keratopathy
cyclin-dependent kinase
CDKI cyclin-dependent kinase
inhibitor
CDK2 cyclin-depenent kinases 2
CDLC continuous double-loop
closure
CDLE chronic discoid lupus
erythematosus
CdLS Cornelia de Lange
syndrome
CDM charge description master
CDP chemical dependence
profile

| | | | |
|---|---|---|---|
| | Chemical Dependency Professional | CDTM | collaborative drug therapy management |
| | Child Development Program | CDU | chemical dependency unit |
| | complete decongestive physiotherapy | | color-coded duplex ultrasonography |
| | crystalline degradation product | CDV | canine distemper virus |
| | | | cardiovascular |
| | cytidine diphosphate | | cyclophosphamide, doxorubicin, and vincristine |
| CDQ | corrected development quotient | | |
| CDR | clinical data repository | CDX | chlordiazepoxide |
| | Clinical Dementia Rating | cdyn | dynamic compliance |
| | continuing disability review | CE | California encephalitis |
| | | | capillary electrophoresis |
| CDRH | Center for Devices and Radiological Health | | carboplatin and etoposide |
| | | | cardiac enlargement |
| CDR(H) | cup-to-disk ratio horizontal | | cardiac enzymes |
| | | | cardioesophageal |
| CDRs | complementary determining regions | | cataract extraction |
| | | | central episiotomy |
| CDR(V) | cup-to-disk ratio vertical | | chemoembolization |
| CDS | Chemical Dependency Specialist | | chest expansion |
| | | | cholesterol ester |
| | Chronic Disease Score | | community education |
| | closed-door seclusion | | consultative examination |
| | color Doppler sonography | | continuing education |
| CDSC | Communicable Disease Surveillance Centre (United Kingdom) | | contrast echocardiology |
| | | C&E | consultation and examination |
| | | | cough and exercise |
| CDSPIES | congestive heart failure, drugs, spasm, pneumothorax, infection, embolism, and secretions (differential diagnosis mnemonic) | | curettage and electrodesiccation |
| | | CEA | carcinoembryonic antigen |
| | | | carotid endarterectomy |
| | | | cost-effectiveness analysis |
| | | CEB | calcium entry blocker |
| CDSR | Cochrane Database of Systematic Reviews | | carboplatin, etoposide, and bleomycin |
| | | CEBV | chronic Epstein-Barr virus |
| CDT | carbohydrate-deficient transferrin | CEC | capillary electrochromatography |
| | Chemical Dependency Technician | | Council for Exceptional Children |
| | complete decongestive therapy (for lymphedema) | CECA | Childhood Experience of Care and Abuse (interview) |
| | connecting discourse tracking (measure of speech perception) | CECD | congenital endothelial corneal dystrophy |
| | | CEc̄/IOL | cataract extraction with intraocular lens |
| | cystic dysplasia of the testis | CECT | contrast-enhanced computed tomography |
| CDTA | cyclohexane-1,2-diaminetetraacetic acid | CED | clinically effective dose |

cystoscopy-endoscopy dilation

CEDS Certified Eating Disorders Specialist

CEE Central European encephalitis

conjugated equine estrogen (Premarin; conjugated estrogen)

CEF chick embryo fibroblast

cyclophosphamide, epirubicin, and fluorouracil

CEFM continuous external fetal monitoring

CEFOT cefotaxime

CEFOX cefoxitin

CEFTAZ ceftazidime

CEFUR cefuroxime

CEI continuous extravascular infusion

converting enzyme inhibitor

CEL cardiac exercise laboratory

CELIP Claims Expansion Line-item Processing

CELP chronic erosive lichen planus

CEM Clinical Event Manager

CEMD consultative examination by physician

CEN Certified (Nurse)– Emergency Room

CENOG computerized electroneuro-ophthalmogram

CEO chief executive officer

CEOT calcifying epithelial odontogenic tumor

CEP cardiac enzyme panel

chronic eosinophilic pneumonia

cognitive evoked potential

congenital erythropoietic porphyria

countercurrent electrophoresis

cyclophosphamide, etoposide, and cisplatin (Platinol)

CEPH cephalic

cephalosporin

CEPH FLOC cephalin flocculation

CEPP (B) cyclophosphamide, etopside, procarbazine, prednisone, and bleomycin

CER conditioned emotional response

CE&R central episiotomy and repair

CERA cortical evoked response audiometry

CERAD Consortium to Establish a Registry for Alzheimer Disease

CERD chronic end-stage renal disease

CERULO ceruloplasmin

CERV cervical

CES Cauda equina syndrome

central excitatory state

cognitive environmental stimulation

estrogen, conjugated (conjugated estrogen substance)

CESB chronic electrical stimulation of the brain

CES-D Center for Epidemiologic Studies – Depression

CESI cervical epidural steroid injection

CET common extensor tendon

CETP cholesterol ester transfer protein

CEV cyclophosphamide, etoposide, and vincristine

CE w/IOL cataract extraction with intraocular lens

CF calcium leucovorin (citrovorum factor)

cancer-free

cardiac failure

Caucasian female

Christmas factor

cisplatin and fluorouracil

complement fixation

contractile force

count fingers

cystic fibrosis

| | | | |
|---|---|---|---|
| C&F | cell and flare | CFT | capillary filling time |
| | chills and fever | | chronic follicular |
| CFA | common femoral artery | | tonsillitis |
| | complete Freund | | complement fixation test |
| | adjuvant | CFTR | cystic fibrosis |
| | cryptogenic fibrosing | | transmembrane |
| | alveolitis | | (conductance) |
| | cystic fibrosis anthropathy | | regulator |
| CFAC | complement-fixing | | cystic fibrosis |
| | antibody consumption | | transmembrane |
| C-factor | cleverness factor | | receptor |
| CFCs | chlorofluorocarbons | CFU | colony-forming units |
| CFD | color-flow Doppler | CFU-E | colony-forming unit– |
| | computational fluid | | erythroid |
| | dynamics | CFU-G | colony-forming |
| CFF | critical fusion (flicker) | | unit–granulocyte |
| | frequency | CFU-G/M | colony-forming unit– |
| CFFT | critical flicker fusion | | granulocyte/macro- |
| | threshold | | phage |
| CFH | chemical fume hood | CFU-M | colony-forming unit– |
| CFI | confrontation fields intact | | macrophage |
| CFIDS | chronic fatigue immune | CFU-S | colony-forming |
| | dysfunction syndrome | | unit–spleen |
| CFL | calcaneofibular ligament | CFV | common femoral vein |
| | cisplatin, fluorouracil, and | CFVR | coronary flow velocity |
| | leucovorin calcium | | reserve |
| CFLX | ciprofloxacin | CFX | circumflex artery |
| | circumflex | CG | cardiogreen (dye) |
| CFM | cerebral function monitor | | caregiver |
| | close fitting mask | | cholecystogram |
| | craniofacial microsomia | | contact guarding |
| | cyclophosphamide, | | contralateral groin |
| | fluorouracil, and | CGA | clonal group A |
| | mitoxantrone | | comprehensive geriatric |
| CFNS | chills, fever, and night | | assessment |
| | sweats | | contact guard assist |
| CFP | cystic fibrosis protein | CGB | chronic gastrointestinal |
| CFPT | cyclophosphamide, | | (tract) bleeding |
| | fluorouracil, | CGCG | central giant-cell |
| | prednisone, and | | granuloma |
| | tamoxifen | CGD | chronic glycogen deficit |
| CFR | case-fatality rates | | chronic granulomatous |
| | *Code of Federal* | | disease |
| | *Regulations* | | cobalt gray equivalent |
| | coronary flow reserve | CGF | continuous gavage feeding |
| CFS | cancer family syndrome | | (infant feeding) |
| | Child and Family Service | CGI | Clinical Global |
| | childhood febrile seizures | | Impressions (scale) |
| | chronic fatigue syndrome | CGIC | Clinical Global |
| | congenital fibrosarcoma | | Impression of Change |
| CFSAN | Center for Food Safety | CGI-S | Clinical Global |
| | and Applied Nutrition | | Impressions, Severity of |
| | (NIH) | | Illness |

| | | | |
|---|---|---|---|
| CGL | chronic granulocytic leukemia | CHAM-OCA | cyclophosphamide, hydroxyurea, |
| | with correction/with glasses | | dactinomycin, methotrexate, |
| CGM | central gray matter | | vincristine, leucovorin, |
| CGMP | Current Good Manufacturing Practices | | and doxorubicin |
| | | CHAM-PUS | Civilian Health and Medical Program of the |
| cGMP | cyclic guanine monophosphate | | Uniformed Services |
| CGN | chronic glomerulonephritis | CHAP | child health associate practitioner |
| cGN | crescentic glomerulonephritis | | cyclophosphamide, altretamine, |
| C-GRD | coffee-ground | | (hexamethylmelamine), |
| CGRP | calcitonin gene-related peptide | | doxorubicin (Adriamycin), and |
| CGS | cardiogenic shock | | cisplatin (Platinol AQ) |
| | catgut suture | CHAQ | childhood health |
| | centimeter-gram-second system | | assessment questionnaire |
| CGTT | cortisol glucose tolerance test | CHARGE | coloboma (of eyes), hearing deficit, choanal |
| cGy | centigray | | atresia, retardation of |
| CH | Caribbean Hispanic | | growth, genital defects |
| | chest | | (males only), and |
| | chief | | endocardial cushion |
| | child (children) | | defect |
| | chronic | CHART | complaint, history, |
| | cluster headache | | assessment, Rx |
| | concentric hypertrophy | | (treatment), transport |
| | congenital hypothyroidism | | continuous hyperfractionated |
| | convalescent hospital | | accelerated radiotherapy |
| | crown-heal | | Craig Handicap |
| $C_h$ | hepatic clearance | | Assessment and |
| $ch^1$ | Christ Church chromosome | | Reporting Technique |
| | | CHB | chronic hepatitis B |
| $CH_{50}$ | total hemolytic complement | | complete heart block |
| | | | congenital heart block |
| C&H | cocaine and heroin | CHBHA | congenital Heinz body hemolytic anemia |
| CHA | compound hypermetropic astigmatism | CHC | concentric hypertrophic cardiomyopathy |
| | congenital hypoplastic anemia | $CH_3-$ CCNU | semustine |
| CHAD | cyclophosphamide, altretamine, | CHCT | caffeine-halothane contracture test |
| | (hexamethylmelamine), | cHct | central hematocrit |
| | doxorubicin (Adriamycin), and | CHD | center hemodialysis |
| | cisplatin (DDP) | | changed diaper |
| CHAI | continuous hepatic artery infusion | | childhood diseases chronic hemodialysis common hepatic duct |

| | | | |
|---|---|---|---|
| | congenital heart disease | ChloMP | chlorambucil, |
| | coordinate home care | | mitoxantrone, and |
| CHE | chronic hepatic | | prednisolone |
| | encephalopathy | ChlVPP | chlorambucil, vinblastine, |
| CHEDDAR | Chief Compliant; History: | | procarbazine, and |
| | social and physical as | | prednisone |
| | well as contributing | CHM | complete hydatidiform |
| | factors; Examination; | | mole |
| | Details of problems and | CHN | central hemorrhagic |
| | complaints; Drugs and | | necrosis |
| | dosage—list current | | Chinese herb nephropathy |
| | meds; Assessment, | | Community Health Nurse |
| | diagnostic process, total | | community nursing home |
| | impression; Return | CHO | carbohydrate |
| | visit information or | | Chemical Hygiene Officer |
| | referral (format of | | Chinese hamster ovary |
| | documentation) | $C_{H_2O}$ | free-water clearance |
| CHEF | clamped homogeneous | $CHO_a$ | cholera vaccine, |
| | electric field | | attenuated live (oral) |
| ChEI | cholinesterase inhibitor | $CHO_{cn^-}$ | cholera vaccine, |
| CHEM 7 | see page 362 | LPS | lipopolysaccharide- |
| CHEMO | chemotherapy | | toxin conjugate |
| ChemoRx | chemotherapy | $C_2 H_5 OH$ | alcohol (ethyl alcohol) |
| CHEOPS | Children's Hospital of | $CHO_{i-w}$ | cholera vaccine, |
| | Eastern Ontario Pain | | inactivated whole |
| | Scale | | cell |
| CHESS | chemical shift | $CHO_{i-w-BS}$ | cholera vaccine, |
| | suppression | | inactivated whole cell, |
| CHF | congestive heart failure | | B subunit |
| | Crimean hemorrhagic | chol | cholesterol |
| | fever | c̄ hold | withhold |
| CHFV | combined high-frequency | $CHO_o$ | cholera, oral vaccine |
| | of ventilation | CHOP | cyclophosphamide, |
| CHG | change | | doxorubicin, vincristine |
| CHI | chikungunya virus vaccine | | (Oncovin), prednisone |
| | closed head injury | CHOP- | cyclophosphamide, |
| | contrast harmonic | Bleo | doxorubicin |
| | imaging | | (hydroxydaunorubicin), |
| | creatinine-height index | | vincristine (Oncovin), |
| CHILD | congenital hemidysplasia | | prednisone, and |
| | with ichthyosiform | | bleomycin |
| | nevus and limb defects | $CHO_{tox}$ | cholera toxin/toxoid |
| | (syndrome) | | vaccine |
| CHIN | community health | CHPB | Canadian Health |
| | information network | | Protection Branch (the |
| CHIP | comprehensive health | | equivalent of the U.S. |
| | insurance plan | | Food and Drug |
| | iproplatin | | Administration) |
| CHIR | Chiron Corporation | CHPX | chickenpox |
| Chix | chickenpox | CHR | Cercaria-Hullen reaction |
| CHL | conductive hearing loss | | chronic |
| CHLC | Cooperative Human | | complete hematological |
| | Linkage Center | | response |

C

CHRPE    congenital hypertrophy of the retinal pigment epithelium

CHRS    congenital hereditary retinoschisis

CHS    Chediak-Higashi syndrome
contact hypersensitivity

CHT    Certified Hand Therapist
Certified Hyperbaric Technician
Certified Hypnotherapist
closed head trauma

ChT    chemotherapy

CHTN    chronic hypertension

CHU    closed head unit

CHUC    Certified Health Unit Coordinator

CHVP    cyclophosphamide, doxorubicin (hydroxydaunorubicin), teniposide (VM26), and prednisone

CHW    community health workers

CHWG    chewing gum

CHX    chlorhexidine

CI    cardiac index
cerebral infarction
cesium implant
Clinical Instructor
cochlear implant
cognitively impaired
colon inertia
commercial insurance
complete iridectomy
confidence interval
continuous infusion
core imprint (cytology)
coronary insufficiency

Ci    curie(s)

CI30    cumulative incidence at 30 years

CIA    calcaneal insufficiency avulsion
chronic idiopathic anhidrosis

CIAA    competitive insulin autoantibodies

CIAED    collagen-induced autoimmune ear disease

CIB    Carnation Instant Breakfast®
crying-induced bronchospasm

cytomegalic inclusion bodies

CIBD    chronic inflammatory bowel disease

CIBI    Clinician Interview-Based Impression (of change)

CIBIC    Clinician Interview-Based Impression of Change

CIBIC-plus    Clinician Interview-Based Impression of Change with Caregiver Input

CIBP    chronic intractable benign pain

C-IBS    constipated predominant irritable bowel syndrome

CIC    cardioinhibitory center
circulating immune complexes
clean intermittent catheterization
completely in-the-canal (hearing aid)
coronary intensive care

CICE    combined intracapsular cataract extraction

CICU    cardiac intensive care unit

CICVC    centrally inserted central venous catheter

CID    Center for Infectious Diseases (CDC)
cervical immobilization device
chemotherapy-induced diarrhea
combined immunodeficiency
cytomegalic inclusion disease

CIDP    chronic inflammatory demyelinating polyradiculoneuropathy (polyneuropathy)

CIDS    cellular immunodeficiency syndrome
continuous insulin delivery system

CIE    capillary immunoelectrophoresis
chemotherapy-induced emesis
congenital ichthyosiform erythroderma

|  |  |  |  |
|---|---|---|---|
|  | counterimmuno-electrophoresis | CIOMS | The Council for International Organization of Medical Sciences |
|  | crossed immunoelectrophoresis |  |  |
| CIEA | continuous infusion epidural analgesia | CIP | Cardiac Injury Panel |
|  |  |  | critical illness polyneuropathy |
| CIEP | counterimmuno-electrophoresis | CIPD | chronic intermittent peritoneal dialysis |
|  | crossed immunoelectrophoresis | CIR | continent intestinal reservior |
| CIFN | chemotherapy-induced fever and neutropenia | Circ | circulation |
|  |  |  | circumcision |
| CIG | cigarettes |  | circumference |
| CIH | Certified in Industrial Health | circ. & sen. | circulation and sensation |
|  | continuous infusion haloperidol | CIRF | cocaine-induced respiratory failure |
| CIHD | chronic ischemic heart disease | CIS | Cancer Information Service (National Cancer Institute) |
| CIHR | Canadian Institutes of Health Research |  |  |
| CII | continuous insulin infusion |  | carcinoma in situ |
| CIIA | common internal iliac artery |  | Commonwealth of Independent States |
| CIL | carbamazepine-induced lupus |  | continuous interleaved sampling |
| CIM | change in menses | CI&S | conjunctival irritation and swelling |
|  | chemotherapy-induced mucositis | CISC | clean intermittent self-catheterization |
|  | constraint-induced movement | CISCA | cisplatin, cyclophosphamide, and doxorubicin (Adriamycin) |
|  | convective interaction media |  |  |
|  | corticosteroid-induced myopathy | CISCOM | The Centralized Information Service for Complementary Medicine |
|  | critical illness myopathy |  |  |
| CIMCU | cardiac intermediate care unit |  |  |
| CIN | cervical intraepithelial neoplasia | CISD | critical incident stress debriefing (used by EMTs) |
|  | chemotherapy-induced neutropenia | Cis-DDP | cisplatin |
|  | chronic interstitial nephritis | CISM | critical incident stress management (debriefing used by EMTs) |
| $C_{IN}$ | insulin clearance |  |  |
| CIND | cognitive impairment, no dementia | CIS-R | Clinical Interview Schedule, Revised |
| CINE | chemotherapy-induced nausea and emesis | CI-Stim | cochlear implant stimulation |
|  | cineangiogram | CIT | chemotherapy-induced toxicities |
| CINV | chemotherapy-induced nausea and vomiting |  | constraint-induced therapy (protocol) |
| CIO | corticosteroid-induced osteoporosis |  |  |

C

| | | | |
|---|---|---|---|
| | conventional immunosuppressive therapy | | congenital lactic acidosis<br>congenital laryngeal atresia<br>conjugated linoleic acid |
| | conventional insulin therapy | C lam | cervical laminectomy |
| CIT IDS | citation identifiers (National Library of Medicine) | CLAMSS | cleavage- and ligation-associated mutation-specific sequencing |
| CITP | capillary isotachophoresis | CLAP | contact laser ablation of prostate |
| CIU | chronic idiopathic urticaria | CLAS | congenital localized absence of skin |
| CIV | common iliac vein<br>continuous intravenous (infusion) | CLASS | computer laser-assisted surgical system |
| CIVI | continuous intravenous infusion | CLASS I | congestive heart failure with no limitation with ordinary activity (New York Heart Association Classification) |
| CIXU | constant infusion excretory urogram | | |
| CIWA-Ar | Clinical Institute Withdrawal Assessment for Alcohol–revised | CLASS II | congestive heart failure with slight limitation of physical activity |
| CJD | Creutzfeldt-Jakob disease | CLASS III | congestive heart failure with marked limitation of physical activity |
| cJET | congenital junctional ectopic tachycardia | | |
| CJR | centric jaw relation | CLASS IV | congestive heart failure with inability to engage in any physical activity without symptoms |
| CK | check<br>conductive keratoplasty<br>creatine kinase | | |
| CK-BB | creatine kinase BB band (primarily in brain) | Clav | clavicle |
| | | CLB | chlorambucil (Leukeran)<br>coccidian-like body |
| CKC | cold-knife conization | | |
| CKD | chronic kidney disease | $CLB_{atx}$ | *Clostridium botulinum* antitoxin |
| CK-ISO | creatine kinase isoenzyme | | |
| CK-MB | creatine kinase MB fraction (primarily in cardiac muscle) | CLBBB | complete left bundle branch block |
| | | CLBD | cortical Lewy body disease |
| CK MM | creatine kinase MM fraction (primarily in skeletal muscle) | CLBP | chronic low back pain |
| | | $CLB_{tox}$ | *Clostridium botulinum* toxoid vaccine |
| CKW | clockwise | CLC | cork leather and celastic (orthotic) |
| Cl | chloride | | |
| CL | central line<br>chemoluminescence<br>clear liquid<br>cleft lip<br>cloudy<br>critical list<br>cycle length<br>lung compliance | CL/CP | cleft lip and cleft palate |
| | | CLD | chronic liver disease<br>chronic lung disease<br>*Clostridium difficile* vaccine |
| | | $Cl_d$ | dialysis clearance |
| $C_L$ | compliance of the lungs | CLE | centrilobular emphysema<br>congenital lobar emphysema<br>continuous lumbar epidural (anesthetic) |
| C-L | consultation-liaison | | |
| CLA | community living arrangements | | |

C

80

| | | | |
|---|---|---|---|
| CLED | cysteine lactose electrolyte-deficient (agar) | clysis | hypodermoclysis |
| | | CLZ | clozapine (Clozaril) |
| | | cm | centimeter |
| CLEIA | chemiluminescent enzyme immunoassay | CM | capreomycin |
| | | | CarboMedics (heart valve prosthesis) |
| CLEP | college level examination program | | cardiac monitor |
| | | | case management |
| CLF | cholesterol-lecithin flocculation | | case manager |
| | | | Caucasian male |
| CLG | clorgyline | | centimeter (cm) |
| CLH | chronic lobular hepatitis | | chondromalacia |
| $C_h$ | hepatic clearance | | cochlear microphonics |
| CLI | central lymphatic irradiation | | common migraine |
| | | | continuous microwave |
| | clomipramine | | continuous murmur |
| | critical leg (limb) ischemia | | contrast media |
| CLIA | Clinical Laboratory Improvement Act | | costal margin |
| | | | cow's milk |
| $Cl_{int}$ | intrinsic clearance | | culture media |
| CLL | chronic lymphocytic leukemia | | cutaneous melanoma |
| | | | cystic mesothelioma |
| CLLE | columnar-lined lower esophagus | | tomorrow morning (this is a dangerous abbreviation) |
| cl liq | clear liquid | | |
| $Cl_{nr}$ | nonrenal clearance | cM | centimorgan (one one-hundredth of a morgan; the unit of distance on a linkage map) |
| CLO | Campylobacter-like organism | | |
| | close | | |
| | cod liver oil | | |
| CLOX | clock-drawing task (cognitive impairment test) | cm1 | circumflex marginal 1 |
| | | cm2 | circumflex marginal 2 |
| | | $cm^2$ | square centimeters |
| CL & P | cleft lip and palate | $cm^3$ | cubic centimeter |
| CL PSY | closed psychiatry | CMA | Certified Medical Assistant |
| $Cl_r$ | renal clearance | | |
| Cl Red | closed reduction | | Certified Movement Analyst |
| CLRO | community leave for reorientation | | compound myopic astigmatism |
| CLS | capillary leak syndrome | | cost-minimization analysis |
| | community living skills | | cow's milk allergy |
| CLSE | calf-lung surfactant extract (Infasurf) | CMAF | centrifuged microaggregate filter |
| CLT | chronic lymphocytic thyroiditis | CMAI | Cohen-Mansfield Agitation inventory |
| | complex lymphedema therapy | CMAPs | compound muscle action potentials |
| | cool lace tent | | |
| $Cl_T$ | total body clearance | $C_{max}$ | maximum concentration of drug |
| CLV | cutaneous leukocytoclastic vasculitis | CMB | carbolic methylene blue |
| CL VOID | clean voided specimen | CMBBT | cervical mucous basal body temperature |
| $CLW_c$ | Clostridium welchii type C (Pigbel) toxoid vaccine | CMC | carboxymethylcellulose |

C

|  |  |  |  |
|---|---|---|---|
|  | carpal metacarpal (joint) | CMID | cytomegalic inclusion disease |
|  | chloramphenicol |  |  |
|  | chronic mucocutaneous candidiasis | $C_{min}$ | minimum concentration of drug |
|  | clinically meaningful change | CMIR | cell-mediated immune response |
|  | closed mitral commissurotomy | CMJ | carpometacarpal joint |
| CMD | congenital muscular dystrophy | CMK | congenital multicystic kidney |
|  | cytomegalic disease | CML | cell-mediated lympholysis |
| CMDRH | Center for Medical Devices and Radiological Health (of the Food and Drug Administration) |  | chronic myelogenous leukemia |
|  |  |  | chronic myeloid leukemia |
|  |  | CML-BP | blastic phase chronic myeloid leukemia |
| CME | cervicomediastinal exploration (examination) | CMM | Comprehensive Major Medical (insurance) |
|  |  |  | continuous metabolic monitor |
|  | continuing medical education |  | cutaneous malignant melanoma |
|  | cystoid macular edema | CMME | chloromethyl methyl ether |
| CMER | current medical evidence of record | CMML | chronic myelomacrocytic leukemia |
| CMF | cyclophosphamide, methotrexate and fluorouracil | CMMS | Columbia Mental Maturity Scale |
| CMFP | cyclophosphamide, methotrexate, fluorouracil, and prednisone | CMN | Certificate of Medical Necessity |
|  |  |  | congenital mesoblastic nephroma |
| CMFT | same as CMF with tamoxifen | CMO | cardiac minute output |
|  |  |  | cetyl myristoleate |
| CMFVP | cyclophosphamide, methotrexate, fluorouracil, vincristine, and prednisone |  | Chief Medical Officer |
|  |  |  | comfort measures only (resuscitation order) |
|  |  |  | consult made out |
|  |  | CMO 1 | corticosterone methyl oxidase type 1 |
| CMG | cystometrogram |  |  |
| CMGM | chronic megakaryocytic granulocytic myelosis | CMOP | cardiomyopathy |
|  |  | C-MOPP | cyclophosphamide, mechlorethamine, vincristine (Oncovin), procarbazine, and prednisone |
| CMGN | chronic membranous glomerulonephritis |  |  |
| CMH | current medical history |  |  |
| CMHC | Certified Mental Health Counselor | CMP | cardiomyopathy |
|  |  |  | chondromalacia patellae |
|  | community mental health center |  | comprehensive (complete) metabolic profile (see page 362) |
| CMHN | Community Mental Health Nurse |  | cushion mouthpiece |
| CMI | case mix index | CMPA | cow's milk protein allergy |
|  | cell-mediated immunity |  |  |
|  | clomipramine |  |  |
|  | Cornell Medical Index | CMPF | cow's milk, protein-free |

C

| | | | |
|---|---|---|---|
| CMPT | cervical mucous penetration test | CMUA | continuous motor unit activity |
| CMR | cerebral metabolic rate | CMV | cisplatin, methotrexate, and vinblastine |
| | chief medical resident | | |
| | child (1-4 years) mortality rates | | controlled mechanical ventilation |
| CMRI | cardiac magnetic resonance imaging | | conventional mechanical ventilation |
| CMRIT | combined modality radioimmunotherapy | | cool mist vaporizer cytomegalovirus |
| CMRNG | chromosomally mediated resistant *Neisseria gonorrhoeae* | CMVIG | cytomegalovirus vaccine cytomegalovirus immune globulin |
| CMRO | chronic multifocal recurrent osteomyelitis | CMVS | culture midvoid specimen |
| CMRO$_2$ | cerebral metabolic rate for oxygen | CN | charge nurse congenital nystagmus |
| CMS | Centers for Medicare and Medicaid Services (replaces Health Care Financing Administration [HCFA]) | | cranial nerve tomorrow night (this is a dangerous abbreviation) |
| | | Cn | cyanide |
| | | C/N | contrast-to-noise ratio |
| | children's medical services | CN II–XII | cranial nerves 2 through 12 |
| | circulation motion sensation | CNA | Certified Nurse Aide chart not available |
| | chocolate milkshake | C$_{Na}$ | sodium clearance |
| | constant moderate suction | CNAG | chronic narrow angle glaucoma |
| | continuous motion syndrome | CNAP | continuous negative airway pressure |
| CMSC | Certified Medical Staff Coordinator | CNB | core-needle biopsy |
| CMSUA | clean midstream urinalysis | CNC | clinical nurse coordinator |
| CMT | carpometatarsal (joint) | | Community Nursing Center |
| | Certified Massage Therapist | CNCbl | cyanocobalamin |
| | Certified Medical Transcriptionist | CND | canned cannot determine |
| | Certified Music Therapist | | chronic nausea and dyspepsia |
| | cervical motion tenderness | | |
| | Charot-Marie-Tooth (phenotype) (disease) | CNDC | chronic nonspecific diarrhea of childhood |
| | Chiropractic manipulative treatment | CNE | chronic nervous exhaustion |
| | choline magnesium trisalicylate (Trilisate) | | could not establish |
| | combined modality therapy | CNEP | continuous negative extrathoracic pressure |
| | continuing medication and treatment | C-NES | conversion nonepileptic seizures |
| | cutis marmorata telangiectasia | CNF | cyclophosphamide, mitoxantrone (Novatantrone), and fluorouracil |
| CMTX | chemotherapy treatment | | |

| | | | |
|---|---|---|---|
| CNH | central neurogenic hypernea | CNTA | combined neurosurgical and transfacial approach |
| | contract nursing home | CNTF | ciliary neurotrophic factor |
| CNHC | chronodermatitis nodularis helicis chronicus | CNV | choroidal neovascularization |
| | community nursing home care | CNVM | choroidal neovascular membrane |
| CNI | calcineurin inhibitors | CO | carbon monoxide |
| CNL | chemonucleolysis | | cardiac output |
| | Connaught Laboratories | | castor oil |
| CNLD | chronic neonatal lung disease | | centric occlusion |
| | | | Certified Orthoptist |
| CNLSD | condensation nucleation light scattering detection | | cervical orthosis |
| | | | corneal opacity |
| | | | corn oil |
| CNM | certified nurse midwife | | court order |
| CNMP | chronic nonmalignant pain | Co | cobalt |
| CNMT | Certified Nuclear Medicine Technologist | C/O | check out |
| | | | complained of |
| CNN | congenital nevocytic nevus | | complaints |
| | | | under care of |
| CNO | Chief Nursing Officer | $^{60}$Co | radioactive isotope of cobalt |
| | community nursing organization | $CO_2$ | carbon dioxide |
| CNOP | cyclophosphamide, mitoxantrone (Novantrone), vincristine (Oncovin), and prednisone | $CO_3$ | carbonate |
| | | COA | children of alcoholic |
| | | | coenzyme A |
| | | | condition on admission |
| | | CoA | coarctation of the aorta |
| CNOR | Certified Nurse, Operating Room | COAD | chronic obstructive airway disease |
| CNP | capillary nonprofusion | | chronic obstructive arterial disease |
| CNPB | continuous negative pressure breathing | COAG | chronic open angle glaucoma |
| CNPS | cardiac nuclear probe scan | COAGSC | coagulation screen |
| CNR | contrast-to-noise ratio (radiology) | COAP | cyclophosphamide, vincristine (Oncovin), cytarabine (ara-C), and prednisone |
| CNRN | Certified Neurosurgical Registered Nurse | COAR | coarctation |
| CNS | central nervous system | COARCT | coarctation |
| | Certified Nutrition Specialist | COB | cisplatin, vincristine (Oncovin), and bleomycin |
| | Clinical Nurse Specialist | | coordination of benefits |
| | coagulase-negative staphylococci | COBE | chronic obstructive bullous emphysema |
| | Crigler-Najjar syndrome | COBRA | Consolidated Omnibus Budget Reconciliation Act of 1985 |
| CNSD | Certified Nutrition Support Dietitian | |
| CNSHA | congenital nonspherocytic hemolytic anemia | COBS | chronic organic brain syndrome |
| CNT | could not tell | | |
| | could not test | | |

84

| COBT | chronic obstruction of biliary tract | COLD | chronic obstructive lung disease |
| COC | calcifying odontogenic cyst | | Computer Output to Laser Disk |
| | chain of custody | COLD A | cold agglutin titer |
| | combination oral contraceptive | Collyr | eye wash |
| | | col/ml | colonies per milliliter |
| | continuity of care | colp | colporrhaphy |
| COCCIO | coccidioidomycosis | COLTRU | *colletotrichum truncatum* |
| COCM | congestive cardiomyopathy | COM | center of mass |
| | | | chronic otitis media |
| COD | carotid occlusive disease | COMBO | combination ultrasound with electrical stimulation |
| | cataract, right eye | | |
| | cause of death | | |
| | chronic oxygen dependency | COMF | comfortable |
| | codeine | COMLA | cyclophosphamide, vincristine (Oncovin), methotrexate, calcium leucovorin, and cytarabine (ara-C) |
| | coefficient of oxygen delivery | | |
| | condition on discharge | | |
| CODAS | chronotherapeutic oral drug absorption system | COMM E | Committee E, a German Federal Health Agency committee for the evaluation of herbal remedies |
| CODE 99 | patient in cardiac or respiratory arrest | | |
| COD-MD | cerebro-oculardysplasia muscular dystrophy | COMP | compensation |
| | | | complications |
| CODO | codocytes | | composite |
| COE | court-ordered examination | | compound |
| COEPS | cortically originating extrapyramidal symptoms | | compress |
| | | | cyclophosphamide, vincristine (Oncovin), methotrexate, and prednisone |
| COER-24 | 24-hour controlled-onset, extended-release (dosage form) | | |
| | | COMS | clinical outcomes management system |
| COFS | cerebro-oculo-facio-skeletal | COMT | catechol-*O*-methyl-transferase |
| COG | center of gravity | | |
| | Central Oncology Group | COMTA | Commission on Message Therapy Accreditation |
| | Children's Oncology Group | | |
| | | CON | catheter over a needle |
| | cognitive function tests | | certificate of need |
| COGN | cognition | | conservatorship |
| COGTT | cortisone-primed oral glucose tolerance test | CON A | concanavalin A |
| | | conc. | concentrated |
| COH | carbohydrate | CONG | congenital |
| | controlled ovarian hyperstimulation | | gallon |
| | | CONJ | conjunctiva |
| COHb | carboxyhemoglobin | CONPA-DRI I | cyclophosphamide, vincristine, doxorubicin, and melphalan |
| Coke | Coca-Cola® | | |
| | cocaine | CONPA-DRI II | conpadri I plus high-dose methotrexate |
| COL | colonoscopy | | |

| CONPA-DRI III | conpadri I plus intensified doxorubicin |
| CoNS | coagulase-negative staphylococci |
| CONT | continuous |
| | contusions |
| CON-TRAL | contralateral |
| CONTU | contusion |
| CONV | conversation |
| Conv. ex. | convergence excess |
| ConvRX | conventional therapy |
| CO-Ox | Co-oximetry |
| COP | center of pressure |
| | change of plaster |
| | cicatricial ocular pemphigoid |
| | *Colibacilosis porcina* vaccine |
| | colloid osmotic pressure |
| | complaint of pain |
| | cycophosphamide, vincristine (Oncovin), and prednisone |
| COP 1 | copolymer 1 |
| COPA | cuffed oropharyngeal airway |
| COP-BLAM | cyclophosphamide, vincristine (Oncovin), prednisone, bleomycin, doxorubicin (Adriamycin), and procarbazine (Matulane) |
| COPD | chronic obstructive pulmonary disease |
| COPE | chronic obstructive pulmonary emphysema |
| COPP | cyclophosphamide, vincristine, procarbazine, and prednisone |
| COPS | community outpatient service |
| COPT | circumoval precipitin test |
| CoQ10 | coenzyme $Q_{10}$ |
| COR | coefficient of reproducibility |
| | conditioned orientation response |
| | coronary |
| CORA | conditioned orientation reflex audiometry |

| CORBA | Common-Object Request Broker Architecture |
| CORE | cardiac or respiratory emergency |
| CORF | Comprehensive Outpatient Rehabilitation Facility |
| COR P | cor pulmonale |
| CORT | Certified Operating Room Technician |
| COS | cataract, left eye |
| | change of shift |
| | Chief of Staff |
| | clinically observed seizure |
| | controlled ovarian stimulation |
| | Crisis Outpatient Services |
| $C_{osm}$ | osmolal clearance |
| COSTART | Coding symbols for a thesaurus of adverse reaction terms |
| COT | content of thought |
| COTA | Certified Occupational Therapy Assistant |
| COTE | comprehensive occupational therapy evaluation |
| COTT CH | cottage cheese |
| COTX | cast-off, to x-ray |
| COU | cardiac observation unit |
| | cataracts, both eyes |
| COV | coefficient of variation |
| COW | circle of Willis |
| COWA | controlled oral word association |
| COWAT | Controlled Oral Word Association Test |
| COWS | cold to the opposite and warm to the same |
| COX | Coxsackie virus |
| | cyclo-oxygenase |
| | cytochrome C oxidase |
| COX-2 | cyclo-oxygenase-2 |
| CP | centric position |
| | cerebral palsy |
| | Certified Paramedic |
| | chemical peel |
| | chemistry profiles |
| | chest pain |
| | chloroquine-primaquine |
| | chondromalacia patella |
| | chronic pain |
| | chronic pancreatitis |
| | cleft palate |

| | | | |
|---|---|---|---|
| | clinical pathway | | coil planet centrifuge |
| | closing pressure | | continue plan of care |
| | cold pack | CPC-H | Certified Procedural |
| | convenience package | | Coder, Hospital-Based |
| | cor pulmonale | CPCR | cardiopulmonary-cerebral |
| | creatine phosphokinase | | resuscitation |
| | cyclophosphamide and | CPCS | clinical pharmacokinetics |
| | cisplatin (Platinol) | | consulting service |
| | cystopanendoscopy | CPD | cephalopelvic |
| $C_p$ | concentration of drug | | disproportion |
| | plasma | | chorioretinopathy and |
| | phosphate clearance | | pituitary dysfunction |
| *Cp* | *Chlamydia pneumoniae* | | chronic peritoneal |
| C/P | carbohydrate-to-protein | | dialysis |
| | ratio | | citrate-phosphate-dextrose |
| C&P | compensation and pension | CPDA-1 | citrate-phosphate- |
| | complete and pain-free | | dextrose-adenine-one |
| | (range of motion) | CPDA-2 | citrate-phosphate-dextrose- |
| | complete and pushing | | adenine-two |
| | cystoscopy and | CPDD | calcium pyrophosphate |
| | pyelography | | deposition disease |
| CPA | cardiopulmonary arrest | CPDG2 | carboxypeptidase-G2 |
| | carotid photoangiography | CPDR | Center for Prostate |
| | cerebellar pontile angle | | Disease Research |
| | chest pain alert | | (Department of |
| | color power angiography | | Defense) |
| | conditioned play | CPE | cardiogenic pulmonary |
| | audiometry | | edema |
| | costophrenic angle | | chronic pulmonary |
| | cyclophosphamide | | emphysema |
| | cyproterone acetate | | Clinical Pastoral Education |
| CPAF | chlorpropamide-alcohol | | clubbing, pitting, or edema |
| | flush | | complete physical |
| $C_{PAH}$ | para-amino hippurate | | examination |
| | clearance | | cytopathic effect |
| CPAP | continuous positive airway | CPE-C | cyclopentenylcytosine |
| | pressure | CPEO | chronic progressive |
| CPB | cardiopulmonary bypass | | external |
| | cisplatin, | | ophthalmoplegia |
| | cyclophosphamide, and | CPER | chest pain emergency |
| | carmustine (BiCNU) | | room |
| | competitive protein | CPET | cardiopulmonary exercise |
| | binding | | testing |
| CPBA | competitive protein- | CPETU | chest pain evaluation and |
| | binding assay | | treatment unit |
| CPBP | cardiopulmonary bypass | CPF | cerebral perfusion |
| CPC | cancer prevention clinic | | pressure |
| | cerebral palsy clinic | CPFT | Certified Pulmonary |
| | Certified Procedural | | Function Technologist |
| | Coder | CPG | clinical practice guidelines |
| | chronic passive congestion | CPG2 | carboxypeptidase G2 |
| | clinicopathologic | CPGN | chronic progressive |
| | conference | | glomerulonephritis |

C

| | | | |
|---|---|---|---|
| CPH | chronic persistent hepatitis | CPO | chief privacy officer |
| | | | continue present orders |
| CPhT | Certified Pharmacy Technician | CPOE | computerized physician (prescriber) order entry |
| CPI | chronic public inebriate | CPOX | chicken pox |
| | constitutionally psychopathia inferior | CPP | central precocious puberty |
| | | | cerebral perfusion pressure |
| CPID | chronic pelvic inflammatory disease | | chronic pelvic pain |
| | | | coronary perfusion pressure |
| CPIP | chronic pulmonary insufficiency of prematurity | | cryo-poor plasma |
| | | CPPB | continuous positive pressure breathing |
| CPK | creatine phosphokinase (BB, MB, MM are isoenzymes) | CPPD | calcium pyrophosphate dihydrate |
| | | | cisplatin |
| CPK-1 | creatine phosphokinase MM fraction | CP & PD | chest percussion and postural drainage |
| CPK-2 | creatine phosphokinase MB fraction | CPPS | chronic pelvice pain syndrome |
| CPK-BB | creatine phosphokinase BB fraction | CPPV | continuous positive pressure ventilation |
| CPKD | childhood polycystic kidney disease | CPQ | Conner Parent Questionnaire |
| CPK-MB | creatine phosphokinase of muscle band | CPR | cardiopulmonary resuscitation |
| CPL | criminal procedure law | | computer-based patient records |
| CPM | cancer pain management | | |
| | central pontine myelinolysis | | computerized patient record |
| | chlorpheniramine maleate | | tablet (French) |
| | chronic progressive myelopathy | CPR-1 | all measures except cardiopulmonary resuscitation |
| | Clinical Practice Model | | |
| | continue present management | CPR-2 | no extraordinary measures (to resuscitate) |
| | continuous passive motion | CPR-3 | comfort measures only |
| | counts per minute | CPRAM | controlled partial rebreathing anesthesia method |
| | cycles per minute | | |
| | cyclophosphamide | | |
| CPmax | peak serum concentration | CP/ROMI | chest pain, rule out myocardial infarction |
| CPMDI | computerized pharmacokinetic model-driven drug infusion | CPRS | Categorical Pain Relief Scale |
| CPmin | trough serum concentration | CPRS-OCS | Comprehensive Psychiatric Rating Scale, Obsessive-Compulsive Subscale |
| CPMM | constant passive motion machine | | |
| CPMP | Committee for Proprietary Medicinal Products (of the European Union) | CPS | carbamyl phosphate synthetase |
| | | | cardiopulmonary support |
| CPN | chronic pyelonephritis | | Center for Prevention Services (CDC) |
| CPNI | common peroneal nerve injury | | |

| | chest pain syndrome | CPU | children's psychiatric unit |
|---|---|---|---|
| | child protective services | | clinical pharmacology unit |
| | Chinese paralytic syndrome | CPUE | chest pain of unknown etiology |
| | chloroquine-pyrimethamine sulfadoxine | CPUM | Certified Professional in Utilization Management |
| | clinical performance score | CPV | cowpox virus |
| | clinical pharmacokinetic service | CPX | complete physical examination |
| | CoaguChek® Plus System | CPZ | chlorpromazine |
| | coagulase-positive staphylococci | | Compazine® (CPZ is a dangerous abbreviation as it could be either) |
| | complex partial seizures | | |
| | counts per second | | |
| | cumulative probability of success | CQDS | cumulative quality disruption score |
| CPs | clinical pathways | CQI | continuous quality improvement |
| CPS I | carbamyl phosphate synthetase I | CR | caloric restrictions |
| cPSA | complexed prostate-specific antigen | | capillary refill |
| CPSC | Consumer Product Safety Commission | | cardiac rehabilitation |
| | | | cardiorespiratory |
| CPSI | Chronic Prostatitis Symptom Index | | case reports |
| | | | chief resident |
| CPSP | central post-stroke pain | | chorioretinal |
| CPT | camptothecin | | clockwise rotation |
| | carnitine palmitoyl transferase | | closed reduction |
| | chest physiotherapy | | colon resection |
| | child protection team | | complete remission |
| | chromo-perturbation | | contact record |
| | cold pressor test | | controlled release |
| | Continuous Performance Test | | cosmetic rhinoplasty |
| | | | creamed |
| | corticosteroid pulse treatment | | credentialing |
| | | | crutches |
| | current perception threshold | | cycloplegia retinoscopy |
| | Current Procedural Terminology (coding system) | Cr | caloric restrictions |
| | | | chromium |
| CPT-2000 | Current Procedural Terminology, 2000 Edition | C/R | conscious, rational |
| | | C & R | convalescence and rehabilitation |
| CPT-11 | irinotecan hydrochloride (Camptosar) | | cystoscopy and retrograde |
| CPTA | Certified Physical Therapy Assistant | $CR_1$ | first cranial nerve |
| | | CRA | central retinal artery |
| | | | chronic rheumatoid arthritis |
| CPT/C | current perception threshold, computerized | | cis-retinoic acid (isotretinion, Accutane®) |
| | | | Clinical Research Associate |
| CPTH | chronic post-traumatic headache | | colorectal anastomosis |
| | | | corticosteroid-resistant asthma |

| | |
|---|---|
| CRABP | cellular retinoic acid binding protein |
| CRAbs | chelating recombinant antibodies |
| CRADA | Cooperative Research and Development Agreement (with NIH) |
| CRAG | cerebral radionuclide angiography |
| CrAg | cryptococcal antigen |
| CRAMS | circulation, respiration, abdomen, motor, and speech |
| CRAN | craniotomy |
| CRAO | central retinal artery occlusion |
| CRAX | crackers |
| CRBBB | complete right bundle branch block |
| CRBIs | catheter-related bloodstream infections |
| CRBP | cellular retinol-binding protein |
| CRBSI | vascular-catheter-related bloodstream infections |
| CRC | case review committee |
| | child-resistant container |
| | clinical research center |
| | Clinical Research Coordinator |
| | colorectal cancer |
| CR & C | closed reduction and cast |
| CrCl | creatinine clearance |
| CRD | childhood rheumatic disease |
| | chronic renal disease |
| | chronic respiratory disease |
| | colorectal distension |
| | cone-rod dystrophy |
| | congenital rubella deafness |
| | crown-rump distance |
| CRE | cumulative radiation effect |
| CREAT | serum creatinine |
| CREF | cycloplegic refraction |
| CRELM | screening tests for Congo-Crimean, Rift Valley, Ebola, Lassa, and Marburg fevers |
| CREP | crepitation |
| CREST | calcinosis, Raynaud disease, esophageal dysmotility, sclerodactyly, and telangiectasia |
| CRF | cardiac risk factors |
| | case report form |
| | chronic renal failure factor |
| CRH | corticotropic-releasing hormone |
| CRFZ | closed reduction of fractured zygoma |
| CRH | corticotropin-releasing hormone |
| CRHCa | cancer-related hypercalcemia |
| CRI | Cardiac Risk Index |
| | catheter-related infection |
| | chronic renal insufficiency |
| CRIB | Clinical Risk Index for Babies |
| CRIE | crossed radioimmuno-electrophoresis |
| CRIF | closed reduction and internal fixation |
| CRIMF | closed reduction/intermaxillary fixation |
| CRIS | controlled-release infusion system |
| crit | hematocrit |
| CRKL | crackles |
| CRL | crown rump length |
| CRM | circumferential resection margins |
| | continual reassessment method |
| | cream |
| | cross-reacting mutant |
| CRM + | cross-reacting material positive |
| CRMD | children with retarded mental development |
| CRN | crown |
| CRNA | Certified Registered Nurse Anesthetist |
| CRNFA | Certified Registered Nurse, First Assistant |
| CRNH | Certified Registered Nurse in Hospice |
| CRNI | Certified Registered Nurse Intravenous |

| | | | |
|---|---|---|---|
| CRNP | Certified Registered Nurse Practitioner | | cryoreductive surgery |
| CRO | cathode ray oscilloscope | | cytokine-release syndrome |
| | contract research organization(s) | CRST | calcification, Raynaud phenomenom, scleroderma, and telangiectasia |
| CROM | cervical range of motion | CRT | cadaver renal transplant |
| | chronic refractory osteomyelitis | | capillary refill time |
| CROMY | chronic refractory osteomyelitis | | Cardiac Rescue Technician |
| CROS | contralateral routing of signals | | cathode ray tube |
| CRP | canalith repositioning procedure | | central reaction time |
| | chronic relapsing pancreatitis | | Certified Rehabilitation Therapist |
| | coronary rehabilitation program | | chemoradiotherapy |
| | C-reactive protein | | choice reaction time |
| C&RP | curettage and root planning | | circuit resistance training |
| CRPA | C-reactive protein agglutinins | | copper reduction test |
| | | | cranial radiation therapy |
| | | Cr Tr | crutch training |
| CRPD | chronic restrictive pulmonary disease | CRTs | case report tabulations |
| CRPF | chloroquine-resistant *Plasmodium falciparum* | CRTT | Certified Respiratory Therapy Technician |
| CRPP | closed reduction and percutaneous pinning | CRTX | cast removed take x-ray |
| CRPS I | complex regional pain syndrome type I | CRU | cardiac rehabilitation unit |
| | | | clinical research unit |
| CRQ | Chronic Respiratory (Disease) Questionnaire | CRV | central retinal vein |
| | | CRVF | congestive right ventricular failure |
| CRR | community rehabilitation residence | CRVO | central retinal vein occlusion |
| CRRT | continuous renal replacement therapy | CRx | chemotherapy |
| CRS | Carroll Self-Rating Scale | CIIRx | Century II Bicarbonate Dialysis Machine |
| | catheter-related sepsis | CRYO | cryoablation |
| | Center for Scientific Review (NIH) | | cryosurgery |
| | Chemical Reference Substances | CRYST | crystals |
| | child restraint system(s) | CS | cardiogenic shock |
| | Chinese restaurant syndrome | | cardioplegia solution |
| | chronic rhinosinusitis | | cat scratch |
| | cocaine-related seizure(s) | | cervical spine |
| | colon-rectal surgery | | cesarean section |
| | congenital rubella syndrome | | chest strap |
| | continuous running suture | | cholesterol stone |
| | | | chlorobenzylidene malononitrile |
| | | | cigarette smoker |
| | | | clinically significant |
| | | | clinical stage |
| | | | close supervision |
| | | | conditionally susceptible |
| | | | congenital syphilis |
| | | | conjunctiva-sclera |

**C**

| | |
|---|---|
| | consciousness |
| | conscious sedation |
| | consultation |
| | consultation service |
| | coronary sinus |
| | corticosteroid(s) |
| | cranial setting |
| | Cushing syndrome |
| | cycloserine |
| | *o*-chlorobenzylidene malononitrile |
| C&S | conjunctiva and sclera |
| | cough and sneeze |
| | culture and sensitivity |
| C/S | cesarean section |
| | consultation |
| | culture and sensitivity |
| CSA | central sleep apnea |
| | compressed spectral activity |
| | Controlled Substances Act |
| | controlled substance analogue |
| | corticosteroid-sensitive asthma |
| CsA | cyclosporine (cyclosporin A) |
| CsA-ME | cyclosporine microemulsion (Neoral) |
| CSAP | cryosurgical ablation of the prostate |
| CSB | caffeine sodium benzoate |
| | Cheyne-Stokes breathing |
| | Children's Services Board |
| CSBF | coronary sinus blood flow |
| CSBO | complete small bowel obstruction |
| CSC | central serous chorioretinopathy |
| | cornea, sclera, and conjunctiva |
| | cryopreserved stem cells |
| CSCI | continuous subcutaneous infusion |
| CSCR | central serous chorioretinopathy |
| CSD | cat scratch disease |
| | celiac sprue disease |
| | cortical spreading depression |
| C S&D | cleaned, sutured, and dressed |
| CSDD | Center for the Study of Drug Development |
| CSDH | chronic subdural hematoma |
| | combined systolic and diastolic hypertension |
| CSE | combined spinal/epidurals |
| | cross-section echocardiography |
| C sect. | cesarean section |
| CSF | cerebrospinal fluid |
| | colony-stimulating factors |
| CSFELP | cerebrospinal fluid electrophoresis |
| CSFP | cerebrospinal fluid pressure |
| CSGIT | continuous-suture graft-inclusion technique |
| C-Sh | chair shower |
| CSH | carotid sinus hypersensitivity |
| | chronic subdural hematoma |
| CSHQ | Children's Sleep Habits Questionnaire |
| CSI | chemical shift imaging |
| | Computerized Severity Index |
| | continuous subcutaneous infusion |
| | coronary stent implantation |
| | craniospinal irradiation |
| CsI | cesium iodide |
| CSICU | cardiac surgery intensive care unit |
| CSID | congenital sucrase-isomaitase deficiency |
| CSII | continuous subcutaneous insulin infusion |
| CS IV | clinical stage 4 |
| CSL | chemical safety level |
| CSLU | chronic status leg ulcer |
| CSM | carotid sinus massage |
| | cerebrospinal meningitis |
| | cervical spondylotic myelopathy |
| | circulation, sensation, and movement |
| | Committee on Safety of Medicines (United Kingdom) |

| | |
|---|---|
| CSME | cotton-spot macular edema |
| CSMN | chronic sensorimotor neuropathy |
| CSN | cystic suppurative necrosis |
| CSNB | congenital stationary night blindness |
| CSNRT | corrected sinus node recovery time |
| CSNS | carotid sinus nerve stimulation |
| CSO | Chief Security Officer |
| | Consumer Safety Officer (FDA) |
| | copied standing orders |
| CSOM | chronic serous otitis media |
| | chronic suppurative otitis media |
| CSP | cellulose sodium phosphate |
| | cervical spine pain |
| | chiral stationary phase |
| C-spine | cervical spine |
| CSR | central supply room |
| | Cheyne-Stokes respiration |
| | corrected sedimentation rate |
| | corrective septorhinoplasty |
| C-S RT | craniospinal radiotherapy |
| CSS | Canadian Stroke Scale (score) |
| | carotid sinus stimulation |
| | Central Sterile Services |
| | chemical sensitivity syndrome |
| | chewing, sucking, and swallowing |
| | child safety seats |
| | Churg-Strauss syndrome |
| $C_{SS}$ | concentration of drug at steady-state |
| CSSD | closed system sterile drainage |
| CST | cardiac stress test |
| | castration |
| | central sensory conducting time |
| | cerebroside sulfotransferase |
| | Certified Surgical Technologist |

**C**

| | |
|---|---|
| | cesarean section prior to labor at term |
| | contraction stress test |
| | convulsive shock therapy |
| | cosyntropin stimulation test |
| | static compliance |
| $C_{STAT}$ | static lung compliance |
| CSU | cardiac surgery unit |
| | cardiac surveillance unit |
| | cardiovascular surgery unit |
| | casualty staging unit |
| | catheter specimen of urine |
| CSVD | cerebral small-vessel disease |
| CSW | cerebral salt-wasting (syndrome) |
| | Clinical Social Worker |
| CSWCM | Certified Social Work Case Manager |
| CSWs | commercial sex workers |
| CSWSS | continuous spike-waves during slow sleep |
| CT | calcitonin |
| | cardiothoracic |
| | carpal tunnel |
| | cellulose triacetate (filter) |
| | cervical traction |
| | chemotherapy |
| | chest tube |
| | *Chlamydia trachomatis* |
| | circulation time |
| | client |
| | clinical trial |
| | clotting time |
| | coagulation time |
| | coated tablet |
| | compressed tablet |
| | computed tomography |
| | Coomb test |
| | corneal thickness |
| | corneal transplant |
| | corrective therapy |
| | cytarabine and thioguanine |
| | cytoxic drug |
| $C_t$ | concentration of drug in tissue |
| C/T | compared to |
| CTA | catamenia (menses) |
| | clear to auscultation |
| | computed tomography angiography |

| | | | |
|---|---|---|---|
| C-TAB | cyanide tablet | CTID | chemotherapy-induced diarrhea |
| CTAP | clear to auscultation and percussion | CTL | cervical, thoracic, and lumbar |
| | computed tomography during arterial portography | | chronic tonsillitis |
| | | | control (subjects) |
| | | | cytotoxic T-lymphocytes |
| CTB | ceased to breathe | CTLSO | cervicothoracic-lumbosacral orthosis |
| | cholera toxin B | | |
| CTC | Cancer Treatment Center | CTM | Chlor-Trimeton |
| | circular tear capsulotomy | | clinical trials materials |
| | Clinical Trial Certificate (United Kingdom's equivalent to the Investigational New Drug Application) | | computed tomographic myelography |
| | | CT/MPR | computed tomography with multiplanar reconstructions |
| | Common Toxicity Criteria | CTN | calcitonin |
| | cyclophosphamide, thiotepa, and carboplatin | C & T N, BLE | color and temperature normal, both lower extremities |
| CTCL | cutaneous T-cell lymphoma (mycosis fungoides) | cTnI | cardiac troponin I |
| | | cTNM | clinical-diagnostic staging of cancer |
| CT & DB | cough, turn & deep breath | | |
| CTD | carpal tunnel decompression | CTP | comprehensive treatment plan |
| | chest tube drainage | CTPA | clear to percussion and auscultation |
| | connective tissue disease | | |
| | corneal thickness depth | CTPN | central total parenteral nutrition |
| | cumulative trauma disorder | | |
| | | CTR | carpal tunnel release |
| CTDW | continues to do well | | carpal tunnel repair |
| CTEP | Cancer Therapy Evaluation Program | | Certified Tumor Registrar |
| | | | cosmetic transdermal reconstruction |
| | Center for Therapy Evaluation Programs (National Cancer Institute) | CTRS | Certified Therapeutic Recreation Specialist |
| | | | Conners Teachers Rating Scale |
| CTF | Colorado tick fever | CT-RT | chemo-radiotherapy |
| | continuous tube feeding | CTS | cardiothoracic surgeon |
| CTG | cardiotocography | | carpal tunnel syndrome |
| C/TG | cholesterol to triglyceride ratio | CTSP | called to see patient |
| | | CTT | cotton-thread test |
| CTGA | complete transposition of the great arteries | CTU | computed tomographic urography |
| | corrected transposition of the great arteries | CTW | central terminal of Wilson |
| CTH | clot to hold | CTX | cerebrotendinous xanthomatosis |
| CTHA | computed tomography hepatic arteriography | | cervical traction |
| | | | chemotherapy |
| CTI | certification of terminal illness | | cyclophosphamide (Cytoxan) |
| CTICU | cardiothoracic intensive care unit | CTXN | contraction |

| | | | |
|---|---|---|---|
| CTZ | chemoreceptor trigger zone | C/V | cervical/vaginal |
| | co-trimoxazole (sulfamethoxazole and trimethoprin) | CVA | cerebrovascular accident costovertebral angle |
| CU | cause undetermined | CVAD | central venous access device |
| | cause unknown | CVAH | congenital virilizing adrenal hyperplasia |
| | chronic undifferentiated clinical units | CVAT | costovertebral angle tenderness |
| | color unit | CVB | chronic villi biopsy |
| | convalescent unit | | group B coxsackievirus |
| | Cuprophan (filter) | CVC | central venous catheter |
| Cu | copper | | chief visual complaint |
| Cu | urea clear clearance | | consonant-vowel-consonant |
| C/U | checkup | | |
| CUA | clean urinalysis | CVD | cardiovascular disease |
| | cost-utility analysis | | collagen vascular disease |
| CUC | chronic ulcerative colitis | CVDU | chronic ventilator-dependent unit |
| | Clinical Unit Clerk | | |
| CUD | cause undetermined | CVEB | cisplatin, vinblastine, etoposide, and bleomycin |
| | controlled unsterile delivery | | |
| CUFCM | Century Ultrafiltration Control Machine | CVENT | controlled ventilation |
| | | CVF | cardiovascular failure |
| CUG | cystourethrogram | | central visual field |
| Cu-IUD | copper intrauterine device | | cervicovaginal fluid |
| CUP | carcinoma of unknown primary (site) | CVG | coronary vein graft |
| | | | cutis verticis gyrata |
| CUPS | carcinoma of unknown primary site | CVHD | chronic valvular heart disease |
| CUR | curettage | CVI | carboplatin, etoposide, ifosfamide, and mesna uroprotection |
| | cystourethrorectocele | | |
| CUS | carotid ultrasound | | cerebrovascular insufficiency |
| | chronic undifferentiated schizophrenia | | |
| | compression ultrasonography | | chronic venous insufficiency |
| | contact urticaria syndrome | | common variable immunodeficiency (disease) |
| CUSA | Cavitron ultrasonic suction aspirator | | |
| CUT | chronic undifferentiated type (schizophrenia) | | continuous venous infusion |
| | | CVICU | cardiovascular intensive care unit |
| CUTA | congenital urinary tract anomaly | CVID | common variable immune deficiency |
| CV | cardiovascular | | |
| | cell volume | CVINT | cardiovascular intermediate |
| | cisplatin and etoposide | | |
| | coefficient of variation | CVL | central venous line |
| | color vision | | cervicovaginal lavage |
| | common ventricle | | clinical vascular laboratory |
| | consonant vowel | | |
| | contrast venography | CVLT | California Verbal Learning Test |
| | *curriculum vitae* | | |

| | | | |
|---|---|---|---|
| CVM | Center for Veterinary Medicine (NIH) | CVVH | continuous venovenous hemofiltration |
| CVMT | cervical-vaginal, motion tenderness | CVVHDF | continuous venovenous hemodiafiltration |
| CVN | central venous nutrient | CW | careful watch |
| CVNSR | cardiovascular normal sinus rhythm | | case worker |
| | | | chest wall |
| CVO | central vein occlusion | | clockwise |
| | conjugate diameter of pelvic inlet | | compare with |
| | | C/W | consistent with |
| CvO₂ | mixed venous oxygen content | | crutch walking |
| | | CWA | chemical warfare agents |
| CVOD | cerebrovascular obstructive disease | CWAF | Chemical Withdrawal Assessment Flowsheet |
| CVOR | cardiovascular operating room | CWAP | continuous wave arthroscopy pump |
| CVP | central venous pressure | CWD | cell wall defective |
| | cyclophosphamide, vincristine, and prednisone | CWE | cotton-wool exudates |
| | | CWL | Caldwell-Luc |
| | | CWM | comprehensive weight management |
| CVPP | lomustine, vinblastine, procarbazine, and prednisone | CWMS | color, warmth, movement, and sensation |
| CVR | cerebral vascular resistance | CWP | centimeters of water pressure |
| | cerebrovascular resuscitation | | childbirth without pain |
| | coronary vascular reserve | | coal worker's pneumoconiosis |
| CVRI | coronary vascular resistance index | | cold wet packs |
| CVRS | Cardiovascular-Respiratory Score | cWPW | concealed Wolff-Parkinson-White syndrome |
| CVS | cardiovascular surgery | CWR | clockwise rotation |
| | cardiovascular system | CWS | Certified Wound Care Specialist |
| | challenge virus standard | | |
| | chorionic villi sampling | | comfortable walking speed |
| | clean voided specimen | | cotton-wool spots |
| | continuing vegetative state | CWT | compensated work training |
| CVSCU | cardiovascular special care unit | CWV | closed wound vacuum |
| CVSD | congenital ventricular septal defecct | CX | cancel |
| | | | cervix |
| CVST | cardiovascular stress test | | chronic |
| | | | circumflex |
| | cerebral venous sinus thrombosis | | circumflex artery |
| | | | culture |
| CVSU | cardiovascular specialty unit | | cylinder axis |
| | | | cystectomy |
| CVT | calf vein thrombosis | CXA | circumflex artery |
| CVTC | central venous tunneled catheter | CxBx | cervical biopsy |
| | | CxMT | cervical motion tenderness |
| CVU | clean voided urine | CXR | chest x-ray |
| CVUG | cysto-void urethrogram | CXTX | cervical traction |

C

| | |
|---|---|
| CY | cyclophosphamide |
| C&Y | Children with Youth (program) |
| CYA | cover your ass |
| CyA | cyclosporine |
| CyADIC | cyclophosphamide, doxorubicin (Adriamycin), and dacarbazine |
| CYC | cyclophosphamide |
| Cyclo C | cyclocytidine HCl |
| CYL | cylinder |
| CYP | cytochrome P-450 system |
| CYP450 | cytochrome P450 system |
| CYRO | cryoprecipitate |
| CYSTA | cystathionine |
| CYSTO | cystogram cystoscopy |
| CYT | cyclophosphamide |
| CYTA | cytotoxic agent |
| CYVA DIC | cyclophosphamide, vincristine, Adriamycin, and dacarbazine |
| CZE | capillary zone electrophoresis |
| CZI | crystalline zinc insulin (regular insulin) |
| CZP | clonazepam (Klonopin) |

# D

| | |
|---|---|
| D | daughter |
| | day |
| | dead |
| | decay |
| | depression |
| | dextrose |
| | dextro |
| | diarrhea |
| | diastole |
| | dictated |
| | dilated |
| | diminished |
| | Dinamap (blood pressure monitor) |
| | diopter |
| | distal |
| | distance |
| | divorced |
| D+ | note has been dictated/ look for report |
| D− | note not dictated, save chart for doctor |
| $D_{0(2/7/00)}$ | Day zero (the day treatment begins, February 7th, 2000) |
| $D_1$ | day one (first day of treatment) |
| | first diagonal branch (coronary artery) |
| D-1 . . . . D-12 | dorsal vertebrae 1 to 12 dorsal nerves 1-12 |
| $D_2$ | second diagonal branch (coronary artery) |
| | ergocalciferol |
| 2/d | twice a day (this is a dangerous abbreviation) |
| 2-D | two-dimensional |
| 3-D | three-dimensional |
| $D_3$ | cholecalciferol |
| D-3+7 | cytarabine and daunorubicin |
| 4D | 4 prism diopters |
| 4-D | four-dimensional |
| D5 | dextrose 5% injection |
| 5xD | five times a day (this is a dangerous abbreviation) |
| D-15 | Farnsworth panel D-15 color vision test |

| | | | |
|---|---|---|---|
| D50 | 50% dextrose injection | DAFNE | dose adjustment for normal eating |
| D<sub>5/.45</sub> | dextrose 5% in 0.45% sodium chloride injection | DAG | diacylglyerol dianhydrogalactitol |
| DA | dark adaptation (test) | DAH | diffuse alveolar hemorrhage |
| | Debtors Anonymous | | disordered action of the heart |
| | degenerative arthritis | | |
| | delivery awareness | DAI | diffuse axonal injury |
| | Dental Assistant | DAIDS | Division of AIDS (of the National Institute of Allergy and Infectious Diseases, NIH) |
| | diagnostic arthroscopy | | |
| | diastolic augmentation | | |
| | direct admission | | |
| | direct agglutination | | |
| | diversional activity | DAL | diffuse aggressive lymphomas |
| | dopamine | | |
| | drug addict | | drug analysis laboratory |
| | drug aerosol | DALE | disability-adjusted life expectancy |
| Da | daltons | | |
| D/A | discharge and advise | DALM | dysplasia-associated lesion or mass |
| DAA | dead after arrival | | |
| | dissection aortic aneurysm | DALY | disability-adjusted life year(s) |
| DA/A | drug/alcohol addiction | DAM | diacetylmonoxine |
| DAB | days after birth | DAMA | discharged against medical advice |
| | diamino benzidine | | |
| DABA | Diplomate of the American Board of Anesthesiology | DANA | drug-induced antinuclear antibodies |
| | | DAo | descending aorta |
| DAC | day activity center | DAOM | depressor anguli oris muscle |
| | disabled adult child | | |
| | Division of Ambulatory Care | DAP | dapsone |
| | | | diabetes-associated peptide |
| DACL | Depression Adjective Checklists | | diastolic augmentation pressure |
| DACS | density-adjusted cell sorting | | distending airway pressure |
| | | | Draw-A-Person |
| DACT | dactinomycin (Cosmegen) | | |
| DAD | diffuse alveolar damage | DAPT | Draw-A-Person Test |
| | diode array detector | DAR | daily affective rhythm |
| | Disability Assessment of Dementia | | data, action, response |
| | | DARE | data, action, response, and evaluation |
| | dispense as directed | | |
| | drug administration device | DARP | drug abuse rehabilitation program |
| | father | | |
| DADS | distal acquired demyelinating symmetrical (neuropathy) | | drug abuse reporting program |
| | | D/ART | depression/awareness, recognition and treatment |
| DAE | diving air embolism | DAS | day of admission surgery |
| DAF | decay-accelerating factor | | developmental apraxia of speech |
| | delayed auditory feedback | | |
| DAFE | Dial-A-Flow Extension® | | |
| DAFM | double-aerosol face mask | | |

| | | | |
|---|---|---|---|
| | died at scene | dBEMCL | decibel effective masking contralateral |
| DAs | daily activities | | |
| DASE | dobutamine-atropine stress echocardiography | D₅BES | dextrose in balanced electrolyte solution |
| DASH | Dietary Approaches to Stop Hypertension (diet) | DBI | documented by initials |
| | | DBI® | phenformin HCl |
| | | DBIL | direct bilirubin |
| DASI | Duke Activity Status Index | DBKT | Diabetes: Basic Knowledge Test |
| DAST | Drug Abuse Screening Test | DBL | double beta-lactam |
| DAT | daunorubicin, cytarabine, (ara-C), and thioguanine | DBM | dibenzoylmethane |
| | definitely abnormal tracing (electrocardiogram) | DBMT | displacement bone marrow transplantation |
| | dementia of the Alzheimer type | DBP | D-binding protein |
| | | | diastolic blood pressure |
| | diet as tolerated | | dibutyl phthalate |
| | diphtheria antitoxin | DBPCFC | double-blind, placebo-controlled food challenge |
| | direct agglutination test | | |
| | direct amplification test | DBPT | dacarbazine (DTIC), carmustine (BCNU), cisplatin (Platinol), and tamoxifen |
| | direct antiglobulin test | | |
| DAU | daughter | | |
| | drug abuse urine | | |
| DAUNO | daunorubicin | DBQ | debrisoquin |
| DAVA | vindesine sulfate (Eldisine; desacetyl vinblastine amide sulfate) | DBS | deep brain stimulation |
| | | | desirable body weight |
| | | | diminished breath sounds |
| DAVM | dural arteriovenous malformation | | dried blood stain |
| DAV SEP | deviated septum | DBT | dialectical behavior therapy |
| DAW | dispense as written | DBW | dry body weight |
| DAWN | Drug Abuse Warning Network | DBZ | dibenzamine |
| dB | decibel | DC | daunorubicin and cytarabine |
| DB | database | | daycare |
| | date of birth | | decrease |
| | deep breathe | | dextrocardia |
| | demonstration bath | | diagonal conjugate |
| | dermabrasion | | direct Coombs (test) |
| | diaphragmatic breathing | | direct current |
| | difficulty breathing | | discharge |
| | direct bilirubin | | discomfort |
| | double blind | | Doctor of Chiropractic |
| DBA | Diamond-Blackfan anemia | D&C | dilatation and curettage |
| | | | direct and consensual |
| DB & C | deep breathing and coughing | D/C | disconnect |
| | | | discontinue |
| DBD | milolactol (dibromodulicitol) | DCA | directional coronary atherectomy |
| | | | disk/condyle adhesion |
| DBE | deep breathing exercise | | double-cup arthroplasty |
| DBED | penicillin G benzathine (for IM use only) | | sodium dichloroacetate |

D

| | | | |
|---|---|---|---|
| DCAG | double-coronary artery graft | DCO | diffusing capacity of carbon monoxide |
| DCAP-BTLS | deformities, contusions, abrasions, and punctures/penetrations, burns, tenderness, lacerations, and swelling (an assessment mnemonic used by EMTs) | DCP | dynamic compression plate |
| | | DCP® | calcium phosphate, dibasic |
| | | DCPM | daunorubicin, cytarabine, prednisolone, and mercaptopurine |
| DC-ART | disease controlling anti-rheumatic therapy | DCPN | direction-changing positional nystagmus |
| DC&B | dilation, currettage, and biopsy | DCR | dacryocystorhinostomy |
| | | | delayed cutaneous reaction |
| DCBE | double-contrast barium enema | DCRC | disseminated colorectal cancer |
| DCC | day care center | DCRF | data case report forms |
| | diabetes care clinic | 3DCRT | three-dimensional conformal radiation therapy |
| | direct current cardioversion | | |
| DCCF | dural carotid-cavernous fistula | DCS | decompression sickness |
| | | | dorsal column stimulator |
| DCCT | Diabetes Control and Complications Trial (questionnaire) | DCSA | double-contrast shoulder arthrography |
| | | DCSW | Diplomate in Clinical Social Work |
| DC'd | discontinued | DCT | daunorubicin, cytarabine, and thioguanine |
| DCE | delayed contrast-enhancement | | decisional conflict theory |
| | designated compensable event | | deep chest therapy |
| DCF | data collection form | | direct (antiglobulin) Coombs test |
| | Denomination Commune Francaise (French-approved nonproprietary name) | DCTM | delay computer tomographic myelography |
| | | DCU | day care unit |
| | pentostatin (Nipent; 2′ deoxycoformycin) | DCUS | duplex-color ultrasonography |
| DCFS | Department of Children and Family Services | DCW | direct care worker |
| | | DCYS | Department of Children and Youth Services |
| DCG | diagnostic cardiogram | DD | delayed diarrhea |
| DCH | delayed cutaneous hypersensitivity | | delivery date |
| | | | dependent drainage |
| DCIA | deep circumflex iliac artery (flap) | | Descemet detachment |
| | | | detrusor dyssynergia |
| DCIS | ductal carcinoma *in situ* | | developmentally delayed |
| DCLHb | diaspirin cross-linked hemoglobin | | developmental disabilities |
| DCM | dementia care mapping | | developmentally disabled |
| | dilated cardiomyopathy | | dialysis dementia |
| DCMXT | dichloromethotrexate | | died of the disease |
| DCN | Darvocet N | | differential diagnosis |
| DCNU | chlorozotocin | | |

| | discharge diagnosis | DDRE | Division of Drug Risk |
| | disk diameter | | Evaluation (FDA) |
| | Doctor of Divinity | DDS | dialysis disequilibrium |
| | double dose (used by | | syndrome |
| | Radiology) | | Doctor of Dental Surgery |
| | down drain | | double-decidual sac |
| | dry dressing | | (sign) |
| | dual disorder | | 4, 4-diaminodiphenyl- |
| | Duchenne dystrophy | | sulfone (dapsone) |
| | due date | DDST | Denver Development |
| | dysthymic disorder | | Screening Test |
| D/D | diarrhea/dehydration | DDT | chlorophenothane |
| D → D | discharge to duty | DDTP | drug dependence |
| D & D | debridement and dressing | | treatment program |
| | diarrhea and dehydration | DDx | differential diagnosis |
| | drilling and drainage | DE | dermal epidermal |
| DDA | dideoxyadenosine | | (junction) |
| DDAH | dimethylarginine | | digitalis effect |
| | dimethylaminohydrolase | $D_5E_{48}$ | 5% Dextrose and |
| DDAVP® | desmopressin acetate | | Electrolyte 48 |
| DDC | zalcitabine (dideoxy- | $D_5E_{75}$ | 5% Dextrose and |
| | cytidine; Hivid) | | Electrolyte 75 |
| DDD | defined daily doses | 2-DE | two-dimensional |
| | degenerative disk disease | | echocardiography |
| | dense deposit disease | | two-dimentional gel |
| | fully automatic pacing | | electrophoresis |
| DDDR | pacemaker code (D = | 3-DE | three-dimensional |
| | chamber paced-**d**ual, | | echocardiography |
| | D = chamber sensed- | D&E | dilation and evacuation |
| | **d**ual, D = response to | DEA# | Drug Enforcement |
| | sensing-**d**ual, R = | | Administration number |
| | programmability-**r**ate | | (physician's federal |
| | modulation) | | narcotic number) |
| DDE | dichlorodiphenylethylene | DEAE | diethylaminoethyl |
| DDGB | double-dose gallbladder | DEB | diepoxybutane (test) |
| | (test) | | dystrophic epidermolysis |
| DDH | developmental dysplasia | | bullosa |
| | of the hip | DEC | deciduous (primary teeth) |
| DDHT | double-dissociated | | decrease |
| | hypertropia | | diethylcarbamazine |
| DDI | didanosine | | (Hetrazan) |
| | (dideoxyinosine; Videx) | | Drug Evaluation and |
| | dressing dry, intact | | Classification (a |
| DDIs | drug-drug interactions | | standardized curriculum |
| DDis | developmental disorder | | to train police officers) |
| DDiv | Doctor of Divinity | DECA | nandrolone decanoate |
| DDMC | diabetes disease | DECAFS | Department of Children |
| | management clinic | | and Family Services |
| DDNS | digestive disease and | DECEL | deceleration |
| | nutrition service | decub | decubitus |
| DDP | cisplatin | DED | diabetic eye disease |
| DDRA | dead despite resuscitation | | died in emergency |
| | attempt | | department |

| | | | |
|---|---|---|---|
| DEEDS | drugs, exercise, education, diet, and self-monitoring | | dexter (right) |
| | | | dexverapamil |
| DEEG | depth electroencephalogram | DEXA | dual-energy x-ray absorptiometry |
| | deteriorating electroencephalogram | DF | day frequency (of voiding) |
| DEET | diethyltoluamide | | decayed and filled |
| DEF | decayed, extracted, or filled | | deferred |
| | | | defibrotide |
| | defecation | | degree of freedom |
| | deficiency | | dengue fever |
| 2-DEF | two-dimensional echo-derived ejection fraction | | dexfenfluramine |
| | | | diabetic father |
| DEFT | defendant | | diastolic filling |
| | driven equilibrium Fourier transform (technique) | | dietary fiber |
| | | | dorsiflexion |
| DEG | diethylene glycol | | drug-free |
| degen | degenerative | | dye-free |
| DEHP | diethylhexyl phthalate | DFA | delayed feedback audiometry |
| DEL | delivered | | |
| | delivery | | diet for age |
| | deltoid | | difficulty falling asleep |
| DEM | drug evaluation matrix | | direct fluorescent antibody |
| DEMRI | dynamic enhanced magnetic resonance imaging | | distal forearm |
| | | DFD | defined formula diets |
| | | | degenerative facet disease |
| DEPs | diesel exhaust particles | | |
| DEP ST SEG | depressed ST segment | DFE | dilated fundus examination |
| DER | disulfiram-ethanol reaction | | distal femoral epiphysis |
| | | DFG | direct forward gaze |
| DERM | dermatology | DFI | disease-free interval |
| DES | desflurane (Supreme) | DFLE | disability-free life expectancy |
| | diethylstilbestrol | | |
| | diffuse esophageal spasm | DFM | decreased fetal movement |
| | disequilibrium syndrome | | deep finger massage |
| | Dissociative Experience Scale | | deep friction massage |
| | | DFMC | daily fetal movement count |
| | dry-eye syndrome | | |
| DESAT | desaturation | DFMR | daily fetal movement record |
| DESF | desflurane (Suprane) | | |
| DESI | Drug Efficacy Study Implementation | DFO | deferoxamine (Desferal) |
| | | DFOM | deferoxamine (Desferal) |
| DET | diethyltryptamine | DFP | diastolic filling period |
| | dipyridamole echocardiography test | | isoflurophate (diisopropyl flurophosphate) |
| DETOX | detoxification | DFR | diabetic floor routine |
| DEV | deviation | DFRC | deglycerolized frozen red cells |
| | duck embryo vaccine | | |
| DEVR | dominant exudative vitreoretinopathy | DFS | disease-free survival |
| | | | Division of Family Services |
| DEX | dexamethasone | | |
| | dexrazoxane (Zinecard) | | Doppler flow studies |

D

| | | | |
|---|---|---|---|
| DFSP | dermatofibrosarcoma protuberans | DHCC | dihydroxycholecalciferol |
| DFT | defibrillation threshold (testing) | DHD | dissociated horizontal deviation |
| DFU | dead fetus in uterus | DHE | dental health education |
| | diabetic foot ulcer | DHE 45® | dihydroergotamine |
| DFV | D'Aoust Fineman virus | | mesylate |
| | dengue fever vaccine | DHEA | dehydroepiandrosterone |
| | diarrhea, fever, and | DHEAS | dehydroepiandrosterone |
| | vomiting | | sulfate |
| DFW | Dexide face wash | DHF | dengue hemorrhagic |
| DFWO | dorsiflexory wedge | | fever |
| | osteotomy | | diastolic heart failure |
| DG | diagnosis | DHFR | dihydrofolate reductase |
| | dorsal glides | DHHS | Department of Health and |
| | downward gaze | | Human Services |
| DGA | DiGeorge anomaly | DHI | Dizziness Handicap |
| DGE | delayed gastric emptying | | Inventory |
| DGF | delayed graft function | | dynamic hyperinflation |
| DGGE | denaturing gradient gel | DHIC | detrusor hyperactivity |
| | electrophoresis | | with impaired |
| DGI | disseminated gonococcal | | contractility |
| | infection | DHL | diffuse histocytic |
| DGL | deglycyrrhizinated licorice | | lymphoma |
| DGR | duodenogastric reflux | DHP | dihydropyridine |
| DGM | ductal glandular | DHP-1 | dehydropeptidase-1 |
| | mastectomy | DHPG | ganciclovir |
| DGs | documentation guidelines | DHPLC | denaturing high- |
| DGT | decaffeinated green tea | | performance liquid |
| DH | delayed hypersensitivity | | chromatography |
| | Dental Hygienist | DHPR | dihydropteridine reductase |
| | dermatitis herpetiformis | DHPS | dihydopteroate synthase |
| | developmental history | DHR | delayed hypersensitivity |
| | diaphragmatic hernia | | reaction |
| D+H | delusions and | DHS | Department of Human |
| | hallucinations | | Services |
| D-H | Dimon-Hughston | | duration of hospital stay |
| | (intertrochanteric | | dynamic hip screw |
| | osteotomy technique) | DHST | delayed hypersensitivity |
| DHA | dihydroxyacetone | | test |
| | docosahexaenoic acid | DHT | dihydrotachysterol |
| DHAC | dihydro-5-azacytidine | | dihydrotestosterone |
| DHAD | mitoxanthrone HCl | | dissociated hypertropia |
| DHANP | Diplomate of the | | Dobhoff tube |
| | Homeopathic Academy | DHTF | Dobhoff tube |
| | of Naturopathic | | feeding |
| | Physicians | DI | (Beck) Depression |
| DHAP | dexamethasone, high-dose | | Inventory |
| | cytarabine, (ara-A) | | date of injury |
| | cisplatin (Platinol AQ) | | Debrix Index |
| DHBV | duck hepatitis B virus | | detrusor instability |
| DHCA | deep hypothermia | | diabetes insipidus |
| | circulatory arrest | | diagnostic imaging |
| | | | dorsal interossei |

**D**

| | | | |
|---|---|---|---|
| | drug interactions | | drug-induced disease |
| D&I | debridement and irrigation | di,di | dichorionic, diamniotic |
| | dry and intact | DIE | died in emergency |
| DIA | drug-induced | | department |
| | agranulocytosis | | drug-induced esophagitis |
| | drug-induced amenorrhea | DIED | died in emergency |
| diag. | diagnosis | | department |
| DIAP-PERS | (causes of transient incontinence) | DIF | differentiation-inducing factor |
| | **d**elirium/confusion, | DIFF | differential blood count |
| | **i**nfection, (urinary), | DIG | digoxin (this is a |
| | **a**trophic | | dangerous |
| | urethritis/vaginitis, | | abbreviation) |
| | **p**harmaceuticals, | DIH | died in hospital |
| | **p**sychological, | DIHS | drug-induced |
| | **e**xcessive excretion | | hypersensitivity |
| | (e.g., CHF, | | syndrome |
| | hyperglycemia) | DIJOA | dominantly inherited |
| | **r**estricted mobility, and | | juvenile optic atrophy |
| | **s**tool impaction | DIL | daughter-in-law |
| DIAS | diastolic | | dilute |
| DIAS BP | diastolic blood pressure | | drug-induced lupus |
| Diath SW | diathermy short wave | DILC | dose-intensity limiting |
| DIAZ | diazepam | | criterium |
| DIB | disability insurance | DILD | diffuse infiltrative lung |
| | benefits | | disease |
| DIBC | drug-induced blood | | drug-induced liver disease |
| | cytopenias | DILE | drug-induced lupus |
| DIBS | dead-in-bed syndrome | | erythematosus |
| DIC | dacarbazine (DTIC-Dome) | DILS | drug-induced lupus |
| | diagnostic imaging center | | syndrome |
| | differential interference | DIM | diminish |
| | contrast | D$_5$IMB | Ionosol MB with 5% |
| | disseminated intravascular | | dextrose injection |
| | coagulation | DIMD | drug-induced movement |
| | drug information center | | disorders |
| DICC | dynamic infusion | DIMOAD | diabetes insipidus, |
| | cavernosometry and | | diabetes mellitus, optic |
| | cavernosography | | atrophy, and deafness |
| DICE | dexamethasone, ifosfamide, | DIMS | disorders of initiating and |
| | cisplatin, and etopside, | | maintaining sleep |
| | with mesna | DIND | delayed ischemic |
| DICLOX | dicloxacillin | | neurologic deficit |
| DICP | demyelinated | DIOS | distal ileal obstruction |
| | inflammatory chronic | | syndrome |
| | polyneuropathy | | distal intestinal |
| DICT | dose-intensive | | obstruction syndrome |
| | chemotherapy | DIP | desquamative interstitial |
| DID | death(s) from intercurrent | | pneumonia |
| | disease | | diphtheria toxoid vaccine |
| | delayed ischemia deficit | | diplopia |
| | dissociative identity | | distal interphalangeal |
| | disorder | | drip infusion pyelogram |

D

|  | drug-induced parkinsonism |
| DIP_ant | diphtheria antitoxin |
| DIPC | dynamic infusion pharmacocavemosometry |
| DIPJ | distal interphalangeal joint |
| DIR | directions |
| DIRD | drug-induced renal disease |
| DIS | Diagnostic Interview Schedule (questionnaire) |
|  | digital imaging spectrophotometer |
|  | dislocation |
| DISC | disabled infectious single cycle (virus) |
|  | dynamic integrated stabilization chair |
| disch. | discharge |
| DISCUS | Dyskinesia Indentification System Condensed User Scale |
| DISH | diffuse idiopathic skeletal hyperostosis |
| DISI | dorsal intercalated segmental (segment) instability |
| DISIDA | diisopropyl iminodiacetic acid |
| D5ISOM | 5% Dextrose and Isolyte M |
| D5ISOP | 5% Dextrose and Isolyte P |
| DISR | drug-induced skin reactions |
| DIST | distal |
|  | distilled |
| DIT | diiodotyrosine |
|  | drug-induced thrombocytopenia |
| DIU | death in utero |
|  | diuretic(s) |
| DIV | double-inlet ventricle |
| DIVA | digital intravenous angiography |
| Div ex | divergence excess |
| DIVP | dilute intravenous Pitocin |
| DJD | degenerative joint disease |
| DK | dark |
|  | diabetic ketoacidosis |
|  | diseased kidney |
| DKA | diabetic ketoacidosis |
|  | didn't keep appointment |
| DKB | deep knee bends |
| DKC | double knee to chest |
|  | dyskeratosis congenita |
| D-K-S | Damus-Kaye-Stansel (operation/procedure) |
| DL | danger list |
|  | deciliter (dL) |
|  | diagnostic laparoscopy |
|  | direct laryngoscopy |
|  | drug level |
|  | dual lumen |
| dL | deciliter (100 mL) |
| D_L | maximal diffusing capacity |
| DLB | dementia with Lewy bodies |
|  | direct laryngoscopy and bronchoscopy |
| DLBCL | diffuse large B-cell lymphoma |
| DLBD | diffuse Lewy body disease |
| DLBL | diffuse large B-cell lymphoma |
| DLC | double lumen catheter |
| DLCL | diffuse large cell lymphoma |
| DLCO sb | diffusion capacity of carbon monoxide, single breath |
| DLD | date of last drink |
| DLE | discoid lupus erythematosus |
|  | disseminated lupus erythematosis |
| DLF | digitalis-like factor |
|  | ductal lavage fluid |
| DLI | donor leukocyte infusions |
| DLIF | digoxin-like immunoreactive factors |
| DLIS | digoxin-like immunoreactive substance |
| DLMP | date of last menstrual period |
| DLNG | dl-norgestrel |
| DLNMP | date of last normal menstrual period |
| DLNs | distant lymph nodes |
| DLP | dislocation of patella |

D

| | | | |
|---|---|---|---|
| | double-limb progression | DMC | dactinomycin, methotrexate, and cyclophosphamide |
| DLPD | diffuse lymphocytic poorly differentiated | | diabetes management center |
| DLPFC | dorsolateral prefrontal cortex | | |
| D5LR | dextrose 5% in lactated Ringer injection | DMD | Descemet membrane detachment |
| DLROW | a test used in mental status examinations (patient is asked to spell WORLD backwards) | | disciform macular degeneration |
| | | | Doctor of Dental Medicine |
| DLS | daily living skills | | drowsiness monitoring device |
| | digitalis-like substances | | Duchenne muscular dystrophy |
| | dynamic light scattering | | |
| DLSC | double-lumen subclavian catheter | DMD w/ SRNM | disciform macular degeneration with subretinal neovascular membrane |
| DLST | drug-induced lymphocyte stimulation test | | |
| DLT | dose-limiting toxicity | DME | diabetic macular edema |
| | double-lung transplant | | Director of Medical Education |
| DLU | diffused lung uptake | | durable medical equipment |
| DLV | delavirdine (Rescriptor) | | |
| DLW | doubly labeled water | | |
| DM | dehydrated and malnourished | DMEC | data-monitoring and ethics committee |
| | dermatomyositis | DMEM | Dulbecco Modified Eagle Medium |
| | dextromethorphan | | |
| | diabetes mellitus | DMEPOS | durable medical equipment, prosthetics, orthotics, and supplies |
| | diabetic mother | | |
| | diastolic murmur | | |
| | disease management | DMERC | Durable Medical Equipment Regional Carrier |
| DM-1 | diabetes mellitus type 1 | | |
| DM-2 | diabetes mellitus type 2 | | |
| DMA | Director of Medical Affairs | DMEs | drug-metabolizing enzymes |
| DMAC | disseminated *Mycobacterium avium* complex | DMETS | Division of Medication Errors and Technical Support (FDA) |
| DMAD | disease-modifying antirheumatic drug | DMF | decayed, missing, or filled |
| | | | dimethylformamide |
| DMAE | dimethylaminoethanol | | Drug Master File |
| DMAIC | disseminated *Mycobacterium avium-intracellulare* complex | DMFS | decayed, missing, or filled surfaces |
| | | DMH | Department of Mental Health |
| DMARD | disease modifying antirheumatic drug | DMI | desipramine (Norpramin) |
| DMAS | Drug Management and Authorization Section | | diaphragmatic myocardial infarction |
| DMAT | disaster medical assistance team | DM Isch | diaphragmatic myocardial ischemia |
| DMB | data monitoring board | DMKA | diabetes mellitus ketoacidosis |
| DMBA | dimethylbenzanthracene | | |

| | | | |
|---|---|---|---|
| DMN | dysplastic melanocytic nevus | DND | died a natural death |
| | | DNE | diabetes nurse educator |
| DMO | dimethadone | DNEPTE | did not exist prior to enlistment |
| DMOADs | disease-modifying osteoarthritis drugs | | |
| | | DNET | dysembryoplastic neuroepithelial tumor |
| DMOOC | diabetes mellitus out of control | | |
| | | DNFC | does not follow commands |
| DMORTs | Disaster Mortuary Operational Response Teams | | |
| | | DNI | do not intubate |
| | | DNIC | diffuse noxious inhibitory control |
| DMP | dimethyl phthalate | | |
| DMPA | depot-medroxypro-gesterone acetate | DNIF | duties not including flying |
| | | DNKA | did not keep appointment |
| DMPC | dimyristoylphosphatidyl choline | DNN | did not nurse |
| | | DNP | did not pay |
| DMPG | dimyristoylphosphatidyl glycerol | | dinitrophenylhydrazine |
| | | | do not publish |
| DMPS | dimercaptopropane-sulfonic acid | DNR | daunorubicin |
| | | | did not respond |
| D-MRI | dynamic magnetic resonance imaging | | do not report |
| | | | do not resuscitate |
| DMS | dimethylsulfide | | dorsal nerve root |
| DMSA | succimer (dimercaptosuccinic acid) | DNS | deviated nasal septum |
| | | | Director of Nursing Services |
| DMSO | dimethyl sulfoxide | | doctor did not see patient |
| DMT | dimethyltryptamine | | do not show |
| DMTU | dimethylthiourea | | dysplastic nevus syndrome |
| DMV | disk, macula, and vessels | $D_5$ 1/4 NS | dextrose 5% in 1/4 normal saline (0.225% sodium chloride) injection |
| | Doctor of Veterinary Medicine | | |
| DMVP | disk, macula, vessel, periphery | $D_5$ 1/2NS | dextrose 5% in 0.45% sodium chloride injection |
| DMX | diathermy, massage, and exercise | | |
| | | $D_5$NS | 5% dextrose in normal saline (0.9% sodium chloride) injection |
| DN | denuded | | |
| | diabetic nephropathy | | |
| | dicrotic notch | DNT | did not test |
| | down | DO | diet order |
| | dysplastic nevus (nevi) | | dissolved oxygen |
| D & N | distance and near (vision) | | distocclusal |
| DNA | deoxyribonucleic acid | | Doctor of Osteopathy |
| | did not answer | | doctor's order |
| | did not attend | D/O | disorder |
| | does not apply | ✓DO | check doctor's order |
| DNA ds | deoxyribonucleic acid double-stranded | $DO_2$ | oxygen delivery |
| | | DOA | date of admission |
| DNA ss | deoxyribonucleic acid single-stranded | | dead on arrival |
| | | | dominant optic atrophy |
| DNCB | dinitrochlorobenzene | | driver of automobile |
| DNC | did not come | | duration of action |
| | dilatation and curettage (usually written as D&C) | DOA-DRA | dead on arrival despite resuscitative attempts |

D

| DOB | dangle out of bed | DOSA | day of surgery admission |
| | date of birth | DOSAK | Central Tumor Registry |
| | Dobrava hantavirus | | operated by the |
| | dobutamine | | German-Austrian-Swiss |
| | doctor's order book | | Association for Head |
| DOC | date of conception | | and Neck Tumors |
| | diabetes out of control | DOSS | docusate sodium (dioctyl |
| | died of other causes | | sodium sulfosuccinate) |
| | diet of choice | DOT | date of transcription |
| | drug of choice | | date of transfer |
| DOCA | desoxycorticosterone | | died on table |
| | acetate | | directly observed |
| DOCP | desoxycorticosterone | | therapy |
| | pivalate | | Directory of Occupational |
| DOD | date of death | | Titles |
| | dead of disease | | Doppler ophthalmic test |
| | Department of Defense | DOTS | directly observed |
| | drug overdose | | treatment, short course |
| DODD | demand oxygen delivery | DOV | date of visit |
| | device | | distribution of ventilation |
| DOE | date of examination | DOX | doxepin |
| | disease-oriented evidence | | doxorubicin (Adriamycin) |
| | dyspnea on exertion | doz | dozen |
| DOES | disorders of excessive | DP | dental prosthesis |
| | somnolence | | diastolic pressure |
| DOH | Department of Health | | disability pension |
| DOI | date of implant | | discharge planning |
| | (pacemaker) | | dorsalis pedis (pulse) |
| | date of injury | DPA | Department of Public |
| DO₂I | oxygen delivery index | | Assistance |
| DOJ | Department of Justice | | dipropylacetic acid |
| DOL | days of life | | dual photon |
| DOL #2 | second day of life | | absorptiometry |
| DOLV | double-outlet left ventricle | | durable power of attorney |
| DOM | Doctor of Oriental | DPAP | diastolic pulmonary artery |
| | Medicine | | pressure |
| | domiciliary | DPB | days postburn |
| | domiciliary care | | diffuse panbronchiolitis |
| DON | Director of Nursing | DPBS | Dulbecco phosphate- |
| DOOC | diabetes out of control | | buffered saline |
| DOP | dopamine | DPC | delayed primary closure |
| DOPS | diffuse obstructive | | discharge planning |
| | pulmonary syndrome | | coordinator |
| | dihydroxyphenylserine | | distal palmar crease |
| | Director of Pharmacy | DPCP | diphenylcyclopropenone |
| | Service(s) | | (diphencyprone) |
| DOR | date of release | DPD | dihydropyrimidine |
| DORV | double-outlet right | | dehydrogenase |
| | ventricle | DPDL | diffuse poorly |
| DORx | date of treatment | | differentiated |
| DOS | date of surgery | | lymphocytic lymphoma |
| | dead on scene | 2,3-DPG | 2,3-diphosphoglyceric |
| | doctor's order sheet | | acid |

| | | | |
|---|---|---|---|
| DPH | Department of Public Health | DPTPM | diphtheria, pertussis, tetanus, poliomyelitis, and measles |
| | diphenhydramine (Benadryl) | DPU | delayed pressure urticaria |
| | Doctor of Public Health | DPUD | duodenal peptic ulcer disease |
| | phenytoin (diphenylhydantoin) | DPVSs | dilated perivascular spaces |
| DPI | dietary protein intake | DPXA | dual-photon x-ray absorptiometry |
| | Doppler perfusion index | D/Q | deep quiet |
| | dry powder inhaler | D&Q | deep and quiet |
| DPIL | dextrose (percentage), protein (grams per kilogram) Intralipid® (grams per kilogram) | DQOL | diabetes quality of life |
| | | Dr | doctor |
| | | DR | delivery room |
| DPL | diagnostic peritoneal lavage | | diabetic retinopathy |
| | | | diagnostic radiology |
| D5PLM | dextrose 5% and Plasmalyte M® injection | | dining room |
| | | | diurnal rhythm |
| DPM | distintegrations per minute (dpm) | | drug resistant |
| | | DRA | distal rectal adenocarcinoma |
| | Doctor of Podiatric Medicine | | drug-related admissions |
| | drops per minute | DRAPE | drug-related adverse patient event |
| DPN | $^{11}$C-diprenorphine | DRC | dose-response curve |
| | diabetic peripheral neuropathy | DRE | digital rectal examination |
| DPOA | durable power of attorney | | Drug Recognition Expert (for detection of impaired drivers) |
| DPOAE | distortion-product otoacoustic emission | DREAM | downstream regulatory element antagonistic modulator (gene) |
| DPOAHC | durable power of attorney for health care | DRESS | depth resolved surface coil spectroscopy |
| DPP | dorsalis pedal pulse | | drug rash with eosinophilia and systemic symptoms |
| | duration of positive pressure | | |
| DPPC | colfosceril palmitate (dipalmitoylphosphatidylcholine) | DREZ | dorsal root entry zone |
| | | DRG | diagnosis-related groups |
| DPR | Department of Professional Regulation | | dorsal root ganglia |
| | | DRGE | drainage |
| | diagnostic procedure room | DRI | defibrillation response interval |
| DPS | disintegration per second | | Dietary Reference Intakes |
| DPSS | Department of Public Social Service | | Discharge Readiness Index |
| DPsy | Doctor of Psychology | | dopamine reuptake inhibitor |
| DPT | Demerol, Phenergan, and Thorazine (this is a dangerous abbreviation) | DRM | drug-related morbidity |
| | | DRN | drug-related neutropenia |
| | | DRP | drug-related problem |
| | diphtheria, pertussis, and tetanus (immunization) | DRPLA | dentatorubral-pallidolluysian atrophy |
| | Driver Performance Test | | |

D

| | | | |
|---|---|---|---|
| DRR | drug regimen review | | Down syndrome child |
| DRS | designated record set | DSD | degenerative spinal |
| | Disability Rating Scale | | disease |
| | disease-related symptoms | | detrusor sphincter |
| | Duane retraction syndrome | | dyssynergia |
| DRSG | dressing | | digital selenium drum |
| DRSI | disease-related symptom | | (radiology) |
| | improvement | | discharge summary |
| DRSP | drug-resistant | | dictated |
| | *Streptococcus* | | dry sterile dressing |
| | *pneumoniae* | DSDB | direct self-destructive |
| DRT | drug-related | | behavior |
| | thrombocytopenia | ds DNA | double-stranded |
| DrTPar | diphtheria toxoid (reduced | | desoxyribonucleic acid |
| | antigen quantity for | DSF | doxorubicin, streptozocin, |
| | adults), tetanus toxoid, | | and fluorouracil |
| | and acellular pertussis | DSG | desogestrel |
| | (reduced antigen | | dressing |
| | quantity for adults) | DSG | deoxyspergualin |
| | vaccine, for adult use | DSHEA | Dietary Supplement |
| DRUB | drug screen-blood | | Health and Education |
| DRUJ | distal or radial ulnar joint | | Act of 1994 |
| dRVVT | diluted Russell viper | DSHR | delayed skin |
| | venom time | | hypersensitivity reaction |
| DS | deep sleep | DSHS | Department of Social and |
| | Dextrostix® | | Health Services |
| | discharge summary | DSI | deep shock insulin |
| | disoriented | | Depression Status |
| | distant supervision | | Inventory |
| | double strength | DSIAR | double-stapled ileoanal |
| | Down syndrome | | reservoir |
| | drug screen | DSM | disease state management |
| D/S | 5% dextrose and 0.9% | | drink skim milk |
| | sodium chloride | DSM-IV | Diagnostic and Statistical |
| | (saline) injection | | Manual of Mental |
| D&S | diagnostic and surgical | | Disorders, 4th edition |
| | dilation and suction | DSMB | Data and Safety |
| D5S | dextrose 5% in 0.9% | | Monitoring Board |
| | sodium chloride | DSMO | Designated Standard |
| | (saline) injection | | Maintenance |
| $D_5$-1/2S | 5% dextrose in 0.45% | | Organization |
| | sodium chloride | DSO | distal subungual |
| | (saline) injection | | onychomycosis |
| DSA | digital subtraction | DSP | digital signal processor |
| | angiography | | distal symmetrical |
| | (angiocardiography) | | polyneuropathy |
| DSAP | disseminated superficial | DSPC | distearoylphosphatidyl |
| | actinic porokeratosis | | choline |
| DSB | drug-seeking behavior | DSPD | dangerous severe |
| DSBs | double-strand (DNA) | | personality disorder |
| | breaks | D-SPINE | dorsal spine |
| DSC | differential scanning | DSPN | distal symmetric |
| | calorimeter | | polyneuropathy |

| | | | |
|---|---|---|---|
| DSPS | delayed sleep phase syndrome | | discharge tomorrow |
| | | | docetaxel (Taxotere) |
| DSRCT | desmoplastic small round cell tumor | D/T | date/time |
| | | | due to |
| DSRF | drainage subretinal fluid | d/t | due to |
| | | d4T | stavudine (Zerit) |
| DSS | dengue shock syndrome | D & T | diagnosis and treatment |
| | Department of Social Services | | dictated and typed |
| | | DTaP | diphtheria and tetanus toxoids with acellular pertussis vaccine |
| | Disability Status Scale | | |
| | discharge summary sheet | | |
| | disease-specific survival | DTBC | tubocurarine (D-tubocurarine) |
| | distal splenorenal shunt | | |
| | docusate sodium (dioctyl sodium sulfosuccinate) | DTBE | Division of Tuberculosis Elimination |
| DSSLR | double, seated straight leg raise | DTC | day treatment center |
| | | | differentiated thyroid cancer |
| DSSN | distal symmetric sensory neuropathy | | direct-to-consumer (advertising) |
| DSSP | distal symmetric sensory polyneuropathy | | diticarb (diethyldiothio-carbamate) |
| DSST | Digit-Symbol Substitution Test | | tubocurarine (D-tubocurarine) |
| DST | daylight saving time | DTD #30 | dispense 30 such doses |
| | dexamethasone suppression test | DTF | deep transverse friction |
| | digit substitution test | DTH | delayed-type hypersensitivity |
| | donor-specific (blood) transfusion | DTI | diffusion-tensor imaging |
| DSU | day stay unit | DTIC | dacarbazine (DTIC-Dome) |
| | day surgery unit | | |
| DSUH | direct suggestion under hypnosis | D TIME | dream time |
| D/Sum | discharge summary | DTM | deep tissue massage |
| DSV | digital subtraction ventriculography | | dermatophyte test medium |
| DSVP | Dietary Supplement Verification Program (United States Pharmacopeia Purity Compliance) | DTO | danger to others |
| | | | deodorized tincture of opium (warning: this is NOT paregoric) |
| | | DTOGV | dextral-transposition of great vessels |
| DSW | Doctorate in Social Work | DTP | differential time to positivity |
| DSWI | deep sternal wound infection | | diphtheria, tetanus toxoids, pertussis (antigens unspecified) vaccine |
| | deep surgical wound infection | | |
| DSX | dysmetabolic syndrome X | | distal tingling on percussion (+Tinel sign) |
| DT | delirium tremens | | |
| | dietary thermogenesis | | |
| | dietetic technician | DTPA | pentetic acid (diethylenetriaminepen-taacetic acid) |
| | diphtheria and tetanus toxoids, adsorbed, pediatric strength | | |

D

DTP$_a$ diphtheria, tetanus toxoids, acellular pertussis vaccine, for pediatric use

DTPa-HIB diphtheria toxoid, tetanus toxoid, acellular pertussis, and *Haemophilus influenzae* type b conjugate vaccine

DTPa-HIB-IPV diphtheria toxoid, tetanus toxoid, acellular pertussis, *Haemophilus influenzae* type b conjugate, and poliovirus inactivated vaccine

DTP$_w$ diphtheria, tetanus toxoids, whole-cell pertussis vaccine

DTR Dance Therapist, Registered
deep tendon reflexes
Dietetic Technician Registered

DTs delirium tremens

DTS danger to self
donor specific transfusion

3D TSE three-dimensional turbo-spin echo (images)

DTT diphtheria tetanus toxoid
dithiothreitol

DTUS diathermy, traction, and ultrasound

DVG double vein graft

DTV due to void

DTVP Developmental Test of Visual Perception

DTwP diphtheria and tetanus toxoids with whole-cell pertussis vaccine

DTX detoxification

DU decubitus ulcer
depleted uranium
developmental unit
diabetic urine
diagnosis undetermined
duodenal ulcer
duroxide uptake

DUB Dubowitz (score)
dysfunctional uterine bleeding

DUD dihydrouracil dehydrogenase

DUE drug use evaluation

D&UE dilation and uterine evacuation

DUF Doppler ultrasonic flowmeter

DUI driving under the influence

DUID driving under the influence of drugs

DUII driving under the influence of intoxicants

DUIL driving under the influence of liquor

DUKM dialysate urea kinetic modeling

DUM drug use monitoring

DUN dialysate urea nitrogen

DUNHL diffuse undifferentiated non-Hodgkins lymphoma

DUO Duotube®

DUR drug utilization review
duration

DUS digital ultrasound
distal urethral stenosis
Doppler ultrasound stethoscope

3DUS three-dimensional ultrasound

DUSN diffuse unilateral subacute neuroretinitis

DV distance vision
domestic violence
double vision

D&V diarrhea and vomiting
disks and vessels

DVA Department of Veterans Affairs
directional vacuum-assisted (biopsy)
distance visual acuity
vindesine (Eldisine; desacetyl vinblastine amide sulfate)

DVC direct visualization of vocal cords

D V® Cream dienestrol vaginal cream

DVD dissociated vertical deviation

| | double-vessel disease | | injection |
|---|---|---|---|
| DVI | atrioventricular sequential pacing | DWDL | diffuse well-differentiated lymphocytic lymphoma |
| | digital vascular imaging | DWI | diffusion-weighted (magnetic resonance) imaging |
| DVIU | direct vision internal urethrotomy | | |
| DVPX | divalproex sodium (Depakote) | | driving while intoxicated |
| | | | driving while impaired |
| DVM | Doctor of Veterinary Medicine | DWI/PI | diffusion-weighted imaging/perfusion imaging |
| DVMP | disks, vessels, and macula periphery | DWMRI | diffusion-weighted magnetic resonance imaging |
| DVPA | daunorubicin, vincristine, prednisone, and asparaginase | | |
| | | DWR | deep water running |
| DVR | Division of Vocational Rehabilitation | DWRT | delayed work recall test |
| | | DWSCL | daily-wear soft contact lens |
| | dose-volume relationship | | |
| | double-valve replacement | DWV | Dandy-Walker variant (a congenital anomaly) |
| DVSA | digital venous subtraction angiography | | |
| | | DWW | dynamic wall walk |
| DVT | deep vein thrombosis | Dx | diagnosis |
| DVTS | deep venous thromboscintigram | | disease |
| | | DXA | dual-energy x-ray absorptiometry |
| DVVC | direct visualization of vocal cords | | |
| | | DXG | dioxalane guanine |
| DW | daily weight | DxLS | diagnosis responsible for length of stay |
| | deionized water | | |
| | detention warrant | DXM | dexamethasone |
| | dextrose in water | | dextromethorphan |
| | diffusion-weighted (imaging) | DXR | delayed xenograft rejection |
| | distilled water | DXT | deep x-ray therapy |
| | doing well | DXRT | deep x-ray therapy |
| | double wrap | DXS | Dextrostix® |
| D/W | dextrose in water | DY | dusky (infant color) |
| | discussed with | | dysprosium |
| D-W | Dandy-Walker (deformity/malformation) | DYF | drag your feet (author's note: see you in court) |
| | Danis-Weber (classification for ankle fractures) | DYFS | Division of Youth and Family Services |
| | | DysD | dysthymic disorder |
| D₅W | 5% dextrose (in water) injection | DYTRO | dynamic tone-reducing orthosis |
| D10W | 10% dextrose (in water) injection | DZ | diazepam (valium) |
| | | | disease |
| D20W | 20% dextrose (in water) injection | | dizygotic |
| | | | dozen |
| D50W | 50% dextrose (in water) injection | DZP | diazepam |
| | | DZT | dizygotic twins |
| D70W | 70% dextrose (in water) injection | DZX | dexrazoxane (Zinecard) |
| 5 DW | 5% dextrose (in water) | | |

D

# E

| | |
|---|---|
| E | East (as in the location e.g., 2E, would be second floor, East wing) |
| | edema |
| | effective |
| | eloper |
| | enema |
| | engorged |
| | eosinophil |
| | *Escherichia* |
| | esophoria for distance |
| | evaluation |
| | evening |
| | expired |
| | eye |
| | methylenedioxyme-thamphetamine (MDMA; Ecstasy) |
| E′ | elbow |
| | esophoria for near |
| $E_1$ | estrone |
| $E_2$ | estradiol |
| $E_3$ | estriol |
| 4E | 4 plus edema |
| E20 | Enfamil 20® |
| E → A | say E,E,E, comes out as A,A,A upon auscultation of lung showing consolidation |
| EA | early amniocentesis |
| | elbow aspiration |
| | electroacoustic analysis |
| | enteral alimentation |
| | epidural anesthesia |
| | episodic ataxia |
| | esophageal atresia |
| E/A | ratio of peak mitral early diastolic and atrial contraction velocity |
| | European-American |
| E&A | evaluate and advise |
| EAA | electrothermal atomic absorption |
| | essential amino acids |
| EAB | elective abortion |
| | Ethical Advisory Board |

| | |
|---|---|
| EAC | erythema annulare centrifugum |
| | esophageal adenocarcinoma |
| | external auditory canal |
| EACA | aminocaproic acid (epsilon-aminocaproic acid) |
| | esophageal adenocarcinoma |
| EADL | extended activities of daily living |
| EADs | early after-depolarizations |
| EAE | experimental allergic encephalomyelitis |
| | experimental autoimmune encephalomyelitis |
| EAEC | enteroaggregative *Escherichia coli* |
| EAggEC | enteroaggregative *Escherichia coli* |
| EAHF | eczema, allergy, and hay fever |
| EAL | electronic artificial larynx |
| EAM | external auditory meatus |
| EAP | Employment (Employee) Assistance Programs |
| | erythrocyte acid phosphatase |
| | etoposide, doxorubicin (Adriamycin), and cisplatin (Platinol) |
| EAR | estimated average requirement |
| EARLIES | early decelerations |
| EART | extended abdominal radiation therapy |
| EAR OX | ear oximetry |
| EAS | external anal sphincter |
| EAST | external rotation, abduction stress test |
| EAT | Eating Attitudes Test |
| | ectopic atrial tachycardia |
| EATL | enteropathy-associated T-cell lymphoma |
| EAU | experimental autoimmune uveitis |
| EB | eosinophilic bronchitis |
| | epidermolysis bullosa |
| | Epstein-Barr (virus) |
| EBA | epidermolysis bullosa acquisita |
| EBB | electron beam boosts |

|        | equal breath bilaterally | EC | ejection click |
|--------|--------------------------|-----|----------------|
| EBBS | equal bilateral breath sounds | | electrical cardioversion |
| EBC | early (stage) breast cancer | | emergency contraception |
| | endoscopic brush cytology | | endocervical |
| | esophageal balloon catheter | | enteric coated |
| | | | *Escherichia coli* |
| EBCPGs | evidence-based clinical practice guidelines | | etopside and carboplatin |
| | | | European Community |
| EBCT | electron-beam computed tomography | | extracellular |
| | | | eye care |
| EBD | endocardial border delineation | | eyes closed |
| | | $E_2C$ | estradiol cypionate |
| | endoscopic balloon dilation | E & C | education and counseling |
| | | ECA | enteric coated aspirin (tablets) |
| | evidence-based decision (making) | | Epidemiological Catchment Area |
| EBE | equal bilateral expansion | | ethacrynic acid |
| EBEA | Epstein-Barr (virus) early antigen | | external carotid artery |
| | | e-CAM | electronic Compilation of Analytical Methods |
| EBF | erythroblastosis fetalis | | |
| EBL | estimated blood loss | ECASA | enteric coated aspirin (tablets) |
| EBL-1 | European bat lyssavirus 1 | | |
| EBM | evidence-based medicine | ECBD | exploration of common bile duct |
| | expressed breast milk | | |
| EBMT | European Bone Marrow Transplant (registry group) | ECBO | enterocytopathogenic bovine orphan (virus) |
| | | ECC | edema, clubbing, and cyanosis |
| EBNA | Epstein-Barr (virus) nuclear antigen | | embryonal cell cancer |
| | | | emergency cardiac care |
| EBO | evidence-based outcomes | | Emergency Communications Center |
| EBOS | early-onset benign occipital seizure | | endocervical curettage |
| | | | estimated creatinine clearance |
| EBP | epidural blood patch | | |
| EBR | external beam radiotherapy | | external cardiac compression |
| | | | extracorporeal circulation |
| EBRs | evidence-based recommendations | | |
| EBRT | external beam radiation therapy | ECCE | extracapsular cataract extraction |
| EBS | epidermolysis bullosa | ECD | endocardial cushion defect |
| EBSB | equal breath sounds bilaterally | | equivalent current dipole |
| | | | Erdheim-Chester disease |
| EBT | electron beam tomography | ECDB | encourage to cough and deep breathe |
| | erythromycin breath test | | |
| EBV | Epstein-Barr virus | ECE | endothelin-converting enzyme |
| EBVCA | Epstein-Barr viral capsid antigen | | extracapsular extension |
| EBVEA | Epstein-Barr virus, early antigen | ECEMG | evoked compound electromyography |
| EBVNA | Epstein-Barr virus, nuclear antigen | ECF | epirubicin, cisplatin, and fluorouracil |

E

|  | extended care facility | ECN | extended care nursery |
|  | extracellular fluid | ecNOS | endothelial constitutive |
| ECF-A | eosinophil chemotactic |  | nitric oxide synthetase |
|  | factors of anaphylaxis | ECochG | electrocochleography |
| ECFV | extracellular fluid volume | ECOG | Eastern Cooperative |
| ECG | electrocardiogram |  | Oncology Group |
| ECGE | extracorporeal gas | ECoG | electrocochleography |
|  | exchange |  | electrocorticogram |
| ECHINO | echinocyte | E coli | *Escherichia coli* |
| ECHO | echocardiogram | ECO$_{tox}$ | *Escherichia coli* (heat- |
|  | enterocytopathogenic |  | labile toxin) vaccine |
|  | human orphan (virus) | ECP | emergency care provider |
|  | etoposide, |  | emergency contraceptive |
|  | cyclophosphamide, |  | pills |
|  | doxorubicin |  | eosinophil cationic protein |
|  | (hydroxydaunomycin), |  | extracorporeal |
|  | and vincristine |  | photochemotherapy |
|  | (Oncovin) |  | extracorporeal |
| ECHO (2D) | echocardiogram (2- |  | photopheresis |
|  | dimensional) | ECPL | endocavitary pelvic |
| EChoG | electrocochleography |  | lymphadenectomy |
| ECHO/ | echocardiography/ | ECPD | external counterpressure |
| RV | radionuclide |  | device |
|  | ventriculography | ECPP | extracorporeal |
| ECI | extracorporeal irradiation |  | photophoresis |
| ECIB | extracorporeal irradiation | ECR | emergency chemical |
|  | of blood |  | restraint |
| ECIC | external carotid and |  | extensor carpi radialis |
|  | internal carotid | ECRB | extensor carpi radialis |
|  | extracranial to intracranial |  | brevis |
|  | (anastamosis) | ECRL | extensor carpi radialis |
| EC/IC | extracranial/intracranial |  | longus |
| ECID | European Centre for | ECS | elective cosmetic surgery |
|  | Infectious Disease |  | electrocerebral silence |
| ECK1 | *Escherichia coli* K1 |  | endometrial-cancer- |
| ECL | electrochemiluminescence |  | specific |
|  | enterochromaffin-like | ECT | electroconvulsive therapy |
|  | extend of cerebral lesion |  | emission computed |
|  | extracapillary lesions |  | tomography |
| ECLA | extracorporeal lung assist |  | enhanced computed |
| ECLP | extracorporeal liver |  | tomography |
|  | perfusion | ECTb | Emory Cardiac Toolbox |
| ECM | erythema chronicum | ECU | electrocautery unit |
|  | migrans |  | emotional care units |
|  | extracellular mass |  | environmental control unit |
|  | extracellular matrix |  | extensor carpi ulnaris |
| ECM/BCM | extracellular mass, body | ECV | emergency center visits |
|  | cell mass ratio |  | external cephalic version |
| ECMO | enterocytopathogenic |  | (obstetrics) |
|  | monkey orphan (virus) | ECVD | extracellular volume |
|  | extracorporeal circulation |  | depletion |
|  | membrane oxygenation | ECVE | extracellular volume |
|  | (oxygenator) |  | expansion |

| | | | |
|---|---|---|---|
| ECW | extracellular water | EDHF | endothelium-derived hyperpolarizing factor |
| ED | eating disorder(s) | | |
| | education | EDI | Eating Disorders Inventory |
| | effective dose | | |
| | elbow disarticulation | | electrodeionization |
| | emergency department | EDITAR | extended-duration topical arthropod repellent |
| | emotional disorder | | |
| | epidural | EDL | extensor digitorum longus |
| | erectile dysfunction | ED/LD | emotionally disturbed and learning disabled |
| | ethynodiol diacetate | | |
| | every day (this is a dangerous abbreviation) | EDLF | endogenous digitalis-like factors |
| | extensive disease | EDLS | endogenous digitalis-like substance |
| | extensor digitorum | | |
| ED$_{50}$ | median effective dose | EDM | early diastolic murmur |
| EDA | elbow disarticulation | | esophageal Doppler monitor |
| EDAM | edatrexate | | |
| EDAP | Emergency Department Approved for Pediatrics | | extensor digiti minimi |
| | | EDMD-AD | autosomal dominate Emery-Dreifuss muscular dystrophy |
| EDAS | encephalodural arterio-synangiosis | | |
| EDAT | Emergency Department Alert Team | EDNO | endothelium-related nitric oxide |
| EDAX | energy-dispersive analysis of x-rays | EDP | emergency department physician |
| EDB | ethylene dibromide | | end-diastolic pressure |
| | extensor digitorum brevis | EDQ | extensor digiti quinti (tendon) |
| EDC | effective dynamic compliance | EDQM | European Directorate for the Quality of Medicines |
| | electrodesiccation and curettage | | |
| | end diastolic counts | EDQV | extensor digiti quinti five |
| | estimated date of conception | EDR | edrophonium (Tensilon) |
| | | | extreme drug resistance |
| | estimated date of confinement | EDRF | endothelium derived relaxing factor (nitric oxide) |
| | estramustine, docetaxel, and carboplatin | | |
| | | EDS | Ehlers-Danlos syndrome |
| | extensor digitorum communis | | excessive daytime somnolence |
| EDCF | endothelium-derived constricting factor | EDSS | Expanded Disability Status Scale (Score) |
| EDCP | eccentric dynamic compression plates | EDT | exposure duration threshold |
| EDD | endothelium-dependent dilation | EDTA | edetic acid (ethylenedi-aminetetraacetic acid) |
| | esophageal detector device | EDTU | emergency diagnostic and treatment unit |
| | expected date of delivery | | |
| EDENT | edentulous | EDU | eating disorder unit |
| EDF | elongation, derotation, and flexion | EDV | end-diastolic volume |
| | | | epidermal dysplastic verruciformis |
| EDH | epidural hematoma | | |
| | extradural hematoma | EDW | estimated dry weight |

E

| | | | |
|---|---|---|---|
| EDX | edatrexate | EFAD | essential fatty acid deficiency |
| EDXRF | energy-dispersive x-ray fluorescence | E-FAP | Emory Functional Ambulation Profile |
| EE | emetic episodes | EFBW | estimate fetal body weight |
| | end to end | EFD | episode free day |
| | energy expenditure | EFE | endocardial fibroelastosis |
| | equine encephalitis | | epidemic fatal |
| | erosive esophagitis | | encephalopathy |
| | esophageal endoscopy | EFF | effacement |
| | ethinyl estradiol | EFR | effective filtration rate |
| | expressed emotion | EFS | event-free survival |
| | external ear | EFHBM | eosinophilic |
| E & E | eyes and ears | | fibrohistiocytic lesion |
| EEA | electroencephalic | | of bone marrow |
| | audiometry | EFM | electronic fetal |
| | elemental enteral | | monitor(ing) |
| | alimentation | | external fetal monitoring |
| | end-to-end anastomosis | EFMM | external fetal maternal |
| | energy expended with | | monitor |
| | activity | EFMT | electric field mediated |
| EEC | ectrodactyly-ectodermal | | transfer |
| | dysplasia (cleft | EFN | effusion |
| | syndrome) | EFV | efavirenz (Sustiva) |
| | endogenous erythroid | EFW | estimated fetal weight |
| | colony | EF/WM | ejection fraction/wall |
| EECP | enhanced external | | motion |
| | counter-pulsation | *e.g.* | for example |
| EEE | eastern equine | EGA | esophageal gastric (tube) |
| | encephalomyelitis | | airway |
| | edema, erythema, and | | estimated gestational age |
| | exudate | EGB | endoscopic grasp biopsy |
| | external eye examination | EGb | extract of *Ginkgo biloba* |
| EEG | electroencephalogram | EGBUS | external genitalia, |
| EELS | electron energy loss | | Bartholin, urethral, and |
| | spectrometry | | Skene glands |
| EEN | estimated energy needs | EGC | early gastric carcinoma |
| EENT | eyes, ears, nose, and | EGCG | epigallocatechin gallate |
| | throat | EGFR | epidermal growth factor |
| EEP | end expiratory pressure | | receptor |
| EER | extended endocardial | EGD | esophagogastroduodeno- |
| | resection | | scopy |
| EES® | erythromycin | EGDT | esophagogastric |
| | ethylsuccinate | | devascularization and |
| EET | early exercise testing | | transection |
| EEV | encircling endocardial | EGF | epidermal growth factor |
| | ventriculotomy | EGF-R | epidermal growth factor |
| EF | eccentric fixation | | receptor |
| | ejection fraction | EGG | electrogastrography |
| | endurance factor | EGJ | esophagogastric junction |
| | erythroblastosis fetalis | EGL | eosinophilic granuloma of |
| | extended-field | | the lung |
| | (radiotherapy) | EGS | ethylene glycol succinate |
| EFA | essential fatty acid | | |

E

| | | | |
|---|---|---|---|
| EGSs | external guide sequences | | exercise-induced asthma |
| EGTA | esophageal gastric tube airway | EIAB | extracranial-intracranial arterial bypass |
| | ethyleneglycoltetracetic acid | EIAV | equine infectious anemia virus |
| EH | eccentric hypertrophy | EIB | exercise-induced bronchospasm |
| | educationally handicapped | | |
| | enlarged heart | EIC | early ischemic change(s) |
| | essential hypertension | | electrical impedance cardiography |
| | extramedullary hematopoiesis | | endometrial intraepithelial carcinoma |
| Eh | *Entamoeba histolytica* | | |
| EHB | elevate head of bed | | epidermal inclusion cyst |
| | extensor hallucis brevis | | extensive intraductal component |
| EHBA | extrahepatic biliary atresia | | |
| EHBF | extrahepatic blood flow | EICA | extra-intracranial artery (bypass) |
| EHC | enterohepatic circulation | | |
| EHD | electronic home detention | EID | electroimmunodiffusion |
| | | | electronic infusion device |
| EHDA | etidronate sodium | EIDC | extreme intervertebral disk collapse |
| EHDP | etidronate disodium (Didronel) | EIEC | enteroinvasive *Escherichia coli* |
| EHE | epithelioid hemangioendothelioma | EIL | elective induction of labor |
| EHEC | enterohemorrhagic *Escherichia coli* | eIND | Electronic Investigational New Drug (application) |
| EHF | epidemic hemorrhagic fever | EIOA | excessive intake of alcohol |
| | extremely high frequency | EIP | elective interruption of pregnancy |
| EHH | episodic hypothermia with hyperhidrosis | | end-inspiratory pressure |
| | esophageal hiatal hernia | | extensor indicis proprius |
| EHI | exertional heat illness | | |
| EHL | electrohydraulic lithotripsy | eIPV | enhanced inactivated polio vaccine |
| | extensor hallucis longus | EIR | entomological inoculation rate |
| EHN | ethotoin | | |
| EHO | extrahepatic obstruction | EIS | endoscopic injection scleropathy |
| EHPH | extrahepatic portal hypertension | EITB | enzyme-linked immunoelectrotransfer blot |
| EHR | electronic health record | | |
| EHS | employee health service | EIV | external iliac vein |
| | exertional heat stroke | EJ | ejection |
| EHT | electrohydrothermosation | | elbow jerk |
| | essential hypertension | | external jugular |
| EI | environmental illness | EJB | ectopic junctional beat |
| | enzyme immunoassay | EJN | extended jaundice of newborn |
| | extensor indicis | | |
| E/I | expiratory to inspiratory (ratio) | EJP | excitatory junction potential |
| E & I | endocrine and infertility | | |
| EIA | enzyme immunoassay | EJV | external jugular vein |

| | | | |
|---|---|---|---|
| EK | Ektachem 400 (see page 358) | Elix | elixir |
| | | ELLIP | elliptocytosis |
| | erythrokinase | ELM | epiluminescent microscopy |
| EKC | epidemic keratoconjunctivitis | | external laryngeal manipulation |
| EKG | electrocardiogram | | |
| EKO | echoencephalogram | ELND | elective lymph node dissection |
| EKY | electrokymogram | | |
| EL | exercise limit | ELOP | estimated length of program |
| | exploratory laparotomy | | |
| E-L | external lids | ELOS | estimated length of stay |
| ELA | Establishment License Application | ELP | electrophoresis |
| | | ELPS | excessive lateral pressure syndrome |
| ELAD | extracorporeal liver-assist device | | |
| | | ELS | Eaton-Lambert syndrome |
| ELAFF | extended lateral arm free flap | ELSD | evaporative light scattering detection |
| ELAM | endothelial leukocyte adhesion molecule | ELSI | ethical, legal, and social implications |
| ELAMS | Electronic Laboratory Animal Monitoring System | ELSS | emergency life support system |
| | | ELT | endoscopic laser therapy |
| ELB | early light breakfast | | euglobulin lysis time |
| | elbow | ELTR | European Liver Transplant Registry |
| ELBW | extremely low birth weight (less than 1000 g) | | |
| | | ELVIS™ | Enzyme-Linked Virus Inducible System |
| ELC | earlobe creases | | |
| ELCA | excimer laser coronary angioplasty | EM | early memory |
| | | | ejection murmur |
| ELD | end-of-life decision | | electron microscope |
| ELEC | elective | | emergency medicine |
| ELF | elective low forceps | | emmetropia |
| | endoscopic laser foraminotomy | | eosinophilia-myalgia (syndrome) |
| | epithelial lining fluid | | erythema migrans |
| | etoposide, leucovorin, and fluorouracil | | erythema multiforme |
| | | | erythromelalgia |
| | extremely low frequency | | esophageal manometry |
| ELFA | enzyme-linked fluorescent immunoassay | | estramustine (Emcyt) |
| | | | extensive metabolizers |
| ELG | endolumenal gastroplication | | external monitor |
| | | E & M | Evaluation and Management (coding system) |
| | endoluminal graft | | |
| ELH | endolymphatic hydrops | | |
| ELI | endomyocardial lymphocytic infiltrates | EMA | early morning awakening |
| | | | endomysial antibody |
| ELIG | eligible | EMA-CO | etoposide, methotrexate, dactinomycin (actinomycin-D), cyclophosphamide, and vincristine (Oncovin) |
| ELISA | enzyme-linked immunosorbent assay | | |
| ELISPOT | enzyme-linked immunospot | | |
| ELITT | endometrial laser intrauterine thermal therapy | | |
| | | EMB | endometrial biopsy |

|  | endomyocardial biopsy | EMo | ear mold |
|  | eosin-methylene blue (agar) | EMP | electromolecular propulsion |
|  | ethambutol (Myambutol) |  | estramustine phosphate (Emcyt) |
|  | Explanation of Medicare Benefits | EMPD | extramammary Paget disease |
| EMC | encephalomyocarditis |  |  |
|  | endometrial currettage | EMR | educable mentally retarded |
|  | essential mixed cryoglobulinemia |  | electrical muscle stimulation |
|  | extraskeletal myxoid chondrosarcoma |  | electronic medical record emergency mechanical |
| EMD | electromechanical dissociation |  | restraint empty, measure, and record |
| EMDA | electromotive drug administration |  | endoscopic mucosal resection |
| EMDR | eye movement desensitization and | EMS | eye-movement recording early morning specimen |
|  | reprocessing |  | early morning stiffness |
| EME | extreme medical emergency |  | electrical muscle stimulation |
| EMEA | European Medicines Evaluation Agency |  | emergency medical services |
| EMF | elective midforceps |  | eosinophilia myalgia syndrome |
|  | electromagnetic field(s) electromagnetic flow | EMSA | electrophoretic mobility shift assay |
|  | electromotive forces endomyocardial fibrosis | EMSU | early morning specimen of urine |
|  | erythrocyte maturation factor | EMT | emergency medical technician |
|  | evaporated milk formula |  | epithelial-mesenchymal |
| EMG | electromyograph emergency |  | transformation estramustine (Emcyt) |
|  | essential monoclonal gammopathy | EMTA | Emergency Medical Technician, Advanced |
| EMI | elderly and mentally infirm | EMTC | emergency medical trauma center |
|  | electromagnetic interference | EMT-D | emergency medical technician-defibrillation |
| EMIC | emergency maternity and infant care | EMTP | Emergency Medical Technician, Paramedic |
| E-MICR | electron microscopy | EMU | early morning urine |
| EMIT | enzyme-multiplied immunoassay technique (test) |  | electromagnetic unit epilepsy monitoring unit |
| EMLA® | eutectic mixture of local anesthetics (lidocaine | EMV | equine morbilli virus eye, motor, verbal (grading for Glasgow |
|  | and prilocaine in an emulsion base) |  | Coma Scale) |
| EMLB | erythromycin lactobionate | EMVC | early mitral valve closure |
| EMMA | eye-movement measuring apparatus | EMW | electromagnetic waves |
| EMMV | extended mandatory minute ventilation | EMZL | extranodal marginal-zone (B-cell) lymphoma |

E

| | | | |
|---|---|---|---|
| EN | enema | | examine, opinion, and |
| | enteral nutrition | | advice |
| | erythema nodosum | | external oblique |
| E/N | eggnog | | aponeurosis |
| E 50% N | extension 50% of normal | EOAE | evoked otoacoustic |
| ENA | extractable nuclear | | emissions |
| | antigen | EOB | edge of bed |
| ENB | esthesioneuroblastoma | | end of bed |
| ENC | encourage | | explanation of benefits |
| eNDA | Electronic New Drug | EOC | Emergency Operations |
| | Application | | Center |
| ENDO | endodontia | | enema of choice |
| | endodontics | | epithelial ovarian cancer |
| | endoscopy | EOD | early-onset disease |
| | endotracheal | | end of day |
| EndoCAB | plasma antiendotoxin | | end organ damage |
| | core antibody | | every other day (this is a |
| ENF | Enfamil | | dangerous abbreviation) |
| ENF c Fe | Enfamil with iron | | extent of disease |
| ENG | electronystagmogram | EOE | Equal Opportunity |
| | engorged | | Employer |
| ENL | enlarged | | extraosseous Ewing |
| | erythema nodosum | | sarcoma |
| | leprosum | EOFAD | early-onset form of |
| ENMG | electroneuromyography | | familial Alzheimer |
| ENMT | ears, nose, mouth, and | | disease |
| | throat | E of I | evidence of insurability |
| ENOG | electroneurography | EOG | electro-oculogram |
| eNOS | endothelial nitric oxide | | Ethrane, oxygen, and gas |
| | synthase | | (nitrous oxide) |
| ENP | extractable nucleoprotein | EOL | end of file |
| ENS | exogenous natural | EOM | error of measurement |
| | surfactant | | external otitis media |
| ENT | ears, nose, throat | | extraocular movement |
| ENTIS | European Network of | | extraocular muscles |
| | Teratology Information | EOMB | explanation of Medicare |
| | Services | | benefits |
| ENTV | enzootic nasal tumor | EOMI | extraocular muscles intact |
| | virus | EOO | external oculomotor |
| ENVD | elevated new vessels on | | ophthalmoplegia |
| | the disk | EOP1 | end-of-phase 1 |
| ENVE | elevated new vessels | EOP2 | end-of-phase 2 |
| | elsewhere | EOR | emergency operating |
| ENVT | environment | | room |
| EO | elbow orthosis | | end of range |
| | embolic occlusion | EORA | elderly onset rheumatoid |
| | eosinophilia | | arthritis |
| | ethylene oxide | EORTC | European Organization for |
| | eyes open | | Research on the |
| E & O | errors and omissions | | Treatment of Cancer |
| EOA | erosive osteoarthritis | EOS | end of study |
| | esophageal obturator | | eosinophil |
| | airway | EP | ectopic pregnancy |

E

electrophysiologic
elopement precaution
endogenous pyrogen
Episcopalian
esophageal pressure
etoposide and cisplatin
(Platinol AQ)
evoked potentials

**E&P** estrogen and progesterone

**EPA** eicosapentaenoic acid
Environmental Protection
Agency

**EPAB** extracorporeal
pneumoperititoneal
access bubble

**E-Panel** electrolyte panel (See
page 362)

**EPAP** expiratory positive airway
pressure

**EPB** extensor pollicis brevis

**EPC** erosive prephloric changes
external pneumatic
compression

**EPCV** engineering, procurement,
construction, and
validation

**EPD** electrode placement
device
equilibrium peritoneal
dialysis

**EPEC** enteropathogen
*Escherichia coli*

**EPEG** etoposide (VePesid)

**EPEs** extrapyramidal effects

**EPF** Enfamil Premature
Formula®

**EPG** electronic pupillography
Episodic Payment Group

**EPI** echoplanar imaging
epinephrine
epirubicin (Ellence)
epitheloid cells
exercise pressure index
exocrine pancreatic
insufficiency
Expanded Program of
Immunizations, (World
Health Organization)
Eysenck Personality
Inventory

**EPIC** etoposide, prednisolone,
ifosfamide, and
cisplatin

**EPID** epidural

**epiDX** epirubicin (4′-
epidoxorubicin; Ellence)

**EPIG** epigastric

**EPIS** epileptic postictal sleep
episiotomy

**epith.** epithelial

**EPL** effective patent life
extensor pollicis longus
(tendon)

**EPM** electronic pacemaker

**EPMR** electronic patient medical
record

**EPN** emphysematous
pyelonephritis
estimated protein needs

**EPO** epoetin alfa
(erythropoietin;
Epogen)
evening primrose oil
exclusive provider
organization

**EPOCH** etoposide, prednisone,
vincristine (Oncovin),
cyclophosphamide,
doxorubicin
(hydroxydaunorubicin)

**EPP** erythropoietic
protoporphyria
extrapleural
pneumonectomy

**EPQ-R** Eysenck Personality
Questionnaire—Revised

**EPR** electronic prescription
record
electron paramagnetic
(spin) resonance
electrophrenic respiration
emergency physical
restraint
epirubicin (Ellence)
estimated protein
requirement

**EPS** electrophysiologic study
expressed prostatic
secretions
extrapulmonary shunt
extrapyramidal syndrome
(symptom)

**EPSA** evoked potential signal
averaging

**EPSCCA** extrapulmonary small cell
carcinoma

E

| | | | |
|---|---|---|---|
| EPSDT | early periodic screening, diagnosis, and treatment | ERL | effective refractory length |
| | | ERLND | elective regional lymph node dissection |
| EPSE | extrapyramidal side effects | ERM | epiretinal membrane |
| | | ERMS | exacerbating-remitting multiple sclerosis |
| EPSP | excitatory postsynaptic potential | | |
| | | ERNA | equilibrium radionuclide angiocardiography |
| EPSS | E point septal separation | | |
| EPT | electroporation therapy endpoint temperature | ERP | effective refractory period emergency room physician endocardial resection procedure endoscopic retrograde pancreatography event-related potentials estrogen receptor protein |
| EPT® | early pregnancy test | | |
| EPTE | existed prior to enlistment | | |
| EPTS | existed prior to service | | |
| ER | emergency room end range estrogen receptors extended release extended external rotation external resistance | | |
| | | ERPF | effective renal plasma flow |
| E & R | equal and reactive examination and report | ER/PR | estrogen receptor/ progesterone receptor |
| ER+ | estrogen receptor-positive | ERS | endoscopic retrograde sphincterotomy evacuation of retained secundines (afterbirth) |
| ER− | estrogen receptor-negative | | |
| ERA | estrogen receptor assay evoked response audiometry | | |
| | | ERSR | Electronic Regulatory Submission and Review |
| %ERAD | eradication rates | | |
| ERAS | Electronic Residency Application Service | ERT | estrogen replacement therapy external radiotherapy |
| erbB1 | estrogen receptor (tyrosine kinase family) type B1 | | |
| | | ERTD | emergency room triage documentation |
| ERBD | endoscopic retrograde biliary drainage | | |
| | | ERUS | endorectal ultrasound |
| ER by ICA | estrogen receptor immunocytochemistry assay | ERV | early revascularization expiratory reserve volume |
| ERC | endoscopic retrograde cholangiography | e-Rx | electronic prescription |
| | | ERYTH | erythromycin |
| ERCP | endoscopic retrograde cholangiopancreatography | ES | electrical stimulation *Eleutherococcus senticosus* (Siberian Ginseng) embryonic stem (cells) emergency service endoscopic sclerotherapy endoscopic sphincterotomy end-to-side Ewing sarcoma ex-smoker extra strength |
| ERCT | emergency room computerized tomography | | |
| ERD | early retirement with disability | | |
| ERE | external rotation in extension | | |
| ERF | external rotation in flexion | | |
| ERFC | erythrocyte rosette forming cells | | |
| ERG | electroretinogram | | |
| ERI | elective replacement indicator | ESA | early systolic acceleration end-to-side anastomosis |

|  | ethmoid sinus adenocarcinoma | ESN | educationally subnormal |
| ESADDI | estimated safe and adequate daily dietary intake | ESN(M) | educationally subnormal-moderate |
|  |  | ESN(S) | educationally subnormal-severe |
| ESAP | evoked sensory (nerve) action potential | ESO | esophagus esotropia |
| ESAS | Edmonton System Assessment System | ESO/D | esotropia at distance |
|  |  | ESO/N | estropia at near |
| ESAT | extrasystolic atrial tachycardia | ESP | endometritis, salpingitis, and peritonitis |
| ESBL | extended-spectrum beta-lactamases |  | end-systolic pressure especially |
| ESBLKP | extended-spectrum beta-lactamase-producing *Klebsiella pneumoniae* |  | extrasensory perception |
|  |  | ESPAC | European Study Group for Pancreatic Cancers |
| ESC | end systolic counts | ES/PNET | Ewing sarcomas and peripheral neuroectodermal tumor |
| ESCC | esophageal squamous cell carcinoma |  |  |
| ESCOP | European Scientific Cooperative on Phytotherapy | ESR | early sheath removal erythrocyte sedimentation rate |
| ESCS | electrical spinal cord stimulation | ESRD | end-stage renal disease |
|  |  | ESRF | end-stage renal failure |
| ESD | Emergency Services Department | ESS | emotional, spiritual, and social |
|  | esophagus, stomach, and duodenum |  | endometrial stromal sarcoma |
| ESE | exon splice enhancer |  | endoscopic sinus surgery |
| ESF | external skeletal fixation |  | Epworth Sleepiness Scale |
| ESFT | Ewing sarcoma family of tumors |  | essential |
|  |  |  | euthyroid sick syndrome |
| ESHAP | etopside, methylprednisolone (Solu-Medrol), high-dose cytarabine (ara-C), and cisplatin (Platinol AQ) | EST | Eastern Standard Time |
|  |  |  | endoscopic spincterotomy |
|  |  |  | electroshock therapy |
|  |  |  | electrostimulation therapy |
|  |  |  | established patient |
|  |  |  | estimated |
| ESI | electrospray ionization epidural steroid injection |  | exercise stress test |
|  |  |  | expressed sequence tag |
| ESI-MS | electrospray ionization-mass spectrometry | E-stim | electrical stimulation |
|  |  | ESTs | expressed sequence tags |
| ESIN | elastic stable intramedullary nailing | ESU | electrosurgical unit |
|  |  | ESWL | extracorporeal shock wave lithotripsy |
| ESKD | end-stage kidney disease |  |  |
| ESL | English as a second language | ESWT | extracorporeal shockwave therapy |
| ESLD | end-stage liver disease | ET | ejection time |
|  | end-stage lung disease |  | embryo transfer |
| ESM | ejection systolic murmur |  | endometrial thickness |
|  | endolymphatic stromal myosis |  | endothelin |
|  |  |  | endotoxin |
|  | ethosuximide (Zarontin) |  | endotracheal |

E

| | endotracheal tube | ETI | ejective time index |
| | enterostomal therapy | | endotracheal intubation |
| | (therapist) | ETKTM | every test known to |
| | epirubicin and paclitaxel | | man |
| | (Taxol) | ETL | echo train length |
| | esotropia | | (radiology) |
| | essential thrombocythemia | ETLE | extratemporal lobe |
| | essential tremor | | epilepsy |
| | eustachian tube | ETO | estimated time of |
| | Ewing tumor | | ovulation |
| | exchange transfusion | | ethylene oxide |
| | exercise treadmill | | etoposide (VePesid) |
| *et* | and | | eustachian tube |
| ET' | esotropia at near | | obstruction |
| E(T) | intermittent esotropia at | EtOH | alcohol |
| | infinity | | alcoholic |
| E(T') | intermittent esotropia at | ETOP | elective termination of |
| | near | | pregnancy |
| ET-1 | endothelin-1 | ETP | elective termination of |
| ET @ 20' | esotropia at 6 meters | | pregnancy |
| | (infinity) | ETS | elevated toilet seat |
| ETA | endotracheal airway | | endoscopic transthoracic |
| | ethionamide | | sympathectomy |
| ETAC | early treatment of the | | endotracheal suction |
| | allergic child | | end-to-side |
| *et al* | and others | | environmental tobacco |
| ETBD | etiology to be determined | | smoke |
| ETC | and so forth | | erythromycin topical |
| | Emergency and Trauma | | solution |
| | Center | ETT | endotracheal tube |
| | endoscopic tissue culture | | esophageal transit time |
| | estimated time of | | exercise tolerance test |
| | conception | | exercise treadmill test |
| ETCO$_2$ | end-tidal carbon dioxide | | (time) |
| ETD | endoscopic | | extrathyroidal thyroxine |
| | transformational | ETT-Tl | exercise treadmill test |
| | diskectomy | | with thallium |
| | eustachian tube | ETU | emergency and trauma |
| | dysfunction | | unit |
| | eye-tracking dysfunction | | emergency treatment unit |
| ETDLA | esophageal-tracheal | ETX | edatrexate |
| | double lumen airway | ETYA | eicosatetraynoic acid |
| ETE | end-to-end | EU | Ehrlich units |
| ETEC | enterotoxigenic | | endotoxin units |
| | *Escherichia coli* | | equivalent units |
| ETF | eustachian tubal | | esophageal ulcer |
| | function | | etiology unknown |
| ETG | Episodic Treatment Group | | European Union |
| ETH | elixir terpin hydrate | | excretory urography |
| | ethanol | EUA | examine under anesthesia |
| | Ethrane | EUCD | emotionally unstable |
| ETHc̄C | elixir terpin hydrate with | | character disorder |
| | codeine | EUD | external urinary device |

126

| | | | |
|---|---|---|---|
| EUG | extrauterine gestation | EVL | endoscopic variceal ligation |
| EUL | extra uterine life | | |
| EUM | external urethral meatus | EVS | endoscopic variceal sclerosis |
| EUP | Experimental Use Permit | EW | expiratory wheeze |
| | extrauterine pregnancy | | elsewhere |
| EUS | endoscopic ultrasonography | EWB | estrogen withdrawal bleeding |
| | esophageal ultrasound | EWCL | extended-wear contact lens |
| | external urethral sphincter | | |
| EUS-FNA | endoscopic ultrasonography with fine-needle aspiration | EWE | Eastern and Western encephalomyelitis vaccine |
| EV | epidermodysplasia verruciformis | EWHO | elbow-wrist-hand orthosis |
| | esophageal varices | EWL | estimated weight loss |
| | etoposide and vincristine | | |
| | eversion | EWSCLs | extended-wear soft contact lenses |
| eV | electron volt (unit of radiation energy) | EWT | erupted wisdom teeth |
| EV71 | enterovirus-71 | ex | examined |
| EVA | Entry and Validation Application | | example |
| | | | excision |
| | ethylene vinyl acetate | | exercise |
| | etoposide, vinblastine, and doxorubicin (Adriamycin) | exam. | examination |
| | | EXECHO | exercise echocardiography |
| EVAC | evacuation | EXEF | exercise ejection fraction |
| EVAc | ethylene-vinyl acetate copolymer | EXGBUS | external genitalia, Bartholin (glands), urethral (glands), and Skene (glands) |
| eval | evaluate | | |
| EVC | Ellis-van Creveld (syndrome) | | |
| EVG | endovascular grafting | EXH VT | exhaled tidal volume |
| EWB | emotional well-being | EXIT 25 | Executive Interview (cognitive impairment test) |
| EWBH | extracorporeal whole body hyperthermia | | |
| EXC | excision | EXL | elixir |
| EVD | external ventricular (ventriculostomy) drain | EXOPH | exophthalmos |
| | | EXP | experienced |
| | | | expired |
| EVE | endoscopic vascular examination | | exploration |
| | | | expose |
| | evening | expect | expectorant |
| EXEC 22 | Executive 22 chemistry profile (see page 362) | exp. lap. | exploratory laparotomy |
| | | EXT | extension |
| EVER | eversion | | extensor (tendon) |
| EVG | endovascular grafting | | external |
| EVH | endoscopic (saphenous) vein harvesting | | extract |
| | | | extraction |
| | | | extremities |
| EVI | Exposure to Violence Interview | | extremity |
| | | Ext mon | external monitor |

E

| | |
|---|---|
| extrav | extravasation |
| ext. rot. | external rotation |
| EXTUB | extubation |
| EX U | excretory urogram |
| EZ | Edmonston-Zagreb (vaccine) |
| EZ-HT | Edmonston-Zagreb high-titer (vaccine) |

| | |
|---|---|
| F | facial |
| | Fahrenheit |
| | fair |
| | false |
| | fasting |
| | father |
| | feces |
| | female |
| | finger |
| | firm |
| | flow |
| | fluoride |
| | French |
| | fundi |
| | fundus |
| F/ | full upper denture |
| /F | full lower denture |
| (F) | final |
| °F | degrees Fahrenheit |
| F= | firm and equal |
| $F_1$ | offspring from the first generation |
| $F_2$ | offspring from the second generation |
| $F_3$ | Fluothane |
| 14 F | 14-hour fast required |
| F II–F XIII | factor 2 through 13 |
| FA | Fanconi anemia |
| | fatty acid |
| | femoral artery |
| | fetus active |
| | first aid |
| | fludarabine (Fludara) |
| | fluorescein angiogram |
| | fluorescent antibody |
| | folic acid |
| | forearm |
| | Friedreich ataxia |
| | functional activities |
| FAA | febrile antigen agglutination |
| | folic acid antagonist |
| FAAH | fatty acid amide hydrolase |
| FAAP | family assessment adjustment pass |
| FAA SOL | formalin, acetic, and alcohol solution |

E

| FAAN | Fellow of the American Academy of Nursing |
|---|---|
| FAAP | Fellow of the American Academy of Pediatrics |
| FAB | digoxin immune Fab (Digibind®) |
| | French-American-British Cooperative group |
| | functional arm brace |
| FABER | flexion, abduction, and external rotation |
| FABF | femoral artery blood flow |
| FAC | ferrite ammonium citrate |
| | fluorouracil, doxorubicin (Adriamycin), and cyclophosphamide |
| | fractional area change |
| | fractional area concentration |
| | functional aerobic capacity |
| FACA | Fellow of the American College of Anaesthetists |
| FACAG | Fellow of the American College of Angiology |
| FACAL | Fellow of the American College of Allergists |
| FACAN | Fellow of the American College of Anesthesiologists |
| FACAS | Fellow of the American College of Abdominal Surgeons |
| FACC | Fellow of the American College of Cardiology |
| FACCP | Fellow of the American College of Chest Physicians |
| FACCPC | Fellow of the American College of Clinical Pharmacology & Chemotherapy |
| FACD | Fellow of the American College of Dentists |
| FACEM | Fellow of the American College of Emergency Medicine |
| FACEP | Fellow of the American College of Emergency Physicians |
| FACES | pain scale for assessing pain intensity |

| FACG | Fellow of the American College of Gastroenterology |
|---|---|
| FACH | forceps to after-coming head |
| FACLM | Fellow of the American College of Legal Medicine |
| FACN | Fellow of the American College of Nutrition |
| FACNP | Fellow of the American College of Neuropsychopharma-cology |
| FACO | Fellow of the American College of Otolaryngology |
| FACOG | Fellow of the American College of Obstetricians & Gynecologists |
| FACOS | Fellow of the American College of Orthopedic Surgeons |
| FACP | Fellow of the American College of Physicians |
| FACPRM | Fellow of the American College of Preventive Medicine |
| FACR | Fellow of the American College of Radiology |
| FACS | Fellow of the American College of Surgeons |
| | fluorescent-activated cell sorter |
| FACSM | Fellow of the American College of Sports Medicine |
| FACT | focused appendix computed tomography |
| FACT-An | Functional Assessment of Cancer Therapy–Anemia |
| FACT-B | ....–Breast |
| FACT-F | ....–Fatigue |
| FACT-G | ....–General |
| FACT-L | ....–Lung |
| FACT-O | ....–Ovarian |
| FACT-P | ....–Prostate |
| FAD | familial Alzheimer disease |
| | Family Assessment Device |
| | fetal abdominal diameter |
| | fetal activity determination |

F

|        | flavin adenine dinucleotide | FARS | Fatality Analysis Reporting System |
|--------|------|------|------|
| FAE | fetal alcohol effect | FAS | fetal alcohol syndrome |
| FAGA | full-term appropriate for gestational age | FASAY | functional analysis of separated alleles in yeast |
| FAH | fumarylacetoacetase hydrolase | FASC | fasciculations |
| FAI | Functional Assessment Inventory | FASHP | Fellow of the American Society of Health-System Pharmacists |
| FAK | focal adhesion kinase | | |
| FAL | femoral arterial line | FASPS | familial advanced sleep-phase syndrome |
| FALL | fallopian | | |
| FALS | familial amyotrophic lateral sclerosis | FAST | fetal acoustic stimulation testing |
| FAM | family | | flow-assisted short-term |
| | fluorouracil, doxorubicin (Adriamycin), and mitomycin | | fluorescent allergosorbent technique |
| | full allosteric modulators | | focused assessment with sonography for trauma |
| FAMA | fluorescent antibody to membrane antigen | FAT | Fetal Activity Test |
| FAME | fluorouracil, doxorubicin (Adriamycin), and semustin (methyl CCNU) | | fluorescent antibody test |
| | | | food awareness training |
| | | FAV | facio-auricular vertebral |
| | | FAZ | foveal avascular zone |
| FAMMM | familial atypical multiple mole melanoma | FB | fasting blood (sugar) |
| | | | finger breadth |
| FAM-S | fluorouracil, doxorubicin (Adriamycin), mitomycin, and streptozotocin | | flexible bronchoscope |
| | | | foreign body |
| | | F/B | followed by |
| | | | forward/backward |
| FAMTX | fluorouracil, doxorubicin (Adriamycin), and methotrexate | | forward bending |
| | | FBC | full (complete) blood count |
| FANA | fluorescent antinuclear antibody | FBCOD | foreign body, cornea, right eye |
| FANG | fluorescent angiography | FBCOS | foreign body, cornea, left eye |
| FANSS&M | fundus anterior, normal size and shape and mobile | FBD | familial British dementia |
| | | | fibrocystic breast disease |
| FAO | fatty acid oxidation | | functional bowel disease |
| | Food and Agriculture Organization | FBF | forearm blood flow |
| | | FBG | fasting blood glucose |
| FAP | familial adenomatous polyposis | | foreign-body-type granulomata |
| | familial amyloid polyneuropathy | FBH | hydroxybutyric dehydrogenase |
| | femoral artery pressure | FBHH | familial benign hypocalciuric hypercalcemia |
| | fibrillating action potential | | |
| FAQ | frequently asked question(s) | FBI | flossing, brushing, and irrigation |
| F-ara-A | fludarabine phosphate (Fludara) | | full bony impaction |

| | | | |
|---|---|---|---|
| FBL | fecal blood loss | FCCA | Final Comprehensive Consensus Assessment |
| FBM | felbamate (Felbatol) | | |
| | fetal breathing motion | FCCC | fracture complete, compound, and comminuted |
| | foreign body, metallic | | |
| FBRCM | fingerbreadth below right costal margin | | |
| | | FCCL | follicular center cell lymphoma |
| FBS | failed back syndrome | | |
| | fasting blood sugar | FCCU | family centered care unit |
| | fetal bovine serum | FCD | feces collection device |
| | foreign body sensation (eye) | | fibrocystic disease |
| | | FCDB | fibrocystic disease of the breast |
| FBSS | failed back surgery syndrome | | |
| | | FCE | fluorouracil, cisplatin, and etoposide |
| FBU | fingers below umbilicus | | |
| FBW | fasting blood work | | functional capacity evaluation |
| FC | family conference | | |
| | febrile convulsion | FCFD | fluorescence capillary-fill device |
| | female child | | |
| | fever, chills | FCH | familial combined hyperlipidemia |
| | film coated (tablets) | | |
| | financial class | | fibrosing cholestatic hepatitis |
| | finger clubbing | | |
| | finger counting | FCHL | familial combined hyperlipemia |
| | flexion contractor | | |
| | flow compensation (radiology) | FCL | fibular collateral ligament |
| | | | |
| | flucytosine (Ancobon) | F-CL | fluorouracil and calcium leucovorin |
| | foam cuffed (tracheal or endotracheal tube) | | |
| | | FCM | flow cytometry |
| | Foley catheter | FCMC | family centered maternity care |
| | follows commands | | |
| | foster care | FCMD | Fukiyama congenital muscular dystrophy |
| | French Canadian | | |
| | functional capacity | FCMN | family centered maternity nursing |
| | functional class | | |
| F/C | film coated (tablet) | FCNV | fever, cough, nausea, and vomiting |
| F + C | flare and cells | | |
| F & C | foam and condom | FCOU | finger count, both eyes |
| 5FC | flucytosine (this is a dangerous abbreviation as it can be seen as 5FU) | FCP | formocresol pulpotomu |
| | | FCR | flexor carpi radialis |
| | | | fractional catabolic rate |
| FCA | Federal False Claims Act | FCRB | flexor carpi radialis brevis |
| | | FCRT | fetal cardiac reactivity test |
| F. cath. | Foley catheter | | focal cranial radiation therapy |
| FCBD | fibrocystic breast disease | | |
| FCC | familial cerebral cavernoma | FCS | fever, chills, and sweating |
| | | FCSNVD | fever, chills, sweating, nausea, vomiting, and diarrhea |
| | familial colonic cancer | | |
| | family centered care | | |
| | femoral cerebral catheter | FCU | flexor carpi ulnaris (tendon) |
| | follicular center cells | | |
| | fracture compound comminuted | FCV | feline calicivirus |
| | | FD | familial dysautonomia |

F

|  |  |  |  |
|---|---|---|---|
|  | fetal demise | FDR | first-dose reaction |
|  | fetal distress | FDS | flexor digitorum |
|  | focal distance |  | superficialis |
|  | forceps delivery |  | for duration of stay |
|  | free drain | FDT | fronto-dextra transversa |
|  | full denture |  | (right frontotransverse) |
|  | fully dilated | FE | field echo (radiology) |
|  | functional deficits |  | frequency encode |
| F & D | fixed and dilated |  | (radiology) |
| FDA | Food and Drug | Fe | female |
|  | Administration |  | iron |
|  | fronto-dextra anterior | F & E | full and equal |
| FDB | first-degree burn | FEB | febrile |
|  | flexor digitorum brevis | FEC | fluorouracil, epirubicin, |
| FDBL | fecal daily blood loss |  | and cyclophosphamide |
| FDC | fixed-dose combination |  | fluorouracil, etoposide, |
|  | (preparations) |  | and cisplatin |
| FDCA | Food, Drug, and Cosmetic |  | forced expiratory capacity |
|  | Act | FECG | fetal electrocardiogram |
| FDCs | follicular dendritic | FeCh | ferrochelatase |
|  | cells | FECP | free erythrocyte |
| FDE | fixed-drug eruption |  | coproporphyrin |
| FDF | flexor digitorum | FECT | fibroelastic connective |
|  | profundus (tendon) |  | tissue |
| FDG | feeding | FED | fish eye disease |
|  | fluorine-18-labeled | FEES | fiberoptic endoscopic |
|  | deoxyglucose |  | evaluation |
|  | ($^{18}$fluorodeoxyglucose) |  | (examination) of |
| FDGB | fall down, go boom |  | swallowing |
| FDG-PET | positron emission | FEF | forced expiratory flow |
|  | tomography with |  | rate |
|  | $^{18}$fluorodeoxyglucose | $FEF_{25\%-75\%}$ | forced expiratory flow |
| FDGS | feedings |  | during the middle half |
| FDI | first dorsal interosseous |  | of the forced vital |
|  | food-drug interaction |  | capacity |
|  | Functional Disability | $FEF_{x-y}$ | forced expiratory flow |
|  | Index |  | between two designated |
| FDIU | fetal death in utero |  | volume points in the |
| FDL | flexor digitorum longus |  | forced vital capacity |
| FDLMP | first day of last menstrual | FEHBP | Federal Employee Health |
|  | period |  | Benefits Plan |
| FDM | fetus of diabetic mother | FEL | familial erythrophagocytic |
|  | flexor digiti minimi |  | lymphohistiocytosis |
| FDP | fibrin-degradation | FeLV | feline leukemia virus |
|  | products | FEM | femoral |
|  | fixed-dose procedure | FEMA | Federal Emergency |
|  | flexor digitorum |  | Management Agency |
|  | profundus | FEM-FEM | femoral femoral (bypass) |
| FDPCA | fixed-dose patient- | FEM-POP | femoral popliteal (bypass) |
|  | controlled analgesia | FEM-TIB | femoral tibial (bypass) |
| FD-PET | fluorodopa-positron | FERGs | focal electroretinograms |
|  | emission tomography | FEN | fluid, electrolytes, and |
| FDQB | flexor digiti quinti brevis |  | nutrition |

**F**

| | | | |
|---|---|---|---|
| FENa | fractional extraction of sodium | | five-minute format |
| | | | flat feet |
| FENIB | familial encephalopathies with neuroserpin inclusion bodies | | force fluids |
| | | | formula fed |
| | | | forward flexion |
| FEN-PHEN | fenfluramine and phentermine | | foster father |
| | | | Fox-Fordyce (disease) |
| FENS | field-electrical neural stimulation | | fundus firm |
| | | | further flexion |
| FEOM | full extraocular movements | F/F | face to face |
| | | F&F | filiform and follower |
| FEP | free erythrocyte porphyrins | | fixes and follows |
| | | F→F | finger to finger |
| | free erythrocyte protoporphorin | FF1/U | fundus firm 1 cm above umbilicus |
| | functional exercise program | FF2/U | fundus firm 2 cm above umbilicus |
| FER | flexion, extension, and rotation | FF@u | fundus firm at umbilicus |
| | | FFA | free fatty acid |
| FERR | serum ferritin | | fundus fluorescein angiogram |
| FES | fat embolism syndrome | | |
| | floppy eyelid syndrome | FFAT | Free Floating Anxiety Test |
| | forced expiratory spirogram | FFB | flexible fiberoptic bronchoscopy |
| | functional electrical stimulation | FFD | fat-free diet |
| | | | focal-film distance |
| FeSO4 | ferrous sulfate | FFDM | freedom from distant metastases |
| FESS | functional endonasal sinus surgery | FFE | free-flow electrophoresis |
| | functional endoscopic sinus surgery | FFF | field-flow fractionation |
| | | | freedom from (biochemical and/or clinical) failure |
| FET | familial essential tremor | | |
| | fixed erythrocyte turnover | FFI | fast food intake |
| FETI | fluorescence (fluorescent) energy transfer immunoassay | | fatal familial insomnia |
| | | FFM | fat-free mass |
| FEUO | for external use only | | five finger movement |
| FEV | familial exudative vitreoretinopathy | | freedom from metastases |
| | | FFP | fresh frozen plasma |
| $FEV_1$ | forced expiratory volume in one second | FFPE | formalin-faxed, paraffin-embedded |
| FEVC | forced expiratory vital capacity | FFQ | food frequency questionnaire |
| $FEV_{1\%VC}$ | forced expiratory volume in one second as percent of forced vital capacity | FFR | freedom from relapse |
| | | FFROM | full, free range of motion |
| | | FFS | failure-free survival |
| FEVR | familial exudative vitreoretinopathy | | fee-for-service |
| | | | Fight For Sight |
| FF | fat free | | flexible fiberoptic sigmoidoscopy |
| | fecal frequency | | |
| | filtration fraction | FFT | fast-Fourier transforms |
| | finger-to-finger | | flicker fusion threshold |

F

| | | | |
|---|---|---|---|
| FFTP | first full-term pregnancy | FHX | fluorouracil, hydroxyurea, and radiotherapy |
| FFU/1 | fundus firm 1 cm below umbilicus | FHx | family history |
| FFU/2 | fundus firm 2 cm below umbilicus | FI | fiscal intermediary |
| | | FIA | familial intracranial aneurysms |
| FG | fibrin glue | | Family Independence Agency (formerly Department of Social Services) |
| FGAs | first-generation antihistamines | | |
| FGC | full gold crown | | |
| FGF | fibroblast growth factor | | |
| FGM | female genital mutilation | FIAC | fiacitabine |
| FGP | fundic gland polyps | FIAU | fialuridine |
| FGS | fibrogastroscopy | FIB | fibrillation |
| | focal glomerulosclerosis | | fibula |
| FH | familial hypercholesterolemia | FICA | Federal Insurance Contributions Act (Social Security) |
| | family history | | |
| | favorable histology | FiCO₂ | fraction of inspired carbon dioxide |
| | fetal head | | |
| | fetal heart | FICS | Fellow of the International College of Surgeons |
| | fundal height | | |
| FH+ | family history positive | FID | father in delivery |
| FH− | family history negative | | free induction decay |
| FHA | filamentous hemagglutinin | FIF | forced inspiratory flow |
| FHB | flexor hallucis brevis | FiF | Functional Intact Fibrinogen (test) |
| FHC | familial hypertrophic cardiomyopathy | | |
| | | FIGE | field inversion gel electrophoresis |
| | family health center | | |
| FHCIC | Fuchs heterochromic iridocyclitis | FIGLU | formiminoglutamic acid |
| | | FIGO | International Federation of Gynecology and Obstetrics |
| FHD | family history of diabetes | | |
| FHF | fulminant hepatic failure | | |
| FHH | familial hypocalciuric hypercalcemia | FIL | father-in-law |
| | | | Filipino |
| | fetal heart heard | FIM | functional independence measure |
| FHI | frontal horn index | | |
| | Fuchs heterochromic iridocyclitis | FIN | flexible intramedullary nail |
| FHL | flexor hallucis longus | FIND | follow-up intervention for normal development |
| FHM | familial hemiplegic migraine | | |
| | | FiO₂ | fraction of inspired oxygen |
| FHN | family history negative | | |
| FHNH | fetal heart not heard | FIP | feline infectious peritonitis |
| FHO | family history of obesity | | |
| FHP | family history positive | | flatus in progress |
| FHR | fetal heart rate | FIRI | fasting insulin resistance index |
| FHRB | fetal heart rate baseline | | |
| FHRV | fetal heart rate variability | FISH | fluorescent (fluorescence) *in situ* hybridization |
| FHS | fetal heart sounds | | |
| | fetal hydantoin syndrome | FISP | fast imaging with steady state precision |
| FHT | fetal heart tone | | |
| FHVP | free hepatic vein pressure | FITC | fluorescein isothiocyanate conjugated |

| | | | |
|---|---|---|---|
| FIV | feline immunodeficiency virus | FLC | follicular large cell lymphoma |
| | *in vitro* fertilization (French) | FLD | fatty liver disease |
| | | | fluid |
| FIVC | forced inspiratory vital capacity | | flutamide and leuprolide acetate depot |
| FIX | factor IX (nine) | | full lower denture |
| FJB | facet joint block | FL Dtr | full lower denture |
| FJN | familial juvenile nephrophthisis | FLE | frontal lobe epilepsy |
| | | FLe | fluorouracil and levamisole |
| FJP | familial juvenile polyposis | | |
| FJROM | full joint range of motion | flexsig | flexible sigmoidoscopy |
| FJS | finger joint size | FLF | funny looking facies (see note under FLK) |
| FJV | first jejunal vein | | |
| FK506 | tacrolimus (Prograf) | FLGA | full-term, large for gestational age |
| FKA | failed to keep appointment | | |
| | formally known as | FLIC | Functional Living Index–Cancer |
| FKBP | FK-506 binding protein (tacrolimus; Prograf) | | |
| | | FLIE | Functional Living Index—Emesis |
| FKD | Kinetic Family Drawing | | |
| FKE | full knee extension | FLK | funny looking kid (should never be used: unusual facial features, is a better expression) |
| FL | fatty liver | | |
| | femur length | | |
| | fetal length | | |
| | fluid | FLM | fetal lung maturity |
| | fluorescein | fl. oz. | fluid ounce |
| | fluorouracil and leucovorin | FLP | fasting lipid profile |
| | | | Functional Limitations Profile |
| | flutamide and leuprolide acetate | | |
| | | FL REST | fluid restriction |
| | focal laser | FLS | fibroblast-like synoviocytes |
| | focal length | | flashing lights and/or scotoma |
| | follicular lymphoma | | |
| | full liquids | | flu-like symptoms |
| | functional limitations | FLT | fluorothymidine |
| fL | femtoliter ($10^{-15}$ liter) | FLU | fluconazole (Diflucan) |
| F/L | father-in-law | | fludarabine (Fludara) |
| FLA | free-living amebic (ameba) | | flunisolide (Aero Bid) |
| | low-friction arthroplasty | | fluoxetine (Prozac) |
| FLAIR | fluid-attenuated inversion recovery | | fluticasone propionate (Flonase) |
| | | | influenza |
| FLAP | fluorouracil, leucovorin, doxorubicin (Adriamycin), and cisplatin (Platinol AQ) | FLU A | influenza A virus |
| | | FLUO | Fluothane |
| | | fluoro | fluoroscopy |
| | 5-lipoxygenase activating protein | FLUT | flutamide (Eulexin) |
| | | FLV | Friend leukemia virus |
| FLASH | fast low-angle shot | FLW | fasting laboratory work |
| FLAVO | flavopiridol | FLZ | flurazepam (Dalmane) |
| FLB | funny looking beat | FM | face mask |
| FLBS | funny looking baby syndrome (see note under FLK) | | fat mass |
| | | | fetal movements |
| | | | fibromyalgia (syndrome) |

F

135

fine motor
floor manager
fluorescent microscopy
foster mother

**F & M** firm and midline (uterus)

**F-MACHOP** fluorouracil, methotrexate, cytarabine (ara-C), cyclophosphamide, doxorubicin (hydroxydaunorubicin), vincristine (Oncovin), and prednisone

**FMC** fetal movement count

**FMD** family medical doctor
fibromuscular dysplasia
flow-mediated dilatation
foot-and-mouth disease

**FMDV** foot-and-mouth disease virus

**FME** Frühsommer-meningoenzephalitis vaccine
full-mouth extraction

**FMEA** failure mode effects analysis

**FMEN-1** familial multiple endocrine neoplasia, type 1

**FMF** familial Mediterranean fever
fetal movement felt
forced midexpiratory flow

**FMG** fine mesh gauze
foreign medical graduate

**FMH** family medical history
fibromuscular hyperplasia

**FmHx** family history

**FML®** fluorometholone

**FMLA** Family and Medical Leave Act of 1993

**FMN** first malignant neoplasm
flavin mononucleotide

**FMOA** full-mouth odontectomy and alveoloplasty

**FMOL** femtomole ($10^{-15}$ mole)

**FMP** fasting metabolic panel
first menstrual period
functional maintenance program

**FMPA** full-mouth periapicals

**FMR** fetal movement record
focused medical review

functional magnetic resonance (imaging)

**FMRD** full-mouth restorative dentistry

**fMRI** functional magnetic resonance imaging

**FMRP** fragile X mental retardation protein(s)

**FMS** fibromyalgia syndrome
fluorouracil, mitomycin, and streptozocin
full-mouth series

**F & MS** frontal and maxillary sinuses

**FMT** functional muscle test

**FMTC** familial medullary thyroid carcinoma

**FMU** first morning urine

**FMV** flow-mediated vasodilation
fluorouracil, semustine (methyl-CCNU), and vincristine

**FMX** full-mouth x-ray

**FMZ** flumazenil (Romazicon)

**FN** facial nerve
false negative
febrile neutropenia
femoral neck
finger-to-nose (test)
flight nurse

**F/N** fluids and nutrition

**F to N** finger-to-nose

**FNA** femoral neck anteversion
fine-needle aspiration

**FNa** filtered sodium

**FNAB** fine-needle aspiration biopsy

**FNAC** fine-needle aspiratory cytology

**FNB** femoral nerve block

**FNCJ** fine-needle catheter jejunostomy

**FND** fludarabine, mitoxantrone (Novantrone), and dexamethasone
focal neurological deficit

**FNF** femoral-neck fracture
finger-nose-finger (test)

**FNH** focal nodular hyperplasia

**FNHL** follicular non-Hodgkin lymphoma

**FNMTC** familial nonmedullary thyroid carcinoma

| | | | |
|---|---|---|---|
| FNP | Family Nurse Practitioner | FOS | fiberoptic sigmoidoscopy |
| | | | fixing left eye |
| FNR | false-negative rate | | fosphenytoin (Cerebyx) |
| FNS | food and nutrition services | | fructooligosaccharides |
| | | | future order screen |
| | functional neuromuscular stimulation | FOSC | freestanding outpatient surgery center |
| F/NS | fever and night sweats | FOT | forced oscillation technique |
| FNT | finger-to-nose (test) | | |
| FNTC | fine-needle transhepatic cholangiography | | form of thought |
| | | | frontal outflow tract |
| FO | foot orthosis | FOV | field of view |
| | foramen ovale | FOVI | field of vision intact |
| | foreign object | FOW | fenestration of oval window |
| | fronto-occipital | | |
| FOB | father of baby | FP | fall precautions |
| | fecal occult blood | | false positive |
| | feet out of bed | | familial porencephaly |
| | fiberoptic bronchoscope | | family planning |
| | foot of bed | | family practice |
| FOBT | fecal occult blood test | | family practitioner |
| FOC | father of child | | family presence |
| | fluid of choice | | fibrous proliferation |
| | fronto-occipital circumference | | flat plate |
| | | | fluorescence polarization |
| FOD | fixing right eye | | fluticasone propionate |
| | free of disease | | food poisoning |
| FOEB | feet over edge of bed | | frozen plasma |
| FOF | fell on floor | F/P | fluid/plasma (ratio) |
| FOG | Fluothane, oxygen and gas (nitrous oxide) | F-P | femoral popliteal |
| | | fpA | fibrinopeptide A |
| | full-on gain | FPAL | full term, premature, abortion, living |
| FOH | family ocular history | | |
| FOI | flight of ideas | FPB | femoral-popliteal bypass |
| FOIA | Freedom of Information Act | | |
| | | | flexor pollicis brevis |
| FOID | fear of impending doom | FPC | familial polyposis coli |
| FOL | fiberoptic laryngoscopy | | family practice center |
| FOM | floor of mouth | FPD | feto-pelvic disproportion |
| FOMi | fluorouracil, Oncovin, (vincristine), and mitomycin | | fixed partial denture |
| | | FPDL | flashlamp-pumped pulsed dye laser |
| FONSI | finding of no significant impact | | |
| | | FPE | first-pass effect |
| | | FPG | fasting plasma glucose |
| FOO | family of origin | FPHx | family psychiatric history |
| FOOB | fell out of bed | | |
| FOOSH | fell on outstretched hand | FPIA | fluorescence-polarization immunoassay |
| FOP | fasting office profile | | |
| | fibrodysplasia ossificans progressiva | FPIES | food protein-induced enterocolitis syndrome |
| FOPS | fiberoptic proctosigmoidoscopy | FPL | flexor pollicis longus (tendon) |
| FORMIL | foreign military | | final printed labeling |

F

137

| | | | |
|---|---|---|---|
| FPLD | familial partial lipodystrophy | FRCSE | Fellow of the Royal College of Surgeons of Edinburgh |
| FPM | full passive movements | | |
| FPNA | first-pass nuclear angiocardiography | FRCSI | Fellow of the Royal College of Surgeons of Ireland |
| FPO | fetal pulse oximetry | FRE | flow-related enhancement |
| FPOR | follicle puncture for oocyte retrieval | FRET | fluoresence resonance energy transfer |
| FPU | family participation unit | FRF | filtration replacement fluid |
| FPZ | fluphenazine | | |
| FPZ-D | fluphenazine decanoate | FRG | Functional Related Groups |
| FQ | fluoroquinolones | | |
| FR | fair | FRJM | full range of joint movement |
| | father | | |
| | Father (priest) | FRN | fetal rhabdomyomatous nephroblastoma |
| | Federal Register | | |
| | first responder | FRNT | focus-reduction neutralization test |
| | flow rate | | |
| | fluid restriction | FROA | full range of affect |
| | fluid retention | FROM | full range of motion |
| | fractional reabsorption | FROMAJE | functioning, reasoning, orientation, memory, arithmetic, judgment, and emotion (mental status evaluation) |
| | freestyle, no head or lower-extremity fixation (aquatic therapy) | | |
| | frequent relapses | | |
| | Friends | | |
| | frothy | FRP | follicle regulatory protein functional refractory period |
| | full range | | |
| Fr | French (catheter gauge) | | |
| F/R | fire/rescue | FRSN | fluoroquinolone-resistant *Streptococcus pneumoniae* |
| F & R | force and rhythm (pulse) | | |
| FRA | fall risk assessment | | |
| | fluorescent rabies antibody | FS | fetoscope |
| FRAC | fracture | | fibromyalgia syndrome |
| FRACTS | fractional urines | | fingerstick |
| FRAG | fragment | | flexible sigmoidoscopy |
| FRAG-X | Fragile X Syndrome | | foreskin |
| FRAP | family risk assessment program | | fractional shortenings |
| | | | frozen section |
| | fluorescence recovery after photobleaching | | full strength |
| | | | functional status |
| FRC | frozen red cells | F & S | full and soft |
| | functional residual capacity | FSA | Family Services Association |
| FRCPC | Fellow of the Royal College of Physicians of Canada | FSAD | female sexual arousal disorder(s) |
| | | FSALO | Fletcher suite after loading ovoids |
| FRCPE | Fellow of the Royal College of Physicians of Edinburgh | FSALT | Fletcher suite after loading tandem |
| | | FSB | fetal scalp blood |
| FRCSC | Fellow of the Royal College of Surgeons of Canada | | full spine board |
| | | FSBG | fingerstick blood glucose |

| | | | |
|---|---|---|---|
| FSBM | full-strength breast milk | FSS | federal supply schedule (cost source) |
| FSBS | fingerstick blood sugar | | fetal scalp sampling |
| FSC | Fatigue Symptom Checklist | | Flinders Symptom Score |
| | flexible sigmoidoscopy | | French steel sound (dilated to #24FSS) |
| | fracture, simple, and comminuted | | frequency-selective saturation |
| | fracture, simple, and complete | | full-scale score |
| FSCC | fracture, simple, complete, and comminuted | FSW | feet of sea water (pressure) |
| FSD | female sexual dysfunction | | field service worker |
| | focal-skin distance | FT | family therapy |
| | fracture, simple, and depressed | | fast-twitch |
| FSE | fast spin-echo | | feeding tube |
| | fetal scalp electrode | | filling time |
| FSF | fibrin stabilizing factor | | finger tip |
| FSG | fasting serum glucose | | flexor tendon |
| | focal and segmental glomerulosclerosis | | fluidotherapy |
| FSGA | full-term, small for gestational age | | follow through |
| | | | foot (ft) |
| FSGN | focal segmental glomerulonephritis | | Fourier transform (radiology) |
| | | | free testosterone |
| FSGS | focal segmental glomerulosclerosis | | full-term |
| | | $F_3T$ | trifluridine (Viroptic) |
| FSH | facioscapulohumeral | $FT_3$ | free triiodothyronine |
| | follicle-stimulating hormone | $FT_4$ | free thyroxine |
| | | $FT_4I$ | free thyroxine index |
| FSHMD | facioscapulohumeral muscular dystrophy | FTA | fluorescent titer antibody |
| | | | fluorescent treponemal antibody |
| FSIQ | Full-Scale Intelligence Quotient (part of Wechsler test) | FTA-ABS | fluorescent treponemal antibody absorption |
| | | FTB | fingertip blood |
| FSL | fasting serum level | FTBD | full-term born dead |
| FSM | functional status measures | FTBI | fractionated total body irradiation |
| F-SM/C | fungus, smear and culture | FTC | emtricitabine (Coviracil) |
| FSME | Frühsommer-meningoencephalitis | | fallopian tube carcinoma |
| | | | Federal Trade Commission |
| FSO | for screws only (prosthetic cups) | | frames to come |
| | | | full to confrontation |
| FSOP | French Society of Pediatric Oncology | FTD | failure to descend |
| | | | frontotemporal degeneration |
| FSP | fibrin split products | | frontotemporal dementia |
| FSR | fractionated stereotactic radiosurgery | | full-term delivery |
| | | FTE | failure to engraft |
| | fusiform skin revision | FTEs | full-time equivalents |
| FSRS | fractionated stereotactic radiosurgery | FTF | finger-to-finger |
| FSRT | fractionated stereotactic radiotherapy | | free thyroxine fraction |

F

| | | | |
|---|---|---|---|
| FTFTN | finger-to-finger-to-nose | FTUPLD | full-term uncomplicated pregnancy, labor, and delivery |
| FTG | full-thickness graft | | |
| FTI | farnesyltransferase inhibitor | FTV | Fortovase (saquinavir, soft gel cap) |
| | force-time integral | | |
| | free thyroxine index | | functional trial visit |
| F TIP | finger tip | FTW | failure to wean |
| FTIUP | full-term intrauterine pregnancy | FU | fraction unbound |
| | | | fluorouracil |
| FTKA | failed to keep appointment | F & U | flanks and upper quadrants |
| FTLB | full-term living birth | F/U | follow-up |
| FTLD | frontotemporal lobar degeneration | | fundus at umbilicus |
| | | F↑U | fingers above umbilicus |
| FTLFC | full-term living female child | F↓U | fingers below umbilicus |
| | | 5-FU | fluorouracil |
| FTLMC | full-term living male child | FUA | flat and upright (x-ray of the) abdomen |
| FTM | fluid thioglycollate medium | FUB | function uterine bleeding |
| | | FUCO | fractional uptake of carbon monoxide |
| FTMH | full-thickness macular hole(s) | FUD | fear, uncertainty, and doubt |
| FTMS | Fourier transform mass spectrometer | | frequency, urgency, and dysuria |
| FTN | finger-to-nose | | full upper denture |
| | full-term nursery | FUDR® | floxuridine |
| FTNB | full-term newborn | FU Dtr | full upper denture |
| FTND | Fagerstrom Test for Nicotine Dependence | FUFA | fluorouracil and leucovorin (folinic acid) |
| | full-term normal delivery | FU/FL | full upper denture, full lower denture |
| FTNSD | full-term, normal, spontaneous delivery | FUFOL | fluorouracil and leucovorin calcium (folinic acid) |
| FTO | full-time occlusion (eye patch) | | |
| FTOZ | frontotemporal orbitozygomatic | Fugl | Fugl-Meyer Assessment of Motor Recovery After Stroke |
| FTOZ1 | one-piece frontotemporal orbitozygomatic | | |
| | | FUL | federal upper limit (price list) |
| FTP | failure to progress | | |
| | full-term pregnancy | FULG | fulguration |
| FTR | father | 5FU/LV | fluorouracil and leucovorin |
| | failed to report | | |
| | failed to respond | FUN | follow-up note |
| | for the record | FUNASA | Fundão Naçional de Sade (Brazil's national health agency) |
| FTRAM | free transverse rectus abdominis myocutaneous (flap) | | |
| | | FUNG-C | fungus culture |
| FTSD | full-term spontaneous delivery | FUNG-S | fungus smear |
| | | FUO | fever of undetermined origin |
| FTSG | full-thickness skin graft | | |
| FTT | failure to thrive | FUOV | follow-up office visit |
| | fetal tissue transplant | FU/LP | full upper denture, partial lower denture |
| | Finger-Tapping Test | | |
| Ftube | feeding tube | | |

| | |
|---|---|
| FUP | follow-up |
| FUS | fusion |
| FUT | fibrinogen update test |
| FUV | follow-up visit |
| FV | femoral vein |
| F & V | fruits and vegetables |
| FVC | false vocal cord(s) |
| | forced vital capacity |
| FVD | fever, vomiting, and diarrhea |
| FVFR | filled voiding flow rate |
| FVH | focal vascular headache |
| F VIII | factor VIII (eight) |
| FVL | factor V-Leiden (mutation) |
| | femoral vein ligation |
| | flow volume loop |
| FVR | feline viral rhinotracheitis |
| | forearm vascular resistance |
| FW | fetal weight |
| F/W | followed with |
| F waves | fibrillatory waves |
| | flutter waves |
| FVWs | flow-velocity waveforms (umbilical artery Doppler) |
| FWB | full weight bearing |
| | functional well-being |
| FWCA | functional work capacity assessment |
| FWD | fairly well developed |
| FWHM | full width at half maximum (radiology) |
| FWS | fetal warfarin syndrome |
| FWW | front wheel walker |
| Fx | fractional urine |
| | fracture |
| Fx-BB | fracture both bones |
| Fx-dis | fracture-dislocation |
| F XI | Factor XI (eleven) |
| FXN | function |
| FXR | fracture |
| FXS | fragile X syndrome |
| FY | fiscal year |
| FYC | facultative yeast carrier |
| FYI | for your information |
| FZ | flutamide and goserelin acetate (Zoladex) |
| FZRC | frozen red (blood) cells |

# G

| | |
|---|---|
| G | gallop |
| | gastrostomy |
| | gauge |
| | gauss (a unit of magnetic flux density in radiology) |
| | gavage feeding |
| | gingiva |
| | good |
| | grade |
| | gram (g) |
| | gravida |
| | guaiac |
| | guanine |
| G + | gram-positive |
| | guaiac positive |
| G − | gram-negative |
| | guaiac negative |
| ↑g | increasing |
| ↓g | decreasing |
| G1–4 | grade 1–4 |
| G-11 | hexachlorophene |
| GA | Gamblers Anonymous |
| | gastric analysis |
| | general anesthesia |
| | general appearance |
| | gestational age |
| | ginger ale |
| | glycyrrhetinic acid |
| | granuloma annulare |
| | glucose/acetone |
| Ga | gallium |
| $^{67}$Ga | gallium citrate Ga 67 |
| GABA | gamma-aminobutyric acid |
| GABHS | group A beta hemolytic streptococci |
| GAD | generalized anxiety disorder |
| | glutamic acid decarboxylase |
| GAF | geographic adjustment factors |
| | Global Assessment of Functioning (scale) |
| GAG | glycosaminoglycan |
| GAGPS | glycosaminoglycan polysulfate |

| GAL | galanthamine hydrobromide |  | ganglionic-blocking agent |
|  | gallon | GBBS | group B beta hemolytic streptococcus |
| G'ale | ginger ale | GBE | *Ginkgo biloba* extract |
| GALI-PUT | galactose-1-phosphate uridye transferase enzyme | GBG | gonadal-steroid binding globulin |
| GALT | galactose-1-phosphate uridyltransferase (gene) | GBH | gamma benzene hexachloride (lindane) |
|  | gut-associated lymphoid tissue | GBIA | Guthrie bacterial inhibition assay |
| GAM | Gamma Knife | GBL | gamma butyrolactone |
|  | gene-activated matrices | GBM | glioblastoma multiforme |
| GAMT | guanidinoacetate methyltransferase |  | glomerular basement membrane |
| GAO | General Accounting Office | GBMI | guilty but mentally ill |
| GAP | GTPase activating protein | GBP | gabapentin (Neurontin) |
| GAP-43 | growth-associated protein-43 |  | gastric bypass |
|  |  |  | gated blood pool (imaging) |
| GAR | gonnococcal antibody reaction | GBPS | gated blood pool scan |
| GARFT | glycinamide ribonucleotide formyl transferase | GBR | gamma band response (audiology) |
|  |  |  | good blood return |
|  |  |  | guided bone regeneration |
| GAS | general adaption syndrome | GBS | gallbladder series |
|  | ginseng-abuse syndrome |  | gastric bypass surgery |
|  | Glasgow Assessment Schedule |  | group B streptococcal (*Streptococcus agalactiae*) disease vaccine |
|  | Global Assessment Scale |  |  |
|  | group A streptococcal (*Streptococcus pyogenes*) disease vaccine |  | group B streptococci |
|  |  |  | Guillain-Barré syndrome |
|  |  | GBV-C | GB virus type C (also known as hepatitis G virus) |
|  | group A streptococci | GBW | generalized body weakness |
| Gas Anal F&T | gastric analysis, free and total | GBX | gall bladder extraction (cholecystectomy) |
| Ga scan | gallium scan | GC | gas chromatography |
| Gastroc | gastrocnemius |  | gastric cancer |
| GAT | geriatric assessment team |  | geriatric chair (Gerichair®) |
|  | group adjustment therapy |  | gingival curettage |
| GATB | General Aptitude Test Battery |  | gonococci (gonorrhea) |
| GAU | geriatric assessment unit |  | good condition |
| GAVE | gastric antral vascular ectasia |  | graham crackers |
| Gaw | airway conductance | G−C | gram-negative cocci |
| GB | gallbladder | G+C | gram-positive cocci |
|  | *Ginkgo biloba* | GCA | ghost cell ameloblastoma |
|  | Guillain-Barré (syndrome) |  | giant cell arteritis |
| G & B | good and bad | GCBP | gated cardiac blood pool |
| GBA | gingivobuccoaxial |  |  |

| GCC | guanylyl cyclase C | GDC | Guglielmi detachable coil |
| GCE | general conditioning exercise | Gd-DTPA | gadopentetate (Magnevist) |
| | | Gd-DTPA-BMA | gadodiamide |
| GCDFP | gross cystic disease fluid protein | GD FA | grandfather |
| GCI | General Cognitive Index | GDH | glutamic dehydrogenase |
| GCIIS | glucose control insulin infusion system | Gd-HPD03A | gadoteridol |
| GCL | generalized congenital lipodystrophy | GDJ | gastroduodenal junction |
| | | g/dl | grams per deciliter |
| GCM | good central maintained | GDM | gestational diabetes mellitus |
| GCMD | generalized cardiovascular metabolic disease | GDM A-1 | gestational diabetes mellitus, insulin controlled, Type I |
| GCMN | giant congenital melanocytic nevus | | |
| GC-MS | gas chromatography-mass spectroscopy | GDM A-2 | gestational diabetes mellitus, diet controlled, Type II |
| GCP | gentamicin, clindamycin, and polymyxin topical preparation | GD MO | grandmother |
| | | Gd-MRI | gadolinium-enhanced magnetic resonance imaging |
| | good clinical practices | | |
| GCR | gastrocolonic response | | |
| | glucocerebrosidase | GDNF | glial-derived neurotrophic factor |
| GCS | Glasgow Coma Scale | | |
| | glucocorticosteroid(s) | GDP | gel diffusion precipitin |
| GCSE | generalized convulsive status epilepticus | GDPs | general dental practitioners |
| G-CSF | filgrastim (granulocyte colony-stimulating factor) | GDR | glucose disposal rate |
| | | GDS | Global Deterioration Scale |
| | | GDx® | a scanning laser polarimeter |
| GCST | Gibson-Cooke sweat test | | |
| GCT | general care and treatment | GE | gainfully employed |
| | germ cell tumor | | gastric emptying |
| | giant cell tumor | | gastroenteritis |
| | granulosa cell tumor | | gastroesophageal |
| GCU | gonococcal urethritis | GEA | gastroepiploic artery |
| GCV | ganciclovir (Cytovene) | GEC | galactose elimination capacity |
| | great cardiac vein | | |
| GCVF | great cardiac vein flow | GED | General Educational Development (Test) |
| GD | gastric distension | | |
| | Gaucher disease | GEE | Global Evaluation of Efficacy |
| | generalized delays | | |
| | gestational diabetes | | glycine ethyl ester |
| | good | | graft-enteric erosion |
| | gravely disabled | GEF | graft-enteric fistula |
| | Graves disease | GEJ | gastroesophageal junction |
| Gd | gadolinium | | |
| G & D | growth and development | GEM | gemcitabine (Gemzar) |
| GDA | gastroduodenal artery | | gemfibrozil (Lopid) |
| GDB | Guide Dogs for the Blind | | generalized erythema multiforme |
| Gd-BOPTA | gadolinium benzyloxypropionic tetra acetate | GEMU | geriatric evaluation and management unit |

G

| | | |
|---|---|---|
| GEN | genital | group G streptococci |
| GEN/ ENDO | general anesthesia with endotracheal intubation | GGT gamma-glutamyl-transferase |
| GENT | gentamicin | GGTP gamma-glutamyl-transpeptidase |
| GENTA/P | gentamicin-peak | |
| GENTA/T | gentamicin-trough | GH general health |
| GEP | gastroenteropancreatic | genetic hemochromatosis |
| GEQ | generic equiavalent | gingival hyperplasia |
| GER | gastroesophageal reflux | glenohumeral |
| GERD | gastroesophageal reflux disease | good health growth hormone |
| GES | gastric emptying scintigraphy | GH₃ Gerovital |
| | | GHAA Group Health Association of America |
| GET | gastric emptying time graded exercise test | GHB gamma hydroxybutyrate (sodium oxybate; Xyrem) |
| GET 1/2 | gastric emptying half-time | |
| GETA | general endotracheal anesthesia | GHb glycosylated hemoglobin |
| GETV | gadolinium-enhancing tumor volume | GHD growth hormone deficiency |
| GEU | geriatric evaluation unit | GHDA growth hormone deficiency (syndrome) in adults |
| GF | gastric fistula gluten free grandfather | |
| | | GHI growth hormone insufficiency |
| GFAAS | graphite furnace atomic absorption spectrometry | GHJ glenohumeral joint |
| GFAP | glial fibrillary acid protein | G-H jt glenohumeral joint |
| GF-BAO | gastric fluid, basal acid output | GHP(S) gated heart pool (scan) |
| | | GHQ General Health Questionnaire |
| GFCL | Goldmann fundus contact lens | GHRF growth hormone releasing factor |
| GFD | gluten-free diet | |
| GFFF | gravitational field-flow fractionation | GI gastrointestinal glycemic index granuloma inguinale |
| GFJ | grapefruit juice | GIA gastrointestinal anastomosis |
| GFM | good fetal movement | |
| GFP | green fluorscent protein | GIB gastric ileal bypass gastrointestinal bleeding |
| GFR | glomerular filtration rate grunting, flaring, and retractions | GIC general immunocompetence |
| GFS | glaucoma filtering surgery | GID gastrointestinal distress gender identity disorder |
| GG | gamma globulin guaifenesin (glyceryl guaiacolate) | GIDA Gastrointestinal Diagnostic Area |
| G=G | grips equal and good | GIFD #3 colonoscope |
| GGE | Gastrografin enema generalized glandular enlargement | GIFT gamete intrafallopian (tube) transfer |
| GGF | great grandfather | GIH gastrointestinal hemorrhage |
| GGM | great grandmother | |
| GGO | ground-glass opacity | GIK glucose-insulin-potassium |
| GGS | glands, goiter, and stiffness | GIL gastrointestinal (tract) lymphoma |

| | | | |
|---|---|---|---|
| GING | gingiva | GLIO | glioblastoma |
| | gingivectomy | GLN | glomerulonephritis |
| G1K | greater than one thousand | GLOC | gravity-induced loss of |
| GIO | glucocorticoid-induced | | consciousness |
| | osteoporosis | GLP | Gambro Liendia Plate |
| GIOP | glucocorticoid-induced | | Good Laboratory Practice |
| | osteoporosis | | (Principles of) |
| GIP | gastric inhibitory peptide | | group-living program |
| | giant cell interstitial | GLP-1 | glucagon-like peptide-1 |
| | pneumonia | GLR | gravity lumbar reduction |
| | glucose-dependent | GLU | glucose |
| | insulinotropic | GLU 5 | five-hour glucose |
| | polypeptide | | tolerance test |
| GIPU | gastrointestinal procedure | GLUC | glucose |
| | unit | GLYCOS | glycosylated hemoglobin |
| GIR | glucose infusion rate | Hb | |
| GIS | gas in stomach | GM | gastric mucosa |
| | gastrointestinal series | | general medicine |
| GISA | glycopeptide intermediate- | | genetically modified |
| | resistant *Staphylococcus* | | geometric mean |
| | *aureus* | | gram (g) |
| GIST | gastrointestinal stromal | | grand mal |
| | tumor | | grandmother |
| GIT | gastrointestinal tract | | gray matter |
| GITS | gastrointestinal therapeutic | G-M | Geiger-Müller (counter) |
| | system | GM + | gram-positive |
| | gut-derived infectious | GM − | gram-negative |
| | toxic shock | gm % | grams per 100 milliliters |
| GITSG | Gastrointestinal Tumor | GmbH | *Gesellschaft mit* |
| | Study Group | | *beschränkter Haftung* |
| GITT | glucose insulin tolerance | | (a corporation with |
| | test | | restricted liability or a |
| GIWU | gastrointestinal work-up | | private limited liability |
| giv | given | | company) |
| GJ | gastrojejunostomy | GMC | general medical clinic |
| | grapefruit juice | | geometric mean |
| GJIC | gap junction intercellular | | concentration |
| | communication | GMCD | grand mal convulsive |
| GJT | gastrojejunostomy tube | | disorder |
| G1K | greater than one thousand | GM-CSF | sargramostim (granulocyte- |
| GK | Gamma Knife | | macrophage colony- |
| GKS | gamma knife surgery | | stimulating factor; |
| GL | gastric lavage | | Leukine) |
| | glaucoma | GME | gaseous microemboli |
| | greatest length | GMF | general medical floor |
| GLA | gamolenic acid | GMFM | gross motor function |
| | gingivolinguoaxial | | measure |
| | glucose-lowering agents | GMH | germinal matrix |
| GLB | Graham-Leach-Bliley Act | | hemorrhage |
| | of 1999 | GMLOS | geometric mean length |
| GLC | gas-liquid chromatography | | of stay |
| GLD | Glanders (*Actinobacillus* | GMOs | genetically modified |
| | *mallei*) vaccine | | organisms |

G

| | | |
|---|---|---|
| GMP | general medical panel (see page 362) | |
| | Good Manufacturing Practices | |
| | guanosine monophosphate | |
| GMR | gallop, murmur or rub | |
| GMS | galvanic muscle stimulation | |
| | general medical services | |
| | general medicine and surgery | |
| | Gomori methenamine silver (stain) | |
| GM&S | general medicine and surgery | |
| GMSPS | Glasgow Meningococcal Septicemia Prognostic Score | |
| GMTs | geometric mean antibody titers | |
| GN | glomerulonephritis | |
| | graduate nurse | |
| | gram-negative | |
| GNA | *Galanthus nivalis* agglutinin | |
| GNB | ganglioneuroblastoma | |
| | gram-negative bacilli | |
| | gram-negative bacteremia | |
| GNBM | gram-negative bacillary meningitis | |
| GNC | gram-negative cocci | |
| GND | gram-negative diplococci | |
| GNID | gram-negative intracellular diplococci | |
| GNP | Geriatric Nurse Practitioner | |
| GNR | gram-negative rods | |
| GnRH | gonadotropin-releasing hormone | |
| GNS | gram-negative sepsis | |
| GnSAF | gonadotropin surge attenuating factor | |
| GNT | Graduate Nurse Technician | |
| GO | Graves ophthalmopathy | |
| | Greek Orthodox | |
| GOAT | Galveston Orientation and Amnesia Test | |
| GOBI | *g*rowth monitoring, *o*ral rehydration, *b*reast feeding, and *i*mmunization | |

| | |
|---|---|
| GOCS | Global Obsessive-Compulsive Scale |
| GOD | glucose oxidase |
| GOG | Gynecologic Oncology Group |
| GOJ | gastro-oesophageal junction (UK and other countries) |
| GOK | God only knows |
| GOMER | get out of my emergency room |
| GON | gonococcal ophthalmia neonatorum |
| | greater occipital neuritis |
| GONA | glaucomatous optic nerve atrophy |
| GONIO | gonioscopy |
| GOO | gastric outlet obstruction |
| GOR | gastro-oesophageal reflux (United Kingdom) |
| | general operating room |
| GORD | gastro-oesophageal reflux disease (United Kingdom) |
| GOS | Glasgow Outcome Scale |
| GOT | glucose oxidase test |
| | glutamic-oxaloacetic transaminase (aspartate aminotransferase) |
| | goals of treatment |
| GOX | glucose oxidation |
| GP | gabapentin (Neurontin) |
| | general practitioner |
| | globus pallidus |
| | glucose polymers |
| | glycoprotein |
| | gram-positive |
| | grandparent |
| | gutta percha |
| G/P | gravida/para |
| $G_4P_{3104}$ | four pregnancies (gravid), 3 went to term, one premature, no abortion (or miscarriage), and 4 living children (p = para) |
| GPA | global program on AIDS |
| G#P#A# | gravida (number of pregnancies) para (number of live births) abortion (number of abortions) |

G

| | | | |
|---|---|---|---|
| GPB | gram-positive bacilli | GRASS | gradient recalled acquisition in a steady state |
| GPC | gel permeation chromatography | | |
| | giant papillary conjunctivitis | Grav. | gravid (pregnant) |
| | | GRC | gastric remnant cancers |
| | glycerophosphorylcholine | GRD | gastroesophageal reflux disease |
| | G-protein coupled | | |
| | gram-positive cocci | GRD DTR | granddaughter |
| GPCL | gas-permeable contact lens | GRD SON | grandson |
| | | GRE | glycopeptide-resistant *Enterococcus* spp |
| GPCR | G protein-coupled receptors | | graded resistive exercise |
| GPC/TP | glycerylphosphorylcholine to total phosphate | | gradient-recalled echo |
| | | | gradient refocused echo |
| G6PD | glucose-6-phosphate dehydrogenase | GR-FR | grandfather |
| | | GRKP | gentamicin-resistant *Klebsiella pneumoniae* |
| GPGL | gamma probe guided lymphoscintigraphy | | |
| GPI | general paralysis of the insane | GR-MO | grandmother |
| | | GRN | granules |
| | | | green |
| | glucose-6-phosphate isomerase | GRO | growth-related oncogene |
| | | GRP | group |
| GPi | globus pallidus interna | $Gr_1P_0AB_1$ | one pregnancy, no births, and one abortion |
| G-PLT | giant platelets | | |
| GPMAL | gravida, para, multiple births, abortions, and live births | GRP HM | group home |
| | | GRT | gastric residence time |
| | | | glandular replacement therapy |
| GPN | graduate practical nurse | | |
| GPO | group purchasing organization | | Graduate Respiratory Therapist |
| | | | grasp and release test |
| GPS | Goodpasture syndrome | | group-randomized trial |
| GPT | glutamic pyruvic transaminase | GRTT | Graduate Respiratory Therapist Technician |
| GPX | glutathione peroxidase | | |
| GR | gastric resection | GS | gallstone |
| | growth rate | | generalized seizure |
| gr | grain (approximately 60 mg) (this is a dangerous abbreviation) | | general surgery |
| | | | Gleason score |
| | | | gliosarcoma |
| G−R | gram-negative rods | | glucosamine sulfate |
| G+R | gram-positive rods | | gluteal sets |
| GRA | granisetron (Kytril) | | Gram stain |
| gravida 6, para 4-0-2-3 | 6 pregnancies resulting in 4-full term deliveries with 0 premature births and 2 abortions or miscarriages and 3 living children | | grip strength |
| | | G/S | 5% dextrose (glucose) and 0.9% sodium chloride (saline) injection |
| | | G & S | gait and stance |
| | | GSAP | greatest single allergen present |
| GRAS | generally recognized as safe | G-SAS | Gambling Symptom Assessment Scale |
| GRASE | Generally Recognized as Safe and Effective | GSCU | geriatric skilled care unit |
| | | GSD | glucogen storage disease |

G

| | | | |
|---|---|---|---|
| GSD-1 | glycogen storage disease, type 1 | GTF | gastrostomy tube feedings |
| | | | glucose tolerance factor |
| GSE | genital self-examination | GTH | gonadotropic hormone |
| | gluten sensitive enteropathy | GTN | gestational trophoblastic neoplasms |
| | grip strong and equal | | glomerulo-tubulo-nephritis |
| GSH | glutathione | | glyceryl trinitrate (name for nitroglycerin in the United Kingdom) |
| GSI | genuine stress incontinence | | |
| GSK | GlaxoSmithKline | GTO | Golgi tendon organ(s) |
| GSM | grey-scale median | GTP | glutamyl transpeptidase |
| GSMD | gestational sack and maternal date | | green tea polyphenols |
| | | | guanosine triphosphate |
| GSP | generalized social phobia | GTR | granulocyte turnover rate |
| | general survey panel | | gross total resection |
| GSPN | greater superficial petrosal neurectomy | | guided tissue regeneration |
| GSR | galvanic skin resistance (response) | GTS | Gilles de la Tourette syndrome |
| | | gtt. | drops |
| | gastrosalivary reflex | GTT | gestational trophoblastic tumor |
| GSS | Gerstmann-Straüssler-Scheinker (syndrome) | | glucose tolerance test |
| GST | glutathione S-transferase | GTT agar | gelatin-tellurite-taurocholate agar |
| | gold sodium thiomalate | | |
| GSTM | gold sodium thiomalate | GTT3H | glucose tolerence test 3 hours (oral) |
| GSUI | genuine stress urinary incontinence | | |
| | | gtts. | drops |
| GSV | greater saphenous vein | G-tube | gastrostomy tube |
| GSW | gunshot wound | GU | gastric upset |
| GSWA | gunshot wound to abdomen | | genitourinary |
| | | | gonococcal urethritis |
| GT | gait | GUAR | guarantor |
| | gait training | GUD | genital ulcer disease |
| | gastrostomy | GUI | genitourinary infection |
| | gastrotomy tube | GUM | Genitourinary Medicine (clinics) |
| | gene therapy | | |
| | glucose tolerance | GUS | genitourinary sphincter |
| | great toe | | genitourinary system |
| | greater trochanter | GUSTO | Global Utilization of Streptokinase and TPA for Occluded Arteries |
| | green tea | | |
| | group therapy | | |
| GTA | glutaraldehyde | GV | gentian violet |
| GTB | gastrointestinal tract bleeding | | growth velocity |
| | | GVF | Goldmann visual fields |
| GTC | generalized tonic-clonic (seizure) | | good visual fields |
| | | GVG | vigabatrin (gamma-vinyl GABA) |
| GTCS | generalized tonic-clonic seizure | | |
| | | GVH | generalized visceral hypersensitivity |
| GTD | gestational trophoblastic disease | | |
| | | GVHD | graft-versus-host disease |
| GTE | general therapeutic exercise | GVL | graft-versus leukemia |
| | | GVN | gentamicin, vancomycin, and nystatin |
| | Green tea extract | | |

| | |
|---|---|
| GVS | gastric vertical stapling |
| GVSDS | growth velocity standard deviation score |
| GVT | graft-versus-tumor |
| G/W | dextrose (glucose) in water |
| G&W | glycerin and water (enema) |
| GWA | gunshot wound of the abdomen |
| GWBI | General Well-Being Index |
| GWD | Guinea worm disease |
| GWS | Gulf war syndrome |
| GWT | gunshot wound of the throat |
| GWX | guide wire exchange |
| GXP | graded exercise program |
| GXT | graded exercise test |
| Gy | gray (radiation unit) |
| GYN | gynecology |
| GZTS | Guilford-Zimmerman Temperament Survey |

# H

| | |
|---|---|
| H | *Haemophilis* |
| | head |
| | heart |
| | height |
| | *Helicobacter* |
| | heroin |
| | Hispanic |
| | hour |
| | husband |
| | hydrogen |
| | hyperopia |
| | hypermetropia |
| | hyperphoria |
| | hypodermic |
| | objective angle |
| | trastuzumab (Herceptin) |
| H′ | hip |
| (H) | hypodermic injection |
| H² | hiatal hernia |
| H$_2$ | hydrogen |
| 3H | high, hot, and a helluva lot |
| HA | headache |
| | hearing aid |
| | heart attack |
| | hemadsorption |
| | hemagglutination |
| | hemolytic anemia |
| | Hispanic American |
| | hospital admission |
| | hyaluronan |
| | hyaluronic acid |
| | hyperalimentation |
| | hypermetropic astigmatism |
| | hypothalmic amenorrhea |
| H/A | head-to-abdomen (ratio) |
| | holding area |
| HA-1A® | nebacumab |
| HAA | hepatitis-associated antigen |
| HAAB | hepatitis A antibody |
| HAART | highly active antiretroviral treatment |
| HABF | hepatic artery blood flow |
| HAc | acetic acid |
| HACA | human antichimeric antibodies |

| | | | |
|---|---|---|---|
| HACCP | Hazard Analysis Critical Control Point(s) | | hip axis length hyperalimentation |
| HACE | hepatic artery chemoembolization | HALN | hand-assisted laparoscopic (radical) nephrectomy |
| | high-altitude cerebral edema | HALO | halothane (Fluothane) hours after light onset |
| HACEK group | *Haemophilus parainfluenzae, H. aphrophilus,* and *H. paraphrophilus, Actinobacillus actinomycetemcomitans, Cardiobacterium hominis, Eikenella corrodens,* and *Kingella kingae* | HALRI | hospital-acquired lower respiratory infections |
| | | HALRN | hand-assisted laparoscopic radical nephrectomy |
| | | HAM | Haldol, Ativan, and morphine |
| | | | high-dose cytarabine (ara-C) and mitoxantrone |
| HACS | hyperactive child syndrome | | HTLV-1-associated myelopathy |
| HAD | HIV (human immunodeficiency virus)-associated dementia | | human albumin microspheres |
| | | HAMA | human antimurine antibody |
| | | HAM-A | Hamilton Anxiety (scale) |
| | human adjuvant disease | HAM D | Hamilton Depression (scale) |
| | hypertonic acetate dextran | HAMS | hamstrings |
| HADH | the reduced form of nicotinamide-adenine dinucleotide (hydride donors in biochemical redox reactions) | HAN | heroin-associated nephropathy |
| | | HANE | hereditary angioneurotic edema |
| | | HAO | hearing aid orientation |
| HADS | Hospital Anxiety and Depression Scale | HAP | hearing aid problem |
| | | | heredopathia atactica polyneuritiformis |
| HAE | hearing aid evaluation | | hospital-acquired pneumonia |
| | hepatic artery embolization | | hydroxyapatite |
| | herb-related adverse event | | |
| | hereditary angioedema | HAPC | hospital-acquired penetration contact |
| HAEC | Hirschprung associated enterocolitis | HAPD | home-automated peritoneal dialysis |
| HAF | hyperalimentation fluid | | |
| HAFM | hospital-acquired *Plasmodium falciparum* malaria | HAPE | high-altitude pulmonary edema |
| HAGG | hyperimmune antivariola gamma globulin | HAPS | hepatic arterial perfusion scintigraphy |
| | | HAPTO | haptoglobin |
| HAH | high-altitude headache | HAQ | Headache Assessment Questionnaire |
| HAI | hemagglutination inhibition assay | | Health Assessment Questionnaire |
| | hepatic arterial infusion | | |
| HAIC | hepatic arterial infusional chemotherapy | HAR | high-altitude retinopathy hyperacute rejection |
| HAK | hyperalimentation kit | | |
| HAL | hemorrhoidal artery ligation | HARH | high-altitude retinal hemorrhage |

150

| | | | |
|---|---|---|---|
| HARP | hypoprebetalipoproteinemia, acanthocytosis, retinitis pigmentosa, and pallidale degeneration (syndrome) | HBAB | hepatitis B antibody |
| | | Hb A$_{1c}$ | glycosylated hemoglobin |
| | | HBAC | hyperdynamic beta-adrenergic circulatory |
| HARS | Hamilton Anxiety Rating Scale | HbAS | sickle cell trait |
| | HIV-associated adipose redistribution syndrome | HBBW | hold breakfast for blood work |
| HAS | Hamilton Anxiety (Rating) Scale | HBC | hereditary breast cancer hit by car |
| | Holmes-Adie syndrome | HBcAb | hepatitis B core antibody (antigen) |
| | home assessment service | HBc AB | hepatitis B core antibody |
| | hyperalimentation solution | HBc Ag | hepatitis B core antigen |
| HASCI | head and spinal cord injury | HbCO | carboxyhemoglobin |
| | | HB core | hepatitis B core antigen |
| HASCVD | hypertensive arteriosclerotic cardiovascular disease | HbCV | *Haemophilus* b conjugate vaccine |
| | | HBD | has been drinking |
| | | | hydroxybutyrate dehydrogenase |
| HASHD | hypertensive arteriosclerotic heart disease | HBDH | hydroxybutyrate dehydrogenase |
| HAT | head, arms, and trunk | HBE | hepatitis B epsilon |
| | heterophile antibody titer | | human bronchial epithelial (cells) |
| | histone acetyltransferase | | hypopharyngoscopy, bronchoscopy, and esophagoscopy |
| | hospital arrival time | | |
| | human African trypanosomiasis (sleeping sickness) | HBeAb | hepatitis Be antibody (antigen) |
| HAV | hallux abducto valgus | HBED | hydroxybenzylethylene-diamine diacetic acid |
| | hepatitis A vaccine | | |
| | hepatitis A virus | HbF | fetal hemoglobin |
| HAV-HBV | hepatitis A virus, and hepatitis B virus vaccine | HBF | hepatic blood flow |
| | | HBGA | had it before, got it again |
| | | HBGM | home blood glucose monitoring |
| HAZWO PER | Hazardous Waste Operations and Emergency Response | HBH | Health Belief Model |
| | | HBHC | hospital based home care |
| HB | heart-beating (donor) | HBI | Harvey-Bradshaw Index |
| | heart block | | hemibody irradiation |
| | heel-to-buttock | HBID | hereditary benign intraepithelial dyskeratosis |
| | hemoglobin (Hb) | | |
| | hepatitis B | | |
| | high calorie | HBIG | hepatitis B immune globulin |
| | hold breakfast | | |
| | housebound | Hb Kansas | mutant hemoglobin with a low affinity for oxygen |
| | hydrocodone bitartrate | | |
| 1$^0$HB | first degree heart block | HBLV | B-lymphotropic virus human |
| HB1° | first degree heart block | | |
| HB2° | second degree heart block | HBM | human bone marrow |
| | | HBNK | heparin-binding neurotrophic factor |
| HB3° | third degree heart block | | |

| | | | |
|---|---|---|---|
| hBNP | human B-type natriuretic peptide (nesiritide [Natrecor]) | 4-HC | 4-hydroperoxycyclo-phosphamide |
| HBO | hyperbaric oxygen (HBO₂ preferred) | H & C | hot and cold |
| | | HCA | health care aide |
| HBO₂ | hyperbaric oxygen | | heterocyclic antidepressant |
| HbO₂ | hemoglobin, oxygenated | | hypercalcemia |
| | hyperbaric oxygen (HBO₂ preferred) | | hypothermic circulatory arrest |
| HBOC | hemoglobin-based oxygen carrier | HCAO | hepatitis C-associated osteosclerosis |
| | hereditary breast and ovarian cancer | H-CAP | altretamine (hexamethyl-melamine), cyclophosphamide, doxorubicin (Adriamycin), and cisplatin (Platinol AQ) |
| HBOT | hyperbaric oxygen treatment/therapy (HBO₂T preferred) | | |
| HBO₂T | hyperbaric oxygen treatment | | |
| | | HCB | hexachlorobenzene |
| HBP | high blood pressure | HCBR | human carbonyl reductase |
| HBPM | home blood pressure monitoring | HCC | hepatocellular carcinoma |
| HBr | hydrobromide | HCD | herniate cervical disk |
| HBS | Health Behavior Scale | | hydrocolloid dressing |
| HbS | sickle cell hemoglobin | HCFA | Health Care Financing Administration |
| HBsAg | hepatitis B surface antigen | HCFC | hydrochlorofluorocarbon |
| HbSC | sickle cell hemoglobin C | hCG | human chorionic gonadotropin |
| HBSS | Hank balanced salt solution | HCH | hexachlorocyclohexane |
| HbSS | sickle cell anemia | | hygroscopic condenser humidifier |
| HBT | hydrogen breath test | | |
| HBV | hepatitis B vaccine | HCI | home care instructions |
| | hepatitis B virus | HCL | hairy cell leukemia |
| | honey-bee venom | HCl | hydrochloric acid |
| HBVig | hepatitis B virus immune globulin | | hydrochloride |
| | | HCLF | high carbohydrate, low fiber (diet) |
| HBVP | high biological value protein | HCLs | hard contact lenses |
| HBW | high birth weight | HCLV | hairy cell leukemia variant |
| H/BW | heart-to-body weight (ratio) | HCM | health care maintenance |
| HC | hairy cell | | heterogeneous cation-exchange membrane |
| | handicapped | | hypercalcemia of malignancy |
| | head circumference | | |
| | heart catheterization | | hypertrophic cardiomyopathy |
| | heel cords | HCMV | human cytomegalovirus |
| | Hickman catheter | HCO₃ | bicarbonate |
| | home care | HCP | handicapped |
| | hot compress | | healthcare provider |
| | housecall | | hearing conservation programs |
| | Huntington chorea | | |
| | hydrocephalus | | |
| | hydrocortisone | | |

H

|  | hereditary coporphyria | | high dose |
| --- | --- | --- | --- |
|  | hexachlorophene | | hip disarticulation |
|  | home chemotherapy | | Hodgkin disease |
|  | program | | hospital day |
|  | hospital chemistry profile | | hospital discharge |
| HCPCS | HCFA (Health Care | | house dust |
|  | Financing | | Huntington disease |
|  | Administration) | HDA | heteroduplex analysis |
|  | Common Procedural | HD-AC | high-dose arm |
|  | Coding System | HD-AC | high-dose cytarabine |
| HCQ | hydroxychloroquine | HD-ara-C | high-dose cytarabine (ara-C) |
|  | (Plaquenil) | | C) |
| HCR | health care review | HDBQ | Hilton Drinking Behavior |
| HCS | heel-cord stretches | | Questionnaire |
|  | human chorionic | HDC | habilitative day care |
|  | somatomammotropin | | high-dose chemotherapy |
| 17-HCS | 17-hydroxycorticosteroids | | histamine dihydrochloride |
| HCSE | horse chestnut seed | HDC-ASCS | high-dose chemotherapy |
|  | extract | | with autologous stem |
| HCSS | hypersensitive carotid | | cell support |
|  | sinus syndrome | HDCC | high-dose combination |
| HCT | head computerized (axial) | | chemotherapy |
|  | tomography | HD-CPA | high-dose |
|  | hematopoietic cell | | cyclophosphamide |
|  | transplantation | HDCPT | high-dose |
|  | hematocrit | | cyclophosphamide |
|  | histamine challenge test | | therapy |
|  | human chorionic | HDC-SCR | high-dose chemotherapy |
|  | thyrotropin | | with stem-cell rescue |
|  | hydrochlorothiazide (this | HDCT | high-dose chemotherapy |
|  | is a dangerous | HDCV | rabies virus vaccine, |
|  | abbreviation) | | human diploid (human |
|  | hydrocortisone | | diploid cell vaccine) |
| HCTU | home cervical traction | HDE | Humanitarian Device |
|  | unit | | Exemption (FDA) |
| HCTZ | hydrochlorothiazide (this | HDF | hemodiafiltration |
|  | is a dangerous | HDG | hydrogel (dressing) |
|  | abbreviation) | HDH | high-density humidity |
| HCV | hepatitis C vaccine | HDI | high-definition image |
|  | hepatitis C virus | HDIs | histone deacetylase |
| HCVD | hypertensive | | inhibitors |
|  | cardiovascular disease | HDL | high-density lipoprotein |
| HCWs | healthcare workers | HDL-C | high-density lipoprotein |
| HCY | homocysteine | | cholesterol |
| HCYS | homocysteine | HDLW | hearing distance for watch |
| HD | haloperidol decanoate | | to be heard in left ear |
|  | Hansen disease | HDM | home-delivered meals |
|  | hearing distance | | house dust mite |
|  | heart disease | HDMEC | human dermal |
|  | Heller-Dor (procedure) | | microvascular |
|  | heloma durum | | endothelial cells |
|  | hemodialysis | HDMP | high-dose |
|  | herniated disk | | methylprednisolone |

H

153

| | | | |
|---|---|---|---|
| HD-MTX | high-dose methotrexate | HEAT | human erythrocyte agglutination test |
| HD-MTX-CF | high-dose methotrexate and leucovorin (citrovorum factor) | HEB | hydrophilic emollient base |
| | | HEC | Health Education Center |
| HD-MTX/LV | high-dose methotrexate and leucovorin | HeCOG | Hellenic Cooperative Oncology Group |
| HDN | hemolytic disease of the newborn | HEDIS | Health Employer Data and Information Set |
| | heparin dosing nomogram | HEENT | head, eyes, ears, nose, and throat |
| | high-density nebulizer | HeFH | heterozygous familial hypercholesterolemia |
| HDNS | Hodgkin disease, nodular sclerosis | | |
| HDP | high-density polyethylene | HEK | human embryonic kidney |
| | hydroxymethyline diphosphonate | HEL | *Helicobacter pylori* vaccine |
| HDPAA | heparin-dependent platelet-associated antibody | | human embryonic lung |
| | | HeLa | Helen Lake (tumor cells) |
| | | HELLP Syndrome | hemolysis, elevated liver enzymes, and low platelet count |
| HDPC | hand piece | | |
| HDPE | high-density polyethylene | HEMA | hydroxyethylmethacrylate |
| HDR | heparin dose response | HEMI | hemiplegia |
| | husband to delivery room | HEMOSID | hemosiderin |
| HDRA | histoculture drug response assay | HEMPAS | hereditary erythrocytic multinuclearity with positive acidified serum test |
| HDRB | high-dose rate brachytherapy | | |
| HDRS | Hamilton Depression Rating Scale | HEMS | helicopter emergency medical services |
| HDRW | hearing distance for watch to be heard in right ear | HEN | hemorrhages, exudates, and nicking |
| HDS | Hamilton Depression (Rating) Scale | | home enteral nutrition |
| | | He-Ne | helium-neon |
| | herniated disk syndrome | HEP | hemoglobin electrophoresis |
| HDSCR | health deviation self-care requisite | | hemorrhage, exudates, and papilledemaa |
| HDT | habilitative day treatment | | heparin |
| | hearing distraction test | | hepatic |
| HDU | hemodialysis unit | | hepatoerythropoietic porphyria |
| | high-dependency unit (an intensive care unit) | | hepatoma |
| HDV | hepatitis D virus | | histamine equivalent prick |
| HDW | hearing distance (with) watch | | home exercise program |
| HDYF | how do you feel | HEPA | hamster egg penetration assay |
| HE | hard exudate | | high-efficiency particulate air (filter) |
| | health educator | | |
| | hepatic encephalopathy | hep cap | heparin cap |
| H&E | hematoxylin and eosin | HERP | human exposure (dose)/rodent potency (dose) |
| | hemorrhage and exudate | | |
| | heredity and environment | | |
| HEA | health | | |
| HEAR | hospital emergency ambulance radio | | |

H

154

| | | | |
|---|---|---|---|
| HES | hetastarch (hydroxyethyl starch; Hespan) | H flu | *Haemophilus influenzae* |
| | | HFM | hand-foot-and-mouth (disease) (often caused by coxsackievirus A16) |
| | hypereosinophilic syndrome | | |
| HEs | hypertensive emergencies | | hemifacial microsomia |
| 20-HETE | 20-hydroxyeicosatetraenoic acid | HFMD | hand-foot-and-mouth disease (often caused by coxsackievirus A16) |
| HETF | home enteral tube feeding | | |
| HEV | hepatitis E vaccine | HFO | high-frequency oscillation |
| | hepatitis E virus | HFOV | high-frequency oscillatory ventilation |
| | high-endothelial venule | | |
| Hex | altretamine (hexamethylmelamine; Hexalen) | HFP | hepatic functional panel (see page 362) |
| | | | Hoffa fat pad |
| Hexa-CAF | altretamine (hexamethylmelamine), cyclophosphamide, methotrexate (amethopterin), and fluorouracil | HFPPV | high-frequency positive pressure ventilation |
| | | HFR | hemorrhagic fever with renal syndrome vaccine |
| | | HFRS | hemorrhagic fever with renal syndrome |
| HF | Hageman factor | HFS | hand-foot syndrome |
| | hard feces | HFSH | human follicle-stimulating hormone |
| | hay fever | | |
| | head of fetus | HFST | hearing-for-speech test |
| | heart failure | HFUPR | hourly fetal urine production rate |
| | high frequency | | |
| | Hispanic female | HFV | high-frequency ventilation |
| | hot flashes | | high-fruit/vegetable (diet) |
| | house formula | HFX RT | hyperfractionated radiation therapy |
| HFA | health facility administrator | | |
| | | HG | handgrasp |
| | hydrofluoroalkane-134a | | handgrip |
| HFAS | hereditary flat adenoma syndrome | | hemoglobin |
| | | Hg | mercury |
| HFB | high-frequency band | HGA | high-grade astrocytomas |
| HFC | hydrofluorocarbon | Hgb | hemoglobin |
| HFCB | horizontal flow clean bench | Hgb ELECT | hemoglobin electrophoresis |
| HFCC | high-frequency chest compression | Hgb F | fetal hemoglobin |
| | | Hgb S | sickle cell hemoglobin |
| HFD | high-fiber diet | HGE | human granulocytic ehrlichiosis |
| | high-forceps delivery | | |
| | high-frequency discharges | HGES | handgrasp equal and strong |
| hFH | heterozygous familial hypercholesterolemia | HGF | hepatocyte growth factor |
| | | | hereditary gingival fibromatosis |
| HFHL | high-frequence hearing loss | | |
| | | HGG | human gamma globulin |
| HFI | hereditary fructose intolerance | HGH | human growth hormone |
| | | HGI | Human Genome Initiative |
| HFIP | hexafluoro-isopropranolol | HGM | home glucose monitoring |
| HFJV | high-frequency jet ventilation | HGN | hypogastric nerve |

H

155

| | | | |
|---|---|---|---|
| HGO | hepatic glucose output | HHNK | hyperglycemic hyperosmolar nonketotic (coma) |
| | hip guidance orthosis | | |
| HGP | Human Genome Project | | |
| HGPIN | high-grade prostatic intraepithelial neoplasia | HHNS | hyperosmolar-hyperglycemic nonketotic syndrome |
| HGPRT | hypoxanthine-guanine phosphoribosyl-transferase | HHRG | Home Health Resource Group (reimbursement categories for home health) |
| HGSIL | high-grade squamous intraepithelial lesion | | |
| HGV | hepatitis G vaccine | HHS | Health and Human Service (US Department of) |
| | hepatitis G virus | | |
| HH | hard of hearing | HHT | hereditary hemorrhagic telangiectasis |
| | head hood | | |
| | hiatal hernia | HHTC | high-humidity trach collar |
| | home health | HHTM | high-humidity trach mask |
| | homonymous hemiopia | HHTS | high-humidity tracheostomy shield |
| | household | | |
| | hyperhomocystinemia | HHV-8 | human herpesvirus 8 |
| | hypogonadotropic hypogonadism | HI | *Haemophilus influenzae* |
| | | | head injury |
| | hypoeninemic hypoaldosteronism | | health insurance |
| | | | hearing impaired |
| H/H | hemoglobin/hematocrit | | hemagglutination inhibition |
| H&H | hematocrit and hemoglobin | | |
| | | | homicidal ideation |
| HHA | health hazard appraisal | | hospital insurance |
| | hereditary hemolytic anemia | | human insulin |
| | | HIA | hemagglutination inhibition antibody |
| | home health agency | | |
| | home health aid | HIAA | hydroxyindoleacetic acid |
| HH Assist | hand held assist | | |
| HHC | home health care | 5-HIAA | 5-hydroxyindoleacetic acid |
| HHCA | home health care agency | | |
| | hypothermic hypokalemic cardioplegic arrest | HIAP | human intracisternal A-type particle |
| HHcy | hyperhomocystinemia | HIB | *Haemophilus influenzae* type b (vaccine) |
| HHD | Doctor of Holistic Health | | |
| | home hemodialysis | HIB_{cn} | *haemophilus influenzae* type b conjugate vaccine |
| | hypertensive heart disease | | |
| HHFM | high-humidity face mask | HIB_{HbOC} | *haemophilus influenzae* type b vaccine, HbOC conjugate vaccine |
| HHH | hypermethionemia, hyperammonemia, and homocitrolinemia (syndrome) | | |
| | | HIB_{PRP-D} | *haemophilus influenzae* type b vaccine, PRP-D conjugate vaccine |
| HHM | high-humidity mask | | |
| | humoral hypercalcemia of malignancy | HIB_{PRP-OMP} | *haemophilus influenzae* type b vaccine, PRP-OMP conjugate vaccine |
| HHN | hand-held nebulizer | | |
| HHNC | hyperosmolar hyperglycemic nonketotic coma | HIB_{PRP-T} | *haemophilus influenzae* type b vaccine, PRP-T conjugate vaccine |

| | | | |
|---|---|---|---|
| HIB$_{ps}$ | *haemophilus influenzae* type b polysaccharide vaccine | HIO | health insuring organization |
| | | | hepatic iron overload |
| HIC | Human Investigation Committee | HIP | health insurance plan |
| | | HIPA | heparin-induced platelet aggregation |
| | Humphriss immediate contrast (astigmatism test) | HIPAA | Health Insurance Portability and Accountability Act of 1996 |
| hi-cal | high caloric | | |
| HID | headache, insomnia, and depression | | |
| | | HIPC | hormone-independent prostate cancer |
| | herniated intervertebral disk | HIPPS | Health Insurance Prospective Payment System |
| HIDA | hepato-iminodiacetic acid (lidofenin) | | |
| HiDAC | high-dose cytarabine (ara-C) | hi-pro | high-protein |
| | | HIR | head injury routine |
| HIDS | hyperimmunoglobulinemia D syndrome | HIS | Hanover Intensive Score |
| | | | Health Intention Scale |
| HIE | hyperimmunoglobulinemia E | | high-intermittent suction |
| | | | histidine |
| | hypoxic-ischemic encephalopathy | | Home Incapacity Scale |
| | | | hospital (healthcare) information system |
| HIF | *Haemophilus influenzae* | | |
| | higher integrative functions | HISMS | How I See Myself Scale |
| | | HISTO | histoplasmin skin test |
| HIFU | high-intensity focused ultrasonography | | histoplasmosis |
| | | HIT | heparin-induced thrombocytopenia |
| HIHA | high impulsiveness, high anxiety | | histamine inhalation test |
| | | | home infusion therapy |
| HIHARS | hyperventilation-induced high-amplitude rhythmic slowing | HITS | high-intensity transient signals |
| HII | hepatic-iron index | HITTS | heparin-induced thrombotic thrombocytopenia syndrome |
| HIIC | heated intraoperative intraperitoneal chemotherapy | | |
| | | HIU | head injury unit |
| HIL | hypoxic-ischemic lesion | HIV | human immunodeficiency virus |
| HILA | high impulsiveness, low anxiety | | human immunodeficiency virus vaccine |
| HILP | hyperthermic isolated limb perfusion | | |
| | | HIV-1 | human immunodeficiency virus type 1 |
| HIM | health information management | HIV-2 | human immunodeficiency virus type 2 |
| | hexyl-insulin monoconjugate | | |
| | | HIVAN | human immunodeficiency virus-associated nephropathy |
| HIN | *haemophilus influenzae* nontypable strain(s) vaccine | | |
| | | HIVAT | home intravenous antibiotic therapy |
| HINI | hypoxic-ischemic neuronal injury | | |
| HINN | Hospital-issued Notice of Noncoverage | HIVD | herniated intervertebral disk |

**H**

| | |
|---|---|
| HIV-D | human immunodeficiency virus-related dementia |
| hi-vit | high-vitamin |
| HIVMP | high-dose intravenous methylprednisolone |
| HJB | Howell-Jolly bodies |
| HJR | hepatojugular reflux |
| HK | hand-to-knee |
| | heel-to-knee |
| | hexokinase |
| HKAFO | hip-knee-ankle-foot orthosis |
| HKAO | hip-knee-ankle orthosis |
| HKMN | Hickman (catheter) |
| HKO | hip-knee orthosis |
| HKS | heel-knee-shin (test) |
| HKT | heterotopic kidney transplant |
| HL | hairline |
| | half-life |
| | hallux limitus |
| | haloperidol |
| | harelip |
| | hearing level |
| | hearing loss |
| | heavy lifting |
| | hemilaryngectomy |
| | heparin lock |
| | hepatic lipase |
| | Hickman line |
| H&L | heart and lung |
| HLA | human leukocyte antigen |
| | human lymphocyte antigen |
| HLA negative | heart, lungs, and abdomen negative |
| HLB | head, limbs, and body |
| HLD | haloperidol decanoate |
| | herniated lumbar disk |
| HLDP | hypoglossia-limb deficiency phenotype |
| HLES | hypertensive lower esophageal sphincter |
| HLGR | high-level gentamicin resistance |
| HLH | hemophagocytic lymphohistiocytosis |
| | human luteinizing hormone |
| HLHS | hypoplastic left-heart syndrome |
| HLK | heart, liver, and kidneys |
| HLM | hemosiderin-laden macrophages |

| | |
|---|---|
| HLOS | hypertensive lower oesophageal sphincter (United Kingdom and other countries) |
| HLP | hyperlipoproteinemia |
| hLS | human lung surfactant |
| HLT | heart-lung transplantation (transplant) |
| HLV | herpes-like virus |
| | hypoplastic left ventricle |
| HM | hand motion |
| | head movement |
| | heart murmur |
| | heavily muscled |
| | heloma molle |
| | Hispanic male |
| | Holter monitor |
| | human milk |
| | human semisynthetic insulin |
| | humidity mask |
| HMA | hemorrhages and microaneurysms |
| | heteroduplex mobility assay |
| HMB | beta-hydroxy-beta methylbutyrate (a leucine metabolite) |
| | homatropine methylbromide |
| HMBA | hexamethylene bisacetamide |
| HMD | hyaline membrane disease |
| HMDP | hydroxymethyline diphosphonate |
| HME | heat and moisture exchanger |
| | heat, massage, and exercise |
| | hereditary multiple exostoses |
| | home medical equipment |
| | human monocytic ehrlichiosis |
| HMEF | heat moisture exchanging filter |
| HMETSC | heavy metal screen |
| HMF | human milk fortifier |
| HMG | human menopausal gonadotropin |
| HMG CoA | hydroxymethyl glutaryl coenzyme A |

| | | | |
|---|---|---|---|
| HMI | healed myocardial infarction | HNCa | head and neck cancer |
| | history of medical illness | HNCCG | Head and Neck Cancer Cooperative Group |
| HMIS | hospital medical information system | HNE | human neutrophil elastase |
| HMK | homemaking | HNI | hospitalization not indicated |
| HM & LP | hand motion and light perception | HNKDC | hyperosomolar nonketotic diabetic coma |
| HMM | altretamine (hexamethyl-melamine) | HNKDS | hyperosmolar nonketotic diabetic state |
| HMO | Health Maintenance Organization | HNLN | hospitalization no longer necessary |
| | hypothetical mean organism | HNN | hybrid neural network |
| HMP | health maintenance plan | HNP | herniated nucleus pulposus |
| | hexose monophosphate | HNPCC | heredity nonpolyposis colorectal cancer |
| | hot moist packs | HNPP | hereditary neuropathy with liability to pressure palsies |
| HMPAO | hexylmethylpropylene amineoxine | | |
| HMR | histocytic medullary reticulosis | HNRNA | heterogeneous nuclear ribonucleic acid |
| | Hoechst Marion Roussel | HNS | 0.45% sodium chloride injection (half-normal saline) |
| [1]H-MRS | proton magnetic resonance spectroscopy | | head and neck surgery |
| HMS | hyper-reactive malarial splenomegaly | | head, neck, and shaft |
| | | HNSCC | squamous cell carcinoma of the head and neck |
| | hypodermic morphine sulfate (this is a dangerous abbreviation) | HNSN | home, no services needed |
| | | HNT | hantaan (hantavirus) vaccine |
| HMS® | medrysone | HNV | has not voided |
| hMSCs | human mesenchymal stem cells | HNWG | has not worn glasses |
| HMSN I | hereditary motor and sensory neuropathy type I | HO | hand orthosis |
| | | | heme oxygenase |
| | | | Hemotology-Oncology |
| HMSR | high medical-social risk | | heterotropic ossification |
| HMSS | hyperactive malarial splenomegaly syndrome | | hip orthosis |
| | | | house officer |
| HMWK | high-molecular weight kininogen | H/O | history of |
| | | $H_2O$ | water |
| HMX | heat massage exercise | $H_2O_2$ | hydrogen peroxide |
| HN | head and neck | HOA | hip osteoarthritis |
| | head nurse | HOB | head of bed |
| | high nitrogen | HOB UPSOB | head of bed up for shortness of breath |
| | home nursing | | |
| H&N | head and neck | HOC | Health Officer Certificate |
| HN2 | mechlorethamine HCl | HOCM | high-osmolality contrast media |
| HNC | head and neck cancer | | |
| | human neutrophil collagenase | | hypertrophic obstructive cardiomyopathy |
| | hyperosmolar nonketotic coma | HOG | halothane, oxygen, and gas (nitrous oxide) |

H

159

| | | | |
|---|---|---|---|
| HOH | hand-over-hand (rehabilitation term) hard of hearing | HPB | Health Protection Branch (the Canadian equivalent of the U.S. Food and Drug Administration) |
| HOI | hospital onset of infection | | |
| HOM | high-osmolar contrast media | | |
| HOMA | homeostatic assessment model algorithm (index) homeostatic model assessment | HPC | hereditary prostate cancer history of present condition (complaint) |
| | | HPCE | high-performance capillary electrophoresis |
| HOME | Home Observation for Measurement of the Environment | HPD | high-protein diet home peritoneal dialysis |
| | | HpD | hematoporphyrin derivative |
| HONK | hyperosmolar nonketotic (coma) | HP&D | hemoprofile and differential |
| HOP | hourly output | HPE | hemorrhage, papilledema, exudate history and physical examination |
| HOPI | history of present illness | | |
| HORF | high-output renal failure | | |
| HORS | Hemiballism/Hemichorea Outcome Rating Score | HPET | *Helicobacter pylori* eradication therapy |
| | | HPF | high-power field |
| HOS | Health Outcomes Survey | HPFH | hereditary persistence of fetal hemoglobin |
| HOSP | hospital hospitalization | | |
| HOTV | letter symbols used in pediatric visual acuity testing | HPG | human pituitary gonadotropin |
| | | HPI | history of present illness |
| HOVT | letter symbols used in pediatric visual acuity testing | HPIP | history, physical, impression, and plan |
| | | HPL | human placenta lactogen hyperplexia |
| HP | hard palate Harvard pump *Helicobacter pylori* hemipelvectomy hemiplegia high-protein (supplement) hot packs house physician hydrogen peroxide hydrophilic petrolatum | HPLC | high-performance (pressure) liquid chromatography |
| | | HPM | hemiplegic migraine |
| | | HPMC | high-performance membrane chromatography hydroxypropyl methylcellulose |
| Hp | *Helicobacter pylori* | HPN | home parenteral nutrition |
| H&P | history and physical | | |
| HPA | hybridization protection assay hypothalamic-pituitary-adrenal (axis) | HPNI | hemodialysis prognostic nutrition index |
| | | HPNS | high-pressure nervous syndrome |
| HPAE-PAD | high-pH anion exchange chromatography coupled with pulsed amperometric detection | HPO | hydrophilic ointment hypertrophic pulmonary osteoarthropathy |
| | | HPOA | hypertrophic pulmonary osteoarthropathy |
| HPAT | home parenteral antibiotic therapy | 2HPP | 2-hour postprandial (blood sugar) |

H

| | | | |
|---|---|---|---|
| 2HPPBS | 2-hour postprandial blood sugar | HRC | Human Rights Committee |
| HPPM | hyperplastic persistent pupillary membrane | HRCT | high-resolution computed tomography |
| hPRL | prolactin, human | HRD | human retroviral disease |
| HPS | hantavirus pulmonary syndrome | HRE | high-resolution electrocardiography |
| | hepatopulmonary syndrome | HRF | Harris return flow |
| | | | health-related facility |
| | hypertrophic pyloric stenosis | | histamine-releasing factor |
| | | | hypertensive renal failure |
| HpSA | *Helicobacter pylori* stool antigen | HRI | HMG-CoA (3-hydroxy-3-methylglutaryl-coenzyme A) reductase inhibitors |
| HPT | heparin protamine titration | | |
| | histamine provocation test | HRIF | histamine inhibitory releasing factor |
| | home pregnancy test | | |
| | hyperparathyroidism | HRL | head rotated left |
| HPTD | highly permeable transparent dressing | HRLA | human reovirus-like agent |
| | | HRLM | high-resolution light microscopy |
| hPTH | human parathyroid hormone $I_{34}$ (teriparatide) | hRLX-2 | synthetic human relaxin |
| | | HRMPC | hormone-refractory metastatic prostate cancer |
| HPTM | home prothrombin time monitoring | | |
| | | HRMS | high-resolution mass spectrometry |
| HPTX | hemopneumothorax | | |
| HPV | human papilloma virus | HRNB | Halstead-Reitan Neuropsychological Battery |
| | human papilloma virus vaccine | | |
| | | | |
| | human parvovirus | HRP | high-risk pregnancy |
| *H pylori* | *Helicobacter pylori* | | horseradish peroxidase |
| HPZ | high-pressure zone | HRP-2 | histidine-rich protein-2 |
| HQC | hydroquinone cream | HRPC | hormone-refractory prostate cancer |
| HQL | health-related quality of life | | |
| | | HRQL | health-related quality of life |
| HR | hallux rigidus | | |
| | Harrington rod | HRQOL | health-related quality of life |
| | hazard ratio | | |
| | heart rate | HRR | head rotated right |
| | hemorrhagic retinopathy | HRRC | Human Research Review Committee |
| | hospital record | | |
| | hour | HRS | Haw River syndrome |
| Hr 0 | zero hour (when treatment starts) | | hepatorenal syndrome |
| | | | Hodgkin-Reed-Sternberg (cells) |
| Hr -2 | minus two hours (two hours prior to treatment) | | |
| | | HRSD | Hamilton Rating Scale for Depression |
| H & R | hysterectomy and radiation | HRST | heat, reddening, swelling, or tenderness |
| HRA | high-right atrium | | |
| | histamine releasing activity | | heavy resistance strength training |
| H2RA | histamine$_2$-receptor antagonist | HRT | heart rate |
| | | | heparin response test |

| | | | |
|---|---|---|---|
| | high-risk transfer | HSD | Honestly Significant |
| | hormone replacement | | Difference (test) |
| | therapy | | (Turkey) |
| | hyperfractioned | | hypoactive sexual desire |
| | radiotherapy | | (disorder) |
| HRV | heart rate variability | HSE | herpes simplex |
| | heterogeneous resistance | | encephalitis |
| | to vancomycin | | human skin equivalent |
| HS | bedtime (must specify if a | | hypertonic saline- |
| | dose is to be given one | | epinephrine |
| | time [HS × 1 dose | HSEES | Hazardous Substances |
| | today] or nightly [HS | | Emergency Events |
| | nightly]) | | Surveillance |
| | half-strength | HSES | hemorrhagic shock and |
| | hamstrings | | encephalopathy |
| | hamstring sets | HSG | herpes simplex genitalis |
| | Hartman solution (lactated | | hysterosalpingogram |
| | Ringers) | HSGYV | heat, steam, gum, yawn, |
| | heart size | | and Valsalva maneuver |
| | heart sounds | | (for otitis media) |
| | heavy smoker | H-SIL | high-grade squamous |
| | heel spur | | intraepithelial lesions |
| | heel stick | HSK | herpes simplex keratitis |
| | hereditary spherocytosis | HSL | herpes simplex labialis |
| | herpes simplex | | hormone sensitive lipase |
| | hidradenitis suppurativa | HSM | hepatosplenomegaly |
| | high school | | holosystolic murmur |
| | hippocampal sclerosis | HSN | Hansen-Street nail |
| | Hurler syndrome | | heart sounds normal |
| H → S | heel-to-shin | | hereditary sensory |
| H&S | hearing and speech | | neuropathy |
| | hemorrhage and shock | HSP | heat shock protein |
| | hysterectomy and | | Henoch-Schönlein purpura |
| | sterilization | | hereditary spastic |
| HSA | Health Services | | paraplegia |
| | Administration | | hysterosalpingography |
| | (Administrator) | HSPC | hydrogenated soy |
| | Health Systems | | phosphatidyl choline |
| | Agency | HSPE | high-strength pancreatic |
| | human serum albumin | | enzymes |
| | hypersomnia-sleep | HSQ | Health Status |
| | apnea | | Questionnaire |
| HSAN | hereditary sensory and | HSR | heated serum reagin |
| | autonomic neuropathy | | hypersensitivity reaction |
| | (types I–IV) | | hypofractionated |
| HSB | husband | | stereotactic |
| HSBS | evening blood sugar | | radiotherapy |
| HSBG | heel-stick blood gas | HSS | half-strength saline |
| HSC | hematopoietic stem cell | | (0.45% Sodium |
| HSCL | Hopkins Symptom-Check | | Chloride) |
| | List | HSSE | high soap suds enema |
| HSCSS | hypersensitive carotid | HS-tk | herpes simplex thymidine |
| | sinus syndrome | | kinase |

H

| | | | |
|---|---|---|---|
| HSV | herpes simplex virus | | human T-cell leukemia |
| | highly selective vagotomy | | human thymic leukemia |
| HSV-1 | herpes simplex virus type 1 | HTLV III | human T-cell |
| | herpes simplex virus | | lymphotrophic virus |
| | type 1 vaccine | | type III |
| HSV₂ | herpes simplex virus | HTM | *Haemophilus* test |
| | type 2 vaccine | | medium |
| HSV₁₂ | herpes simplex virus | | high threshold |
| | types 1, 2 vaccine | | mechanoceptors |
| HSV-2 | herpes simplex virus type 2 | HTML | hypertext markup |
| HSVE | herpes simplex virus | | language |
| | encephalitis | HTN | hypertension |
| HT | hammertoe | HTO | high tibial osteotomy |
| | head trauma | HTP | House-Tree-Person-test |
| | hearing test | 5-HTP | serotonin (5- |
| | heart | | hydroxytryptophan) |
| | heart transplant | HTR | hard tissue replacement |
| | height | hTRT | human telomerase reverse |
| | heparin trap (hep-trap; | | transcriptase |
| | heparin lock; a venous | HTS | head traumatic syndrome |
| | access device) | | heel-to-shin (test) |
| | high temperature | | Hematest® stools |
| | hormonotherapy | | high-throughput |
| | Hubbard tank | | screening |
| | hypermetropia | HTSCA | human tumor stem cell |
| | hyperopia | | assay |
| | hypertension | HtSDS | height standard deviation |
| | hyperthermia | | score |
| | hyperthyroid | H-TSH | human thyroid-stimulating |
| H/T | heel and toe (walking) | | hormone |
| H&T | hospitalization and | HTT | hand thrust test |
| | treatment | HTV | herpes-type virus |
| H(T) | intermittent hypertropia | HTVD | hypertensive vascular |
| HT-1 | hereditary tyrosinemia | | disease |
| | type 1 | HTX | hemothorax |
| 5-HT₁ | serotonin | HTx | heart transplant |
| | (5-hydroxytryptamine) | HU | head unit |
| HTA | hypertension (French) | | hydroxyurea |
| ht. aer. | heated aerosol | | hypertensive urgencies |
| HTAT | human tetanus antitoxin | Hu | Hounsfield units |
| HTB | hot tub bath | HUAEC | human umbilical |
| HTC | heated tracheostomy collar | | endothelial cells |
| | hypertensive crisis | HUCB | human umbilical cord |
| HTE | highly treatment | | blood |
| | experienced (patients) | HUH | Humana Hospital |
| hTERT | human telomerase reverse | HUI | Health Utilities Index |
| | transcriptase | HUI2 | Health Utilities Index |
| HTF | house tube feeding | | Mark 2 |
| HTGL | hepatic triglyceride lipase | HUIFM | human leukocyte |
| HTK | heel-to-knee (test) | | interferon meloy |
| HTL | hearing threshold level | HUK | human urinary kallikrein |
| | honey-thick liquid (diet | HUM | heat, ultrasound, and |
| | consistency) | | massage |

H

| | | | |
|---|---|---|---|
| HUM 70/30 | human insulin, regular 30 units/mL with human insulin isophane suspension 70 units/mL (Humulin® 70/30 insulin) | HVOO | hepatic venous outflow obstruction |
| | | HVPC | high-voltage pulsed current |
| | | HVPG | hepatic venous pressure gradient |
| HUMARA | human androgen receptor assay | HYPT | hyperventilation provocation test |
| HUM L | human insulin zinc suspension (Humulin® L Insulin) | HVR | hypoxic ventilatory response |
| | | HVS | hyperventilation syndrome |
| HUM N | human insulin isophane suspension (Humulin® N Insulin) | HVS-TK | herpes simplex virus thymidine kinase |
| | | HW | heparin well |
| HUM R | human insulin, regular (Humulin® R Insulin) | | homework |
| | | | housewife |
| HUR | hydroxyurea | HWB | hot water bottle |
| HUS | head ultrasound | HWFE | housewife |
| | hemolytic uremic syndrome | HWG | has worn glasses |
| | | HWH | halfway house |
| | husband | HWP | hot wet pack |
| husb | husband | HWPG | has worn prescription glasses |
| HUT | head-upright tilt (test) | | |
| | hyperplasia of usual type | Hx | history |
| HUVEC | human umbilical vein endothelial cells | | hospitalization |
| | | HXM | altretamine (hexamethylmelamine) |
| HV | hallux valgus | | |
| | Hantavirus | Hx & Px | history and physical (examination) |
| | has voided | | |
| | Hemovac® | Hy | hypermetropia |
| | hepatic vein | HYDRO | hydronephrosis |
| | herpesvirus | | hydrotherapy |
| | home visit | HYG | hygiene |
| H&V | hemigastrecotomy and vagotomy | HYPER | above |
| | | | higher than |
| HVII | hypervariable segment II | Hyper Al | hyperalimentation |
| HVA | homovanillic acid | Hyper K | hyperkalemia |
| HVD | hypertensive vascular disease | HYPER T & A | hypertrophic tonsils and adenoids |
| HVDO | hypovitaminosis D osteopathy | HYPO | below |
| | | | hypodermic injection |
| | | | lower than |
| HVE | high-voltage electrophoresis | Hypo K | hypokalemia |
| HVES | high-voltage electrical stimulation | hypopit | hypopituitarism |
| | | HYs | healthy years of life |
| HVF | Humphrey visual field | Hyst | hysterectomy |
| HVGS | high-voltage galvanic stimulation | Hz | Hertz |
| | | HZ | herpes zoster |
| HVI | hollow viscus injury | HZD | herpes zoster dermatitis |
| HVL | half-value layer | HZO | herpes zoster ophthalmicus |
| | hippocampal volume loss | | |
| HVOD | hepatic veno-occlusive disease | HZV | herpes zoster virus |

# I

| | |
|---|---|
| I | impression |
| | incisal |
| | incontinent |
| | independent |
| | initial |
| | inspiration |
| | intact (bag of waters) |
| | intermediate |
| | iris |
| | one |
| $I_2$ | iodine |
| $I^{131}$ | radioactive iodine |
| I-3+7 | idarubicin and cytarabine |
| IA | ideational apraxia |
| | incidental appendectomy |
| | incurred accidentally |
| | intra-amniotic |
| | intra-arterial |
| | invasive aspergillosis |
| I & A | irrigation and aspiration |
| IAA | ileoanal anastomosis |
| | insulin autoantibodies |
| | interrupted aortic arch |
| IAB | incomplete abortion |
| | induced abortion |
| | intermittent androgen blockade |
| IABC | intra-aortic balloon counterpulsation |
| IABCP | intra-aortic balloon counterpulsation |
| IABP | intra-aortic balloon pump |
| | intra-arterial blood pressure |
| IAC | internal auditory canal |
| | intra-arterial chemotherapy |
| | isolated adrenal cell |
| IAC-CPR | interposed abdominal compressions—cardiopulmonary resuscitation |
| IACG | intermittent angle-closure glaucoma |
| IACNS | isolated angiitis of central nervous system |

| | |
|---|---|
| IACP | intra-aortic counterpulsation |
| IAD | implantable atrial defibrillator |
| | intermittent androgen deprivation |
| | intractable atopic dermatitis |
| | intraoperative autologous (blood) donation |
| IADHS | inappropriate antidiuretic hormone syndrome |
| IADL | Instrumental Activities of Daily Living |
| IA DSA | intra-arterial digital subtraction arteriography |
| IAET | International Association for Enterostomal Therapy (Standards of Care Dermal Wounds: Pressure Ulcers)—see WOCN |
| IAF | intra-abdominal fat |
| IAGT | indirect antiglobulin test |
| IAHA | immune adherence hemagglutination |
| IAHC | intra-arterial hepatic chemotherapy |
| IAHD | idiopathic acquired hemolytic disease |
| IAI | intra-abdominal infection |
| | intra-abdominal injury |
| | intra-amniotic infection |
| IALD | instrumental activities of daily living |
| IAM | internal auditory meatus |
| IAN | indinavir (Crixivan)-associated nephrolithiasis |
| | intern's admission note |
| IAO | immediately after onset |
| IAP | independent adjudicating panel |
| | intermittent acute porphyria |
| | intra-abdominal pressure |
| | intracarotid amobarbital procedure |
| IARC | International Agency for Research on Cancer |
| IART | intra-atrial reentrant tachycardia |

I

| IAS | idiopathic ankylosing spondylitis | | infectious bovine rhinotracheitis |
| | intermittent androgen suppression | IBRS | Inpatient Behavior Rating Scale |
| | internal anal sphincter | IBS | irritable bowel syndrome |
| IASD | interatrial septal defect | IBT | ink blot test (Rorschach test) |
| IAT | immunoaugmentive therapy | | interblinking time |
| | indirect antiglobulin test | | immune-based therapy |
| | intracarotid amobarbital test | IBTR | intrabreast-tumor recurrence |
| | intraoperative autologous transfusion | | ipsilateral breast tumor recurrence |
| IATT | intra-arterial thrombolytic therapy | IBU | ibuprofen |
| IAV | intermittent assist ventilation | IBW | ideal body weight |
| IB | ileal bypass | IC | between meals |
| | insulin receptor binding test | | iliac crest |
| | | | immune complex |
| | isolation bed | | immunocompromised |
| IB1A | interferon beta-1a (Avonex) | | incipient cataract (grade 1+ to 4+) |
| IBAM | idiopathic bile acid malabsorption | | incomplete |
| | | | indirect calorimetry |
| IBBB | intra-blood-brain barrier | | indirect Coombs (test) |
| IBBBB | incomplete bilateral bundle branch block | | individual counseling |
| | | | informed consent |
| IBC | Institutional Biosafety Committee | | inspiratory capacity |
| | | | intensive care |
| | invasive bladder cancer | | intercostal |
| | iron binding capacity | | intercourse |
| IBD | infectious bursal disease | | intermediate care |
| | inflammatory bowel disease | | intermittent catheterization |
| | | | intermittent claudication |
| | isosulfan blue dye | | interstitial changes |
| IBDQ | Inflammatory Bowel Disease Questionnaire | | interstitial cystitis |
| | | | intracerebral |
| IBG | iliac bone graft | | intracranial |
| IBI | intermittent bladder irrigation | | intraincisional |
| | | | ion chromatography |
| *ibid* | at the same place | | irritable colon |
| IBILI | indirect bilirubin | I/C | imipenem-cilastatin (Primaxin) |
| IBM | ideal body mass | ICA | ileocolic anastomosis |
| | inclusion body myositis | | intermediate care area |
| IBMI | initial body mass index | | internal carotid artery |
| IBMTR | International Bone Marrow Transplant Registry | | intracranial abscess |
| | | | intracranial aneurysm |
| IBNR | incurred but not reported | | islet-cell antibody |
| IBOW | intact bag of waters | ICa | calcium, ionized |
| IBP | ibuprofen | ICAAC | Interscience Conference on Antimicrobial Agents and Chemotherapy |
| IBPS | Insall-Burstein posterior stabilizer | | |
| IBR | immediate breast reconstruction | | |

| ICAM | intracellular adhesion molecule | ICD-10-PCS | International Statistical Classification of Diseases, Tenth Revision, Procedure Coding Classification System |
| ICAM-1 | intercellular adhesion molecule-1 | | |
| ICAO | internal carotid artery occlusion | ICDO | International Classification of Diseases for Oncology |
| ICAS | intermediate coronary artery syndrome | ICE | ice, compression, and elevation |
| ICAT | infant cardiac arrest tray | | ifosfamide, carboplatin, and etoposide |
| ICB | intracranial bleeding | | individual career exploration |
| ICBG | iliac crest bone graft | | interleukin-1 alpha converting enzyme |
| ICBT | intercostobronchial trunk | | interleukin-1 beta converting enzyme |
| ICC | immunocytochemistry | | intracardiac echocardiography |
| | Indian childhood cirrhosis | | |
| | Infection Control Committee | + ice | add ice |
| | intracluster correlation coefficient | ICER | incremental cost-effectiveness ratio |
| | intraclass correlation coefficient | ICES | ice, compression, elevation, and support |
| | invasive cervical carcinoma | ICF | intermediate care facility |
| | islet cell carcinoma | | intracellular fluid |
| ICCD | intensified charge-coupled device | ICG | indocyanine green |
| ICCE | intracapsular cataract extraction | ICGA | indocyanine green angiography |
| ICCU | intensive coronary care unit | ICH | immunocompromised host |
| | intermediate coronary care unit | | International Council on Harmonization (of Technical Requirements for Registration of Pharmaceuticals for Human Use) |
| ICD | implantable cardioverter defibrillator | | |
| | indigocarmine dye | | |
| | informed consent document | | |
| | instantaneous cardiac death | | intracerebral hemorrhage |
| | | | intracranial hemorrhage |
| | isocitrate dehydrogenase | ICI | intracranial injury |
| | irritant contact dermatitis | ICIT | intensified conventional insulin therapy |
| ICDA | International Classification of Disease, Adapted | ICL | intracorneal lens |
| | | | isocitrate lyase |
| ICDB | incomplete database | ICLE | intracapsular lens extraction |
| ICDC | implantable cardioverter defibrillator catheter | ICM | intercostal margin |
| | | | intercostal muscle |
| ICD 9 CM | International Statistical Classification of Diseases, 9th Revision, Clinical Modification | ICN | infection control nurse |
| | | | intensive care nursery |
| | | ICN2 | neonatal intensive care unit level II |

I

| ICP | inductively coupled plasma |
| | intercostal position (for chest lead) |
| | intracranial pressure |
| | intrahepatic cholestasis of pregnancy |
| ICP-MS | inductively-coupled plasma—mass spectrometer |
| ICP-OES | inductively-coupled plasma—optical emission spectrometry |
| ICPP | intubated continuous positive pressure |
| ICR | intercostal retractions |
| | intrastromal corneal ring |
| ICRC | International Committee of the Red Cross |
| ICRF-159 | razoxane |
| ICRS | intrastromal corneal ring segments |
| ICS | ileocecal sphincter |
| | inhaled corticosteroid(s) |
| | intercostal space |
| ICSC | idiopathic central serous choroidopathy |
| ICSH | interstitial cell-stimulating hormone |
| ICSI | intracytoplasmic sperm injection |
| ICSR | Individual Case Safety Reports |
| | intercostal space retractions |
| ICT | icterus |
| | indirect Coombs test |
| | inflammation of connective tissue |
| | intensive conventional therapy |
| | intermittent cervical traction |
| | intracranial tumor |
| | intracutaneous test |
| | islet cell transplant |
| ICTX | intermittent cervical traction |
| ICU | intensive care unit |
| | intermediate care unit |
| ICV | intracerebroventricular |
| ICVH | ischemic cerebrovascular headache |

| ICW | in connection with |
| | intercellular water |
| ID | identification |
| | identify |
| | idiotype |
| | ifosfamide, mesna uroprotection, and doxorubicin |
| | immunodiffusion |
| | induction delivery |
| | infectious disease (physician or department) |
| | initial diagnosis |
| | initial dose |
| | intellectual disability |
| | internal derangement |
| | intradermal |
| id | the same |
| I & D | incision and drainage |
| IDA | idarubicin (Idamycin) |
| | iron deficiency anemia |
| IDAM | infant of drug abusing mother |
| IDB | incomplete database |
| IDC | idiopathic dilated cardiomyopathy |
| | invasive ductal cancer |
| IDCF | immunodiffusion complement fixation |
| IDCM | idiopathic dilated cardiomyopathy |
| IDD | insulin-dependent diabetes |
| | iodine-deficiency disorders |
| IDDD | Interview for Deterioration in Daily life in Dementia |
| IDDM | insulin-dependent diabetes mellitus |
| IDDS | implantable drug delivery system |
| IDE | Investigational Device Exemption |
| IDEA | Individuals with Disabilities Education Act |
| IDET | intradiskal electrothermal therapy |
| IDFC | immature dead female child |

| IDH | isocitric dehydrogenase | | intradiskal electrothermal coagulation |
| IDI | Interpersonal Dependency Inventory | IEF | isoelectric focusing |
| | intrathecal drug infusion | IEI | idiopathic environmental intolerance |
| IDK | internal derangement of knee | IEL | internal elastic lamina |
| IDL | intermediate-density lipoprotein | | intestinal-intraepithelial lymphocyte |
| | ischemic digital loss | IEM | immune electron microscopy |
| IDM | infant of a diabetic mother | | inborn errors of metabolism |
| IDMC | immature dead male child | | |
| IDNA | iron-deficient, not anemic | | |
| IDP | initiate discharge planning | iEMG | integrated electromyography |
| | inosine diphosphate | | |
| IDPN | intradialytic parenteral nutrition | IEMR | integrated electronic medical records |
| IDR | idarubicin | IEP | immunoelectrophoresis |
| | idiosyncratic drug reaction | | Individualized Education Plan |
| | intradermal reaction | IEPA | immunoelectrophoresis analysis |
| IDS | infectious disease service | | |
| | integrated delivery system | I:E ratio | inspiratory to expiratory time ratio |
| IDSA | Infectious Disease Society of America (guidelines) | IES | Impact of Event Scale |
| IDT | intensive diabetes treatment | IET | infantile estropia |
| | | IF | idiopathic flushing |
| | interdisciplinary team | | ifosfamide (Ifex) |
| | intradermal test | | immunofluorescence |
| IDTP | immunodiffusion tube precipitin | | injury factor |
| | | | interferon |
| IDU | idoxuridine | | interfrontal |
| | infectious disease unit | | intermaxillary fixation |
| | injecting drug user | | internal fixation |
| IDV | indinavir (Crixivan) | | intrinsic factor |
| | intermittent demand ventilation | | involved field (radiotherapy) |
| IDVC | indwelling venous catheter | IFA | immunofluorescent assay |
| IE | ifosfamide, and etoposide with mesna | | indirect fluorescent antibody |
| | immunoelectrophoresis | IFAT | immunofluorescence antibody test (technique) |
| | induced emesis | IFC | interferential current |
| | infective endocarditis | IFE | immunofixation electrophoresis |
| | inner ear | | |
| | internal/external (rotation) | | in-flight emergency |
| | international unit | IFG | impaired fasting glucose |
| | (European abbreviation) | IFL | indolent follicular lymphoma |
| I & E | ingress and egress (tubes) | | |
| | internal and external | IFM | internal fetal monitoring |
| i.e. | that is | IFN | interferon |
| IEC | independent ethics committee inpatient exercise center | IFNB | interferon beta-1 b (Betaseron) |
| | | IFO | ifosfamide (Ifex) |

|        | in front of | | immunohistochemistry |
| IFOS | ifosfamide (Ifex) | | inner hair cell |
| IFP | inflammatory fibroid | | (in cochlea) |
|        | polyps | IHD | intermittent hemodialysis |
| IFPMA | International Federation of | | intraheptic duct (ule) |
|        | Pharmaceutical | | ischemic heart disease |
|        | Manufacturers | IHDN | integrated health delivery |
|        | Associations | | network |
| IFSAC | Inventory of Functional | IHH | idiopathic |
|        | Status After Childbirth | | hypogonadotrophic |
| IFSE | internal fetal scalp | | hypogonadism |
|        | electrode | IHO | idiopathic hypertrophic |
| IFSP | individualized family | | osteoarthropathy |
|        | service plan | IHP | idiopathic |
| IgA | immunoglobulin A | | hypoparathyroidism |
| IGCS | inpatient geriatric | | inferior hypogastric plexus |
|        | consultation services | | isolated hepatic perfusion |
| IgD | immunoglobulin D | IHPH | intrahepatic portal |
| IGDE | idiopathic gait disorders | | hypertension |
|        | of the elderly | IHPS | infantile hypertrophic |
| IGDM | infant of gestational | | pyloric stenosis |
|        | diabetic mother | IHR | inguinal hernia repair |
| IgE | immunoglobulin E | | intrinsic heart rate |
| IGF-I | insulin-like growth | IHS | Indian Health Service |
|        | factor I | | integrated healthcare |
| IGFA | indocyanine-green fundus | | system |
|        | angiography | | International Headache |
| IGFBP-3 | insulin-like growth factor- | | Society (criteria) |
|        | binding protein 3 | | Iodiopathic Headache |
| IgG | immunoglobulin G | | Score |
| IGIM | immune globulin | IHs | iris hamartomas |
|        | intramuscular | IHSA | iodinated human serum |
| IGIV | immune globulin | | albumin |
|        | intravenous | IHSS | idiopathic hypertrophic |
| IgM | immunoglobulin M | | subaortic stenosis |
| IGP | interstitial glycoprotein | IHT | insulin hypoglycemia test |
| IGR | intrauterine growth | IHU | inpatient hospice unit |
|        | retardation | IHW | inner heel wedge |
| IGT | impaired glucose | II | internal iliac (artery) |
|        | tolerance | IIA | internal iliac artery |
| IGTN | ingrown toenail | IICP | increased intracranial |
| IH | indirect hemagglutination | | pressure |
|        | infectious hepatitis | IICU | infant intensive care unit |
|        | inguinal hernia | IID | infectious intestinal |
|        | in-house | | disease |
| IHA | immune hemolytic anemia | IIEF | International Index of |
|        | indirect hemagglutination | | Erectile Function |
|        | infusion hepatic | IIF | indirect |
|        | arteriography | | immunofluorescence |
|        | intrahepatic arterial | IIH | idiopathic infantile |
| IHC | idiopathic hypercalciuria | | hypercalcemia |
|        | immobilization | | iodine-induced |
|        | hypercalcemia | | hyperthyroidism |

I

| | |
|---|---|
| IIHT | iodide-induced hyperthyroidism |
| IIM | idiopathic inflammatory myopathies |
| | intracortical interaction mapping |
| IINB | iliohypogastric ilioinguinal nerve block |
| IIP | idiopathic interstitial pneumonitis |
| IIPF | idiopathic interstitial pulmonary fibrosis |
| IJ | ileojejunal |
| | internal jugular |
| I&J | insight and judgment |
| IJC | internal jugular catheter |
| IJD | inflammatory joint disease |
| IJO | idiopathic juvenile osteoporosis |
| IJP | internal jugular pressure |
| IJR | idiojunctional rhythm |
| IJT | idiojunctional tachycardia |
| IJV | internal jugular vein |
| IK | immobilized knee |
| | interstitial keratitis |
| IKDC | International Knee Documentation Committee (evaluation; score; form) |
| IL | immature lungs |
| | interleukin (1, 2, etc.) |
| | intralesional |
| | Intralipid® |
| IL-2 | aldesleukin (Proleukin; interleukin-2) |
| IL-11 | oprelvekin (Neumega; interleukin-11) |
| ILA | inferior lateral angle |
| | insulin-like activity |
| ILB | incidental Lewy body |
| ILBBB | incomplete left bundle branch block |
| ILBW | infant, low birth weight (less than 2,500 g) |
| ILC | interstitial laser coagulation |
| | invasive lobular cancer |
| ILD | immature lung disease |
| | indentation load deflection |
| | intermediate density lipoproteins |
| | interstitial lung disease |

| | |
|---|---|
| | ischemic leg disease |
| ILE | infantile lobar emphysema |
| ILF | indicated low forceps |
| ILFC | immature living female child |
| ILHP | ipsilateral hemidiaphragmatic paresis |
| ILI | influenza-like illness |
| ILM | internal limiting membrane |
| ILMC | immature living male child |
| ILMI | inferolateral myocardial infarct |
| ILP | interstitial laser photocoagulation |
| | isolated limb perfusion |
| ILQTS | idiopathic long QT (interval) syndrome |
| ILS | intralabyrinthine schwannomas |
| ILT | interstitial laser therapy |
| ILVEN | inflammatory linear verrucal epidermal nevus |
| IM | ice massage |
| | infectious mononucleosis |
| | intermetatarsal |
| | internal medicine |
| | intramedullary |
| | intramuscular |
| IMA | inferior mesenteric artery |
| | internal mammary artery |
| IMAC | ifosfamide, mesna uroprotection, doxorubicin (Adriamycin), and cisplatin |
| | immobilized metal affinity chromatography |
| IMAE | internal maxillary artery embolization |
| IMAG | internal mammary artery graft |
| IMARD | immunomodulating antirheumatic drugs |
| IMB | intermenstrual bleeding |
| IMBP | immobilized mismatch binding protein |
| IMC | intermittent catheterization |
| | intramedullary catheter |
| IMCI | Integrated Management of Childhood Illness |

I

| | | | |
|---|---|---|---|
| IMCU | intermediate care unit | | intensity-modulated radiation therapy |
| IME | important medical event | | intensity-modulated radiosurgery |
| | independent medical examination (evaluation) | IMS | immunosuppressants incurred in military service |
| IMF | idiopathic myelofibrosis | IMT | inspiratory muscle training |
| | ifosfamide, mesna uroprotection, methotrexate, and fluorouracil | | intimal medial thickness |
| | | IMU | intermediate medicine unit |
| | immobilization mandibular fracture | IMV | inferior mesenteric vein |
| | inframammary fold | | intermittent mandatory ventilation |
| | intermaxillary fixation | | intermittent mechanical ventilation |
| IMG | internal medicine group | | |
| IMGU | insulin-mediated glucose uptake | IMVP-16 | ifosfamide, mesna uroprotection, methotrexate, and etoposide |
| IMH | idiopathic myocardial hypertrophy | IN | insulin intranasal |
| IMH test | indirect microhemagglutination test | In | indium |
| | | in. | inch |
| IMI | imipramine | INAD | in no apparent distress |
| | impending myocardial infarction | | Investigational New Animal Drug |
| | inferior myocardial infarction | INB | intercostal nerve blockade |
| | intramuscular injection | INC | incisal |
| $^{131}$I-MIBG | iodine$^{131}$-metaiodobenzyl-guanidine (iobenguane $^{131}$I) | | incision |
| | | | incomplete |
| IMIG | intramuscular immunoglobulin | | incontinent |
| | | | increase |
| IMLC | incomplete mitral leaflet closure | | inside-the-needle catheter |
| | | INCC | Institut National du Cancer du Canada |
| IMM | immune modulating nutrition (immunonutrition) | Inc Spir | incentive spirometer |
| | | IND | indinavir (Crixivan) |
| | immunizations | | induced |
| IMN | idiopathic membranous nephropathy | | Investigational New Drug (application) |
| | internal mammary (lymph) node | INDA | Investigational New Drug Application |
| IMP | impacted | INDIGO | interstitial laser ablation of the prostate |
| | important | | |
| | impression | INDM | infant of nondiabetic mother |
| | improved | | |
| | inosine monophoshate | INDO | indomethacin |
| IMPX | impaction | $^{111}$In-DTPA | indium pentetate |
| IMR | infant mortality rate | | |
| IMRA | immunoradiometric assay | INE | infantile necrotizing encephalomyelopathy |

| | | | |
|---|---|---|---|
| INEX | inexperienced | INST | instrumental delivery |
| INF | infant | INT | intermittent needle therapy |
| | infarction | | internal |
| | infected | Int mon | internal monitor |
| | infection | INTERP | interpretation |
| | inferior | Int Med | internal medicine |
| | influenza virus vaccine, not otherwise specified | intol | intolerance |
| | information | int-rot | internal rotation |
| | infused | int trx | intermittent traction |
| | infusion | intub | intubation |
| | intravenous nutritional fluid | INV | Invirase (saquinavir, hard gel cap) |
| INF$_a$ | influenza virus, attenuated live vaccine | inver | inversion |
| INFas | influenza virus attenuated live vaccine, intranasal | INVOS | *in vivo* optical spectroscopy |
| INFC | infected | IO | inferior oblique |
| | infection | | initial opening |
| INFi | influenza virus inactivated vaccine | | intestinal obstruction |
| | | | intraocular pressure |
| INFs | influenza virus vaccine, split viron | | intra-Ommaya |
| | | | intraoperative |
| | | | intraosseous |
| INFs-AB3 | influenza virus inactivated vaccine, split virion, types A and B, trivalent | I&O | intake and output |
| | | IOA | intact on admission |
| | | IOC | intern on call |
| INF$_w$ | influenza virus vaccine, whole viron | | intraoperative cholangiogram |
| ING | inguinal | IOCG | intraoperative cholangiogram |
| ✓ing | checking | | |
| INH | isoniazid | IOD | implant-supported overdenture |
| INI | intranuclear inclusion | | |
| inj | injection | | interorbital distance |
| | injury | IODM | infant of diabetic mother |
| INK | injury not known | | |
| INN | International Nonproprietary Name | IOF | intraocular fluid |
| | | IOFB | intraocular foreign body |
| INO | inhaled nitrous oxide | IOFNA | intraoperative fine needle aspiration |
| | internuclear ophthalmoplegia | IOH | idiopathic orthostatic hypotension |
| INOP | internodal ophthalmoplegia | IO-HDRBT | intraoperative high-dose-rate brachytherapy |
| iNOS | inducible nitric oxide synthase | IOI | idiopathic orbital inflammation |
| inpt | inpatient | | intraosseous infusion |
| INQ | inferior nasal quadrant | IOL | intraocular lens |
| INR | international normalized ratio (for anticoagulant monitoring) | IOLI | intraocular lens implantation |
| INS | idiopathic nephrotic syndrome | IOLM | intraoperative lymphatic mapping |
| | inspection | IOM | Institute of Medicine |
| | insurance | ION | ischemic optic neuropathy |

| | | | |
|---|---|---|---|
| IONIS | indirect optic nerve injury syndrome | | intraperitoneal chemotherapy |
| IONTO | iontophoresis | IPCD | idiopathic paroxysmal cerebral dysrhythmia |
| IOOA | inferior oblique overaction | | infantile polycystic disease |
| IOP | intraocular pressure intraosseous puncture | IPCK | infantile polycystic kidney (disease) |
| IOR | ideas of reference immature oocyte retrieval | IPCT | intraperitoneal chemotherapy |
| | inferior oblique recession | IPD | idiopathic Parkinson disease |
| IO-RB | intraocular retinoblastoma | | immediate pigment darkening |
| IORT | intraoperative radiation therapy | | inflammatory pelvic disease |
| IOS | intraoperative sonography | | intermittent peritoneal dialysis |
| IOT | intraocular tension | | interpupillary distance |
| IOTEE | intraoperative transesophageal echocardiography | | invasive pneumococcal disease |
| IOTT | intensification-of-treatment trigger (criteria) | IPEX | immune dysregulation, polyendocrinopathy, enteropathy, X-linked (syndrome) |
| IOUS | intraocular ultrasound | IPF | idiopathic pulmonary fibrosis |
| IOV | initial office visit | | interstitial pulmonary fibrosis |
| IP | ice pack incubation period | IPFD | intrapartum fetal distress |
| | individualized plan Infrapatellar | IPG | immobilized pH gradient |
| | inpatient | | impedance plethysmography |
| | in plaster interphalangeal | | individually polymerized grass |
| | interstitial pneumonia intestinal permeability | IPH | idiopathic pulmonary hemosiderosis |
| | intraperitoneal | | interphalangeal |
| | invasive procedures | | intraparenchymal hemorrhage |
| | inverted (inverting) papilloma | | intraperitoneal hemorrhage |
| I/P | iris/pupil | IPHC | intraperitoneal hyperthermic chemotherapy |
| IP3 | inositol triphosphate | | |
| IPA | independent practice association | IPHEP | independent progressive home exercise program |
| | interpleural analgesia | | |
| | invasive pulmonary aspergillosis | IPHP | intraperitoneal hyperthermic chemotherapy |
| | isopropyl alcohol | | |
| IPAA | ileo-pouch anal anastamosis | | |
| IPAP | inspiratory positive airway pressure | IPI | International Prognostic Index |
| IPB | infrapopliteal bypass | | |
| IPC | indirect pulp cavity | IPJ | interphalangeal joint |
| | intermittent pneumatic compression (boots) | | |

| | | | |
|---|---|---|---|
| IPK | intractable plantar keratosis | IPT | intermittent pelvic traction |
| IPM | intrauterine pressure monitor | iPTH | parathyroid hormone by radioimmunoassay |
| | interventional pain management | IPTX | intermittent pelvic traction |
| IPMI | inferoposterior myocardial infarct | IPV | inactivated poliovirus vaccine |
| IPN | infantile periarteritis nodosa | IPVC | interpolated premature ventricular contraction |
| | intern's progress note | IPW | interphalangeal width |
| | interstitial pneumonia | IQ | intelligence quotient |
| IPOF | immediate postoperative fitting | IQR | interquartile range |
| | | IR | immediate-release (tablets) |
| IPOM | intraperitoneal onlay mesh | | immunoreactive |
| IPOP | immediate postoperative prosthesis | | inferior rectus |
| IPP | inflatable penile prosthesis | | infrared |
| | intrapleual pressure | | insulin resistance |
| | isolated pelvic perfusion | | internal reduction |
| IPPA | inspection, palpation, percussion, and auscultation | | internal resistance |
| | | | internal rotation |
| | | I&R | insertion and removal |
| | | IRA | infarct-related artery |
| IPPB | intermittent positive-pressure breathing | IRAAF | intraoperative radiofrequency ablation for chronic atrial fibrillation |
| IP-PDT | intraperitoneal photodynamic therapy | IRA-EEA | ileorectal anastomoses with end-to-end anastomosis |
| IPPF | immediate postoperative prosthetic fitting | | |
| IPPI | interruption of pregnancy for psychiatric indication | IRAP | interleukin-1 receptor antagonist protein |
| | | IRB | Institutional Review Board |
| IPPV | intermittent positive pressure ventilation | IRBBB | incomplete right bundle branch block |
| IPS | idiopathic pneumonia syndrome | IRBC | immature red blood cell |
| | infundibular pulmonic stenosis | | irradiated red blood cells |
| | | IRBP | interphotoreceptor retinoid-binding protein |
| | initial prognostic score | IRC | indirect radionuclide cystography |
| | intermittent photic stimulation | | |
| IPSCs | islet-producing stem cells | | infrared coagulation |
| IPSF | immediate postsurgical fitting | | Institutional Review Committee (Board) |
| IPSID | immunoproliferative small intestinal disease | IRCU | intensive respiratory care unit |
| IPSP | inhibitory postsynaptic potential | IRD | immune renal disease(s) |
| | | IRDM | insulin-resistant diabetes mellitus |
| IPSS | inferior petrosal sinus sampling | IRDS | idiopathic respiratory distress syndrome |
| I-PSS | International Prostate Symptom Score | | infant respiratory distress syndrome |
| I PSY | intermediate psychiatry | | |

| | | | |
|---|---|---|---|
| IRE | internal rotation in extension | | *in situ* |
| | | | intercostal space |
| IRED | infrared emission detection | | inventory of systems |
| | | | ipecac syrup |
| IRF | inpatient rehabilitation facilities | I-S | Ionescu-Shiley (prosthetic heart valve) |
| | internal rotation in flexion | I & S | intact and symmetrical |
| IRH | intraretinal hemorrhage | I/S | instruct/supervise |
| IRI | immunoreactive insulin | ISA | ileosigmoid anastomosis |
| IRIV | immunopotentiating reconstituted influenza virosomes | | Incest Survivors Anonymous |
| | | | intrinsic sympathomimetic activity |
| IRM | magnetic resonance imaging (French) | ISAAC | International Study of Asthma and Allergies in Childhood (questionnaire; protocol) |
| IRMA | immediate response mobile analysis (blood analysis system) | | |
| | | ISADH | inappropriate secretion of antidiuretic hormone |
| | immunoradiometric assay | ISB | incentive spirometry breathing |
| | intraretinal microvascular abnormalities | | |
| | | ISBP | interscalen brachial plexus |
| IRMS | isotope-ratio mass spectrometry | ISC | carcinoma *in situ* (also CIS) |
| IRN | iterated rippled noise | | indwelling subclavian catheter |
| IROS | ipsilateral routing of signals | | infant servo-control |
| IRP | intellectual property rights | | infant skin control |
| IRR | infrared radiation | | intermittent self-catheterization |
| | intrarenal reflux | | |
| | irregular rate and rhythm | | intermittent straight catheterization |
| IRRC | Institutional Research Review Committee | | |
| | | | isolette servo-control |
| irreg | irregular | ISCM | intramedullary spinal cord metastases |
| IRR HYDRO | irreversible hydrocolloid | | |
| | | I/SCN | urinary iodine/thiocyanate ratio |
| IRRs | incidence rate ratios | | |
| IRS | Information and Referral Society | ISCOM | immunostimulating complex |
| | insulin-resistance syndrome | ISCP | infection surveillance and control program |
| IRSB | intravenous regional sympathetic block | | |
| | | ISCs | irreversible sickle cells |
| IRSG | Intergroup Rhabdomyosarcoma Study Group | ISCU | infant special care unit |
| | | ISD | inhibited sexual desire |
| IRT | immunoreactive trypsin | | initial sleep disturbance |
| | incident response team | | intrinsic (urethral) sphincter deficiency |
| IRV | inspiratory reserve volume | | |
| | | | isosorbide dinitrate |
| | inverse ratio ventilation | ISDN | isosorbide dinitrate |
| IS | incentive spirometer | ISE | ion-sensitive electrode |
| | induced sputum | ISEL | *in situ* end labeling |
| | Information Services (Department) | ISF | interstitial fluid |

| | | | |
|---|---|---|---|
| ISFET | ion-selective field effect transistor | IST | injection sclerotherapy |
| | | | insulin sensitivity test |
| ISG | immune serum globulin (immune globulin) | | insulin shock therapy |
| | | ISU | intermediate surgical unit |
| ISH | isolated systolic hypertension | ISW | interstitial water |
| | | IS10W | 10% invert sugar injection (in water) |
| ISHH | *in situ* hybridization histochemistry | ISWI | incisional surgical wound infection |
| ISHLT | International Society for Heart and Lung Transplantation | IT | incentive therapy |
| | | | individual therapy |
| | | | inferior-temporal |
| ISHT | isolated systolic hypertension | | information technology |
| | | | Inhalation Therapist |
| ISI | International Sensitivity Index | | inhalation therapy |
| | | | inspiratory time |
| ISK | isokinetic | | intensive therapy |
| ISMA | infantile spinal muscular atrophy | | intermittent traction |
| | | | interpreted |
| ISMN | isosorbide mononitrate | | intertrochanteric |
| ISMO® | isosorbide mononitrate | | intertuberous |
| ISMP | Institute for Safe Medication Practices | | intrathecal (dangerous abbreviation) |
| ISNA | iron-sufficient, not anemic | | intratracheal (dangerous, could be interupted as intrathecal) |
| ISO | isodose | | |
| | isolette | | |
| | isoproterenol | | intratumoral |
| ISOE | isoetharine | ITA | individual treatment assessment |
| ISOF | isoflurane (Florane) | | |
| ISOK | isokinetic | | inferior temporal artery |
| ISOM | isometric | | itasetron |
| ISOs | isoenzymes | ITAG | internal thoracic artery graft |
| ISP | inferior spermatic plexus | | |
| | interspace | | |
| *ISQ* | as before; continue on (*in status quo*) | ITAL | intrathoracic artificial lung |
| | | ITB | iliotibial band |
| ISR | injection site reaction | | intrathecal baclofen |
| | integrated secretory response | ITBC | intraluminal typical bronchial carcinoid |
| ISS | idiopathic short stature | ITBS | iliotibial band syndrome |
| | Individual Self-Rating Scale | | Iowa Tests of Basic Skills |
| | | ITC | Incontinence Treatment Center |
| | Injury Severity Score | | |
| | irritable stomach syndrome | | in-the-canal (hearing aid) |
| | | | isothermal titration calorimetry |
| | Integrated Summary of Safety | | |
| IS10S | 10% invert sugar in 0.9% sodium chloride (saline) injection | ITCP | idiopathic thrombocytopenic purpura |
| | | ITCU | intensive thoracic cardiovascular unit |
| ISSP | Infant Support Services Program | ITE | insufficient therapeutic effect |
| IST | immunosuppressive therapy | | in-the-ear (hearing aid) |

I

| | | | |
|---|---|---|---|
| ITF | inpatient treatment facility | IUDR | idoxuridine (Herplex) |
| ITFF | intertrochanteric femoral fracture | IUFB | intrauterine foreign body |
| ITGV | intrathoracic gas volume | IUFD | intrauterine fetal death (demise) |
| ITM | Institute of Tropical Medicine, Antwerp, Belgium | | intrauterine fetal distress |
| | | IUFT | intrauterine fetal transfusion |
| ITMTX | intrathecal methotrexate | IUGR | intrauterine growth retardation (restriction) |
| ITN | irinotecan (Camptosar) | | |
| ITNs | insecticide treated nets | IUI | intrauterine insemination |
| ITOC | intratracheal oxygen catheter | IULN | institutional upper limit of normal |
| ITOP | intentional termination of pregnancy | IUP | intrauterine pregnancy |
| | | IUPC | intrauterine pressure catheter |
| ITOU | intensive therapy observation unit | IUPD | intrauterine pregnancy delivered |
| ITP | idiopathic thrombocy-topenic purpura | IUP,TBCS | intrauterine pregnancy, term birth, cesarean section |
| | interim treatment plan | | |
| ITPA | Illinois Test of Psycholinguistic Ability | IUP,TBLC | intrauterine pregnancy, term birth, living child |
| ITQ | inferior temporal quadrant | IUR | intrauterine retardation |
| ITR | isotretinoin (Accutane) | IUS | intrauterine system |
| ITRA | itraconazole (Sporanox) | IUT | intrauterine transfusion |
| ITS | internal transcribed spacer | IUTD | immunizations up to date |
| | | IV | four |
| | isometric trunk stabilization | | interview |
| | | | intravenous (i.v.) |
| ITSCU | infant-toddler special care unit | | intravertebral |
| | | | invasive |
| ITT | identical twins (raised) together | | inversion |
| | | | symbol for class 4 controlled substances |
| | insulin tolerance test | | |
| | intention-to-treat (analysis) | IVA | Intervir-A |
| | | IVAD | implantable venous access device |
| ITU | infant-toddler unit | | |
| | intensive therapy unit | | implantable vascular access device |
| | intensive treatment unit | | |
| ITVAD | indwelling transcutaneous vascular access device | IVBAT | intravascular bronchoalveolar tumor |
| ITX | immunotoxin(s) | IVC | inferior vena cava |
| ITZ | itraconazole (Sporanox) | | inspiratory vital capacity |
| IU | international unit (this is a dangerous abbreviation as it is read as intravenous; use "units") | | intravenous chemotherapy |
| | | | intravenous cholangiogram |
| | | | intraventricular catheter |
| IUC | intrauterine catheter | | intraventricular conduction |
| IUCD | intrauterine contraceptive device | IVCD | intraventricular conduction defect (delay) |
| IUD | intrauterine death | | |
| | intrauterine device | | |

| IVCF | inferior vena cava filter | IVOX | intravascular oxygenator (oxygenation) |
| IVCI | intravenous continuous infusion | IVP | intravenous push (this is a dangerous meaning as it is read as intravenous pyelogram) |
| IVCP | inferior vena cava pressure | | |
| IVCV | inferior venacavography | | intravenous pyelogram |
| IVD | intervertebral disk intravenous drip *in vitro* diagnostic | IVPB | intravenous piggyback |
| | | IVPF | isovolume pressure flow |
| IVDA | intravenous drug abuse | IVPU | intravenous push |
| IVDSA | intravenous digital subtraction angiography | IVR | idioventricular rhythm interactive voice-response (system) intravaginal ring intravenous retrograde intravenous rider (this is a dangerous abbreviation as it has been read as IVP-intravenous push) isovolumic relaxation (time) |
| IVDU | intravenous drug user | | |
| IVET | *in vivo* expression technology | | |
| IVF | intervertebral foramina intravenous fluid(s) *in vitro* fertilization | | |
| IVFA | intravenous fluorescein angiography | | |
| IVFE | intravenous fat emulsion | IVRA | intravenous regional anesthesia |
| IVF-ET | *in vitro* fertilization-embryo transfer | IVRAP | intravenous retrograde access port |
| IVFT | intravenous fetal transfusion | IVRG | intravenous retrograde |
| IVGG | intravenous gamma globulin | IV-RNV | intravenous radionuclide venography |
| IVGTT | intravenous glucose tolerance test | IVRO | intraoral vertical ramus osteotomy |
| IVH | intravenous hyperalimentation intraventricular hemorrhage | IVRT | isovolumic relation time |
| | | IVS | intraventricular septum irritable voiding syndrome |
| IVID | intravenous iron dextran (INFeD; DexFerrum) | IVSD | intraventricular septal defect |
| IVIG | intravenous immunoglobulin | IVSE | interventricular septal excursion |
| IVJC | intervertebral joint complex | IVSO | intraoral vertical segmental osteotomy |
| IVL | intravascular lymphomatosis intravenous lock | IVSS | intravenous Soluset® |
| | | IVST | interventricular septum thickness |
| IVLBW | infant of very low birth weight (less than 1,500 g) | IVT | intravenous transfusion intraventricular |
| IVMP | intravenously administered methylprednisolone | IVTTT | intravenous tolbutamide tolerance test |
| | | IVU | intravenous urography (urogram) |
| IVNC | isolated ventricular noncompaction | IVUC | intravenous ultrasound catheter |
| IVO | intraoral vertical osteotomy | IVUS | intravascular ultrasound |
| | | IW | inspiratory wheeze |

| | |
|---|---|
| IWD | individual with a disability |
| IWI | inferior wall infarction |
| IWL | insensible water loss |
| IWMI | inferior wall myocardial infarct |
| IWML | idiopathic white matter lesion |
| IWT | ice-water test |
| | impacted wisdom teeth |

# J

| | |
|---|---|
| J | Jaeger measure of near vision with 20/20 about equal to J1 |
| | jejunostomy |
| | Jewish |
| | joint |
| | joule |
| | juice |
| J 1-16 | Jaeger near acuity notation (1 to 16 scale) |
| JA | joint aspiration |
| Jack | jacknife position |
| JAFAR | Juvenile Arthritis Functional Assessment Report |
| JAMA | *Journal of the American Medical Association* |
| JAMG | juvenile autoimmune myasthenia gravis |
| JAN | Japanese Accepted Name |
| JAR | junior assistant resident |
| JARAN | junior assistant resident admission note |
| JBE | Japanese B encephalitis |
| JBS | Johanson Blizzard syndrome |
| JC | junior clinicians (medical students) |
| JCA | juvenile chronic arthritis |
| JCAHO | Joint Commission on Accreditation of Healthcare Organizations |
| JCC | Jackson cross cylinder (astigmatism test) |
| JCOG | Japanese Clinical Oncology Group |
| JCQ | Job Content Questionnaire |
| JD | Doctor of Jurisprudence (a law degree) |
| | jaundice |
| JDG | jugulodigastric |
| JDM | juvenile diabetes mellitus |
| JDMS | juvenile dermatomyositis |
| JE | Japanese encephalitis |
| JEB | junctional escape beat |
| JEJ | jejunum |

| | | | |
|---|---|---|---|
| JEN | Japanese encephalitis vaccine | | joint protection |
| JER | junctional escape rhythm | JPB | junctional premature beats |
| JET | jejunal extension tube | JP BS | Jackson-Pratt to bulb suction |
| | junctional ectopic tachycardia | JPC | junctional premature contraction |
| JEV | Japanese encephalitis virus | JPS | joint position sense |
| JF | joint fluid | JR | junctional rhythm |
| JFS | Jewish Family Service | JRA | juvenile rheumatoid arthritis |
| JGCT | juvenile granulosa cell tumor | JRAN | junior resident admission note |
| JHR | Jarisch-Herxheimer reaction | Jr BF | junior baby food |
| JI | jejunoileal | JRC | joint replacement center |
| JIA | juvenile idiopathic arthritis | JSF | Japanese spotted fever |
| JIB | jejunoileal bypass | JSRV | jaagziekte sheep retrovirus |
| JIS | juvenile idiopathic scoliosis | JT | jejunostomy tube |
| | | | joint |
| JJ | jaw jerk | | junctional tachycardia |
| J & J | Johnson & Johnson Health Care Systems, Inc. | JTF | jejunostomy tube feeding |
| | | JTJ | jaw-to-jaw (position) |
| | | JTP | joint projection |
| JLO | Judgment of Line Orientation (test) | JTPS | juvenile tropical pancreatitis syndrome |
| JLP | juvenile laryngeal papillomatosis | J-Tube | jejunostomy tube |
| | | JUV | juvenile |
| JM-9 | iproplatin | JV | jugular vein |
| JME | juvenile myoclonic epilepsy | JVC | jugular venous catheter |
| | | JVD | jugular venous distention |
| JMS | junior medical student | JVI | jugular-valve incompetencce |
| JNA | juvenile nasopharyngeal angiofibroma | JVP | jugular venous pressure |
| | | | jugular venous pulsation |
| JNB | jaundice of newborn | | jugular venous pulse |
| JNCL | juvenile-onset neuronal ceroid lipofuscinosis | JVPT | jugular venous pulse tracing |
| JND | just noticeable difference | JW | Jehovah's Witness |
| JNT | joint | Jx | joint |
| JNVD | jugular neck vein distention | JXG | juvenile xanthogranuloma |
| JODM | juvenile-onset diabetes mellitus | | |
| JOMAC | judgment, orientation, memory, abstraction, and calculation | | |
| JOMACI | judgment, orientation, memory, abstraction, and calculation intact | | |
| JOR | jaw-opening reflex | | |
| JP | Jackson-Pratt (drain) | | |
| | Jobst pump | | |

J

# K

| | | | |
|---|---|---|---|
| | | | keratoconus |
| | | | knees-to-chest |
| | | | Korean conflict |
| | | kcal | kilocalorie |
| | | KCCT | kaolin cephalin clotting time |
| K | cornea | | |
| | kelvin | KChIPs | potassium channel-interacting proteins |
| | ketamine (Ketalar, Vitamin K, Special K, and Super K) | kCi | kilocurie |
| | | KCl | potassium chloride |
| | kilodalton | KCS | keratoconjunctivitis sicca |
| | Kosher | KCZ | ketoconazole (Nizoral) |
| | potassium | KD | Kawasaki disease |
| | thousand | | Keto Diastix® |
| | vitamin K | | ketogenic diet |
| K' | knee | | kidney donors |
| $K^+$ | potassium | | knee disarticulation |
| $K_1$ | phytonadione | | knowledge deficit |
| $K_2$ | menatetrenone | Kd | kilodalton |
| $K_3$ | menadione | KDA | known drug allergies |
| $K_4$ | menadiol sodium diphosphate | KDC® | brand name of infant warmer |
| 17K | 17-ketosteroids | KDQ | Kidney Disease Questionnaire |
| 510(k) | Medical Device Premarket Notification | KDU | Kidney Dialysis Unit |
| KA | kainic acid | KE | first order elimination rate constant in hr.$^{-1}$ |
| | keratoacanthoma | | |
| | ketoacidosis | KED | Kendrick extrication device |
| Ka | first order absorption constant in hr.$^{-1}$ | $k_{el}$ | elimination rate constant |
| | | KET | ketoconazole (Nizoral) |
| KAB | knowledge, attitude, and behavior | | ketones |
| | | KETO | ketoconazole (Nizoral) |
| K-ABC | Kaufman Assessment Battery for Children | 17 Keto | 17 ketosteroids |
| | | keV | kilo-electron volts |
| KABINS | knowledge, attitude, behavior, and improvement in nutritional status | KEVD | Krupin eye valve with disk |
| | | KF | kidney function |
| | | KFA | kinetic fibrinogen assay |
| | | KFAB | kidney-fixing antibodies |
| KACT | kaolin-activated clotting time | KFAO | knee-foot-ankle orthosis |
| | | KFD | Kyasanur Forrest disease |
| KAFO | knee-ankle-foot orthosis | KFR | Kayser-Fleischer ring |
| KAO | knee-ankle orthosis | KFS | Klippel-Feil syndrome |
| KAS | Katz Adjustment Scale | kg | kilogram |
| KASH | knowledge, abilities, skills, and habits | K-G | Kimray-Greenfield (filter) |
| | | KGF | keratinocyte growth factor |
| kat | katal | KGC | Keflin, gentamicin, and carbenicillin |
| K-A units | King-Armstrong units | | |
| KB | ketone bodies | 17-KGS | 17-ketogenic steroids |
| | kilobase | KGy | kiloGray |
| | knee-bearing | KHF | Korean hemorrhagic fever |
| KBD | Kashin-Beck disease | K24H | potassium, urine 24-hour |
| KC | kangaroo care | kHz | kilohertz |
| | keratoconjunctivitis | KI | karyopyknotic index |

K

| | | | |
|---|---|---|---|
| | knee immobilizer | KQI | key quality indicators |
| | potassium iodide | Kr | krypton |
| KID | keratitis, ichthyosis, and deafness (syndrome) | K-rod | Küntscher rod |
| | | KS | Kawasaki syndrome |
| | kidney | | Kaposi sarcoma |
| kilo | kilogram | | kidney stone |
| | thousand | | Klinefelter syndrome |
| KIN | kinetic | 17-KS | 17-ketogenic steroids |
| KISS | saturated solution of | | 17-ketosteroids |
| | potassium iodide | KSA | knowledge, skills, and |
| KIT | Kahn Intelligence Test | | abilities |
| KIU | kallikrein inhibitor units | K-SADS | Kiddie Schedule for |
| KJ | kilojoule | | Affective Disorders and |
| | knee jerk | | Schizophrenia |
| KJR | knee jerk reflex | KSE | knee sling exercises |
| KK | knee kick | KSHV | Kaposi sarcoma- |
| | knock-knee | | associated herpesvirus |
| KKS | kallikrein-kinin system | KS/OI | Kaposi sarcoma and |
| K & L | Kellgren and Lawrence | | opportunistic infections |
| | (scale for osteoarthritis | KSP | Karolinska Scales of |
| | assessment) | | Personality |
| KLB | klebsiella vaccine | KSR | potassium chloride |
| KL-BET | Kleihauer-Betke | | sustained release |
| Kleb | *Klebsiella* | | (tablets) |
| KLH | keyhole limpet hemocyanin | KSS | Kearns-Sayre syndrome |
| K-Lor® | potassium chloride tablets | KSW | knife stab wound |
| KLS | kidneys, liver, and spleen | KT | kidney transplant |
| | Kleine-Levin syndrome | | kinesiotherapy |
| KM | kanamycin | | known to |
| KMG | kangaroo-mother care | KTC | knee-to-chest |
| KMnO4 | potassium permanganate | KTP | potassium-titanyl- |
| KMO | Kaiser-Meyer-Olkin | | phosphate (laser) |
| | (measure of statistical | KTS | Klippel-Trenaunay |
| | sampling adequacy) | | syndrome |
| KMV | killed measles vaccine | KTU | kidney transplant unit |
| KN | knee | | known to us |
| KNO | keep needle open | KTZ | ketoconazole (Nizoral) |
| KNSA | Kron Nutritive Sucking | KUB | kidney(s), ureter(s), and |
| | Apparatus | | bladder |
| KO | keep open | | kidney ultrasound biopsy |
| | knee orthosis | KUS | kidney(s), ureter(s), |
| | knocked out | | and spleen |
| KOH | potassium hydroxide | KV | kilovolt |
| KOR | keep open rate | KVO | keep vein open |
| KP | hot pack | KVP | kilovolt peak |
| | keratoprecipitate | KW | Keith-Wagener |
| | kinetic perimetry | | (ophthalmoscopic |
| kPa | kilopascal | | finding, graded I-IV) |
| KPE | Kelman | | Kimmelstiel-Wilson |
| | phacoemulsification | KWB | Keith, Wagener, Barker |
| KPM | kilopounds per minute | KWIC | keyword in context |
| KPS | Karnofsky performance status (scores) (scale) | K-wire | Kirschner wire |

K

# L

| | |
|---|---|
| L | fifty |
| | left |
| | lente insulin (this is a dangerous abbreviation, since there is also a Lantus insulin available) |
| | levorotatory |
| | lingual |
| | *Listeria* |
| | liter |
| | liver |
| | lumbar |
| | lung |
| l | levorotatory |
| L′ | lumbar |
| Ⓛ | left |
| L₁...L₅ | lumbar nerve 1 through 5 |
| | lumbar vertebra 1 through 5 |
| L1-2 | lumbar spine, between first and second vertebrae (the disk space) |
| LA | language age |
| | latex agglutination |
| | Latin American |
| | left arm |
| | left atrial |
| | left atrium |
| | leukoaraiosis (a radiologic finding) |
| | light adaptation |
| | linguoaxial |
| | linoleic acid |
| | local anesthesia |
| | long acting |
| | lupus anticoagulant |
| L + A | light and accommodation |
| | living and active |
| LAA | large artery atherosclerosis |
| | left atrium and its appendage |
| LAAM | levomethadyl acetate (L-alpha acetylmeth-adol, Orlaam) |
| LAAs | leukemia-associated antigens |

| | |
|---|---|
| LAB | laboratory |
| | left abdomen (LAb) |
| LABA | laser-assisted balloon angioplasty |
| LABBB | left anterior bundle branch block |
| LABC | locally advanced breast cancer |
| LABD | linear immunoglobulin A bullous dermatosis |
| LAC | laceration |
| | *lactobacillus acidophilus* vaccine |
| | laparoscopic-assisted colectomy |
| | left antecubital |
| | left atrial catheter |
| | locally advanced cancer |
| | long arm cast |
| | lupus anticoagulant |
| LAc | Licensed Acupuncturist |
| LACC | locally advanced cervical carcinoma |
| LACI | lacunar circulation infarct |
| | lipoprotein-associated coagulation inhibitor |
| LACT-ART | lactate arterial |
| LAD | left anterior descending |
| | left axis deviation |
| | leukocyte adhesion deficiency |
| | ligament augmentation device |
| LADA | left anterior descending (coronary) artery |
| LADCA | left anterior descending coronary artery |
| LADD | left anterior descending diagonal |
| LAD-MIN | left axis deviation minimal |
| LADPG | laparoscopically assisted distal partial gastrectomy |
| LAE | left atrial enlargement |
| | long above elbow |
| LAEC | locally advanced esophageal cancer |
| LAF | laminar air flow |
| | Latin American female |
| | low animal fat |
| | lymphocyte-activating factor |

| | | | |
|---|---|---|---|
| LAFB | left anterior fascicular block | LAPA | locally-advanced pancreatic adenocarcinoma |
| LAFF | lateral arm free flap | | |
| LAFM | locally acquired *Plasmodium falciparum* malaria | LAP-APPY | laparoscopic appendectomy |
| | | LAPC | locally-advanced prostate cancer |
| LAFR | laminar airflow room | | |
| LAG | lymphangiogram | LAP CHOLE | laparoscopic cholecystectomy |
| LAH | left anterior hemiblock left atrial hypertrophy | | |
| | | LAPMS | long arm posterior molded splint |
| LAHB | left anterior hemiblock | | |
| LAI | left atrial isomerism | LAPW | left atrial posterior wall |
| LAIT | latex agglutination inhibition test | LAQ | long arc quad |
| | | LAR | left arm, reclining long-acting release low anterior resection |
| LAK | lymphokine-activated killer | | |
| LAL | left axillary line limulus amebocyte lysate | LARM | left arm |
| | | LARS | laparoscopic antireflux surgery |
| LALLS | low-angle laser light scattering | | |
| | | LARSI | lumbar anterior-root stimulator implants |
| LALT | larynx-associated lymphoid tissue low air loss therapy (mattress) | | |
| | | LAS | lactic acidosis syndrome laxative abuse syndrome left arm, sitting leucine acetylsalicylate long arm splint low-amplitude signal lymphadenopathy syndrome lymphangioscintigraphy lysine acetylsalicylate |
| LAM | lactational anovulatory method (birth control) laminectomy laminogram Latin American male lymphangioleiomyomatosis | | |
| lam✓ | laminectomy check | | |
| LAMA | laser-assisted microanastomosis | LASA | Linear Analogue Self-Assessment (scales) lipid-associated sialic acid |
| LAMB | mucocutaneous lentigines, atrial myxoma, and blue nevus (syndrome) | | |
| | | LASCC | locally advanced squamous cell carcinoma |
| L-AMB | liposomal amphotericin B | LASEC | left atrial spontaneous echo contrast |
| LAMMA | laser microprobe mass analysis | | |
| | | LASER | light amplification by stimulated emission of radiation |
| LAN | lymphadenopathy | | |
| LANC | long arm navicular cast | | |
| LA-NSCLC | locally advanced nonsmall-cell lung cancer | LASIK | laser *in situ* keratomileusis |
| | | L-ASP | asparaginase (Elspar) |
| LAO | left anterior oblique | LAST | left anterior small thoracotomy |
| LAP | laparoscopy laparotomy left abdominal pain left atrial pressure leucine amino peptidase leukocyte alkaline phosphatase lower abdominal pain | | |
| | | LASW | Licensed Advanced Social Worker |
| | | LAT | lateral latex agglutination test left anterior thigh |
| | | LATCH | literature attached to chart |
| | | lat.men. | lateral meniscectomy |

185

| | | | |
|---|---|---|---|
| LATS | long-acting thyroid stimulator | LBNP | lower-body negative pressure |
| LAUP | laser-assisted uvula-palatoplasty | LBO | large bowel obstruction |
| | | LBOTC | laryngeal and base-of-tongue carcinomas |
| LAV | lymphadenopathy associated virus | LBP | low back pain |
| LAVA | laser-assisted vasal anastomosis | | low blood pressure |
| | | LBQC | large base quad cane |
| LAVH | laparoscopically assisted vaginal hysterectomy | LBS | low back syndrome |
| | | | pounds |
| LAW | left atrial wall | LBT | low back tenderness |
| LAWER | life-terminating acts without the explicit request | | low back trouble |
| | | LBV | left brachial vein |
| | | | low biological value |
| LAX | laxative | LBVO | left brachial vein occlusion |
| LB | large bowel | | |
| | lateral bend | LBW | lean body weight |
| | left breast | | low birth weight (less than 2,500 g) |
| | left buttock | | |
| | live births | LBWI | low birth weight infant |
| | low back | LC | Laënnec cirrhosis |
| | lung biopsy | | laparoscopic cholecystectomy |
| | lymphoid body | | |
| | pound | | left circumflex |
| L&B | left and below | | leisure counseling |
| LB3 | colonoscope | | level of consciousness |
| LBA | laser balloon angioplasty | | levocarnitine (Carnitor) |
| | lower body adiposity | | living children |
| LBB | left breast biopsy | | low calorie |
| | long back board | | lung cancer |
| LBBB | left bundle branch block | L & C | lids and conjunctivae |
| | | 3LC | triple-lumen catheter |
| LBBx | left breast biopsy | LCA | Leber congenital amaurosis |
| LBCD | left border of cardiac dullness | | left circumflex artery |
| | | | left coronary artery |
| L/B/Cr | electrolytes, blood urea nitrogen, and serum creatinine (see page 362) | | light contact assist |
| | | LCAD | long-chain acyl-coenzyme A dehydrogenase |
| | | LCAH | life-care at home |
| LBD | large bile duct | LCAL | large-cell anaplastic lymphoma |
| | left border dullness | | |
| | Lewy body dementia | LCAT | lecithin cholesterol acyltransferase |
| | low back disability | | |
| LBE | long below elbow | LCB | left costal border |
| LBG | Landry-Guillain-Barré (syndrome) | LCCA | left circumflex coronary artery |
| LBH | length, breadth, and height | | left common carotid artery |
| LBM | last bowel movement | | leukocytoclastic angiitis |
| | lean body mass | LCCS | low cervical cesarean section |
| | loose bowel movement | | |
| LBMI | last body mass index | LCD | coal tar solution (*liquor carbonis detergens*) |
| LBNA | lysis bladder neck adhesions | | |

L

|  | localized collagen dystrophy | LCS | Leydig cell stimulation |
|  | low-calcium diet |  | lids, conjunctiva, and sclera |
| LCDC | Laboratory Centre for Disease Control (Canada) |  | low constant suction |
|  |  |  | low continuous suction |
|  |  |  | Lung Cancer Subscale |
| LCDCP | low-contact dynamic compression plate | LCSG | left cardiac sympathetic ganglionectomy |
| LCDE | laparoscopic common duct exploration |  | lost child support group |
|  |  | LCSS | Lung Cancer Symptom Score |
| LCE | laparoscopic cholecystectomy | LCSW | Licensed Clinical Social Worker |
|  | left carotid endarterectomy |  | low continuous wall suction |
| LCF | left circumflex | LCT | long-chain triglyceride |
| LCFA | long-chain fatty acid |  | low cervical transverse |
| LCFM | left circumflex marginal |  | lymphocytotoxicity |
| LCGU | local cerebral glucose utilization | LCTA | lungs clear to auscultation |
| LCH | Langerhans cell histiocytosis | LCTCS | low cervical transverse cesarean section |
|  | local city hospital | LCTD | low-calcium test diet |
| LCIS | lobular cancer *in situ* | LCV | leucovorin |
| LCL | lateral collateral ligament |  | leukocytoclastic vasculitis |
| LCLC | large-cell lung carcinoma |  | low cervical vertical |
| LCM | laser-capture microdissection | LCX | left circumflex coronary artery |
|  | left costal margin | LD | lactic dehydrogenase (formerly LDH) |
|  | lower costal margin |  | laser Doppler |
|  | lymphocytic choriomeningitis |  | last dose |
| LCMI | left ventricular mass index |  | latissimus dorsi |
| LC-MS-MS | liquid chromatography coupled to tandem mass spectrometry |  | learning disability |
|  |  |  | learning disorder |
|  |  |  | left deltoid |
| LCN | lidocaine |  | Legionnaires disease |
| LCNB | large-core needle biopsy |  | lethal dose |
| LCO | low cardiac output |  | levodopa |
| LCP | long, closed, posterior (cervix) |  | Licensed Dietician |
| LCPD | Legg-Calvé-Perthes disease |  | liver disease |
|  |  |  | living donor |
| LCPUFAs | long-chain polyunsaturated fatty acids |  | loading dose |
|  |  |  | long dwell |
|  |  |  | low density |
| LCR | cerebrospinal fluid (French) |  | low dosage |
|  |  |  | Lyme disease |
|  | late cortical response | L&D | labor and deliver |
|  | late cutaneous reaction | L/D | labor and delivery |
|  | ligase chain reaction |  | light to dark (ratio) |
|  | locus control region | LD-1 | lactic dehydrogenase 1 |
| LCRS | Living Conditions Rating Scale | LD-5 | lactic dehydrogenase 5 |
|  |  | LD$_{50}$ | median lethal dose |

| | | | |
|---|---|---|---|
| LDA | laser-Doppler anemometry | LE | left ear |
| | low density areas | | left eye |
| | low-dose arm | | lens extraction |
| LDB | Legionnaires disease | | leptin |
| | bacterium | | live embryo |
| LDCOC | low-dose combination | | lower extremities |
| | oral contraceptive | | lupus erythematosus |
| LDD | laser disk decompression | LEA | lower extremity |
| | Lee and Desu D (test) | | amputation |
| | light-dark discrimination | | lumbar epidural |
| LDDS | local dentist | | anesthesia |
| LDEA | left deviation of electrical | LEAD | lower extremity arterial |
| | axis | | disease |
| LDF | laser-Doppler flowmetry | LEAP | Lower Extremity |
| LDH | lactic dehydrogenase | | Amputation Prevention |
| LDIH | left direct inguinal hernia | | (program) |
| LDIR | low-dose of ionizing | LEB | lumbar epidural block |
| | radiation | LEC | lens epithelial cell |
| LDI-TOF-MS | laser desorption/ionization time-of-flight-mass | LECBD | laparoscopic exploration of the common bile duct |
| | spectrometer | LED | liposomal encapsulated |
| LDL | low-density lipoprotein | | doxorubicin (Doxil) |
| LDL-C | low-density lipoprotein | | lowest effective dose |
| | cholesterol | | lupus erythematosus |
| LDLT | living donor liver | | disseminatus |
| | transplantation | LEEP | loop electrosurgical |
| LDM | lorazepam, | | excision procedure |
| | dexamethasone, and | LEF | lower extremity fracture |
| | metoclopramide | LEH | liposome-encapsulated |
| LDMRT | low-dose mediastinal | | hemoglobin |
| | radiation therapy | LEHPZ | lower esophageal high |
| LDNF | lung-derived | | pressure zone |
| | neurotrophic factor | LEJ | ligation of the |
| LDO | Licensed Dispensing | | esophagogastric |
| | Optician | | junction |
| l-dopa | levodopa | LEL | low-energy laser |
| LD-PCR | limiting dilution | LEM | lateral eye movements |
| | polymerase chain | | light electron microscope |
| | reaction | LEMS | Lambert-Eaton myasthenic |
| LDR | labor, delivery, and | | syndrome |
| | recovery | LENT-SOMA | Late Effect of Normal Tissue—Subjective |
| | length-to-diameter ratio | | Objective Management |
| | long-duration response | | Analytic (toxicity table) |
| LDR/P | labor, delivery, recovery, | LEP | leptospirosis |
| | and postpartum | | liposome-encapsulated |
| LDT | left dorsotransverse | | paclitaxel |
| LD-T | lactic dehydrogenase total | | lower esophageal pressure |
| LDUB | long double upright | LEP 2 | leptospirosis 2 |
| | brace | LE prep | lupus erythematosus |
| LDUH | low-dose unfractionated | | preparation |
| | heparin | L-ERX | leukoerythroblastic |
| LDV | laser-Doppler | | reaction |
| | velocimetry | | |

L

| | | | |
|---|---|---|---|
| LES | local excitatory state | LFL | left frontolateral |
| | lower esophageal sphincter | LFM | lateral force microscopy |
| | | LFP | left frontoposterior |
| | lumbar epidural steroids | LFS | leukemia-free survival |
| | lupus erythematosus systemic | | Li-Fraumeni syndrome |
| | | | liver function series |
| LESEP | lower extremity somatosensory evoked potential | LFT | latex flocculation test |
| | | | left fronto-transverse |
| | | | liver function tests |
| LESG | Late Effects Study Group | | low-flap transverse |
| LESI | lumbar epidural steroid injection | LFU | limit flocculation unit |
| | | | lost to follow-up |
| LESP | lower esophageal sphincter pressure | LG | large |
| | | | laryngectomy |
| LET | left esotropia | | left gluteal |
| | leukocyte esterase test | | linguogingival |
| | lidocaine, epinephrine and tetracaine gel | | lymphography |
| | | L-G | Lich-Gregoire (ureteroneocystostomy) |
| | linear energy transfer | | |
| LEU | leucine | LGA | large for gestational age |
| LEV | levamisole (Ergamisol) | | left gastric artery |
| | levator muscle | LGG | low-grade gliomas |
| LEVA | levamisole (Ergamisol) | L-GG | *Lactobacillus rhamnosus* strain GG |
| LF | laparoscopic fundoplications | LGI | lower gastrointestinal (series) |
| | Lassa fever | | |
| | left foot | LGIOS | low-grade intraosseous-type osteosarcoma |
| | left frontal | | |
| | living female | LGL | large granular lymphocyte |
| | low fat | | low-grade lymphoma(s) |
| | low forceps | | Lown-Ganong-Levine (syndrome) |
| | low frequency | | |
| LFA | left femoral artery | LGLS | Lown-Ganong-Levine syndrome |
| | left forearm | | |
| | left fronto-anterior | LGM | left gluteus medius (maximus) |
| | leukocyte function-associated antigen | | |
| | | LGN | lateral geniculate leaflet |
| | low-friction arthroplasty | | lobular glomerulonephritis |
| | lymphocyte function-associated antigen | LG-NHL | low-grade non-Hodgkin lymphoma |
| LFA-1 | leukocyte function-associated antigen-1 | LGS | Lennox-Gastaut syndrome |
| | | | low-Gomco suction |
| LFB | low-frequency band | LGSIL | low-grade squamous intraepithelial lesion |
| LFC | living female child | | |
| | low-fat and cholesterol | LGV | lymphogranuloma venerum |
| LFCS | low-flap cesarean section | | |
| LFD | lactose-free diet | LH | learning handicap |
| | low-fat diet | | left hand |
| | low-fiber diet | | left hemisphere |
| | low-forceps delivery | | left hyperphoria |
| | lunate fossa depression | | luteinizing hormone |
| LFGNR | lactose fermenting gram-negative rod | | lymphoid hyperplasia |
| | | LHA | left hepatic artery |

**L**

| | | | |
|---|---|---|---|
| LHC | left heart catheterization | | liver (migration) inhibitory factor |
| LHD | left-hand dominant | | |
| LHF | left heart failure | LIFE | laser-induced fluorescence emission |
| LHG | left hand grip | | |
| LHH | left homonymous hemianopsia | | lung imaging fluorescence endoscopy |
| LHI | Labor Health Institute | LIG | ligament |
| LHL | left hemisphere lesions | | lymphocyte immune globulin |
| | left hepatic lobe | | |
| LHON | Leber hereditary optic neuropathy | LIGHTS | phototherapy lights |
| | | LIH | laparoscopic inguinal herniorrhaphy |
| LHP | left hemiparesis | | |
| LHR | legal health record | | left inguinal hernia |
| | leukocyte histamine release | LIHA | low impulsiveness, high anxiety |
| LHRH | luteinizing hormone-releasing hormone | LIJ | left internal jugular |
| | | LILA | low impulsiveness, low anxiety |
| LHRH-A | luteinizing hormone-releasing hormone analogue | LILT | low-intensity laser therapy |
| | | LIM | limited toxicology screening |
| LHRT | leukocyte histamine release test | LIMA | left internal mammary artery (graft) |
| LHS | left hand side | | |
| | long-handled sponge | LIMS | laboratory information management system(s) |
| LHSH | long-handled shoe horn | | |
| LHT | left hypertropia | LINDI | lithium-induced nephrogenic diabetes insipidus |
| LI | lactose intolerance | | |
| | lamellar ichthyosis | | |
| | large intestine | LING | lingual |
| | laser iridotomy | LIO | laser-indirect ophthalmoscope |
| | learning impaired | | |
| | linguoincisal | | left inferior oblique (muscle) |
| | liver involvement | | |
| Li | lithium | LIOU | laparoscopic intraoperative ultrasound |
| LIA | laser interference acuity | | |
| | left iliac artery | LIP | lithium-induced polydipsia |
| LIB | left in bottle | | |
| LIC | left iliac crest | | lymphocytic interstitial pneumonia |
| | left internal carotid | | |
| | leisure interest class | LIPV | left inferior pulmonary vein |
| LICA | left internal carotid artery | | |
| | | LIQ | liquid |
| LICD | lower intestinal Crohn disease | | liquor |
| | | | lower inner quadrant |
| LICM | left intercostal margin | LIR | left iliac region |
| Li$_2$CO$_3$ | lithium carbonate | | left inferior rectus |
| LICS | left intercostal space | LIS | left intercostal space |
| Lido | lidocaine | | locked-in syndrome |
| LIF | laser-induced fluorescence | | low intermittent suction |
| | left iliac fossa | | |
| | left index finger | | lung injury score |
| | leukemia-inhibiting factor | LISS | low ionic strength saline |

L

| | | | |
|---|---|---|---|
| LISW | Licensed Independent Social Worker | LLAs | lipid-lowering agents |
| | | LLAT | left lateral |
| LIT | literature | LLB | last living breath |
| | liver injury test | | left lateral bending |
| LITA | left internal thoracic artery | | left lateral border |
| | | | long leg brace |
| LITH | lithotomy | LLC | laparoscopic laser cholecystectomy |
| LITHO | lithotripsy | | |
| LITT | laser-induced thermotherapy | | Lewis lung carcinoma |
| | | | long leg cast |
| LIV | left innominate vein | LLBCD | left lower border of cardiac dullness |
| L-IVP | limited intravenous pyelogram | | |
| | | LLD | left lateral decubitus |
| LIVB | live birth | | left length discrepancy |
| LIVC | left inferior vena cava | | leg length differential |
| LIVPRO | liver profile (see page 362) | LLE | left lower extremity |
| | | | little league elbow |
| LIWS | low intermittent wall suction | LLETZ | large-loop excision of the transformation zone |
| LJ | left jugular | LLFG | long leg fiberglas (cast) |
| LJL | lateral joint line | LLG | left lateral gaze |
| LJM | limited joint mobility | LL-GXT | low-level graded exercise test |
| LK | lamellar keratoplasty | | |
| | left kidney | LLL | left lower lid |
| LKA | Lazare-Klerman-Armour (Personality Inventory) | | left lower lobe (lung) |
| | | LLLE | lower lid, left eye |
| LKM-3 | liver-kidney microsomal antibodies type 3 | LLLNR | left lower lobe, no rales |
| | | LLLT | low-level laser therapy |
| LKS | Landau-Kleffner syndrome | LLN | lower limit of normal |
| | | LLO | Legionella-like organism |
| | liver, kidneys, spleen | LLOD | lower lid, right eye |
| LKSB | liver, kidneys, spleen, and bladder | | lower limit of detection |
| | | LLOS | lower lid, left eye |
| LKSNP | liver, kidneys, and spleen not palpable | LLP | Limited Liability Partnership |
| LL | large lymphocyte | | long leg plaster |
| | left lateral | LLPDD | late luteal phase dysphoric disorder |
| | left leg | | |
| | left lower | LLPS | low-load prolonged stress |
| | left lung | | |
| | lid lag | LLQ | left lower quadrant (abdomen) |
| | long leg (brace or cast) | | |
| | lower lid | LLR | left lateral rectus |
| | lower lip | LLRE | lower lid, right eye |
| | lower lobe | LLS | lazy leukocyte syndrome |
| | lumbar laminectomy | LLSB | left lower sternal border |
| | lumbar length | LLSD | laser light scattering detector |
| | lymphocytic leukemia | | |
| | lymphoblastic lymphoma | LLT | left lateral thigh |
| L&L | lids and lashes | | lowest level term |
| LL2 | limb lead two | LLWC | long leg walking cast |
| LLA | lids, lashes, and adnexa | LLX | left lower extremity |
| | limulus lysate assay | LM | left main |

L

| | | | |
|---|---|---|---|
| | light microscopy | LMS | lateral medullary syndrome |
| | linguomesial | | leiomyosarcomas |
| | living male | | left main trunk |
| | lung metastases | LMT | left mentotransverse |
| L/M | liters per minute | | Licensed Massage Therapist |
| LMA | laryngeal mask airway | | light moving touch |
| | left mentoanterior | LMW | low molecular weight |
| | liver membrane autoantibody | LMWD | low molecular weight dextran |
| LMAM | left message on answering machine | LMWH | low molecular weight heparins |
| LMB | Laurence-Moon-Biedl syndrome | LN | latent nystagmus |
| | left main bronchus | | left nostril (nare) |
| LMC | living male child | | lymph nodes |
| LMCA | left main coronary artery | $LN_2$ | liquid nitrogen |
| | left middle cerebral artery | LNA | alpha-linolenic acid |
| LMCAT | left middle cerebral artery thrombosis | LNB | lymph node biopsy |
| LMCL | left midclavicular line | LNCs | lymph node cells |
| LMD | local medical doctor | LND | light-near dissociation |
| | low molecular weight dextran | | lonidamine |
| | | | lymph node dissection |
| LME | left mediolateral episiotomy | LNE | lymph node enlargement |
| | | | lymph node excision |
| LMEE | left middle ear exploration | LNF | laparoscopic Nissen fundoplication |
| LMF | left middle finger | | |
| | melphalan (L-PAM), methotrexate, and fluorouracil | LNG | levonorgestrel |
| | | LNM | lymph node metastases |
| LMFT | Licensed Marriage and Family Therapist | LNMC | lymph node mononuclear cells |
| LMHC | Licensed Mental Health Counselor | LNMP | last normal menstrual period |
| LMI | large multivalent immunogen | LNNB | Luria-Nebraska Neuropsychological Battery |
| L/min | liters per minute | LNS | lymph node sampling |
| LML | left medial lateral | LNT | late neurological toxicity |
| | left middle lobe | LO | lateral oblique (x-ray view) |
| LMLE | left mediolateral episiotomy | | linguo-occlusal |
| LMM | lentigo maligna melanoma | | lumbar orthosis |
| LMN | letter of medical necessity | 5-LO | 5-lipoxygenase |
| | lower motor neuron | LOA | late-onset agammaglobulinemia |
| LMNL | lower motor neuron lesion | | leave of absence |
| LMP | last menstrual period | | left occiput anterior |
| | left mentoposterior | | looseness of associations |
| | low malignant potential | | lysis of adhesions |
| LMR | left medial rectus | LOAD | late-onset Alzheimer disease |
| LMRM | left modified radical mastectomy | | |
| LMRP | Local Medical Review Policy | LOAEL | lowest observed adverse effect level |

| LOB | loss of balance | LoNa | low sodium |
| LOC | laxative of choice | LOO | length of operation |
| | level of care | LOP | laparoscopic orchiopexy |
| | level of comfort | | leave on pass |
| | level of concern | | left occiput posterior |
| | level of consciousness | | level of pain |
| | local | LOQ | limit(s) of quantitation |
| | loss of consciousness | | lower outer quadrant |
| LOCF | last observation carried | LOR | loss of resistance |
| | forward (used for | LORS-I | Level of Rehabilitation |
| | inputting data missing | | Scale-I |
| | due to dropouts in | LOS | length of stay |
| | longitudinal clinical | | loss of sight |
| | trials) | | low-output syndrome |
| LOCM | low-osmolality contrast | LOT | left occiput transverse |
| | media | | Licensed Occupational |
| LOD | limit of detection | | Therapist |
| | line of duty | LOV | loss of vision |
| LOE | left otitis externa | LOVA | loss of visual acuity |
| LOEL | lowest-observed-effect | LOX | lipid oxidation |
| | level | LOZ | lozenge |
| LOF | leaking of fluids | LP | Licensed Psychologist |
| | leave on floor | | light perception |
| LOFD | low outlet forceps | | linguopulpal |
| | delivery | | lipid panel (see page 362) |
| LOG | Logmar chart | | lipoprotein |
| LOH | loss of heterozygosity | | low protein |
| LOHF | late-onset hepatic failure | | lumbar puncture |
| LOHP | oxaliplatin (Eloxatin) | L/P | lactate-pyruvate ratio |
| LOIH | left oblique inguinal | LP5 | Life-Pak 5 |
| | hernia | LPA | left pulmonary artery |
| LOI | level of injury | Lp(a) | lipoprotein (a) |
| | Leyton Obsessional | LPA% | left pulmonary artery |
| | Inventory | | oxygen saturation |
| | loss of imprinting | L-PAM | melphalan (Alkeran) |
| LOINC | Logical Observation | LPC | laser photocoagulation |
| | Identifier Names and | | Licensed Professional |
| | Codes | | Counselor |
| LOL | laughing out loud | LPCC | Licensed Professional |
| | left occipitolateral | | Certified Counselor |
| | little old lady | LPC-L | lymphoplasmacytoid |
| LOLINAD | little old lady in no | | lymphoma |
| | apparent distress | LPcP | light perception with |
| LOM | left otitis media | | projection |
| | limitation of motion | LPD | leiomyomatosis |
| | little old man | | peritonealis |
| | loss of motion | | disseminata |
| | low-osmolar (contrast) | | low potassium dextran |
| | media | | low-protein diet |
| LOMSA | left otitis media, | | luteal phase defect |
| | suppurative, acute | | luteal phase deficiency |
| LOMSC | left otitis media, | | lymphoproliferative |
| | suppurative, chronic | | disease |

L

| | | | |
|---|---|---|---|
| LPDA | left posterior descending artery | LPV | left portal vein |
| | | | left pulmonary vein |
| LPEP | left pre-ejection period | | lopinavir |
| LPF | liver plasma flow | LQTS | long QT (interval) syndrome |
| | low-power field | | |
| | lymphocytosis-promoting factor | LR | labor room |
| | | | lactated Ringer (injection) |
| LPFB | left posterior fascicular block | | laser resection |
| | | | lateral rectus |
| LPH | left posterior hemiblock | | left-right |
| | lumbar puncture headache | | light reflex |
| LPHB | left posterior hemiblock | | likelihood ratios |
| LPI | laser peripheral iridectomy | L&R | left and right |
| | | L → R | left to right |
| | leukotriene pathway inhibitor | LR1A | labor room 1A |
| | | LRA | left radial artery |
| LPICA | left posterior internal carotid artery | | left renal artery |
| | | LRC | locoregional control |
| LPIH | left-posterior-inferior hemiblock | | lower rib cage |
| | | LRCP | Licentiate of the Royal College of Physicians |
| LPL | laparoscopic pelvic lymphadenectomy | LRCS | Licentiate of the Royal College of Surgeons |
| | left posterolateral | LRD | limb reduction defects |
| | lipoprotein lipase | | living-related donor |
| LPLC | low-pressure liquid chromatography | | living renal donor |
| | | LRDT | living-related donor transplant |
| LPLND | laparoscopic pelvic lymph node dissection | | |
| | | LRE | localization-related epilepsy |
| LPM | latent primary malignancy | LREH | low-renin essential hypertension |
| | liters per minute | | |
| LPN | Licensed Practical Nurse | LRF | left rectus femoris |
| LPO | left posterior oblique | | left ring finger |
| | light perception only | | local-regional failure |
| LPPC | leukocyte-poor packed cells | L&R gtt | Levophed and Regitine drip (infusion) |
| LPPH | late postpartum hemorrhage | LRHT | living-related hepatic transplantation |
| LPR | leprosy (Hansen disease) vaccine | LRI | lower respiratory infection |
| LPS | last Pap smear | | |
| | lipopolysaccharide | LRLT | living-related liver transplantation |
| LP SHUNT | lumboperitoneal shunt | | |
| | | LRM | left radical mastectomy |
| LPsP | light perception without projection | | local regional metastases |
| | | LRMP | last regular menstrual period |
| LPT | leptospirosis (Leptospira-Leptospires sp.) vaccine | LRND | left radical neck dissection |
| | | LRO | long range objective |
| | Licensed Physical Therapist | Lrot | left rotation |
| | | LRP | laparoscopic radical prostatectomy |
| LPTN | Licensed Psychiatric Technical Nurse | | lung-resistance protein |

| | | | |
|---|---|---|---|
| LRQ | lower right quadrant | | liquid scintillation |
| LROU | lateral rectus, both eyes | | counting |
| LRR | light reflection | LSCA | left scapuloanterior |
| | rheography | LSCC | laryngeal squamous cell |
| LRRT | locoregional radiotherapy | | carcinoma |
| LRS | lactated Ringer solution | LSCCB | limited-state small-cell |
| LRT | living renal transplant | | cancer of the bladder |
| | local radiation therapy | LSCM | laser-scanning confocal |
| | lower respiratory tract | | microscopy |
| LRTD | living relative transplant | LSCP | left scapuloposterior |
| | donor | LSCS | lower segment cesarean |
| LRTI | ligament reconstruction | | section |
| | with tendon | LSD | least significant difference |
| | interposition | | low-salt diet |
| | lower respiratory tract | | lumbosacral derangement |
| | infection | | lysergide |
| LRV | left renal vein | LSE | local side effects |
| | log reduction value | LSed | level of sedation |
| LRZ | lorazepam (Ativan) | LSF | low-saturated fat |
| LS | left side | LSFA- | low-saturated fatty acid |
| | legally separated | | (diet) |
| | Leigh syndrome | LSH | laparoscopic supracervical |
| | liver scan | | hysterectomy |
| | liver-spleen | | leishmaniasis vaccine |
| | low salt | LSI | levonorgestrel subdermal |
| | lumbosacral | | implant |
| | lung sounds | L-SIL | low-grade squamous |
| L/S | lecithin-sphingomyelin | | intraepithelial lesions |
| | ratio | LSK | liver, spleen, and |
| L&S | ligation and stripping | | kidneys |
| | liver and spleen | LSKM | liver-spleen-kidney- |
| L5-S1 | lumbar fifth vertebra to | | megalgia |
| | sacral first vertebra | LSL | left sacrolateral |
| | (where the lumbar and | | left short leg (brace) |
| | sacral spines join) | LSLF | low sodium, low fat (diet) |
| LSA | left sacrum anterior | LSM | laser scanning microscope |
| | lipid-bound sialic acid | | late systolic murmur |
| | lymphosarcoma | | least squares mean |
| LSB | left scapular border | | limited sampling model |
| | left sternal border | | liver, spleen masses |
| | local standby | LSMFT | liposclerosing |
| | lumbar spinal block | | myxofibrous tumor |
| | lumbar sympathetic | LSMT | life-sustaining medical |
| | block | | treatment |
| LS BPS | laparoscopic bilateral | LSO | left salpingo- |
| | partial salpingectomy | | oophorectomy |
| LSC | last sexual contact | | left superior oblique |
| | late systolic click | | lumbosacral orthosis |
| | least significant change | LSP | left sacrum posterior |
| | left subclavian (artery) | | liver-specific (membrane) |
| | (vein) | | lipoprotein |
| | lichen simplex | L–Spar | Elspar (asparaginase) |
| | chronicus | L-SPINE | lumbar spine |

| | | | |
|---|---|---|---|
| LSQ | Life Situation Questionnaire | LTCBDE | laparoscopic transcystic common bile duct exploration |
| LSR | left superior rectus | | |
| L/S ratio | lecithin/sphingomyelin ratio | LTCCS | low transverse cervical cesarean section |
| LSS | limb-sparing surgery | LTCF | long-term care facility |
| | liver-spleen scan | LTCH | long-term care hospital |
| | lumbar spinal stenosis | LTC-IC | long-term culture-initiating cells |
| LSSS | Liverpool Seizure Severity Scale | LTCS | low-transverse cesarean section |
| LST | left sacrum transverse | LTD | largest tumor dimension |
| LSTC | laparoscopic tubal coagulation | | leg transfer device |
| | | | long-term disability |
| LSTL | laparoscopic tubal ligation | $LTD_4$ | leukotriene $D_4$ |
| L's & T's | lines and tubes | LTE | less than effective |
| LSU | life support unit | $LTE_4$ | leukotriene $E_4$ |
| LSV | left subclavian vein | LTED | long-term estrogen deprivation |
| LSVC | left superior vena cava | | |
| LSW | left-side weakness | LTFU | long-term follow-up |
| | Licensed Social Worker | LTG | lamotrigine (Lamictal) |
| LT | laboratory technician | | long-term goal |
| | left | | low-tension glaucoma |
| | left thigh | LTGA | left transposition of great artery |
| | left triceps | | |
| | leukotrienes | LTH | left total hip (arthroplasty) |
| | Levin tube | | luteotropic hormone |
| | light | LTK | laser thermal keratoplasty |
| | light touch | | left total knee (arthroplasty) |
| | low transverse | LTL | laparoscopic tubal ligation |
| | lumbar traction | | |
| | lung transplantation | LTM | long-term memory |
| | lunotriquetral | | long-term monitoring |
| | lymphotoxin | LTNPs | long-term nonprogressors (AIDS patients) |
| L&T | lettuce and tomato | | |
| LT4 | levothyroxine | LTOT | long-term oxygen therapy |
| LTA | laryngotracheal applicator | LTP | laser trabeculoplasty |
| | | | long-term plan |
| | laryngeal tracheal anesthesia | | long-term potentiation |
| | | LTPA | leisure-time physical activity |
| | lateral thoracic arteries | | |
| | local tracheal anesthesia | LTR | long terminal repeats |
| LTAC | long-term acute care | | lower trunk rotation |
| LTAS | left transatrial septal | LTRA | leukotriene receptor antagonist |
| LTB | laparoscopic tubal banding | | |
| | laryngotracheobronchitis | LTS | laparoscopic tubal sterilization |
| $LTB_4$ | leukotriene $B_4$ | | |
| LTBI | latent tuberculosis infection | | long-term survivors |
| LTC | left to count | LTT | lactose tolerance test |
| | long-term care | | lymphocyte transformation test |
| | long thick closed | | |
| $LTC_4$ | leukotriene $C_4$ | LTUI | low transverse uterine incision |
| LTC-101 | long-term care form-101 | | |

| LTV | long-term variability | LVAD | left ventricular assist |
| | Luche tumor virus | | device |
| LTV+ | long-term variability– | LV Angio | left ventricular angiogram |
| | average to moderate | L-VAM | leuprolide acetate, |
| LTV 0 | long-term | | vinblastine, doxorubicin |
| | variability–absent | | (Adriamycin), and |
| LTVC | long-term venous | | mitomycin |
| | catheter | LVAS | left ventricular assist |
| LTWN | long-term low-level white | | system |
| | noise | LVAT | left ventricular activation |
| LTZ | letrozole (Femara) | | time |
| LU | left upper | LVBP | left ventricle bypass pump |
| | left ureteral | LVD | left ventricular dimension |
| | living unit | | left ventricular |
| | Lutheran | | dysfunction |
| L & U | lower and upper | LVDd | left ventricular end- |
| LUA | left upper arm | | diastolic diameter |
| LUD | left uterine displacement | LVDP | left ventricular diastolic |
| LUE | left upper extremity | | pressure |
| Lues I | primary syphilis | LVDs | left ventricular systolic |
| Lues II | secondary syphilis | | diameter |
| Lues III | tertiary syphilis | LVDT | linear variable differential |
| LUL | left upper lid | | transformer |
| | left upper lobe (lung) | LVDV | left ventricular diastolic |
| LUNA | laparoscopic uterosacral | | volume |
| | nerve ablation | LVE | left ventricular enlargement |
| LUOB | left upper outer buttock | LVEDD | left ventricular end- |
| LUOQ | left upper outer quadrant | | diastolic diameter |
| LUQ | left upper quadrant | LVEDP | left ventricular end |
| LURD | living-unrelated donor | | diastolic pressure |
| LUS | laparoscopic | LVEDV | left ventricular end- |
| | ultrasonography | | diastolic volume |
| | lower uterine segment | LVEF | left ventricular ejection |
| LUSB | left upper scapular border | | fraction |
| | left upper sternal border | LVEP | left ventricular end |
| LUST | lower uterine segment | | pressure |
| | transverse | LVESD | left ventricular end- |
| LUT | lower urinary tract | | systolic dimension |
| LUTD | lower urinary tract | LVESVI | left ventricular end- |
| | dysfunction | | systolic volume index |
| LUTS | lower urinary tract | LVET | left ventricular ejection |
| | symptoms | | time |
| LUTT | lower urinary tract tumor | LVF | left ventricular failure |
| LUW | lungworm vaccine | | left visual field |
| LUX | left upper extremity | LVFP | left ventricular filling |
| LV | leave | | pressure |
| | left ventricle | LVFU | leucovorin and |
| | leucovorin | | fluorouracil |
| | live virus | LVG | left ventrogluteal |
| LVA | left ventricular aneurysm | LVH | left ventricular |
| LVC | laser vision correction | | hypertrophy |
| | low viscosity cement | LVID | left ventricular internal |
| | low vision clinic | | diameter |

**L**

| | | | |
|---|---|---|---|
| LVIDd | left ventricle internal diameter at end-diastole | LW | lacerating wound |
| | | | living will |
| LVIDs | left ventricle internal dimension systole | L & W | Lee and White (coagulation) |
| LVL | large volume leukapheresis | | living and well |
| | | LWAQ | Living with Asthma Questionnaire |
| | left vastus lateralis | | |
| LVM | left ventricular mass | LWCT | Lee-White clotting time |
| LVMI | left ventricular mass index | LWBS | left without being seen |
| LVMM | left ventricular muscle mass | LWC | leave without consent |
| | | LWCT | left without completing treatment |
| LVN | Licensed Visiting Nurse | | |
| | Licensed Vocational Nurse | LWOP | leave without pay |
| LVO | left ventricular overactivity | LWOT | left without treatment |
| | | LWP | large whirlpool |
| LVOT | left ventricular outflow tract | LX | larynx local irradiation |
| | | | lower extremity |
| LVOTO | left ventricular outflow tract obstruction | LXC | laxative of choice |
| | | LXT | left exotropia |
| LVP | large volume parenteral | LYCD | live yeast cell derivative |
| | left ventricular pressure | LYEL | lost years of expected life |
| LVPW | left ventricular posterior wall | LYG | lymphomatoid granulomatosis |
| LVR | leucovorin | LYM | Lyme disease vaccine |
| LVRS | lung-volume reduction surgery | | lymphocytes |
| | | lymphs | lymphocytes |
| LVRT | liver-volume replaced by tumor | LYS | large yellow soft (stools) |
| | | | life-year saved (cost of) |
| LVS | laryngeal videostroboscopy | | lysine |
| | | lytes | electrolytes (Na, K, Cl, etc.) |
| | left ventricular strain | | |
| LVS EMI | left ventricular subendocardial myocardial ischemia | | electrolyte panel (see page 362) |
| | | LZ | landing zone |
| LVSI | lymph-vascular space invasion | LZP | lorazepam (Ativan) |
| LVSP | left ventricular systolic pressure | | |
| LVSW | left ventricular stroke work | | |
| LVSWI | left ventricular stroke work index | | |
| LVT | levetiracetam (Keppra) | | |
| LVV | left ventricular volume | | |
| | live varicella vaccine | | |
| LVW | left ventricular wall | | |
| LVWI | left ventricular work index | | |
| LVWMA | left ventricular wall motion abnormality | | |
| LVWMI | left ventricular wall motion index | | |
| LVWT | left ventricular wall thickness | | |

L

# M

M    male
manual
marital
married
masked (audiology)
mass
medial
memory
mesial
meta
meter (m)
mild
million
minimum
molar
Monday
monocytes
mother
mouth
murmur
muscle
*Mycobacterium*
*Mycoplasma*
myopia
myopic
thousand

Ⓜ    murmur

$M_1$    first mitral sound

M1    left mastoid
tropicamide 1%
ophthalmic solution
(Mydriacyl)

M1 to M7    categories of acute
nonlymphoblastic
leukemia

$M_2$    second mitral sound

$m^2$    square meters (body
surface)

M2    right mastoid

M-2    vincristine, carmustine,
cyclophosphamide,
melphalan, and
prednisone

$M_3$    third mitral sound

M-3    medical student 3rd year

3M    mitomycin, mitoxantrone,
and methotrexate

M-3+7    mitoxantrone and
cytarabine

M-4    medical student 4th year

MA    machine
Master of Arts
mean arterial (blood
pressure)
medical assistance
medical authorization
megestrol acetate
menstrual age
mental age
meter angle
Mexican American
microalbuminuria
metabolic acidosis
microaneurysms
Miller-Abbott (tube)
milliamps
monoclonal antibodies
motorcycle accident

M/A    mood and/or affect

MA-1    Bennett volume
ventilator

MAA    macroaggregates of
albumin
Marketing Authorization
Application (European
Union)

MAAS    Motor Activity
Assessment Scale

MAB    Massachusetts Biologic
Laboratories
maximum androgen
blockade

Mab    monoclonal antibody

MABP    mean arterial blood
pressure

MAC    macrocytic erythrocytes
macrophage
macula
maximal allowable
concentration
medial arterial
calcification
membrane attack complex
Mental Adjustment to
Cancer (scale)
methotrexate,
dactinomycin
(Actinomycin D), and
cyclophosphamide
mid-arm circumference

minimum alveolar concentration

monitored anesthesia care

multi-access catheter

*Mycobacterium avium complex*

**MACC** methotrexate, doxorubicin, (Adriamycin) cyclophosphamide, and lomustine (Cee Nu)

**MACCC** Master Arts, Certified Clinical Competence

**MACE** Malon antegrade continence enema

**MACOP-B** methotrexate, doxorubicin, (Adriamycin) cyclophosphamide, vincristine (Oncovin), prednisone, and bleomycin with leucovorin rescue

**MACRO** macrocytes

**MACS** magnetic activated cell sorting

**MACs** malignancy-associated changes

**MACTAR** McMaster-Toronto Arthritis Patient Reference (Disability Questionnaire)

**MAD** major affective disorder

mind altering drugs

moderate atopic dermatitis

**MADD** Mothers Against Drunk Driving

**MADL** mobility activities of daily living

**MADRS** Montgomery-Åsburg Depression Rating Scale

**MAE** medical air evacuation

moves all extremities

**MAES** moves all extremities slowly

**MAEEW** moves all extremities equally well

**MAEW** moves all extremities well

**MAF** malignant ascites fluid

metabolic activity factor

Mexican-American female

**MAFAs** movement-associated fetal (heart rate) accelerations

**MAFO** molded ankle/foot orthosis

**MAFP** maternal alpha-fetoprotein

**MAG** medication administration guideline (record)

**mag cit** magnesium citrate

**MAGP** meatal advancement glanduloplasty

**mag sulf** magnesium sulfate

**MAHA** macroangiopathic hemolytic anemia

**MAI** maximal aggregation index

minor acute illness

*Mycobacterium avium-intracellulare*

**MAID** mesna, doxorubicin (Adriamycin), ifosfamide, and dacarbazine

**MAL** malaria vaccine

malignant

midaxillary line

Motor Activity Log

**MALDI** matrix-assisted laser desorption ionization

**MALDI-TOFMS** matrix-assisted laser desorption ionization–time-of-flight mass spectrometry

**MALG** Minnesota antilymphoblast globulin

**malig** malignant

**MALT** mucosa-associated lymphoid tissue

**MALToma** lymphoma of mucosa-associated lymphoid tissue

**MAM** mammogram

Mexican-American male

monitored administration of medication

**MAMC** mid-arm muscle circumference

**Mammo** mammography

**MAMP** milliampere

**m-AMSA** amsacrine

**MAMTT** minimal active muscle tendon tension

| | |
|---|---|
| MAN | malignancy associated neutropenia |
| Mand | mandibular |
| MANE | Morrow Assessment of Nausea and Emesis |
| MANOVA | multivariate analysis of variance |
| MAO | maximum acid output |
| MAO-A | monoamine oxidase type A |
| MAO-B | monoamine oxidase type B |
| MAOI | monoamine oxidase inhibitor |
| MAOP | Mid-Atlantic Oncology Program |
| MAP | magnesium, ammonium, and phosphate (Struvite stones) |
| | mean airway pressure |
| | mean arterial pressure |
| | Medical Assistance Program |
| | megaloblastic anemia of pregnancy |
| | Miller Assessment for Preschoolers (test for developmental delays) |
| | mitogen-activated protein |
| | mitomycin, doxorubicin (Adriamycin), and cisplatin (Platinol) |
| | morning after pill (oral contraceptives) |
| | muscle-action potential |
| MAPC | multipotent adult progenitor cell |
| MAPI | Millon Adolescent Personality Inventory |
| MAPS | Make a Picture Story |
| MAR | marital |
| | medication administration record |
| | mineral apposition rates |
| MARE | manual active-resistive exercise |
| MARSA | methicillin-aminoglycoside-resistant *Staphylococcus aureus* |
| MAS | macrophage activation syndrome |
| | meconium aspiration syndrome |
| | Memory Assessment Scale |
| | minimum-access surgery |
| | mobile arm support |
| | Modified Ashworth Scale |
| MASA | mutant allele-specific amplification |
| MASDA<sup>SM</sup> | Multiple-Allele-Specific Diagnostic Assay |
| MASER | microwave amplification (application) by stimulated emission of radiation |
| MASH POT | mashed potatoes |
| MAST | mastectomy |
| | medical antishock trousers |
| | Michigan Alcoholism Screening Test |
| | military antishock trousers |
| MAT | manual arts therapy |
| | maternal |
| | maternity |
| | mature |
| | medication administration team |
| | Miller-Abbott tube |
| | multifocal atrial tachycardia |
| MATHS | muscle pain, allergy, tachycardia and tiredness, and headache syndrome |
| MAU | microalbuminuria |
| MAVR | mitral and aortic valve replacement |
| max | maxillary |
| | maximal |
| MAX A | maximum assistance (assist) |
| MAXCONT | maximum contrast method |
| MAxL | midaxillary line |
| MAYO | mayonnaise |
| MB | buccal margin |
| | mandible |
| | Mallory body |
| | Medical Board |
| | medulloblastoma |
| | mesiobuccal |
| | methylene blue |
| | myocardial bands |

| M/B | mother/baby | | medullary bone pain |
| MBA | Master of Business Administration | | mesiobuccopulpal |
| | | | myelin basic protein |
| M-BACOD | methotrexate (high-dose), bleomycin, doxorubicin (Adriamycin), cyclophosphamide, vincristine (Oncovin), and dexamethasone with leucovorin rescue | MBq | megabecquerels |
| | | MBS | modified barium swallow |
| | | MBT | maternal blood type |
| | | | multiple blunt trauma |
| | | MC | male child |
| | | | medium-chain (triglycerides) |
| MBC | male breast cancer | | metacarpal |
| | maximum bladder capacity | | metatarso - cuneiform |
| | | | microcalcifications (breast) |
| | maximum breathing capacity | | mini-laparotomy cholecystectomy |
| | metastatic breast cancer | | mitoxantrone and cytarabine |
| | methotrexate, bleomycin, and cisplatin | | mitral commissurotomy |
| | minimal bactericidal concentration | | mixed cellularity |
| MB-CK | a creatinine kinase isoenzyme | | molluscum contagiosum |
| | | | monocomponent highly purified pork insulin |
| MBD | metabolic bone disease | | *Moraxella catarrhalis* |
| | methylene blue dye | | mouth care |
| MBEST | modulus blipped echo-planar single-pulse technique | | myocarditis |
| | | m + c | morphine and cocaine |
| MBD | minimal brain damage | MCA | Medicines Control Agency (United Kingdom) |
| | minimal brain dysfunction | | |
| MBE | may be elevated | | megestrol, cyclophosphamide, and doxorubicin (Adriamycin) |
| | medium below elbow | | |
| MBF | meat-base formula | | metacarpal amputation |
| | myocardial blood flow | | micrometastases clonogenic assay |
| MBFC | medial brachial fascial compartment | | middle cerebral aneurysm |
| MBHI | Millon Behavioral Health Inventory | | middle cerebral artery |
| | | | monoclonal antibodies |
| MBI | methylene blue installation | | motorcycle accident |
| | | | multichannel analyzer |
| MBL | mannose-binding lectin | | multiple congenital anomalies |
| | menstrual blood loss | | |
| MBM | mind-body medicine | 2-MCA | 2-methyl citric acid |
| | mother's breast milk | MCAD | medium-chain acyl-CoA dehydrogenase |
| MBNW | multiple-breath nitrogen washout | | |
| | | MCAF | monocyte chemoattractant and activity factor |
| MBO | mesiobuccal occulusion | | |
| MBOT | mucinous borderline ovarian tumors | MCAO | middle cerebral artery occlusion |
| MBP | malignant brachial plexopathy | MCAP | middle cerebral artery pressure |
| | mannan-binding protein | | |
| | mannose-binding protein | | |

| | | | |
|---|---|---|---|
| MCAT | Medical College Admission Test | MCL | mantle cell lymphoma |
| | | | maximum comfort level |
| MCB | Medicines Control Board (United Kingdom's equivalent to the United States Food and Drug Administration) | | medial collateral ligament |
| | | | midclavicular line |
| | | | midcostal line |
| | | | modified chest lead |
| | | | most comfortable level |
| | midcycle bleeding | mcL | microliter (1/1,000 of an mL) |
| | middle chamber bubbling | | |
| McB pt | McBurney point | MCLL | most comfortable listening level |
| MCC | meningococcal serogroup C conjugate | | |
| | | MCLNS | mucocutaneous lymph node syndrome |
| | Merkel cell carcinoma | | |
| | microcrystalline cellulose | MCMI | Millon Clinical Multiaxial Inventory |
| | midstream clean-catch | | |
| MCCU | mobile coronary care unit | mcmol | micromoles (one millionth $[10^{-6}]$ of a mole) |
| MCD | malformation of cortical development | | |
| | | MCN | minimal change nephropathy |
| | mean cell diameter | | |
| | minimal-change disease | MCNS | minimal change nephrotic syndrome |
| | multicystic dysplasia | | |
| MCDK | multicystic dysplasia of the kidney | MCO | managed care organization |
| | | | mupirocin calcium ointment (Bactroban Nasal) |
| MCDT | mast cell degranulation test | | |
| MCE | major coronary event | MCP | mean carotid pressure |
| MCF | multicentric foci | | metacarpophalangeal joint |
| MCFA | medium-chain fatty acid | | metoclopramide (Reglan) |
| mcg | microgram (do not hand write μg, as it is mistakenly read as milligram [mg]) | | monocyte chemotactic protein |
| | | MCR | Medicare |
| | | | metabolic clearance rate |
| MCG | magnetocardiogram | | myocardial revascularization |
| | magnetocardiography | | |
| MCGN | minimal-change glomerular nephritis | MC=R | moderately constricted and equally reactive |
| MCH | mean corpuscular hemoglobin | MCRC | metastatic colorectal cancer |
| | microfibrillar collagen hemostat | MCS | manufacturer cannot supply |
| | muscle contraction headache | | mental component summary |
| MCHC | mean corpuscular hemoglobin concentration | | microculture and sensitivity |
| | | | moderate constant suction |
| MCHL | medial head of the coracohumeral ligament | | multiple chemical sensitivity |
| | | | myocardial contractile state |
| MCI | mild cognitive impairment | | |
| mCi | millicurie | MCSA | minimal cross-sectional area |
| MCID | minimum clinically important difference(s) | | |
| mckat | microkatal (1 millionth $[10^{-6}]$ of a katal) | M-CSF | macrophage colony-stimulating factor |

| | | | |
|---|---|---|---|
| MC-SR | moderately constricted and slightly reactive | | Multichannel Discrete Analyzer |
| MCT | manual cervical traction | MDAC | multiple-dose activated charcoal |
| | mean circulation time | | |
| | medial canthal tendon | MDACC | MD Anderson Cancer Center |
| | medium chain triglyceride | | |
| | medullary carcinoma of the thyroid | MDA LDL | malondialdehydeconjugated low-density lipoprotein |
| | microwave coagulation therapy | MDC | Major Diagnostic Category |
| MCTC | metrizamide computed tomography cisternogram | | medial dorsal cutaneous (nerve) |
| MCTD | mixed connective tissue disease | MDCM | mildly dilated congestive cardiomyopathy |
| MCTZ | methyclothiazide (Enduron) | MDD | major depressive disorder manic-depressive disorder |
| MCU | micturating cystourethrogram | MDE | major depressive episode |
| MCV | mean corpuscular volume | MDF | myocardial depressant factor |
| MCVRI | minimal coronary vascular resistance index | MDGF | macrophage-derived growth factor |
| MCYLS | marginal cost per year of life saved | MDI | manic-depressive illness |
| MD | macula degeneration | | mental developmental index |
| | maintenance dialysis | | metered-dose inhaler |
| | maintenance dose | | methylenedioxyindenes |
| | major depression | | multiple daily injection |
| | mammary dysplasia | | multiple dosage insulin |
| | manic depression | | |
| | mean deviation | MDIA | Mental Development Index, Adjusted |
| | medical doctor | | |
| | mediodorsal | MDII | multiple daily insulin injection |
| | Menière disease | | |
| | mental deficiency | MDIS | metered-dose inhaler-spacer (device) |
| | mesiodistal | | |
| | movement disorder | MDiv | Master of Divinity |
| | multiple dose | MDM | mid-diastolic murmur |
| | muscular dystrophy | | minor determinant mix (of penicillin) |
| | myocardial damage | | |
| MD-50® | diatrizoate sodium injection 50% | MDMA | methylenedioxy-methamphetamine (ecstasy) |
| MDA | malondialdehyde | | |
| | manual dilation of the anus | MDNT | midnight |
| | | MDO | mentally disordered offender |
| | Medical Devises Agency (United Kingdom) | | |
| | methylenedioxyamphet-amine | MDOT | modified directly observed therapy |
| | | MDP | methylene diphosphonate |
| | micrometastases detection assay | MDPH | Michigan Department of Public Health |
| | motor discriminative acuity | MDPI | maximum daily permissible intake |

| | | | |
|---|---|---|---|
| MDR | Medical Device Reporting (regulation) | | middle ear |
| | minimum daily requirement | | myalgic encephalomyelitis |
| | | M/E | metabloic/endocrine |
| | multidrug resistance | | myeloid-erythroid (ratio) |
| MD=R | moderately dilated and equally reactive | M&E | Mecholyl and Eserine |
| | | | mucositis and enteritis |
| MDR-1 | multidrug resistance gene | MEA | microwave endometrial ablation |
| MDRE | multiple-drug-resistant enterococci | | measles virus vaccine |
| MDREF | multidrug resistant enteric fever | MEA-I | multiple endocrine adenomatosis type I |
| MDRSP | multidrug resistant *Streptococcus pneumoniae* | MEB | Medical Evaluation Board |
| | | | methylene blue |
| | | MEC | meconium |
| | | | middle ear canal(s) |
| MDRTB | multidrug resistant tuberculosis | MeCCNU | semustine |
| | | MECG | maternal electrocardiogram |
| MDS | maternal deprivation syndrome | MeCP | semustine (methyl CCNU) cyclophosphamide, and prednisone |
| | Miller-Dieker syndrome | | |
| | Minimum Data Set | | |
| | myelodysplastic syndromes | MED | male erectile dysfunction |
| | | | medial |
| MD-SR | moderately dilated and slightly reactive | | median erythrocyte diameter |
| MDSU | medical day stay unit | | medical |
| MDT | maggot debridement therapy | | medication |
| | | | medicine |
| | Mechanical Diagnostic Therapist | | medium |
| | | | medulloblastoma |
| | motion detection threshold | | minimal erythema dose |
| | | | minimum effective dose |
| | multidisciplinary team | | |
| | multidrug therapy | MEd | Master of Education |
| MDTM | multidisciplinary team meeting | MEDAC | multiple endocrine deficiency Addison disease (autoimmune) candidiasis |
| MDTP | multidisciplinary treatment plan | | |
| MDU | maintenance dialysis unit | MEDCO | Medcosonolator |
| | microvascular Doppler ultrasonography | MedDRA | Medical Dictionary for Regulatory Activities |
| MDUO | myocardial disease of unknown origin | MEDEX | medication administration record |
| MDV | Marek disease virus | MED-LARS | Medical Literature Analysis and Retrieval System |
| | multiple dose vial | | |
| MDY | month, date, and year | | |
| ME | macular edema | MEDLINE | National Library of Medicine medical database |
| | manic episode | | |
| | medical events | | |
| | medical evidence | MED NEC | medically necessary |
| | medical examiner | MEDS | medications |
| | mestranol | MEE | maintenance energy expenditure |
| | Methodist | | |

|  |  |  |  |
|--|--|--|--|
| | measured energy expenditure | | *meningitidis*) serogroup B conjugate vaccine |
| | middle ear effusion | MEN<sub>ps</sub> | meningococcal (*Neisseria meningitidis*) polysaccharide vaccine, not otherwise specified |
| MEE/OC | middle ear exploration with ossicular chain reconstruction | | |
| MEF | maximum expired flow rate | MEN<sub>ps-ACYW</sub> | meningococcal (*Neisseria meningitidis*) serogroups A, C, Y, W-135 polysaccharide vaccine |
| | middle ear fluid | | |
| MEFR | mid expiratory flow rate | MEN<sub>ps-B</sub> | meningococcal (*Neisseria meningitidis*) serogroup B polysaccharide vaccine |
| MEFV | maximum expiratory flow-volume | | |
| MEG | magnetoencephalogram magnetoencephalography | MENS | microcurrent electrical neuromuscular stimulation mini-electrical nerve stimulator |
| Meg-CSF | megakaryocytic colony-stimulating factor | | |
| MEGX | monoethylglycinexylidide | | |
| MeHg | methylmercury | MEO | malignant external otitis |
| MEI | magnetic endoscope imaging | MeOH | methyl alcohol |
| | | MEOS | microsomal ethanol oxidizing system |
| | medical economic index | MEP | maximal expiratory pressure |
| MEIA | microparticle enzyme immunoassay | | meperidine motor-evoked potential multimodality-evoked potential |
| MEKC | micellar electrokinetic chromatography | | |
| MEL | melatonin | | |
| MELAS | mitochondrial encephalomyopathy with lactic acidosis, and stroke-like episodes (syndrome) | MEPS | Medical Expenditure Panel Survey |
| | | mEq | milliequivalent |
| | | mEq/24 H | milliequivalents per 24 hours |
| MEL B | melarsoprol (Arsobal) | mEq/L | milliequivalents per liter |
| MEM | memory | MER | medical evidence of record |
| | monocular estimate method (near retinoscopy) | | methanol-extracted residue (of phenol-treated BCG) |
| MEMB | modified eosin-methylene blue (agar) | | |
| MEN | meningeal meninges | M/E ratio | myeloid/erythroid ratio |
| | | MERRF | myoclonic epilepsy and ragged red fibers |
| | meningitis | | |
| | meningococcal (*Neisseria meningitidis*) (serogroups unspecified) vaccine | MES | mesial |
| | | MeSH | Medical Subject Headings of the National Library of Medicine |
| MEN (II) | multiple endocrine neoplasia (type II) | | |
| MEN<sub>cn-AC</sub> | meningococcal (*Neisseria meningitidis*) serogroups A, C conjugate vaccine | MESS | Mangled Extremity Severe Score |
| | | MET | medical emergency treatment |
| MEN<sub>cn-B</sub> | meningococcal (*Neisseria* | | metabolic |

|  | metamyelocytes |  | midforceps delivery |
|  | metastasis |  | milk-free diet |
|  | metronidazole |  | multiple fractions per day |
| meT | methyltestosterone | MFEM | maximal forced expiratory |
| META | metamyelocytes |  | maneuver |
| METH | methicillin | MFFT | Matching Familiar |
| MetHb | methemoglobin |  | Figures Test |
|  | methemoglobinemia | MFH | malignant fibrous |
| methyl CCNU | semustine |  | histiocytoma |
| methyl G | mitroguazone | MFI | mean fluorescent intensity |
|  | dihydrochloride | MFM | multifidus muscle |
|  | (Zyrkamine) | MFNS | mometasone furoate nasal |
| methyl GAG | mitroguazone |  | spray (Nasonex) |
|  | dihydrochloride | MFPS | myofascial pain |
|  | (Zyrkamine) |  | syndrome |
| METS | metabolic equivalents | MFR | mid-forceps rotation |
|  | (multiples of resting |  | myofascial release |
|  | oxygen uptake) | MFS | Marfan syndrome |
|  | metastases |  | maternal-fetal surgery |
| METT | maximum exercise |  | Miller-Fisher syndrome |
|  | tolerance test |  | mitral first sound |
|  |  |  | monofixation syndrome |
| MEV | million electron volts | MFT | muscle function test |
| MEWDS | multifocal evanescent | MFU | medical follow-up |
|  | white dot syndrome | MFVNS | middle fossa vestibular |
| MEX | Mexican |  | nerve section |
| MF | Malassezia folliculitis | MFVPT | Motor Free Visual |
|  | *Malassezia furfur* |  | Perception Test |
|  | masculinity/femininity | MFVR | minimal forearm vascular |
|  | meat-free |  | resistance |
|  | mesial facial | MG | Marcus Gunn |
|  | methotrexate and |  | Michaelis-Gutmann |
|  | fluorouracil |  | (bodies) |
|  | midcavity forceps |  | milligram (mg) |
|  | midforceps |  | myasthenia gravis |
|  | mother and father | mg | milligram |
|  | mycosis fungoides | Mg | magnesium |
|  | myelofibrosis | mG | milligauss |
|  | myocardial fibrosis | μg | microgram (1/1000 of a |
| M/F | male-female ratio |  | milligram) (This is a |
| M & F | male and female |  | dangerous abbreviation |
|  | mother and father |  | when hand written, as |
| MFA | malaise, fatigue, and |  | it is read as mg. |
|  | anorexia |  | Use mcg) |
| MFAT | multifocal atrial | M&G | myringotomy and |
|  | tachycardia |  | grommets |
| MFB | metallic foreign body | mg% | milligrams per 100 |
|  | multiple-frequency |  | milliliters |
|  | bioimpedance | MGBG | mitoguazone (Zyrkamine) |
| MFC | medial femoral condyle | MGCT | malignant glandular cell |
| MFCU | Medicaid Fraud Control |  | tumor |
|  | Unit | MGD | meibomian gland |
| MFD | Memory for Designs |  | dysfunction |

| | | | |
|---|---|---|---|
| MGd | motexafin gadolinium (Xcytrin) | mGy | milligray (radiation unit) |
| | | MH | macular hemorrhage |
| MGDF | megakaryocyte growth and development factor | | malignant hyperthermia |
| | | | marital history |
| mg/dl | milligrams per 100 milliliters | | medical history |
| | | | menstrual history |
| MGF | macrophage growth factor | | mental health |
| | | | moist heat |
| | mast cell growth factor | MHA | Mental Health Assistant |
| | maternal grandfather | | methotrexate, hydrocortisone, and cytarabine (ara-C) |
| MGG | May-Grünwald-Giemsa (stain) | | |
| | | | microangiopathic hemolytic anemia |
| MGGM | maternal great grandmother | | |
| | | | microhemagglutination |
| MGHL | middle glenohumeral ligament | MHA-TP | microhemagglutination-*Treponema pallidum* |
| mg/kg | milligram per kilogram | | |
| mg/kg/d | milligram per kilogram per day | MHB | maximum hospital benefits |
| | | MHb | methemoglobin |
| mg/kg/hr | milligram per kilogram per hour | MHBSS | modified Hank balanced salt solution |
| MGM | maternal grandmother | MHC | major histocompatibility complex |
| | milligram (mg is correct) | | |
| MGMA | Medical Group Management Association | | mental health center (clinic) |
| | | | mental health counselor |
| MGN | membranous glomerulonephritis | M/hct | microhematocrit |
| MGO | methylglyoxal | MHD | 10-hydroxycarbazepine (oxcarbazepine metabolite) |
| MgO | magnesium oxide | | |
| MG/OL | molecular genetics/oncology laboratory | | maintenance hemodialysis |
| | | mHg | millimeters of mercury |
| MGP | Marcus Gunn pupil | MHH | mental health hold |
| | medical group practice | MHI | Mental Health Index (information) |
| MGR | murmurs, gallops, or rubs | | |
| MGS | malignant glandular schwannoma | MHL | mesenchymal hamartoma of the liver |
| MgSO$_4$ | magnesium sulfate (Epsom salt) | MHIP | mental health inpatient |
| | | MH/MR | mental health and mental retardation |
| MGT | management | | |
| mgtt | minidrop (60 minidrops = 1 mL) | MHN | massive hepatic necrosis |
| | | MHO | medical house officer |
| MGUS | monoclonal gammopathy of undetermined significance | MHP | moist heat packs |
| | | MHRI | Mental Health Research Institute |
| MGW | multiple gunshot wound | MHS | major histocompatibility system |
| MGW enema | magnesium sulfate, glycerin, and water enema | | malignant hyperthermia susceptible |
| | | | monomethyl hydrogen sulfate |
| M-GXT | multistage graded exercise test | | multihospital system |

| | | | |
|---|---|---|---|
| MHT | malignant hypertension | MICU | medical intensive care |
| | mental health team | | unit |
| | Mental Health Technician | | mobile intensive care unit |
| MHTAP | microhemagglutination | MID | mesioincisodistal |
| | assay for antibody to | | microvillus inclusion |
| | *Treponema pallidum* | | disease |
| MHV | mechanical heart valves | | minimal ineffective dose |
| | middle hepatic vein | | multi-infarct dementia |
| MHW | medial heel wedge | MIDCAB | minimally invasive direct |
| | mental health worker | | coronary artery bypass |
| MHX | methohexital sodium | MID EPIS | midline episiotomy |
| MHx | medical history | Mid I | middle insomnia |
| MHxR | medical history review | MIE | maximim inspiratory |
| MHz | megahertz | | effort |
| MI | membrane intact | | meconium ileus equivalent |
| | mental illness | | (cystic fibrosis) |
| | mental institution | | medical improvement |
| | mesial incisal | | expected |
| | mitral insufficiency | MIEI | medication-induced |
| | myocardial infarction | | esophageal injury |
| MIA | medically indigent adult | MIF | Merthiolate, iodine, |
| | missing in action | | and formalin |
| MIBI | technetium Tc99m | | mifepristone (RU 486; |
| | sestamibi (a | | Mifeprex) |
| | myocardial perfusion | | migration inhibitory factor |
| | agent; Cardiolite) | MIFR | midinspiratory flow rate |
| MIBG | iobenguane sulfate I 123 | MIF | midinspiratory flow at |
| | (meta-iodobenzyl | 50% VC | 50% of vital capacity |
| | guanidine I 123) | MIG | measles immune globulin |
| MIBK | methylisobutylketone | MIGET | multiple inert gas |
| MIC | maternal and infant care | | elimination technique |
| | methacholine inhalation | MIH | medication-induced |
| | challenge | | headache |
| | medical intensive care | | migraine with |
| | microscope | | interparoxysmal |
| | microcytic erythrocytes | | headache |
| | minimum inhibitory | | myointimal hyperplasia |
| | concentration | MIL | military |
| MICA | mentally ill, chemical | | mesial incisal lingual |
| | abuser | | (surface) |
| MICAR | Mortality Medical | | mother-in-law |
| | Indexing, Classification, | MIMCU | medical intermediate care |
| | and Retrieval | | unit |
| MICE | mesna, ifosfamide, | MIN | mammary intraepithelial |
| | carboplatin, and | | neoplasia |
| | etoposide | | melanocytic |
| MICN | mobile intensive care | | intraepidermal |
| | nurse | | neoplasia |
| MICR | methacholine inhalation | | mineral |
| | challenge response | | minimum |
| MICRO | microcytes | | minor |
| MICS | minimally invasive | | minute (min) |
| | cardiac surgery | MIN A | minimal assistance (assist) |

| | | | |
|---|---|---|---|
| MIME | mitoguazone, ifosfamide, methotrexate, and etoposide with mesna | | Modified Injury Severity Score (Scale) |
| | | MIT | meconium in trachea |
| MINE | Medical Information Network of Europe | | miracidia immobilization test |
| | mesna, ifosfamide, mitoxantrone (Novantrone), and etoposide | | multiple injection therapy (of insulin) |
| | | MITO-C | mitomycin (Mutamycin) |
| | | MITOX | mitoxantrone (Novantrone) |
| | medical improvement not expected | MIU | million international units |
| MINI | Mini International Neuropsychiatric Interview | mIU | milli-international unit (one-thousandth of an International unit) |
| MIO | minimum identifiable odor | MIVA | mivacurium (Mivacron) |
| | | MIW | mental inquest warrant |
| | monocular indirect ophthalmoscopy | mix mon | mixed monitor |
| | | MJ | marijuana |
| MIP | macrophage inflammatory protein | | megajoule |
| | | MJD | Machado-Joseph Disease |
| | maximum inspiratory pressure | MJL | medial joint line |
| | | MJS | medial joint space |
| | maximum-intensity projection (radiology) | MJT | Mead Johnson tube |
| | | μkat | microkatal (micro-moles/sec) |
| | mean intrathoracic pressure | MKAB | may keep at bedside |
| | mean intravascular pressure | MKB | married, keeping baby |
| | | MK-CSF | megakaryocyte colony-stimulating factor |
| | medical improvement possible | MKI | mitotic-karyorrhectic index |
| | metacarpointerphalangeal | MKM | microgram per kilogram per minute |
| | Michigan Biologic Products Institute | | |
| MIRD | medical internal radiation dose | ML | malignant lymphoma |
| | | | mediolateral |
| MIRP | myocardial infarction rehabilitation program | | middle lobe |
| | | | midline |
| MIRS | Medical Improvement Review Standard | mL | milliliter |
| | | M/L | monocyte to lymphocyte (ratio) |
| MIS | management information systems | | mother-in-law |
| | minimally invasive surgery | MLA | medical laboratory assay |
| | mitral insufficiency | | mento-laeva anterior |
| | moderate intermittent suction | MLAC | minimum local analgesic concentration |
| MISC | miscarriage | MLAP | mean left atrial pressure |
| | miscellaneous | MLBW | moderately low birth weight |
| M Isch | myocardial ischemia | | |
| MISH | multiple in situ hybridization | MLC | metastatic liver cancer |
| | | | minimal lethal concentration |
| MISO | misonidazole | | |
| MISS | minimally invasive spine surgery | | mixed lymphocyte culture |
| | | | multilevel care |

| | | |
|---|---|---|
| | multilumen catheter | MLT | melatonin |
| | myelomonocytic leukemia, chronic | | mento-laeva transversa |
| MLD | manual lymph drainage | MLU | mean length of utterance |
| | masking level difference | MLV | monitored live voice |
| | melioidosis (*Pseudomonas pseudomallei*) vaccine | MLWHF | Minnesota Living with Heart Failure (questionnaire) |
| | metachromatic leukodystrophy | MM | major medical (insurance) malignant melanoma |
| | microlumbar diskectomy | | malignant mesothelioma |
| | microsurgical lumbar diskectomy | | Marshall-Marchetti medial malleolus |
| | minimal lethal dose | | member months |
| MLDT | Manual Lymph Drainage Therapist | | meningococcic meningitis mercaptopurine and methotrexate |
| MLE | maximum likelihood estimation | | methadone maintenance micrometastases |
| | midline (medial) episiotomy | | millimeter (mm) mismatch (ing) |
| MLF | median longitudinal fasciculus | | mist mask morbidity and mortality |
| MLN | manifest latent nystagmus | | motor meal |
| | mediastinal lymph node | | mucous membrane |
| | melanoma vaccine | | multiple myeloma |
| | mesenteric lymph node | | muscle movement |
| MLNS | minimal lesions nephrotic syndrome | mM. | myelomeningocele millimole (mmol) |
| | mucocutaneous lymph node syndrome (Kawasaki syndrome) | mm M&M | millimeter milk and molasses morbidity and mortality |
| MLO | mesiolinguo-occlusal | MMA | methylmalonic acid |
| MLP | mento-laeva posterior | | methylmethacrylate |
| | mesiolinguopulpal | MMC | mitomycin (mitomycin C) |
| | midlevel provider | | myelomeningocele |
| MLPN | Medical Licensed Practical Nurse | MMD | malignant metastatic disease |
| MLPP | maximum loose-packed position | | moyamoya disease mucus membranes dry |
| MLR | middle latency response | | myotonic muscular dystrophy |
| | mixed lymphocyte reaction | MMECT | multiple monitor electroconvulsive therapy |
| | multiple logistic regression | MMEFR | maximal mid-expiratory flow rate |
| MLRA | multiple linear-regression analysis | MMF | mean maximum flow mycophenolate mofetil (CellCept) |
| MLS | macrolides, lincosamides, and streptogramins | MMFR | maximal mid-expiratory flow rate |
| | Maroteaux-Lamy syndrome | MMG | mammography mechanomyography |
| | maximum likelihood score | | |
| | mediastinal B-cell lymphoma with sclerosis | | |

| | | | |
|---|---|---|---|
| mm Hg | millimeters of mercury | | number, |
| MMI | maximal medical improvement | | **r**ed hair or freckles, **i**nability to tan, sunburn, **k**indred |
| MMK | Marshall-Marchetti-Krantz (cystourethropexy) | | |
| MML | minimal masking level (audiology) | MMRS | Metropolitan Medical Response System |
| MMM | metastatic malignant melanoma | MMR-VAR | measles virus, mumps virus, rubella virus, and varicella virus vaccine |
| | mitoxantrone, methotrexate, and mitomycin | MMS | Mini-Mental State (examination) |
| | mucous membrane | | Mohs micrographic surgery |
| | moist | | |
| | myelofibrosis with myeloid metaplasia | MMSE | Mini-Mental State Examination |
| mMMSE | modified version of the mini mental status examination | MMT | malignant mesenchymal tumors |
| MMMT | malignant mixed mesodermal tumor | | manual muscle test meal-tolerance test medial meniscal tear methadone maintenance treatment |
| | metastatic mixed müllerian tumor | | |
| MMN | multifocal motor neuropathy | | Mini Mental Test mixed müllerian tumors |
| MMOA | maxillary mandibular odontectomy alveolectomy | MMTP | Methadone Maintenance Treatment Program |
| mmol | millimole | MMTV | malignant mesothelioma of the tunica vaginalis |
| μmol | micromole | | |
| MMP | matrix metalloproteinase | | monomorphic ventricular tachycardia |
| | multiple medical problems | | mouse mammary tumor virus |
| | multiplexed molecular profiling (system) | MMV | mandatory minute volume |
| MMP-8 | metalloproteinase-8 | MMWR | *Morbidity and Mortality Weekly Report* |
| MMPI | matrix metalloproteinase inhibitor | MN | midnight |
| | Minnesota Multiphasic Personality Inventory | | mononuclear |
| | | Mn | manganese |
| MMPI-D | Minnesota Multiphasic Personality Inventory-Depression Scale | M&N | morning and night Mydriacyl and Neo-Synephrine |
| 6-MMPR | 6-methylmercaptopurine riboside | MNC | monomicrobial necrotizing cellulitis |
| MMR | measles, mumps, and rubella | | mononuclear leukocytes |
| | | MNCV | motor nerve conduction velocity |
| | midline malignant reticulosis | MND | modified neck dissection |
| | mismatch repair | | motor neuron disease |
| MMRISK | a skin cancer mnemonic; **m**oles that are atypical, **m**oles that are many in | MNF | myelinated nerve fibers |
| | | MNG | multinodular goiter |
| | | MNM | mononeuritis multiplex |

| | | | |
|---|---|---|---|
| MNMCB | motor neuropathy with multifocal conduction block | MOCI | Maudsley Obsessive-Compulsive Inventory |
| MNNB | Monas-Nitz Neuropsychological Battery | MOD | maturity onset diabetes |
| | | | medical officer of the day |
| | | | mesio-occlusodistal |
| MNPRT | mixed neutron and photon radiotherapy | | moderate |
| | | | mode of death |
| MNR | marrow neutrophil reserve | | moment of death |
| MNSc | Master of Nursing Science | | multiorgan dysfunction |
| MnSOD | manganese superoxide dismutase | MOD A | moderate assistance (assist) |
| Mn SSEPS | median-nerve somatosensory-evoked potentials | MODM | mature-onset diabetes mellitus |
| | | MODS | multiple-organ dysfunction syndrome |
| MNTB | medial nucleus of the trapezoid body | MODY | maturity-onset diabetes of youth |
| MNX | meniscectomy | MOE | movement of extremities |
| MNZ | metronidazole | MOEMs | micro-opto-electro-mechanical systems |
| MO | medial oblique (x-ray view) | MOF | mesial occlusal facial |
| | menhaden oil | | methotrexate, vincristine (Oncovin), and fluorouracil |
| | mesio-occlusal | | |
| | mineral oil | | |
| | month (mo) | | methoxyflurane (Penthrane) |
| | months old | | |
| | morbidly obese | | multiple-organ failure |
| | mother | MOFS | multiple-organ failure syndrome |
| | myositis ossificans | | |
| Mo | molybdenum | MOG | myelin oligodendrocyte glycoprotein |
| M/O | morning of | | |
| MOA | mechanism of action | MOH | Ministry of Health |
| | metronidazole, omeprazole, and amoxicillin | Mohs | Mohs technique; serial excision and microscopic examination of skin cancers |
| MoAb | monoclonal antibody | | |
| MOAHI | mixed obstructive apnea and hypopnea index | MOI | mechanism of injury |
| MOB | medical office building | | multiplicity of infection |
| | mobility | MoICU | mobile intensive care unit |
| | mobilization | MOJAC | mood orientation, judgement, affect, and content |
| MOB-PT | mitomycin, vincristine (Oncovin), bleomycin, and cisplatin (Platinol AQ) | | |
| | | MOM | milk of magnesia |
| | | | mother |
| MOC | medial olivocochlear | | mucoid otitis media |
| | Medical Officer on Call | MoM | multiples of the median |
| | metronidazole, omeprazole, and clarithromycin | MOMP | major outer membrane protein |
| | | MON | maximum observation nursery |
| | mother of child | | monitor |

213

| | | | |
|---|---|---|---|
| MONO | infectious mononucleosis | | motor potential |
| | monocyte | | mouthpiece |
| | monospot | | myocardial perfusion |
| mono, di | monochorionic, diamniotic | M & P | Millipore and phase |
| mono, mono | monochorionic, monoamniotic | 4 MP | methylpyrazole (fomepizole; Antizol) |
| MOP | medical outpatient | 6-MP | mercaptopurine |
| 8 MOP | methoxsalen | | (Purenthol) |
| MOPP | mechlorethamine, vincristine (Oncovin), procarbazine, and prednisone | MPA | main pulmonary artery Medical Products Agency (Sweden) medroxyprogesterone acetate |
| MOPV | monovalent oral poliovirus vaccine | MPa | megapascal |
| MOR | morphine | MPAC | Memorial Pain Assessment Card |
| MOS | Medical Outcome Study | | |
| | mirror optical system | MPA/E₂C | medroxyprogesterone |
| | months | | acetate; estradiol |
| mOsm | milliosmol | | cypionate (Lunelle) |
| MOSF | multiple-organ system failure | MPAP | mean pulmonary artery pressure |
| MOS sf-20 | Medical Outcomes Study, short form 20 items | MPAQ | McGill Pain Assessment Questionnaire |
| MOS sf-36 | Medical Outcomes Study, short form, 36 items | MPB | male-pattern baldness mephobarbital |
| mOsmol | milliosmole | MPBFV | mean pulmonary-blood- |
| MOT | motility examination | | flow velocity |
| MOTS | mucosal oral therapeutic system | MPBNS | modified Peyronie bladder neck suspension |
| MOTT | mycobacteria other than tubercle | MPC | meperidine, promethazine, and chlorpromazine |
| MOU | medical oncology unit | | mucopurulent cervicitis |
| | memorandum of understanding | MPCN | microscopically positive and culturally negative |
| MOUS | multiple occurrences of unexplained symptoms | M-PCR | multiplex polymerase chain reaction |
| MOV | minimum obstructive volume | MPCU | medical progressive care unit |
| | multiple oral vitamin | MPD | maximum permissable |
| MOW | Meals on Wheels | | dose |
| MP | malignant pyoderma | | methylphenidate (Ritalin) |
| | melphalan and prednisone | | moisture permeable dressing |
| | menstrual period | | multiple personality |
| | mercaptopurine (Purinethol) | | disorder |
| | | | myeloproliferative disorder |
| | metacarpal phalangeal joint | | myofascial pain dysfunction (syndrome) |
| | mitoxantrone and prednisone | mPD | minimal peripheral dose |
| | moist park | MPE | malignant pleural effusion |
| | monitor pattern | | massive pulmonary |
| | monophasic | | embolism |

| | | | |
|---|---|---|---|
| | mean prediction error | MPPT | methylprednisolone pulse therapy |
| | multiphoton excitation | | |
| MPEC | multipolar electrocoagulation | MPR | massive periretinal retraction |
| MPEG | methoxypolyethylene glycol | MPS | mean particle size |
| | | | mononuclear phagocyte system |
| MPF | methylparaben free | | |
| m-PFL | methotrexate, cisplatin (Platinol), fluorouracil, and leucovorin | | mucopolysaccharidosis |
| | | | multiphasic screening |
| | | MPS-1 | mucopolysaccharidosis I |
| MPGN | membranoproliferative glomerulonephritis | MPSS | massively parallel signature sequencing |
| MPH | massive pulmonary hemorrhage | | methylprednisolone sodium succinate |
| | Master of Public Health | MPT | multiple parameter telemetry |
| | methylphenidate (Ritalin) | | |
| | miles per hour | MPTRD | motor, pain, touch, and reflex deficit |
| MPHD | multiple pituitary hormone deficiencies | MPU | maternal pediatric unit |
| MPI | master patient index | MPV | mean platelet volume |
| | Maudsley Personality Inventory | MQ | memory quotient |
| | | MR | Maddox rod |
| | myocardial perfusion imaging | | magnetic resonance |
| | | | manifest refraction |
| MPIF-1 | myeloid progenitor inhibitory factor-1 | | may repeat |
| | | | measles-rubella |
| MPJ | metacarpophalangeal joint | | medial rectus |
| MPK | milligram per kilogram | | medical record |
| MPL | maximum permissable level | | mental retardation |
| | | | milliroentgen |
| | mesiopulpolingual | | mitral regurgitation |
| MPL® | monophosphoryl lipid A | | moderate resistance |
| MPLC | medium pressure liquid chromatography | M&R | measure and record |
| | | MR × 1 | may repeat times one (once) |
| MPM | malignant peritoneal mesothelioma | MRA | magnetic resonance angiography |
| | malignant pleural mesothelioma | | main renal artery |
| | Mortality Prediction Model | | medical record administrator |
| MPN | monthly progress note | | medical research associate |
| | most probable number | | midright atrium |
| | multiple primary neoplasms | | multivariate regression analysis |
| MPO | male-pattern obesity | mrad | millirad |
| | myeloperoxidase | MRAN | medical resident admitting note |
| MPOA | medial preoptic area | | |
| MPP | massive periretinal proliferation | MRAP | mean right atrial pressure |
| | | MRAS | main renal artery stenosis |
| | maximum pressure picture | MRC | Master of Rehabilitation Counseling |
| MPP | multiple presentation phenotype | | |
| | | MRCA | magnetic resonance coronary angiography |
| MPQ | McGill Pain Questionnaire | | |

| | |
|---|---|
| MRCC | metastatic renal cell carcinoma |
| MRCP | magnetic resonance cholangiopancreatography |
| | Member of the Royal College of Physicians |
| | mental retardation, cerebral palsy |
| MRCPs | movement-related cortical potentials |
| MRCS | Member of the Royal College of Surgeons |
| MRD | margin reflex distance |
| | Medical Records Department |
| | Minimal Record of Disability |
| | minimal residual disease |
| MRDD | maximum recommended daily dose |
| | Mental Retardation and Development Disabilities |
| | mentally retarded and developmentally disabled |
| MRDM | malnutrition-related diabetes mellitus |
| MRE | manual resistance exercise |
| | most recent episode |
| MRFC | mouse rosette-forming cells |
| MR FIT | Multiple Risk Factor Intervention Trial |
| MRG | murmurs, rubs, and gallops |
| MRH | Maddox rod hyperphoria |
| MRHD | maximum recommended human dose |
| MRHT | modified rhyme hearing test |
| MRI | magnetic resonance imaging |
| M & R I & O | measure and record input and output |
| MRK | Merck & Co., Inc. |
| MRL | minimal response level |
| | moderate rubra lochia |
| MRLVD | maximum residue limits of veterinary drugs |
| MRLT | mesalamine-related lung toxicity |

| | |
|---|---|
| MRM | modified radical mastectomy |
| MRN | magnetic resonance neurography |
| | malignant renal neoplasm |
| | medical record number |
| | medical resident's note |
| mRNA | messenger ribonucleic acid |
| MROU | medial rectus, both eyes |
| MRP | multidrug resistance-associated protein |
| MP-RAGE | magnetization prepared rapid acquisition gradient-echo |
| MRPN | medical resident progress note |
| MRPs | medication-related problems |
| MRR | medical record review |
| MRS | magnetic resonance spectroscopy |
| | mental retardation syndrome |
| | methicillin-resistant *Staphylococcus aureus* |
| MRSA | methicillin-resistant *Staphylococcus aureus* |
| MRSE | methicillin-resistant *Staphylococcus epidermidis* |
| MRSI | magnetic resonance spectroscopic imaging |
| MRSS | methicillin-resistant *Staphylococcus* species |
| MRT | magnetic resonance tomography |
| | malignant rhabdoid tumor |
| | modified rhyme test |
| MRTA | magnetic resonance tomographic angiography |
| MRU | medical resource utilization |
| MRV® | mixed respiratory vaccine |
| MRX | *Moraxella catarrhalis* vaccine |
| MR × 1 | may repeat once |
| MS | mass spectroscopy |
| | Master of Science |
| | medical student |
| | mental status |
| | milk shake |

| | | | |
|---|---|---|---|
| | minimal support | MSCT | multislice computed tomography |
| | mitral sounds | | |
| | mitral stenosis | MSCU | medical special care unit |
| | moderately susceptible | MSCWP | musculoskeletal chest wall pain |
| | morning stiffness | | |
| | morphine sulfate | MSD | male sexual dysfunction |
| | motile sperm | | microsurgical diskectomy |
| | multiple sclerosis | | midsleep disturbance |
| | muscle spasm | | musculoskeletal disorder |
| | muscle strength | MSDBP | mean sitting diastolic blood pressure |
| | musculoskeletal | | |
| M & S | microculture and sensitivity | MSDS | material safety data sheet |
| 3MS | Modified Mini-Mental Status (examination) | MSE | Mental Status Examination |
| MS III | third-year medical student | Msec | milliseconds |
| MSA | Medical Savings Accounts | MSEL | myasthenic syndrome of Eaton-Lambert |
| | membrane-stabilizing activity | MSER | mean systolic ejection rate |
| | methane sulfonic acid | | Mental Status Examination Record |
| | metropolitan statistical area | MSF | meconium-stained fluid |
| | microsomal autoantibodies | | Médicins Sans Frontières (Doctors Without Borders) |
| | multiple system atrophy | | |
| MSAF | meconium-stained amniotic fluid | | megakaryocyte stimulating factor |
| MSAFP | maternal serum alpha-fetoprotein | MSG | massage |
| MSAP | mean systemic arterial pressure | | methysergide (Sansert) |
| | | | monosodium glutamate |
| MSAS | Mandel Social Adjustment Scale | MSH | melanocyte-stimulating hormone |
| MSAS-SF | Memorial Symptom Assessment Scale – short form | MSHA | mannose-sensitive hemagglutinin |
| | | MSI | magnetic source imaging |
| MSB | mainstem bronchus | | mass sociogenic illness |
| MSBOS | maximum surgical blood order schedule | | microsatellite instability |
| | | | multiple subcortical infarction |
| MSBP | Munchausen syndrome by proxy | | musculoskeletal impairment |
| MSC | major symptom complex | MSIA | mass spectrometric immunoassay |
| | midsystolic click | | |
| | MS Contin® | MSIR® | morphine sulfate immediate release tablets |
| MSCA | McCarthy Scales of Children's Abilities | | |
| MSCC | malignant spinal cord compression | MSIS | Multiple Severity of Illness System |
| | midstream clean-catch (urine culture) | MSK | medullary sponge kidney |
| | | | musculoskeletal |
| MSCCC | Master Sciences, Certified Clinical Competence | MSKCC | Memorial Sloan-Kettering Cancer Center |
| MSCs | mesenchymal stem cells | | |

| | | | |
|---|---|---|---|
| MSL | midsternal line | | mean survival time |
| | multiple symmetrical lipomatosis | | median survival time |
| | | | mental stress test |
| MSLT | multiple sleep latency test | | multiple subpial |
| MSM | magnetic starch microspheres | | transection |
| | | MSTA® | mumps skin test antigen |
| | men who have sex with men | MSTI | multiple soft tissue injuries |
| | methsuximide (Celontin) | MSTS | American Musculoskeletal |
| | methylsulfonylmethane | | Tumor Society |
| | midsystolic murmur | | (functional rating |
| MSN | Master of Science in Nursing | | system) |
| | | MSU | maple-syrup urine |
| MSNA | muscle sympathetic nerve activity | | midstream urine |
| | | | monosodium urate |
| MSO | managed services organization | MSUD | maple-syrup urine disease |
| | | MSUS | musculoskeletal |
| | mentally stable and oriented | | ultrasound |
| | | MSUs | midstream specimens of |
| | mental status, oriented | | urine |
| | most significant other | mSv | millisievert (radiation unit) |
| MSO₄ | morphine sulfate (this is a dangerous abbreviation) | MSW | Master of Social Work |
| | | | multiple stab wounds |
| | multisystem organ dysfunction | MT | empty |
| | | | macular target |
| MSOF | multisystem organ failure | | maggot therapy |
| MSPN | medical student progress notes | | maintenance therapy |
| | | | malaria therapy |
| MSPU | medical short procedure unit | | malignant teratoma |
| | | | Medical Technologist |
| MSQ | Mental Status Questionnaire | | metatarsal |
| | | | middle turbinate |
| | meters squared | | monitor technician |
| MSR | muscle stretch reflexes | | mucosal thickening |
| MSRPP | Multidimensional Scale for Rating Psychiatric Patients | | muscles and tendons |
| | | | muscle tone |
| | | | music therapy (Therapist) |
| MSS | Marital Satisfaction Scale | | myringotomy tube(s) |
| | mean sac size | M/T | masses of tenderness |
| | microsatellite stable | | myringotomy with tubes |
| | minor surgery suite | M & T | *Monilia* and *Trichomonas* |
| MSSA | methicillin-susceptible *Staphylococcus aureus* | | muscles and tendons |
| | | | myringotomy and tubes |
| MSS-CR | mean sac size and crown-rump length | MTA | Medical Technical Assistant |
| | | | metatarsal adduction |
| MSSP | Maternal Support Services Program | | multi-targeted antifolate (pemetrexed disodium [Alimta]) |
| MSSU | midstream specimen of urine | | |
| | | MTAD | tympanic membrane of the right ear |
| MST | maladies sexuellement transmissibles (French for sexually transmitted diseases) | | |
| | | MT/AK | music therapy/ audiokinetics |

| MTAS | tympanic membrane of the left ear |
|---|---|
| MTAU | tympanic membranes of both ears |
| MTB | *Mycobacterium tuberculosis* |
| MTBC | Music Therapist-Board Certified |
| MTBE | methyl tert-butyl ether |
| MTC | magnetization transfer contrast (radiology) |
| | medullary thyroid carcinoma |
| | metoclopramide |
| | mitomycin |
| MTCT | mother-to-child transmission |
| MTD | maximum tolerated dose |
| | metastatic trophoblastic disease |
| | minimum toxic dose |
| | Monroe tidal drainage |
| | *Mycobacterium tuberculosis* direct (test) |
| MTDDA | Minnesota Test for Differential Diagnosis of Aphasia |
| MTDI | maximum tolerable daily intake |
| MTDT | *Mycobacterium tuberculosis* direct test |
| MTE | multiple trace elements |
| MTE-4® | trace metal elements injection (there is also a #5, #6, and #7) |
| MTET | modified treadmill exercise testing |
| MTF | medical treatment facility |
| MTG | middle temporal gyrus (gyri) |
| | midthigh girth |
| MTHFR | methylene tetrahydrofolate reductase |
| MTI | magnetization transfer imaging |
| | malignant teratoma intermediate |
| MTJ | midtarsal joint |
| MTL | Metropolitan Life (Insurance Company) Table (for desirable weight) |

| MTLE | medial (mesial) temporal-lobe epilepsy |
|---|---|
| MTM | modified Thayer-Martin medium |
| | mouth-to-mouth (resuscitation) |
| MTNX | methylnaltrexone |
| mTOR | mammalian target of rapamycin |
| MTP | master treatment plan |
| | medical termination of pregnancy |
| | metatarsophalangeal |
| | microsomal triglyceride transfer protein |
| MTPJ | metatarsophalangeal joint |
| MTR | mother |
| MTR-Ō | no masses, tenderness, or rebound |
| MTRS | Licensed Master Therapeutic Recreation Specialist |
| MTS | mesial temporal sclerosis |
| MTST | maximal treadmill stress test |
| MTT | mamillothalamic tract |
| | mean transit time |
| | methylthiotetrazole |
| MTU | malignant teratoma undifferentiated |
| | methylthiouracil |
| MTX | methotrexate |
| MTZ | mirtazapine (Remeron) |
| | mitoxantrone (Novantrone) |
| MU | million units |
| | Murphy unit |
| mU | milliunits |
| MUA | manipulation under anesthesia |
| MUAC | middle upper arm circumference |
| MUD | matched-unrelated donor |
| MUDDLES | miosis, urination, diarrhea, diaphoresis, lacrimation, excitation of central nervous system, and salivation (effects of cholinesterase inhibitors) |
| MUDPILES | *m*ethanol, *m*etformin; *u*remia; *d*iabetic ketoacidosis; |

*p*henformin, paraldehyde; *i*ron, *i*soniazid, ibuprofen; *l*actic acidosis; *e*thanol, ethylene glycol; and *s*alicylates, sepsis (causes of metabolic acidosis)

**MUE** medication use evaluation

**MUFA** monounsaturated fatty acid

**MUGA** multigated (radionuclide) angiogram
multiple gated acquisition (scan)

**MUGX** multiple gated acquisition exercise

**MULE** microcomputer upper limb exerciser

**MuLV** murine leukemia virus

**MUM** mumps virus vaccine

**MUNSH** Memorial University of Newfoundland Scale of Happiness

**MUO** metastasis of unknown origin

**MUPAT** multiple-site perineal applicator technique

**MUSE®** Medicated Urethral System for Erection (alprostadil urethral suppository)

**mus-lig** musculoligamentous

**MUU** mouse uterine units

**MV** manual ventilation
mechanical ventilation
millivolts
minute volume
mitoxantrone and etoposide
mitral valve
mixed venous
multivesicular

**MVA** malignant vertricular arrhythmias
manual vacuum aspiration
mitral valve area
motor vehicle accident

**M-VAC** methotrexate, vinblastine doxorubicin (Adriamycin), and cisplatin

**MVB** methotrexate and vinblastine
mixed venous blood

**MVC** maximal voluntary contraction
motor vehicle collision (crash)

**MVc** mitral valve closure

**MVD** microvascular decompression
microvessel density
mitral valve disease
multivessel disease

**MVE** mitral valve (leaflet) excursion
Murray Valley encephalitis

**MV Grad** mitral valve gradient

**MVI** malignant vascular injury
multiple vitamin injection

**MVI®** brand name for parenteral multivitamins

**MVI 12®** brand name for parenteral multivitamins

**MVO** mixed venous oxygen saturation

**MVO$_2$** myocardial oxygen consumption

**MVP** mean venous pressure
mitomycin, vinblastine, and cisplatin (Platinol AQ)
mitral valve prolapse

**MVPA** moderate-to-vigorous physical activity

**MVPP** mechlorethamine, vinblastine, procarbazine, and prednisone

**MVPS** mitral valve prolapse syndrome

**MVR** massive vitreous retraction
micro-vitreoretinal (blade)
mitral valve regurgitation
mitral valve replacement

**MVRI** mixed vaccine respiratory infections

**MVS** mitral valve stenosis
motor, vascular, and sensory

| | |
|---|---|
| MVT | movement |
| | multiform ventricular tachycardia |
| | multivitamin |
| MVU | Montevideo units |
| MVV | maximum ventilatory volume |
| | maximum voluntary ventilation |
| | mixed vespid venom |
| MWB | minimal weight bearing |
| MWD | maximum walking distance |
| | microwave diathermy |
| M-W-F | Monday-Wednesday-Friday |
| MWI | Medical Walk-In (Clinic) |
| MWOA | migraine without aura |
| MWS | Mickety-Wilson syndrome |
| MWT | maintenance of wakefulness test |
| | Mallory-Weiss tear |
| | malpositioned wisdom teeth |
| Mx | manifest refraction |
| | mastectomy |
| | maxilla |
| | movement |
| | myringotomy |
| My | myopia |
| MYD | mydriatic |
| myelo | myelocytes |
| | myelogram |
| MyG | myasthenia gravis |
| MYOP | myopia |
| MYR | myringotomy |
| MYS | medium yellow soft (stools) |
| MZ | monozygotic |
| M/Z | mass/charge |
| MZL | marginal zone lymphocyte |
| MZT | monozygotic twins |

## N

| | |
|---|---|
| N | nausea |
| | negative |
| | Negro |
| | *Neisseria* |
| | nerve |
| | neutrophil |
| | never |
| | newton |
| | night |
| | nipple |
| | nitrogen |
| | no |
| | nodes |
| | nonalcoholic |
| | none |
| | normal |
| | North (as in the location 2N, would be second floor, North wing) |
| | not |
| | notified |
| | noun |
| | NPH insulin |
| | size of sample |
| N I .... N XII | first through twelfth cranial nerves |
| 0.1 N | tenth-normal |
| N₂ | nitrogen |
| N 2.5 | phenylephrine HCl 2.5% ophthalmic solution (Neo-Synephrine) |
| n-3 | omega-3 |
| 5'-N | 5'-nucleotidase |
| NA | Narcotics Anonymous |
| | Native American |
| | Negro adult |
| | new admission |
| | nicotinic acid |
| | nonalcoholic |
| | norethindrone acetate |
| | normal axis |
| | not admitted |
| | not applicable |
| | not available |
| | nurse aide |
| | nurse's aid |
| | Nurse Anesthetist |
| | nursing assistant |

| | | | |
|---|---|---|---|
| Na | sodium | NADE | New Animal Drug Evaluation |
| Na$^+$ | sodium | | |
| N & A | normal and active | NADPH | nicotinamide adenine dinucleotide phosphate |
| NAA | N-acetylaspartate | | |
| | National Average Allowance (federal physician office visit cost guide) | NADSIC | no apparent disease seen in chest |
| | | NaE | exchangeable sodium |
| | | NAF | nafcillin |
| | neutron activation analysis | | Native-American female |
| | no apparent abnormalities | | |
| | nucleic acid amplification | | Negro adult female |
| NAAC | no apparent anesthesia complications | | normal adult female |
| | | | Notice of Adverse Findings (FDA post-audit letter) |
| NAA/Cr | N-acetylaspartate/creatine ratio | | |
| | | NaF | sodium fluoride |
| NAAT | nucleic acid amplification techniques (testing) | NAFLD | nonalcoholic fatty liver disease |
| NAATPT | not available at the present time | NAG | narrow angle glaucoma |
| | | NaHCO$_3$ | sodium bicarbonate |
| NAB | not at bedside | NAHI | nonaccidental head injury |
| NABS | normoactive bowel sounds | NAI | no action indicated |
| NABT | normal-appearing brain tissue | | no acute inflammation |
| | | | nonaccidental injury |
| NABTC | North American Brain Tumor Consortium | | Nuremberg Aging Inventory |
| | | NaI | sodium iodide |
| NABX | needle aspiration biopsy | NAION | nonarteritic ischemic optic neuropathy |
| NAC | acetylcysteine (N-acetylcysteine; Mucomyst) | | |
| | | NAIT | neonatal alloimmune thrombocytopenia |
| | neoadjuvant chemotherapy | NAL | nasal angiocentric lymphoma |
| | nipple-areola complex | | |
| | no acute changes | NAM | nail-apparatus melanoma |
| | no anesthesia complications | | |
| | | | Native-American male |
| NACD | no anatomical cause of death | | no abnormal masses |
| | | | normal adult male |
| NaClO | sodium hypochlorite | NANB | non-A, non-B (hepatitis) (hepatitis C) |
| NaCl | sodium chloride (salt) | | |
| NaCMC | sodium carboxymethyl cellulose | NANBH | non-A, non-B hepatitis (hepatitis C) |
| NACS | Neurologic and Adaptive Capacity Score | NANC | nonadrenergic, noncholinergic |
| NACT | neoadjuvant chemotherapy | NANDA | North American Nursing Diagnosis Association (taxonomy) |
| NAD | nicotinamide adenine dinucleotide | | |
| | no active disease | NANSAIDs | nonaspirin, nonsteroidal anti-inflammatory drugs |
| | no acute distress | | |
| | no apparent distress | NAP | narrative, assessment, and plan |
| | no appreciable disease | | |
| | normal axis deviation | | nosocomial acquired pneumonia |
| | nothing abnormal detected | | |
| NADA | New Animal Drug Application | | |

| | | | |
|---|---|---|---|
| NAPA | N-acetyl procainamide | NBC | newborn center |
| NAPD | no active pulmonary disease | | nonbed care |
| | | | nuclear, biological, and chemical |
| Na Pent | Pentothal Sodium | | |
| NAR | no action required | NBCCS | nevoid basal-cell carcinoma syndrome |
| | no adverse reaction | | |
| | nonambulatory restraint | NBD | neurologic bladder dysfunction |
| | not at risk | | |
| NARC | narcotic(s) | | no brain damage |
| NaRI | noradrenaline reuptake inhibitor | NBF | not breast fed |
| | | NBH | new bag (bottle) hung |
| NART | National Adult Reading Test (United Kingdom) | NBHH | newborn helpful hints |
| | | NBI | no bone injury |
| NAS | nasal | NBICU | newborn intensive care unit |
| | neonatal abstinence syndrome | | |
| | | nBiPAP | nasal bilevel (biphasic) positive airway pressure |
| | no abnormality seen | | |
| | no added salt | NBIs | nosocomial bloodstream infections |
| NASBA | nucleic-acid sequencing based amplification | | |
| | | NBL/OM | neuroblastoma and opsoclonus-myoclonus |
| NaSCN | sodium thiocyanate | | |
| NASH | nonalcoholic steatohepatitis | NBM | no bowel movement |
| | | | normal bone marrow |
| NAS-NRC | National Academy of Sciences – National Research Council | | normal bowel movement |
| | | | nothing by mouth |
| | | NBN | newborn nursery |
| NaSSA | noradrenergic and specific serotonergic antidepresssant | NBP | needle biopsy of prostate |
| | | | no bone pathology |
| | | NBQC | narrow base quad cane |
| NASTT | nonspecific abnormality of ST segment and T wave | NBR | no blood return |
| | | NBS | newborn screen (serum thyroxine and phenylketonuria) |
| NAT | N-acetyltransferase | | |
| | no action taken | | Nijmegen breakage syndrome |
| | no acute trauma | | |
| | nonaccidental trauma | | no bacteria seen |
| | nonspecific abnormality of T wave | | normal bowel sounds |
| | | NBT | nitroblue tetrazolium reduction (tests) |
| | nucleic acid test (testing) | | |
| $Na^{99m}$ $TcO_4^-$ | sodium pertechnetate Tc 99m | | normal breast tissue |
| | | NBTE | nonbacterial thrombotic endocarditis |
| NAUC | normalized area under the curve | NBTNF | newborn, term, normal female |
| NAW | nasal antral window | NBTNM | newborn, term, normal, male |
| NAWM | normal-appearing white matter | | |
| | | NBW | normal birth weight (2,500–3,999 g) |
| NB | nail bed | | |
| | needle biopsy | NC | nasal cannula |
| | neuroblastomas | | Negro child |
| | newborn | | neurologic check |
| | nitrogen balance | | no change |
| | note well | | no charge |

| | | | |
|---|---|---|---|
| | no complaints | NCDB | National Cancer Data Base |
| | noncontributory | | |
| | normocephalic | NCE | new chemical entity |
| | nose clamp | NCEH | National Center for Environmental Health (CDC) |
| | nose clips | | |
| | not classified | | |
| | not completed | NCEP | National Cholesterol Education Program |
| | not cultured | | |
| 9 NC | rubitecan (9-nitrocamptothecin) | NCF | neutrophilic chemotactic factor |
| NCA | neurocirculatory asthenia | | no cold fluids |
| | no congenital abnormalities | NCHGR | National Center for Human Genome Research (NIH) |
| N/CAN | nasal cannula | | |
| NCAP | nasal continuous airway pressure | NCHS | National Center for Health Statistics |
| NCAS | zinostatin (neocarzinostatin) | NCI | National Cancer Institute |
| | | NCIC | National Cancer Institute of Canada |
| NC/AT | normocephalic atraumatic | NCI-CTC | National Cancer Institute Common Toxicity Criteria |
| NCB | natural childbirth | | |
| | no code blue | | |
| NCC | no concentrated carbohydrates | NCIC-CTG | National Cancer Institute of Canada Clinical Trials Group |
| | nursing care card | | |
| NCCAM | National Center for Complementary and Alternative Medicine (NIH) | NCID | National Center for Infectious Diseases (CDC) |
| NCCDPHP | National Center for Chronic Disease and Prevention and Health Promotion (CDC) | NCIPC | National Center for Injury Prevention and Control (CDC) |
| | | NCIS | nursing care information sheet |
| NCCI | National Correct Coding Initiative | NCIT | Nursing Care Intervention Tool |
| NCCLS | National Committee for Clinical Laboratory Standards | NCJ | needle catheter jejunostomy |
| | | NCL | neuronal ceroid lipofuscinosis |
| NCCN | National Comprehensive Cancer Network | | no cautionary labels |
| NCCP | noncardiac chest pain | | nuclear cardiology laboratory |
| NCCTG | North Central Cancer Treatment Group | | |
| NCCU | neurosurgical continuous care unit | NCLD | neonatal chronic lung disease |
| NCD | neck-capsule distance | NCM | nailfold capillary microscope |
| | no congenital deformities | | nonclinical manager |
| | normal childhood diseases | NCNC | normochromic, normocytic |
| | not considered disabling | | |
| | not considered disqualifying | NCNR | National Center for Nursing Research (NIH) |
| | Nursing-Care Dependency (scale) | | |

| | | | |
|---|---|---|---|
| NCO | no complaints offered | | no data |
| | noncommissioned officer | | no disease |
| NCOG | North California | | nondisabling |
| | Oncology Group | | nondistended |
| NCP | no caffeine or pepper | | none detectable |
| | nursing care plan | | normal delivery |
| NCPAP | nasal continuous positive | | normal development |
| | airway pressure | | nose drops |
| NCPB | neurolytic celiac plexus | | not detected |
| | block | | not diagnosed |
| NcpPCu | nonceruloplasmin plasma | | not done |
| | copper | | nothing done |
| NCPR | no cardiopulmonary | | Nursing Doctorate |
| | resuscitation | N&D | nodular and diffuse |
| NCQA | National Commission for | Nd | neodymium |
| | Quality Assurance | NDA | New Drug Application |
| nCR | nodular complete response | | no data available |
| NCRA | National Cancer | | no demonstrable |
| | Registrars Association | | antibodies |
| NCRC | nonchild-resistant | | no detectable activity |
| | container | NDC | National Drug Code |
| NCRR | National Center for | NDD | no dialysis days |
| | Research Resources | NDE | near-death experience |
| | (NIH) | NDEA | no deviation of electrical |
| NCS | nerve conduction studies | | axis |
| | no concentrated sweets | NDF | neutral density filter (test) |
| | noncontact supervision | | no disease found |
| | not clinically significant | NDGA | nordihydroguaiaretic acid |
| | zinostatin | NDI | National Death Index |
| | (neocarzinostatin) | | nephrogenic diabetes |
| NCSE | nonconvulsive status | | insipidus |
| | epilepticus | NDIR | nondispersive infrared |
| NCT | neoadjuvant chemotherapy | NDIRS | nondispersive infrared |
| | neutron capture therapy | | spectrometer |
| | noncontact tonometry | NDM | neonatal diabetes mellitus |
| | Nursing Care Technician | Nd/NT | nondistended, nontender |
| NCV | nerve conduction velocity | NDP | nedaplatin |
| | nuclear venogram | | net dietary protein |
| NCVHS | National Committee on | | Nurse Discharge Planner |
| | Vital and Health | NDR | neurotic depressive |
| | Statistics | | reaction |
| ND | Doctor of Naturopathy | | normal detrusor reflex |
| | (Naturopathic | NDS | Neurologic Disability |
| | Physician) | | Score |
| | nasal deformity | | neuropathy disability score |
| | nasal discharge | NDST | neurodevelopmental |
| | nasoduodenal | | screening test |
| | natural death | NDT | nasal duodenostomy tube |
| | neck dissection | | neurodevelopmental |
| | neonatal death | | techniques |
| | neurological development | | neurodevelopmental |
| | neurotic depression | | treatment |
| | Newcastle disease | | noise detection threshold |

| | | | |
|---|---|---|---|
| NDV | Newcastle disease virus | NEO | necrotizing external otitis |
| Nd:YAG | neodymium:yttrium-aluminum-garnet (laser) | NEOH | neonatal high risk |
| | | NEOM | neonatal medium risk |
| Nd:YLF | neodymium:yttrium-lithium-fluoride (laser) | NEP | needle-exchange program |
| | | | neutral endopeptidase |
| NE | nausea and emesis | | no evidence of pathology |
| | nephropathica epidemica | NEPD | no evidence of pulmonary disease |
| | neurological examination | | |
| | never exposed | NEPHRO | nephrogram |
| | no effect | NEPPK | nonepidermolytic palmoplantar keratoderma |
| | no enlargement | | |
| | norethindrone | | |
| | norepinephrine | NER | no evidence of recurrence |
| | not elevated | NERD | no evidence of recurrent disease |
| | not examined | | |
| NEAA | nonessential amino acids | | nonerosive reflux disease |
| NEAC | norethindrone acetate | NES | nonepileptic seizure |
| NEAD | nonepileptic attack disorder | | nonstandard electrolyte solution |
| NEAT | .nonexercise activity thermogenesis | | not elsewhere specified |
| | | NESP | novel erythropoiesis stimulating protein (darbepoetin [Aranesp]) |
| NEB | hand-held nebulizer | | |
| NEC | necrotizing entercolitis | | |
| | noise equivalent counts | NET | choroidal or subretinal neovascularization |
| | nonesterified cholesterol | | |
| | not elsewhere classified | | Internet |
| NED | no evidence of disease | | naso-endotracheal tube |
| NEDSS | National Electronic Disease Surveillance System | | neuroectodermal tumor |
| | | NETA | norethindrone acetate (Aygestin) |
| | | | |
| NEEG | normal electroencephalogram | NETSS | National Electronic Telecommunications System for Surveillance |
| NEEP | negative end-expiratory pressure | | |
| | | NETT | nasal endotracheal tube |
| NEF | negative expiratory force | NEVA | nocturnal electrobioimpedance volumetric assessment (penile measurement) |
| NEFA | nonesterified fatty acid(s) | | |
| NEFG | normal external female genitalia | | |
| NEFT | nasoenteric feeding tube | NEX | nose-to-ear-to-xiphoid |
| NEG | negative | | number of excitations (radiology) |
| | neglect | | |
| NEI | National Eye Institute (NIH) | NETZ | needle (diathermy) excision of the transformation zone |
| NEJM | *New England Journal of Medicine* | | |
| | | NF | necrotizing fasciitis |
| NEM | neurotrophic enhancing molecule | | Negro female |
| | | | neurofibromatosis |
| | no evidence of malignancy | | night frequency (of voiding) |
| NEMD | nonexudative macular degeneration | | none found |
| | | | not found |
| | nonspecific esophageal motility disorder | | nursed fair |
| NENT | nasal endotracheal tube | | nursing facility |

| Nf | *Naegleria fowleri* | NGT | nasogastric tube |
| NF1 | neurofibromatosis type 1 | | normal glucose tolerance |
| NF2 | neurofibromatous type 2 | NgTD | negative to date |
| NFA | Nerve Fiber Analyzer® | NGU | nongonococcal urethritis |
| NFALO | Nerve Fiber Analyzer laser oththalmoscope | NH | normal-hearing nursing home |
| NFAP | nursing facility-acquired pneumonia | NHA | no histologic abnormalities |
| NFAR | no further action required | NHB | nonheart-beating (donor) |
| NFCS | Neonatal Facial Coding System | NHBD | nonheart-beating donor |
| NFD | no family doctor | NHC | neighborhood health center |
| NFFD | not fit for duty | | neonatal hypocalcemia |
| NFI | nerve-function impairment | | nursing home care |
| | no-fault insurance | $NH_3$ | ammonia |
| | no further information | $NH_4Cl$ | ammonium chloride |
| | normal female infant | NHCU | nursing home care unit |
| NFL | nerve fiber layer | NHD | normal hair distribution |
| NFLX | norfloxacin (Noroxin) | NHE | sodium/hydrogen exchanger |
| NFP | natural family planning | | |
| | no family physician | NHGRI | National Human Genome Research Institute (NIH) |
| | not for publication | | |
| NFT | no further treatment | | |
| NFTD | normal full-term delivery | NHL | nodular histiocytic lymphoma |
| NFTE | not found this examination | | non-Hodgkin lymphomas |
| | | nHL | normalized hearing level |
| NFTs | neurofibrillary tangles | NHLBI | National Heart, Lung, and Blood Institute (NIH) |
| NFTSD | normal full-term spontaneous delivery | | |
| | | NHLPP | hereditary neuropathy with liability for pressure palsy |
| NFTT | nonorganic failure to thrive | | |
| | | NHM | no heroic measures |
| NFV | nelfinavir (Viracept) | NHO | notify house officer |
| NFW | nursed fairly well | NHP | Nottingham Health Profile |
| NG | nanogram (ng) $(10^{-9}$ gram) | | nursing home placement |
| | | NHS | National Health Service (UK) |
| | nasogastric | | |
| | night guard | NHT | neoadjuvant hormonal therapy |
| | nitroglycerin | | |
| | no growth | | nursing home transfer |
| | norgestrel | NHTR | nonhemolytic transfusion reaction |
| ng | nanogram | | |
| NGB | neurogenic bladder | NHW | nonhealing wound |
| NGF | nerve growth factor | NI | neurological improvement |
| n giv | not given | | no improvement |
| NGJ | nasogastro-jejunostomy | | no information |
| NGM | norgestimate | | none indicated |
| NGOs | nongovernmental organizations | | not identified |
| | | | not isolated |
| NGR | nasogastric replacement | NIA | National Institute on Aging (NIH) |
| NGRI | not guilty by reason of insanity | | |
| | | | no information available |
| NGSF | nothing grown so far | | |

NIAAA National Institute on Alcohol Abuse and Alcoholism (NIH)

NIADDK National Institute of Arthritis, Diabetes, and Digestive and Kidney Diseases (NIH)

NIAID National Institute of Allergy and Infectious Diseases (NIH)

NIAL not in active labor

NIAMS National Institute of Arthritis and Musculoskeletal and Skin Diseases (NIH)

NIA-RI National Institute on Aging–Reagan Institute

NIBP noninvasive blood pressure

NIBPM noninvasive blood pressure measurement

NIC Nursing Intervention Classification

NICC neonatal intensive care center
noninfectious chronic cystitis

NICE National Institute for Clinical Excellence (United Kingdom)
new, interesting, and challenging experiences

NICHD National Institute of Child Health and Human Development (NIH)

NICO neuralgia-inducing cavitational osteonecrosis
noninvasive cardiac output (monitor)

NICS noninvasive carotid studies

NICU neonatal intensive care unit
neurosurgical intensive care unit

NID no identifiable disease
not in distress

NIDA National Institute of Drug Abuse (NIH)

NIDA five National Institute on Drug Abuse screen for cannabinoids, cocaine metabolite, amphetamine/methamphetamine, opiates, and phencyclidine

NIDCD National Institute of Deafness and other Communication Disorders (NIH)

NIDCR National Institute of Dental and Craniofacial Research (NIH)

NIDD noninsulin-dependent diabetes

NIDDK National Institute of Diabetes and Digestive and Kidney Diseases (NIH)

NIDDM noninsulin-dependent diabetes mellitus

NIDR National Institute of Dental Research (NIH)

NIEHS National Institute of Environmental Health Sciences (NIH)

NIF negative inspiratory force
neutrophil inhibitory factor
not in file

NIFS noninvasive flow studies

NIG NSAIA (nonsteroidal anti-inflamatory agent) induced gastropathy

NIGMS National Institute of General Medical Sciences (NIH)

NIH National Institutes of Health

NIHD noise-induced hearing damage

NIHL noise-induced hearing loss

NIHSS National Institutes of Health Stroke Scale

NIID neuronal intranuclear inclusion disease

NIL not in labor

NIMAs noninherited maternal antigens

NIMH National Institute of Mental Health (NIH)

| | | | |
|---|---|---|---|
| NIMHDIS | National Institute for Mental Health Diagnostic Interview Schedule (NIH) | NJ | nasojejunal |
| | | NK | natural killer (cells) |
| | | | not known |
| | | NKA | no known allergies |
| NINDS | National Institute of Neurological Disorders and Stroke (NIH) | nkat | nanokatal (nanomole/sec) |
| | | NKB | no known basis |
| | | | not keeping baby |
| NINR | National Institute for Nursing Research (NIH) | | neurokinin B |
| | | NKC | nonketotic coma |
| | | NKD | no known diseases |
| NINU | neuro intermediate nursing unit | NKDA | no known drug allergies |
| | | NKFA | no known food allergies |
| NINVS | noninvasive neurovascular studies | NKH | nonketotic hyperglycemia |
| | | NKHA | nonketotic hyperosmolar acidosis |
| NIOPCs | no intraoperative complications | NKHHC | nonketotic hyperglycemic-hyperosmolar coma |
| NIOSH | National Institute of Occupational Safety and Health (NIH) | NKHOC | nonketotic hyperosmolar coma |
| NIP | catnip | NKHS | nonketotic hyperosmolar syndrome |
| | no infection present | | |
| | no inflammation present | NKMA | no known medication (medical) allergies |
| NIPAs | noninherited paternal antigens | NL | nasolacrimal |
| | | | nonlatex |
| NIPD | nocturnal intermittent peritoneal dialysis | | normal |
| | | | normal libido |
| NIPPV | noninvasive positive-pressure ventilation | NLB | needle liver biopsy |
| | | NLC | nocturnal leg cramps |
| NIPS | Neonatal Infant Pain Scale | NLC & C | normal libido, coitus, and climax |
| NIP/S | noninvasive programming stimulation | | |
| | | NLD | nasolacrimal duct |
| NIPSV | noninvasive pressure support ventilation | | necrobiosis lipoidica diabeticorum |
| NIR | near infrared | | no local doctor |
| | nitroprusside-induced relaxation | NLDO | nasolacrimal duct obstruction |
| NIRCA | nonisotopic RNase cleavage assay | NLE | neonatal lupus erythematosus |
| NISH | nonradioactive in situ hybridization | | nursing late entry |
| NISS | New Injury Severity Score | NLEA | Nutrition Labeling and Education Act of 1990 |
| NISs | no-impact sports | | |
| NISV | nonionic surfactant vesicle | NLF | nasolabial fold |
| NITD | neuroleptic-induced tardive dyskinesia | | nelfinavir (Viracept) |
| | | NLFGNR | nonlactose fermenting gram-negative rod |
| Nitro | nitroglycerin (this is a dangerous abbreviation) | NLM | National Library of Medicine |
| | sodium nitroprusside (this is a dangerous abbreviation) | | no limitation of motion |
| | | NLMC | nocturnal leg muscle cramp |
| NIV | noninvasive ventilation | | |
| NIVLS | noninvasive vascular laboratory studies | NLN | no longer needed |
| | | NLO | nasolacrimal occlusion |

**N**

| | | | |
|---|---|---|---|
| NLP | natural language processing | NMM | nodular malignant melanoma |
| | nodular liquifying panniculitis | NMN | no middle name |
| | no light perception | NMNKB | not married, not keeping baby |
| NLS | neonatal lupus syndrome | nmol | nanomole (one billionth [$10^{-9}$] of a mole) |
| NLs | neuroimmunophilin ligands | NMOH | no medical ocular history |
| NLT | not later than | NMP | normal menstrual period |
| | not less than | NMR | nuclear magnetic resonance (same as magnetic resonance imaging) |
| NLV | nelfinavir (Viracept) | | |
| NM | nanometer (nm) ($10^{-9}$ meters) | | |
| | Negro male | NMRS | nuclear magnetic resonance spectroscopy |
| | neuromuscular | | |
| | neuronal microdysgenesis | NMRT (R) | Nuclear Medicine Radiologic Technologist (Registered) |
| | nodular melanoma | | |
| | nonmalignant | | |
| | not measurable | NMS | neonatal morphine solution |
| | not measured | | |
| | not mentioned | | neuroleptic malignant syndrome |
| | nuclear medicine | | |
| | nurse manager | NMSC | nonmelanoma skin cancer |
| N & M | nerves and muscles | NMSE | normalized mean square root |
| | night and morning | | |
| NMBA | neuromuscular blocking agent | NMSIDS | near-miss sudden infant death syndrome |
| NMC | no malignant cells | NMT | nebulized mist treatment |
| NMD | Doctor of Naturopathic Medicine | | no more than |
| | | NMTB | neuromuscular transmission blockade |
| | neuromuscular disorders | | |
| | neuronal migration disorders | NMTCB | Nuclear Medicine Technology Certification Board |
| | Normosol M and 5% Dextrose® | NMT(R) | Nuclear Medicine Technologist Registered |
| NMDA | N-methyl-D-aspartate | | |
| NMDP | National Marrow Donor Pool | NMU | nitrosomethylurea |
| | | NN | narrative notes |
| NME | new molecular entity | | Navajo neuropathy |
| NMES | neuromuscular electrical stimulation | | neonatal |
| | | | neural network |
| NMF | neuromuscular facilitation | | normal nursery |
| NMH | neurally mediated hypotension | | nurses' notes |
| | | N/N | negative/negative |
| NMHH | no medical health history | NNB | normal newborn |
| NMI | no manifest improvement | NNBC | node-negative breast cancer |
| | no mental illness | | |
| | no middle initial | NND | neonatal death |
| | no more information | | number needed to detain |
| | normal male infant | | |
| NMJ | neuromuscular junction | NNE | neonatal necrotizing enterocolitis |
| NML | normal | | |
| NMKB | not married, keeping baby | NNH | number needed to harm |

| | | | |
|---|---|---|---|
| NNIS | National Nosocomial Infections Surveillance | NOED | no observed effect dose |
| NNM | Nicolle-Novy-MacNeal (media) | NOEL | no observable effect level |
| | | NOF | National Osteoporosis Foundation (treatment criteria) |
| NNL | no new laboratory (test orders) | | |
| NNN | normal newborn nursery | NOFT | nonorganic failure to thrive |
| NNO | no new orders | | |
| NNP | Neonatal Nurse Practitioner | NOFTT | nonorganic failure to thrive |
| | non-nociceptive pain | NOGM | nonoxidative glucose metabolism |
| N:NPK | grams of nitrogen to non-protein kilocalories | | |
| | | NOH | neurogenic orthostatic hypotension |
| NNR | not necessary to return | | |
| NNRTI | non-nucleoside reverse transcriptase inhibitor | NOI | nature of illness |
| | | NOK | next of kin |
| | | NOL | not on label |
| NNS | neonatal screen (hematocrit, total bilirubin, and total protein) | NOM | nonsuppurative otitis media |
| | | NOMI | nonocclusive mesenteric infarction |
| | nicotine nasal spray | NOMS | not on my shift |
| | non-nutritive sucking | NO/N$_2$ | nitric oxide; nitrogen |
| | number needed to screen | NONMEM | nonlinear mixed-effects model (modeling) |
| NNT | number needed to treat | | |
| NNTB | number needed to treat to benefit | non pal | not palpable |
| | | non-REM | nonrapid eye movement (sleep) |
| NNTH | number needed to treat to harm | | |
| | | *non rep* | do not repeat |
| NNU | net nitrogen utilization | NON VIZ | not visualized |
| NO | nasal oxygen | NOOB | not out of bed |
| | nitric oxide | NOP | not on patient |
| | nitroglycerin ointment | NOR | norethynodrel |
| | none obtained | | normal |
| | nonobese | | nortriptyline |
| | number (no.) | NOR-EPI | norepinephrine |
| | nursing office | norm | normal |
| NO$_2$ | nitrogen dioxide | NOS | neonatal opium solution (diluted deodorized tincture of opium) |
| N$_2$O | nitrous oxide | | |
| NOAA | National Oceanic and Atmospheric Administration | | new-onset seizures |
| | | | nitric oxide synthase |
| NOAEL | no observed adverse effect level | | no organisms seen |
| | | | not on staff |
| N$_2$O:O$_2$ | nitrous oxide to oxygen ratio | | not otherwise specified |
| | | NOSI | nitric oxide synthase inhibitors |
| NOC | nonorgan-confined | | |
| | Nursing Outcome Classification | NOSIE | Nurse's Observation Scale (Schedule) for Inpatient Evaluation |
| noc. | night | | |
| noct | nocturnal | NOSPECS | categories for classifying eye changes in Graves ophthalmopathy: **n**o |
| NOD | nonobese diabetic | | |
| | notice of disagreement | | |
| | notify of death | | |

signs or symptoms,
**o**nly signs, **s**oft tissue
involvement with
symptoms and signs,
**p**roptosis, **e**xtraocular
muscle involvement,
**c**orneal involvement,
and **s**ight loss (visual
acuity)

NOT   nocturnal oxygen
therapy

NOTT   nocturnal oxygen therapy
trial

NOU   not on unit

NOV   Novartis

NOV
70/30   human insulin, regular 30
units/mL with human
insulin isophane
suspension 70 units/mL
(Novolin 70/30)

NOV L   human insulin zinc
suspension (Novolin L)

NOV N   human insulin isophane
suspension
(Novolin N)

NOV R   human insulin regular
(Novolin R)

NP   nasal prongs
nasopharyngeal
near point
neuropathic pain
neurophysin
neuropsychiatric
neutrogenic precautions
newly presented
nonpalpable
no pain
not performed
not pregnant
not present
nuclear pharmacist
nuclear pharmacy
nursed poorly
nurse practitioner

NPA   nasal pharyngeal airway
nasopharyngeal aspirate
near point of
accommodation
no previous admission

NPAT   nonparoxysmal atrial
tachycardia

NPBC   node-positive breast
cancer

NPC   nasopharyngeal carcinoma
near-point convergence
Niemann-Pick disease
Type C (sphingomyelin
lipidosis)
nodal premature
contractions
nonpatient contact
nonproductive cough
nonprotein calorie
no prenatal care
no previous complaint(s)

NPCC   nonprotein carbohydrate
calories

NPCPAP   nasopharyngeal
continuous positive
airway pressure

NPD   Niemann-Pick disease
nonprescription drugs
no pathological diagnosis

NPDL   nodular poorly
differentiated
lymphocytic

NPDR   nonproliferative diabetic
retinopathy

NPE   neurogenic pulmonary
edema
neuropsychologic
examination
no palpable enlargement
normal pelvic
examination

NPEM   nocturnal penile erection
monitoring

NPF   nasopharyngeal fiberscope
no predisposing factor

N-PFMSO$_4$   nebulized preservative-
free morphine sulfate

NPFS   nonpenetrating filtering
surgery

NPG   nonpregnant
normal-pressure glaucoma

NPH   isophane insulin (neutral
protamine Hagedorn)
no previous history
normal-pressure
hydrocephalus

NPhx   nasopharynx

NPI   Neuropsychiatric
Inventory
no present illness
Nottingham Prognostic
Index

| | | | |
|---|---|---|---|
| NPIS | Numeric Pain Intensity Scale | | nothing per vagina |
| | | NPY | neuropeptide Y |
| NPJT | nonparoxysmal junctional tachycardia | NPZ | neuropsychologic text z |
| | | NQECN | nonqueratinizing epidermoid carcinoma |
| NPL | insulin lispro protamine component suspension | | |
| | | NQMI | non-Q wave myocardial infarction |
| NPLSM | neoplasm | | |
| NPK | nonprotein kilocalories | NQWMI | non-Q wave myocardial infarction |
| NPM | nothing per mouth | | |
| NPN | nonprotein nitrogen | NR | do not repeat |
| NPNC | no prenatal care | | newly reformulated |
| NPNT | nonpalpable, nontender | | none reported |
| n.p.o. | nothing by mouth | | nonreactive |
| NPOC | nonpurgeable organic carbon | | nonrebreathing |
| | | | no refills |
| NPOD | Neuropsychiatric Officer of the Day | | no report |
| | | | no response |
| NPP | nonphysician practitioner normal postpartum | | no return |
| | | | normal range |
| NPPI | nonpeptidic protease inhibitor | | normal reaction |
| | | | not reached |
| NPPNG | nonpenicillinase-producing *Neisseria gonorrhoeae* | | not reacting |
| | | | not remarkable |
| | | | not resolved |
| NPPV | noninvasive positive-pressure ventilation | | number |
| | | NRAF | nonrheumatic atrial fibrillation |
| NPR | normal pulse rate nothing per rectum | NRB | Noninstitutional Review Board |
| NPRL | normal pupillary reaction to light | | nonrebreather (oxygen mask) |
| NPS | National Pharmaceutical Stockpile | | |
| | | NRBC | normal red blood cell nucleated red blood cell |
| | new patient set-up | | |
| NPSA | nonphysician surgical assistant | NRBS | nonrebreathing system |
| NPSD | nonpotassium-sparing diuretics | NRC | National Research Council |
| | | | normal retinal correspondence |
| NPSF | National Patient Safety Foundation | | Nuclear Regulatory Commission |
| NPSG | nocturnal polysomnography | | |
| NPSLE | neuropsychiatric systemic lupus erythematosus | NREH | normal renin essential hypertension |
| | | NREM | nonrapid eye movement |
| NPT | near-patient tests neopyrithiamin hydrochloride | NREMS | nonrapid eye movement sleep |
| | | NREMT-P | National Registry of Emergency Medical Technicians–Paramedic level |
| | nocturnal penile tumescence | | |
| | no prior tracings | | |
| | normal pressure and temperature | NRF | normal renal function |
| NPU | net protein utilization | NRI | nerve root involvement |
| NPV | negative predictive value | | nerve root irritation |

| | | | |
|---|---|---|---|
| | no recent illnesses | | Adjuvant Breast |
| | norepinephrine reuptake | | Project |
| | inhibitor | NSAD | no signs of acute disease |
| N-RLX | nonrelaxed | NSAIA | nonsteroidal anti- |
| NRM | nonrebreathing mask | | inflammatory agent |
| | no regular medicines | NSAID | nonsteroidal anti- |
| | normal range of motion | | inflammatory drug |
| | normal retinal movement | NSAP | nonspecific abdominal |
| NRN | no return necessary | | pain |
| NRNST | nonreassuring-nonstress | NSBGP | nonspecific bowel gas |
| | test | | pattern |
| NRO | neurology | NSC | no significant change |
| NROM | normal range of motion | | nonservice-connected |
| NRP | nonreassuring patterns | NSCC | nonsmall cell carcinoma |
| NRPR | nonbreathing pressure | NSCD | nonservice-connected |
| | relieving | | disability |
| NRS | Neurobehavioral Rating | NSCFPT | no significant change |
| | Scale | | from previous tracing |
| NRT | neuromuscular | NSCIDRC | National Spinal Cord |
| | reeducation techniques | | Injury Data Research |
| | nicotine-replacement | | Center |
| | therapy | NSCLC | nonsmall-cell–lung |
| NRTI | nucleoside reverse | | cancer |
| | transcriptase inhibitor | NSCST | nipple stimulation |
| NRTs | nitron radical traps | | contraction stress test |
| NS | nephrotic syndrome | NSD | nasal septal deviation |
| | neurological signs | | nominal standard dose |
| | neurosurgery | | nonstructural deterioration |
| | nipple stimulation | | normal spontaneous |
| | nodular sclerosis | | delivery |
| | no-show | | no significant disease |
| | nonsmoker | | (difference, defect, |
| | normal saline solution | | deviation) |
| | (0.9% sodium chloride | NSDA | nonsteroid dependent |
| | solution) | | asthmatic |
| | normospermic | NSDU | neonatal stepdown unit |
| | no sample | NSE | neuron-specific enolase |
| | not seen | | normal saline enema |
| | not significant | | (0.9% sodium chloride) |
| | nuclear sclerosis | N s E | nausea without emesis |
| | nursing service | NSF | no significant findings |
| | nutritive sucking | NSFTD | normal spontaneous full- |
| | nylon suture | | term delivery |
| NSA | neck-shaft angle | NSG | nursing |
| | normal serum albumin | NSGCT | nonseminomatous germ- |
| | (albumin, human) | | cell tumors |
| | no salt added | NSGCTT | nonseminomatous germ- |
| | no significant | | cell tumor of the testis |
| | abnormalities | NSGI | nonspecific genital |
| | number of signals | | infection |
| | averaged (radiology) | NSGT | nonseminomatous germ- |
| NSAA | nonsteroidal antiandrogen | | cell tumor |
| NSABP | National Surgical | NSHD | nodular sclerosing |

| | Hodgkin disease | NST | nonmyeloablative stem-cell transplant |
| NSI | negative self-image | | nonstress test |
| | no signs of infection | | normal sphincter tone |
| | no signs of inflammation | | not sooner than |
| NSICU | neurosurgery intensive care unit | | nutritional support team |
| NSILA | nonsuppressible insulin-like activity | NSTD | nonsexually transmitted disease |
| NSIP | nonspecific interstitial pneumonia | NSTEMI | non-ST-segment elevation myocardial infarction |
| NSMMVT | nonsustained monomorphic ventricular tachycardia | NSTGCT | nonseminomatous testicular germ cell tumor |
| NSN | Neo-Synephrine nephrotoxic serum nephritis | NSTI | necrotizing soft-tissue infection |
| NSO | Neosporin® ointment | NSTT | nonseminomatous testicular tumors |
| NSOM | near field scanning optical microscope | NSU | neurosurgical unit nonspecific urethritis |
| NSOP | no soft organs palpable | NSV | nonspecific vaginitis |
| NSP | neck and shoulder pain | NSVD | nonstructural valve deterioration |
| NSPs | nonstarch polysaccharides | | |
| NSPVT | nonsustained polymorphic ventricular tachycardia | | normal spontaneous vaginal delivery |
| NSR | nasoseptal repair | NSVT | nonsustained ventricular tachycardia |
| | nonspecific reaction | | |
| | normal sinus rhythm | NSX | neurosurgical examination |
| | not seen regularly | | |
| NSRP | nerve-sparing radical prostatectomy | NSY | nursery |
| | | NT | nasotracheal |
| NSS | nephron-sparing surgery | | next time |
| | neurological signs stable | | Nordic Track® |
| | neuropathy symptom score | | normal temperature |
| | | | normotensive |
| | normal size and shape | | nortriptyline |
| | not statistically significant | | not tender |
| | nutritional support service | | not tested |
| | | | nourishment taken |
| | sodium chloride 0.9% (normal saline solution) | | numbness and tingling |
| 1/2 NSS | sodium chloride 0.45% (1/2 normal saline solution) | | nursing technician |
| | | N&T | nose and throat |
| | | | numbness and tingling |
| NSSC | normal size, shape and consistency (uterus) | N Tachy | nodal tachycardia |
| NSSL | normal size, shape, and location | NT-ANP | N-terminal atrial natriuretic peptide |
| NSSP | normal size, shape, and position | NTBR | not to be resuscitated |
| | | NTC | neurotrauma center |
| NSSTT | nonspecific ST and T-wave | NTCS | no tumor cells seen |
| NSST-TWCs | nonspecific ST-T wave changes | NTD | negative to date neural-tube defects nitroblue tetrazolium dye (test) |

| | | | |
|---|---|---|---|
| NTE | neutral thermal environment | NTT | nasotracheal tube |
| | not to exceed | | nonthrombocytopenic term (infant) |
| NTED | neonatal toxic-shock-syndrome-like exanthematous disease | NTTP | no tenderness to palpation |
| NTF | neurotrophic factor | NTU | nephelometric turbidity units |
| | normal throat flora | NTX | naltrexone (ReVia) |
| NTG | nitroglycerin | NTZ | nitazoxanide |
| | nontoxic goiter | NTZ Long-acting® | oxymetazoline nasal spray |
| | nontreatment group | | |
| | normal tension glaucoma | NU | name unknown |
| NTGO | nitroglycerin ointment | NUD | nonulcer dyspepsia |
| NTI | narrow therapeutic index | NUG | necrotizing ulcerative gingivitis |
| | no treatment indicated | | |
| NTIS | National Technical Information Service (U.S. Department of Commerce) | nullip | nullipara |
| | | NUN | nonurea nitrogen |
| | | NV | naked vision |
| | | | nausea and vomiting |
| NTL | nectar-thick liquid (diet consistency) | | near vision |
| | | | negative variation |
| | nortriptyline | | neovascularization |
| | no time limit | | neurovascular |
| NTLE | neocortical temporal-lobe epilepsy | | new vessel |
| | | | next visit |
| NTM | nocturnal tumescence monitor | | nonvenereal |
| | | | nonveteran |
| | nontuberculous mycobacterium | | normal value |
| | | | not vaccinated |
| NTMB | nontuberculous myobacteria | | not verified |
| | | N&V | nausea and vomiting |
| NTMI | nontransmural myocardial infarction | NVA | near visual acuity |
| | | NVAF | nonvalvular atrial fibrillation |
| NTND | not tender, not distended | | |
| NTP | narcotic treatment program | NVB | Navelbine (vinorelbine tartrate) |
| | | NVBo | oral vinorelbine |
| | National Toxicology Program | NVC | neurovascular checks |
| | Nitropaste® (nitroglycerin ointment) | nvCJD | new-variant Creutzfeldt-Jakob disease |
| | nonthrombocytopenic preterm (infant) | NVD | nausea, vomiting, and diarrhea |
| | | | neck vein distention |
| | normal temperature and pressure | | neovascularization of the (optic) disk |
| | sodium nitroprusside | | neurovesicle dysfunction |
| NTPD | nocturnal tidal peritoneal dialysis | | normal vaginal delivery |
| | | | no venereal disease |
| NTS | nasotracheal suction | | no venous distention |
| | nicotine transdermal system | | nonvalvular disease |
| | | NVDC | nausea, vomiting, diarrhea, and constipation |
| | nontyphoidal salmonellae | | |
| | nucleus tractus solitarii | | |

| NVE | native |
| | native valve endocarditis |
| | neovascularization elsewhere |
| NVG | neovascular glaucoma |
| | neoviridogrisein |
| NVL | neurovascular laboratory |
| NVM | neovascular membrane |
| NVP | nausea and vomiting of pregnancy |
| | nevirapine (Viramune) |
| NVS | neurological vital signs |
| | neurovascular status |
| NVSS | normal variant short stature |
| NW | naked weight |
| | nasal wash |
| | not weighed |
| NWB | nonweight bearing |
| NWBL | nonweight bearing, left |
| NWBR | nonweight bearing, right |
| NWC | number of words chosen |
| NWD | neuroleptic withdrawal |
| | normal well developed |
| NWS | New World screwworm (*Cochliomyia hominivorax* [Coquerel]) |
| NWTS | National Wilms Tumor Study (rating scale) |
| NWTSG | National Wilms Tumor Study Group |
| Nx | nephrectomy |
| | next |
| NX211 | liposomal lurtotecan |
| NYB | New York Blood Center |
| NYD | not yet diagnosed |
| NYHA | New York Heart Association (classification of heart disease) |
| NYST | nystagmus |
| NZ | enzyme |

# O

| O | eye |
| | objective findings |
| | obvious |
| | occlusal |
| | often |
| | open |
| | oral |
| | ortho |
| | other |
| | oxygen |
| | pint |
| | zero |
| $\bar{o}$ | negative |
| | no |
| | none |
| | pint |
| | without |
| O+ | blood type O positive (O positive is preferred) |
| O− | blood type O negative (O negative is preferred) |
| Ⓞ | orally (by mouth) |
| $_1O_2$ | singlet oxygen |
| $O_2$ | both eyes |
| | oxygen |
| $O_2^-$ | superoxide |
| $O_3$ | ozone |
| O157 | *Escherichia coli* O157 |
| OA | occipital artery |
| | occipitoatlantal |
| | occiput anterior |
| | old age |
| | on admission |
| | on arrival |
| | ophthalmic artery |
| | oral airway |
| | oral alimentation |
| | osteoarthritis |
| | Overeaters Anonymous |
| O/A | on or about |
| O & A | observation and assessment |
| | odontectomy and alveoloplasty |
| OAA | Old Age Assistance |
| OAA/S | Observer's Assessment of Alertness/Sedation |

O

| | | | |
|---|---|---|---|
| OAB | overactive bladder | OBG | obstetrics and gynecology |
| OAC | omeprazole, amoxicillin, and clarithromycin | Ob-Gyn | obstetrics and gynecology |
| | | Obj | objective |
| | oral anticoagulant(s) | obl | oblique |
| | overaction | OB marg | obtuse marginal |
| OAD | obstructive airway disease | OB-ND | obstetrics-not delivered |
| | occlusive arterial disease | OBP | office blood pressure |
| | overall diameter | OBRR | obstetric recovery room |
| OAE | otoacoustic emissions | OBS | obstetrical service |
| OAF | oral anal fistula | | organic brain syndrome |
| | osteoclast activating factor | OBT | obtained |
| OAG | open angle glaucoma | OBTM | omeprazole, bismuth subcitrate, tetracycline, and metronidazole |
| OAP | old age pension | | |
| OAR | Ottawa Ankle Rules | | |
| OAS | Older Adult Services | OBUS | obstetrical ultrasound |
| | oral allergy syndrome | OBW | open bed warmer |
| | organic anxiety syndrome | OC | obstetrical conjugate |
| | outpatient assessment service | | office call |
| | | | on call |
| | overall survival | | only child |
| | Overt Aggression Scale | | open cholecystectomy |
| OASDHI | Old Age, Survivors, Disability, and Health Insurance | | open colectomy |
| | | | optical chromatography |
| | | | oral care |
| OASI | Old Age and Survivors Insurance | | oral contraceptive |
| | | | osteocalcin |
| OASIS | Outcomes and Assessment Information Set | | osteoclast |
| | | | OxyContin (oxycodone) |
| OASO | overactive superior oblique | O & C | onset and course |
| OASR | overactive superior rectus | OCA | oculocutaneous albinism |
| OASS | Overt Agitation Severity Scale | | open care area |
| | | | oral contraceptive agent |
| OAT | ornithine aminotransferase | OCAD | occlusive carotid artery disease |
| OATP | organic anion-transporting polypeptide | | |
| | | OCB | obstructive chronic bronchitis |
| OATS | osteochondral autograft transfer system | | |
| | | OCBZ | oxcarbazepine (Trileptal) |
| OAV | oculoauriculovertebral (dysplasia) | | |
| | | OCC | occasionally |
| OAW | oral airway | | occlusal |
| OB | obese | | old chart called |
| | obesity | OCCC | open chest cardiac compression |
| | obstetrics | | |
| | occult blood | | ovarian clear cell carcinoma |
| | osteoblast | | |
| OBA | office-based anesthesia | occl | occlusion |
| | Office of Biotechnology Activities (NIH) | OCCM | open chest cardiac massage |
| OB-A | obstetrics-aborted | OCC PR | open chest cardiopulmonary resuscitation |
| OB-Del | obstetrics-delivered | | |
| OBE | out-of-body experience | | |
| OBE-CALP | placebo capsule or tablet | OCC Th | occupational therapy |
| | | Occup Rx | occupational therapy |

238

| | | | |
|---|---|---|---|
| OCD | obsessive-compulsive disorder | | overdose |
| | | | right eye |
| | osteochondritis dissecans | Δ OD 450 | deviation of optical density at 450 |
| OCE | outpatient code editor | | |
| OCG | oral cholecystogram | ODA | occipitodextra anterior |
| OCI | Obsessive-Compulsive Inventory | | once-daily aminoglycoside |
| | | | osmotic driving agent |
| OCL® | oral colonic lavage | ODAC | Oncologic Drugs Advisory Committee (of the US Food and Drug Administration) |
| OCN | obsessive-compulsive neurosis | | |
| | | | |
| | Oncology Certified Nurse | | |
| | | | on-demand analgesia computer |
| OCNS | Obsessive-Compulsive Neurosis Scale | | |
| | | ODAT | one day at a time |
| O-CNV | occult choroidal neovascularization | ODC | oral disease control |
| | | | ornithine decarboxylase |
| OCOR | on-call to operating room | | outpatient diagnostic center |
| OCP | ocular cicatricial pemphigoid | ODCH | ordinary diseases of childhood |
| | oral contraceptive pills | ODD | oculodentodigital (dysplasia) |
| | ova, cysts, parasites | | |
| OCR | oculocephalic reflex | | opposition defiance disorder |
| | optical character recognition | OD'd | overdosed |
| | | ODed | overdosed |
| OCS | Obsessive-Compulsive Scale | ODM | occlusion dose monitor |
| | | | ophthalmodynamometry |
| | oral cancer screening | ODN | optokinetic nystagmus |
| 11-OCS | 11-oxycorticosteroid | ODP | occipitodextra posterior |
| OCT | octreotide (Sandostatin) | | offspring of diabetic parents |
| | optical coherence tomograph (tomography) | | |
| | | OD/P | right eye patched |
| | | ODQ | on direct questioning |
| | oral cavity tumors | ODS | Office of Drug Safety (FDA) |
| | ornithine carbamyl transferase | | |
| | | | organized delivery system |
| | oxytocin challenge test | ODSS | Office of Disability Support Services |
| OCU | observation care unit | | |
| OCVM | occult cerebrovascular malformations | ODSU | oncology day stay unit |
| | | | One-Day Surgery Unit |
| OCX | oral cancer examination | ODT | occipitodextra transverse |
| OD | Doctor of Optometry | | orally disintegrating tablet |
| | Officer-of-the-Day | OE | on examination |
| | once daily (this is a dangerous abbreviation as it is read as right eye; use "once daily") | | orthopedic examination |
| | | | otitis externa |
| | | O-E | standard observed minus expected |
| | on duty | O&E | observation and examination |
| | optic disk | | |
| | oral-duodenal | OEC | outer ear canal |
| | outdoor | OEI | opioid escalation index |
| | outside diameter | O₂EI | oxygen extraction index |
| | ovarian dysgerminoma | | |

O

| | | | |
|---|---|---|---|
| OENT | oral endotracheal tube | | ocular hypertension |
| OEP | Office of Emergency Preparedness | | on hand |
| | | | open-heart |
| | oil of evening primrose (evening primrose oil) | | oral hygiene |
| | | | orthostatic hypotension |
| OEPA | vincristine (Oncovin), etoposide, prednisone, and doxorubicin (Adriamycin) | | outside hospital |
| | | 17-OH | 17-hydroxycorticosteroids |
| | | OHA | oral hypoglycemic agents |
| | | OHC | outer hair cell (in cochlea) |
| OER | oxygen extraction ratios | | |
| O₂ER | oxygen extraction ratio | OH Cbl | hydroxycobalamine |
| OERR | order entry/results-reports (Veterans Administration's physician computer order entry system) | 17-OHCS | 17-hydroxycorticosteroids |
| | | OHD | hydroxy vitamin D |
| | | | organic heart disease |
| | | 25(OH)D₃ | 25-hydroxy vitamin D (calcifediol, Calderol) |
| OET | oral esophageal tube | | |
| OETT | oral endotracheal tube | OHF | old healed fracture |
| OF | occipital-frontal | | Omsk hemorrhagic fever |
| | optic fundi | | overhead frame |
| | osteitis fibrosa | OHFA | hydroxy fatty acid |
| OFC | occipital-frontal circumference | OHFT | overhead frame and trapeze |
| | orbitofacial cleft | OHG | oral hypoglycemic |
| OFF | shoes off during weighing | OHI | oral hygiene instructions |
| | | OHIAA | hydroxyindolacetic acid |
| OFI | other febrile illness | OHL | oral hairy leukoplakia |
| OFLOX | ofloxacin (Floxin) | OHNS | Otolaryngology, Head, and Neck Surgery (Dept.) |
| OFLX | ofloxacin (Floxin) | | |
| OFM | open-face mask | | |
| OFNE | oxygenated fluorocarbon nutrient emulsion | OHP | obese hypertensive patient |
| | | | oxygen under hyperbaric pressure |
| OFPF | optic fundi and peripheral fields | 17 OHP | 17-hydroxyprogesterone |
| OFR | oxygen-free radicals | OHRP | open-heart rehabilitation program |
| OFTT | organic failure to thrive | | |
| OG | Obstetrics-Gynecology | OHRR | open-heart recovery room |
| | orogastric (feeding) | OHS | obesity hypoventilation syndrome |
| | outcome goal (long-term goal) | | occupational health service |
| OGC | oculogyric crisis | | ocular histoplasmosis syndrome |
| OGCT | ovarian germ cell tumor | | |
| OGD | oesophagogastro-duodenoscopy (United Kingdom and other countries) | | ocular hypoperfusion syndrome |
| | | | open-heart surgery |
| | Office of Generic Drugs (of the Food and Drug Administration) | OHSS | ovarian hyperstimulation syndrome |
| | | OHT | ocular hypertension |
| OGT | orogastric tube | | overhead trapeze |
| OGTT | oral glucose tolerance test | OHTN | ocular hypertension |
| OH | occupational history | OHTx | orthotopic heart transplantation |
| | ocular history | | |

**240**

| OI | opportunistic infection | | ophthalmic laser |
|---|---|---|---|
| | osteogenesis imperfecta | | microendoscope |
| | otitis interna | OLNM | occult lymph node |
| OIF | oil-immersion field | | metastases |
| OIG | Office of the Inspector | OLP | abnormal lipoprotein |
| | General | OLR | optic labyrinthine righting |
| OIH | orthoiodohippurate | | otology, laryngology, and |
| OIHA | orthoiodohippuric acid | | rhinology |
| OI&I | occupational injury and | OLS | ordinary least squares |
| | illness | | ouabain-like substance |
| OINT | ointment | OLT | occipitolaevoposterior |
| OIRDA | occipital intermittent | | orthotopic liver |
| | rhythmical delta activity | | transplantation |
| OIS | ocular ischemic syndrome | OLTP | online transaction |
| | optical intrinsic signal | | processing |
| | (imaging) | OLTx | orthotopic liver |
| | optimum information size | | transplantation |
| OIs | opportunistic infections | OLV | one-lung ventilation |
| OIT | ovarian immature | OLZ | olanzapine (Zyprexa) |
| | teratoma | OM | every morning (this is a |
| OIU | optical internal | | dangerous abbreviation) |
| | urethrotomy | | obtuse marginal |
| OJ | orange juice (this is a | | ocular melanoma |
| | dangerous abbreviation | | oral motor |
| | as it is read as OS-left | | oral mucositis |
| | eye) | | organomegaly |
| | orthoplast jacket | | osteomalacia |
| OK | all right | | osteomyelitis |
| | approved | | otitis media |
| | correct | $O_2M$ | oxygen mask |
| OKAN | optokinetic after | $OM_1$ | first obtuse marginal |
| | nystagmus | | (branch) |
| OKC | odontogenic keratocyst | $OM_2$ | second obtuse marginal |
| | open kinetic chain | | (branch) |
| OKN | optokinetic nystagmus | OMA | older maternal age |
| OKT | Ortho Kung T-cell, | OMAC | otitis media, acute, |
| | designation for a series | | catarrhal |
| | of antigens | OMAS | otitis media, acute, |
| OL | left eye | | suppurating |
| | open label (study) | OMB | obtuse marginal branch |
| OLA | occiput left anterior | $OMB_1$ | first obtuse marginal |
| | occipitolaevoanterior | | branch |
| OLAP | online analytical | $OMB_2$ | second obtuse marginal |
| | processing | | branch |
| OLB | open-liver biopsy | OMC | open mitral |
| | open-lung biopsy | | commissuortomy |
| OLBPQ | Oswestry Low Back Pain | | ostiomeatal complex |
| | Questionnaire | OMCA | otitis media, catarrhalis, |
| OLC | ouabain-like compound | | acute |
| OLD | obstructive lung | OMCC | otitis media, catarrhalis, |
| | disease | | chronic |
| OLF | ouabain-like factor | OMD | organic mental |
| OLM | ocular larva migrans | | disorder |

| | | | |
|---|---|---|---|
| OME | Office of Medical Examiner | ONSD | optic nerve sheath decompression |
| | otitis media with effusion | ONSF | optic nerve sheath fenestration |
| 7-OMEN | menogaril | ONTD | open neural tube defect(s) |
| OMFS | oral and maxillofacial surgery | ONTR | orders not to resuscitate |
| OMG | ocular myasthenia gravis | OO | ophthalmic ointment |
| OMI | old myocardial infarct | | oral order |
| OMP | oculomotor (third nerve) palsy | | other |
| | open mediastinal biopsy | o/o | on account of |
| OMPA | otitis media, purulent, acute | O&O | off and on |
| | | OOB | out of bed |
| OMPC | otitis media, purulent, chronic | OOBL | out of bilirubin light |
| | | OOBBRP | out of bed with bathroom privileges |
| OMR | operative mortality rate | | |
| OMS | oral morphine sulfate | OOC | onset of contractions |
| | organic mental syndrome | | out of cast |
| | organic mood syndrome | | out of control |
| OMSA | otitis media secretory (or suppurative) acute | OO Con | out of control |
| | | OOD | outer orbital diameter |
| OMSC | otitis media secretory (or suppurative) chronic | | out of doors |
| | | OOF | out of facility |
| OMT | oral mucosal transudate | OOH | out of hospital |
| | Osteopathic manipulative technique | OOH&NS | ophthalmology, otorhinolaryngology, and head and neck surgery |
| OMVC | open mitral valve commissurotomy | | |
| | | OOI | out of isolette |
| OMVD | optimized microvessel density (analysis) | OOL | onset of labor |
| | | OOLR | ophthalmology, otology, laryngology, and rhinology |
| OMVI | operating motor vehicle intoxicated | | |
| | | OOM | onset of menarche |
| ON | every night (this is a dangerous abbreviation) | OOP | out of pelvis |
| | | | out of plaster |
| | optic nerve | | out on pass |
| | optic neurophathy | OOPS | out of program status |
| | oronasal | OOR | out of room |
| | Ortho-Novum® | OORW | out of radiant warmer |
| | overnight | OOS | out of sequence |
| ONC | over-the-needle catheter | | out of specification (deviation from standard) |
| | vincristine (Oncovin) | | |
| OND | ondansetron (Zofran) | | out of splint |
| | other neurologic disorder(s) | | out of stock |
| ONH | optic nerve head | OOT | out of town |
| | optic nerve hypoplasia | OOW | out of wedlock |
| ONM | ocular neuromyotonia | OP | oblique presentation |
| ON RR | overnight recovery room | | occiput posterior |
| | | | open |
| ONS | Office for National Statistics (United Kingdom) | | operation |

| | organophosphorous | OPL | oral premalignant lesion |
| | oropharynx | | other party liability |
| | oscillatory potentials | OPLL | ossification of posterior |
| | osteoporosis | | latitudinal ligament |
| | outpatient | OPM | occult primary |
| | overpressure | | malignancy |
| O&P | ova and parasites (stool | | oral and pharyngeal |
| | examination) | | mucositis |
| OPA | oral pharyngeal | OPN | osteopontin |
| | airway | OPO | organ procurement |
| | outpatient anesthesia | | organizations |
| OPAC | opacity (opacification) | OPOC | oral pharynx, oral cavity |
| OPAT | outpatient parenteral | OPP | opposite |
| | antibiotic therapy | OPPG | oculopneumoplethysmog- |
| OPB | outpatient basis | | raphy |
| OPC | operable pancreatic | OPPOS | opposition |
| | carcinoma | OPPS | Outpatient Prospective |
| | oropharyngeal candidiasis | | Payment System |
| | outpatient care | OPQRST | onset, provocation, |
| | outpatient catheterization | | quality, radiation, |
| | outpatient clinic | | severity, and time (an |
| OPCA | olivopontocerebellar | | EMT mnemonic used |
| | atrophy | | in initial patient |
| OPCAB | off-pump coronary artery | | questioning) |
| | bypass (grafting) | OPRDU | outpatient renal dialysis |
| *op cit* | in the work cited | | unit |
| OPCS-4 | Classification of Surgical | OPS | Objective Pain Scores |
| | Operations and | | operations |
| | Procedures (4th | | Orpington prognostic |
| | revision) | | scale |
| OPD | oropharyngeal dysphagia | | orthogonal polarization |
| | Orphan Products | | spectral (imaging) |
| | Development (office of) | | outpatient surgery |
| | outpatient department | OPSI | overwhelming |
| O'p'-DDD | mitotane (Lysodren) | | postsplenectomy |
| OPDRA | Office of Postmarketing | | infection |
| | Drug Risk Assessment | OPSU | outpatient surgical unit |
| | (FDA) (name changed | O PSY | open psychiatry |
| | to Office of Drug | OPT | optimum |
| | Safety [ODS]) | | outpatient treatment |
| OPDUR | on-line prospective drug | OPT c CA | Ohio pediatric tent with |
| | utilization review | | compressed air |
| OPE | oral peripheral | OPT c O₂ | Ohio pediatric tent with |
| | examination | | oxygen |
| | outpatient evaluation | OPTN | Organ Procurement and |
| OPEN | vincristine (Oncovin), | | Transplantation |
| | prednisone, etoposide, | | Network |
| | and mitoxantrone | OPT-NSC | outpatient treatment, |
| | (Novantrone) | | nonservice-connected |
| OPERA | outpatient endometrial | OPT-SC | outpatient treatment, |
| | resection/ablation | | service-connected |
| OPG | ocular plethysmography | OPV | oral polio vaccine |
| | osteoprotegerin | | outpatient visit |

| | | | |
|---|---|---|---|
| OR | odds ratio | | occipitosacral |
| | oil retention | | oligospermic |
| | open reduction | | opening snap |
| | operating room | | ophthalmic solution (this |
| | Orthodox | | is a dangerous |
| | own recognizance | | abbreviation as it is |
| ORA | occiput right anterior | | read as left eye) |
| ORC | outpatient rehabilitation | | oral surgery |
| | centers | | Osgood-Schlatter (disease) |
| ORCH | orchiectomy | | osmium |
| ORD | orderly | | osteosarcoma |
| OREF | open reduction, external | | overall survival |
| | fixation | OSA | obstructive sleep apnea |
| ORF | open reading frame | | off-site anesthesia |
| OR&F | open reduction and | | osteosarcoma |
| | fixation | OSA/HS | obstructive sleep apnea/ |
| ORIF | open reduction internal | | hypopnea syndrome |
| | fixation | OSAS | obstructive sleep apnea |
| ORL | oblique retinacular | | syndrome |
| | ligament | OSCAR | On-line Survey |
| | otorhinolaryngology | | Certification and |
| | (otology, rhinology and | | Reporting |
| | laryngology) | OSCC | oral squamous cell |
| ORMF | open reduction metallic | | carcinoma |
| | fixation | OSCE | Objective Structured |
| ORN | operating room nurse | | Clinical Examination |
| | osteoradionecrosis | OSD | Osgood-Schlatter disease |
| OROS | ostomotic release oral | | overseas duty |
| | system | | overside drainage |
| ORP | occiput right posterior | OSE | ovarian surface epithelium |
| ORR | overall response rate | OSESC | opening snap ejection |
| ORS | olfactory reference | | systolic click |
| | syndrome | OSFT | outstretched fingertips |
| | oral rehydration salts | OSH | outside hospital |
| ORT | oestrogen (estrogen)- | OSHA | Occupational Safety & |
| | replacement therapy | | Health Administration |
| | operating room | OSM S | osmolarity serum |
| | technician | OSM U | osmolarity urine |
| | oral rehydration therapy | OSN | off-service note |
| | Registered Occupational | OSP | outside pass |
| | Therapist | OS/P | left eye patched |
| OR XI | oriented to time | OSS | osseous |
| OR X2 | oriented to time and | | over-shoulder strap |
| | place | OSSI | orthognathic surgery |
| OR X3 | oriented to time, place, | | simulating instrument |
| | and person | OST | optimal sampling theory |
| OR X4 | oriented to time, place, | OT | occiput transverse |
| | person, and objects | | occupational therapy |
| | (watch, pen, book) | | old tuberculin |
| OS | left eye | | on-treatment |
| | mouth (this is a dangerous | | oral transmucosal |
| | abbreviation as it is | | orotracheal |
| | read as left eye) | | outlier threshold |

|       | oxytocin (Pitocin) | OVAL | ovalocytes |
| O/T | oral temperature | OVF | Octopus® visual field |
| OTA | open to air | OVLT | organum vasculosum of lamina terminalis |
| OTC | occult tumor cell | OVR | Office of Vocational Rehabilitation |
|       | ornithine transcarbamoylase | OVS | obstructive voiding symptoms (syndrome) |
|       | Orthopedic Technician, Certified | OW | once weekly (this is a dangerous abbreviation) |
|       | over-the-counter (sold without prescription) |       | open wound |
| OTCD | ornithine-transcarbamylase deficiency |       | oral warts |
|       |       |       | outer wall |
| OTD | optimal therapeutic dose |       | out of wedlock |
|       | organ tolerance dose |       | ova weight |
|       | out-the-door | O/W | oil in water |
| OTE | (McMaster) Overall Treatment Evaluation |       | otherwise |
| OTFC | oral transmucosal fentanyl citrate (Fentanyl Oralet; Actiq) | OWL | out of wedlock |
|       |       | OWNK | out of wedlock, not keeping (baby) |
| OTH | other | OWR | Osler-Weber-Rendu (disease) |
| OTHS | occupational therapy home service | OWT | zero work tolerance |
| OTIS | Organization of Teratology Information Services | OX | oximeter |
|       |       | O×1 | oriented to time |
|       |       | O×2 | oriented to time and place |
| OTJ | on-the-job (injury) | O×3 | oriented to time, place, and person |
| OTO | one-time only | O×4 | oriented to time, place, person, and objects (watch, pen, book) |
|       | otolaryngology |       |       |
|       | otology |       |       |
| OTPT | oral triphasic tablets (contraceptive) | OXA | oxacillinase |
| OTR | Occupational Therapist, Registered |       | oxaliplatin (Eloxatin) |
|       |       | OXC | oxcarbazepine (Trileptal) |
| OTRL | Occupational Therapist, Registered Licensed | Oxi | oximeter (oximetry) |
|       |       | Ox-LDL | oxidized low-density lipoprotein |
| OT/RT | occupational therapy/ recreational therapy | OXPHOS | oxidative phosphorylation |
|       |       | OxPt | oxaliplatin (Eloxatin) |
| OTS | orotracheal suction | OXM | pulse oximeter |
| OTT | oral transit time | OXT | oxytocin (Pitocin) |
|       | orotracheal tube | Oxy-5® | benzoyl peroxide |
| OTW | off-the-wall | OXZ | oxazepam (Serax) |
| OU | each eye | OZ | optical zone |
| OUES | oxygen uptake efficiency slope |       | ounce |
| OULQ | outer upper left quadrant |       |       |
| OU/P | both eyes patched |       |       |
| OURQ | outer upper right quadrant |       |       |
| OUS | obstetric ultrasound |       |       |
| OV | office visit |       |       |
|       | ovary |       |       |
|       | ovum |       |       |

O

# P

| | | | |
|---|---|---|---|
| P | para | | phenol and alcohol (procedure for of toenail) |
| | peripheral | | position and alignment |
| | phosphorus | $P_2 > A_2$ | pulmonic second heart |
| | pint | | sound greater than |
| | plan | | aortic second heart |
| | *Plasmodium* | | sound |
| | poor | PAAA | para-anastomotic |
| | protein | | aneurysm of the |
| | Protestant | | aorta |
| | pulse | PAB | premature atrial beat |
| | pupil | | pulmonary artery banding |
| *P* | statistical probability | PABA | aminobenzoic acid (para-aminobenzoic acid) |
| | value | | |
| p̄ | after | PABD | preoperative autologous |
| /P | partial lower denture | | blood donation |
| P/ | partial upper denture | PAC | cisplatin (Platinol), |
| P1 | pilocarpine 1% | | doxorubicin |
| | ophthalmic solution | | (Adriamycin), and |
| $P_2$ | pulmonic second heart | | cylcophosphamide |
| | sound | | phenacemide |
| P20 | Ocusert® P20 | | Physical Assessment |
| $^{32}P$ | radioactive phosphorus | | Center |
| P40 | Ocusert® P40 | | Physician Assistant, |
| P53 | tumor suppressive | | Certified |
| | gene | | picture archiving |
| PA | panic attack | | communication |
| | paranoid | | (system) |
| | periapical (x-ray) | | Port-a-cath® |
| | pernicious anemia | | premature atrial |
| | phenol alcohol | | contraction |
| | physical activity | | prophylactic |
| | Physician Assistant | | anticonvulsants |
| | pineapple | | pulmonary artery catheter |
| | platelet aggregometry | PA-C | Physician Assistant, |
| | posterior-anterior | | Certified |
| | (posteroanterior) (x-ray) | PACATH | pulmonary artery catheter |
| | premature adrenarche | PACE | population-adjusted |
| | presents again | | clinical epidemiology |
| | professional association | PACG | primary angle-closure |
| | (similar to a | | glaucoma |
| | corporation) | PACH | pipers to after coming |
| | *Pseudomonas aeruginosa* | | head |
| | psychiatric aide | PACI | partial anterior cerebral |
| | psychoanalysis | | infarct |
| | pulmonary artery | $PACO_2$ | partial pressure (tension) |
| Pa | pascal | | of carbon dioxide, |
| P&A | percussion and | | alveolar |
| | auscultation | $PaCO_2$ | partial pressure (tension) of carbon dioxide, artery |
| | | PACS | picture archiving and |

|  | communications systems |  | polynuclear aromatic hydrocarbon |
|---|---|---|---|
| PACT | prism and alternate cover test |  | predicted adult height |
|  |  |  | primary adrenal hyperplasia |
|  | Program of Assertive Community Treatment |  | pulmonary arterial hypertension |
| PAC-V | cisplatin (Platinol), doxorubicin (Adriamycin), and cyclophosphamide | PAHO | Pan American Health Organization |
|  |  | PAI | plasminogen activator inhibitor |
| PACU | postanesthesia care unit |  | platelet accumulation index |
| PAD | pelvic adhesive disease |  |  |
|  | peripheral artery disease | PAIDS | pediatric acquired immunodeficiency syndrome |
|  | pharmacologic atrial defibrillator |  |  |
|  | preliminary anatomic diagnosis | PAIgG | platelet-associated immunoglobulin G |
|  | preoperative autologous donation | PAIVMs | passive accessory intervertebral movements |
|  | primary affective disorder |  |  |
| PADP | pulmonary arterial diastolic pressure | PAIVS | pulmonary atresia with intact ventricle septum |
|  |  | PAK | pancreas and kidney |
|  | pulmonary artery diastolic pressure | PAL | physical activity levels |
| PADS | Post Anesthesia Discharge Scoring System |  | posterior axillary line |
|  |  |  | posteroanterior and lateral |
| PAE | percutaneous angiographic embolization | PALA | N-phosphoacetate-L aspartate |
|  | postanoxic encephalopathy | Pa Line | pulmonary artery line |
|  |  | PALN | para-aortic lymph node |
|  | postantibiotic effect | PALP | palpation |
|  | pre-admission evaluation | PALS | pediatric advanced life support |
|  | progressive assistive exercise |  |  |
| PAEDP | pulmonary artery and end-diastole pressure |  | periarterial lymphatic sheath |
| PAF | paroxysmal atrial fibrillation | PAM | partial allosteric modulators |
|  |  |  | potential acuity meter |
|  | platelet-activating factor |  | primary acquired melanosis |
| PA&F | percussion, auscultation, and fremitus |  | primary amebic meningoencephalitis |
| PAFE | postantifungal effect |  | protein A mimetic |
| PAGA | premature appropriate for gestational age | 2-PAM | pralidoxime (Protopam) |
| PAGE | polyacrylamide gel electrophoresis | PAMP | pulmonary arterial (artery) mean pressure |
| PAH | para-aminohippurate | PAN | pancreas |
|  | partial abdominal hysterectomy |  | pancreatic |
|  | phenylalanine hydroxylase |  | pancuronium (Pavulon) |
|  | polycyclic aromatic hydrocarbons |  | panoral x-ray examination |
|  |  |  | periodic alternating nystagmus |

| | | | |
|---|---|---|---|
| | polyacrylonitrile (filter) | PAR | parafin |
| | polyarteritis nodosa | | parainfluenza |
| pANCA | perinuclear antineutrophil | | (paramyxovirus) |
| | cytoplasmic antibody | | vaccine |
| PANDAS | pediatric autoimmune | | parallel |
| | neuropsychiatric | | perennial allergic rhinitis |
| | disorders associated | | platelet aggregate ratio |
| | with streptococcal | | possible allergic reaction |
| | infections | | postanesthetic recovery |
| PANENDO | panendoscopy | | procedures, alternatives, |
| PANESS | physical and neurological | | and risks |
| | examination for soft | | pulmonary arteriolar |
| | signs | | resistance |
| PANP | pelvic autonomic nerve | PARA | number of pregnancies |
| | preservation | | producing viable |
| PANSS | Positive and Negative | | offspring |
| | Syndrome Scale | | paraplegic |
| PAO | peak acid output | | parathyroid |
| | peripheral arterial | PARA 1 | having borne one child |
| | occlusion | Paraflu | Parainfluenza |
| PAO$_2$ | alveolar oxygen pressure | PARC | perennial allergic |
| | (tension) | | rhinoconjunctivitis |
| PaO$_2$ | arterial oxygen pressure | PAROM | passive assistance range |
| | (tension) | | of motion |
| PAOD | peripheral arterial | PARR | postanesthesia recovery |
| | occlusive disease | | room |
| PAOP | pulmonary artery | PARS | postanesthesia recovery |
| | occlusion pressure | | score |
| PAP | passive-aggressive | PARU | postanesthetic recovery |
| | personality | | unit |
| | patient assistance program | PAS | aminosalicylic acid (para- |
| | peroxidase-anti-peroxidase | | aminosalicylic acid) |
| | pokeweed antiviral protein | | periodic acid-Schiff |
| | positive airway pressure | | (reagent) |
| | primary atypical | | peripheral anterior |
| | pneumonia | | synechia |
| | prostatic acid phosphatase | | physician-assisted suicide |
| | pulmonary alveolar | | pneumatic antiembolic |
| | proteinosis | | stocking |
| | pulmonary artery pressure | | postanesthesia score |
| PAPS | primary antiphospholipid | | premature auricular |
| | syndrome | | systole |
| Pap smear | Papanicolaou smear | | Professional Activities |
| PA/PS | pulmonary atresia/ | | Study |
| | pulmonary stenosis | | pulmonary artery stenosis |
| PAPVC | partial anomalous | | pulsatile antiembolism |
| | pulmonary venous | | system (stockings) |
| | connection | PA-S | Physician Assistant, |
| PAPVR | partial anomalous | | Student |
| | pulmonary venous | PASA | aminosalicylic acid (para- |
| | return | | aminosalicylic acid) |
| PAQLQ | Pediatric Asthma Quality | PA/S/D | pulmonary artery |
| | of Life Questionnaire | | systolic/diastolic |

P

| | | | |
|---|---|---|---|
| Pas Ex | passive exercise | | protein-bound |
| PASG | pneumatic antishock garment | | pudendal block |
| PASI | Psoriasis Area and Severity Index | Pb | pyridostigmine bromide (Mestinon) lead |
| PASK | peripheral anterior stromal keratopathy | p/b | phenobarbital postburn |
| PASP | pulmonary artery systolic pressure | P&B | pain and burning Papanicolaou and breast (examinations) |
| PASS | Pain Anxiety Symptoms Scale | | phenobarbital and belladonna |
| PAT | paroxysmal atrial tachycardia | PBA | percutaneous bladder aspiration |
| | passive alloimmune thrombocytopenia | PBAL | protected bronchoalveolar lavage |
| | patella patient | PbB | whole blood lead |
| | percent acceleration time peripheral arterial tone | PBC | point of basal convergence |
| | platelet aggregation test preadmission testing | | prebed care primary biliary cirrhosis |
| | pregnancy at term | PBD | percutaneous biliary drainage |
| PATH | pituitary adrenotropic hormone | | postburn day |
| | pathology | | proliferative breast disease |
| PATP | preadmission testing program | PBE | partial breech extraction power building exercise |
| PATS | payment at time of service | PBF | placental blood flow pulmonary blood flow |
| PAV | Pavulon (pancuronium bromide) | PBFS PBG | penile blood flow study porphobilinogen |
| PAVe | procarbazine, melphalan (Alkeran), and vinblastine (Velban) | PBI PBK | protein-bound iodine pseudophakic bullous keratopathy |
| PAVF | pulmonary arteriovenous fistula | PBL | peripheral blood lymphocyte |
| PAVM | pulmonary arteriovenous malformation | | primary breast lymphoma primary brain lymphoma |
| PAVNRT | paroxysmal atrial ventricular nodal re-entrant tachycardia | PBLC | problem-based learning premature birth live child |
| PAWP | pulmonary artery wedge pressure | PBM | pharmacy benefit management (manager) |
| PAX | periapical x-ray | PBMC | peripheral blood mononuclear cell |
| PB | barometric pressure British Pharmacopeia | PBMNC | peripheral blood mononuclear cell |
| | parafin bath phenylbutyrate piggyback | PBN | polymyxin B sulfate, bacitracin, and neomycin |
| | powder board power building | PB:ND | problem: nursing diagnosis |
| | premature beat Presbyterian | PBNS | percutaneous bladder neck stabilization |

P

| | | | |
|---|---|---|---|
| PBO | placebo | | patient care assistant (aide) |
| PBP | penicillin-binding protein | | patient-controlled analgesia |
| | phantom breast pain | | penicillamine |
| | protein-bound polysaccharide | | porous coated anatomic (joint replacement) |
| PBPC | peripheral blood progenitor cell | | postcardiac arrest |
| PBPCT | peripheral blood progenitor cell transplant | | postciliary artery |
| | | | postconceptional age |
| PBPI | penile-brachial pulse index | | posterior cerebral artery |
| | | | posterior communicating artery |
| PBPs | penicillin-binding proteins | | procainamide |
| PBS | phosphate-buffered saline | | procoagulation activity |
| | prune-belly syndrome | | prostate cancer |
| PBSC | peripheral blood stem cells | PCa | prostate cancer |
| PBT | primary brain tumor | PCAC | Physical Care Assessment Center |
| PBT$_4$ | protein-bound thyroxine | | |
| PbtO$_2$ | brain tissue partial pressure of oxygen | P-CAC | preparative continuous annular chromatography |
| PBV | percutaneous balloon valvuloplasty | PCAD | posterior circulation arterial dissection |
| PBZ | phenoxybenzamine | PCASSO | patient-centered access to secure systems online |
| | phenylbutazone | | |
| | pyribenzamine | PCB | pancuronium bromide |
| ΦBZ | phenylbutazone | | para cervical block |
| PC | after meals (*p.c.* preferred) | | placebo |
| | cisplatin (Platinol) and cyclophosphamide | | postcoital bleeding |
| | | | prepared childbirth |
| | packed cells | | procarbazine (Matulane) |
| | palliative care | | *Pseudomonas cepacia* bacteremia |
| | pancreatic carcinoma | | |
| | pathologic consultation | PCBH | personal care boarding home |
| | photocoagulation | | |
| | placebo-controlled (study) | PCBMN | palmar cutaneous branch of the median nerve |
| | platelet concentrate | | |
| | *Pneumocystis carinii* | PCBs | polychlorinated biphenyls |
| | poor condition | | |
| | politically correct | PCBUN | palmar cutaneous branch of the ulnar nerve |
| | popliteal cyst | | |
| | posterior canals (vestibular) | PCC | patient care coordinator |
| | | | petrous carotid canal |
| | posterior chamber | | pheochromocytoma |
| | premature contractions | | pneumatosis cystoides coli |
| | present complaint | | poison control center |
| | productive cough | | precipitated calcium carbonate |
| | professional corporation | | |
| | psychiatric counselor | | progressive cardiac care |
| | pubococcygeus (muscle) | PCCC | pediatric critical care center |
| *p.c.* | after meals | | |
| PCA | passive cutaneous anaphylaxis | PCCI | penetrating craniocerebral injuries |

| | | | |
|---|---|---|---|
| PCCM | primary care case management | PC&HS | after meals and at bedtime |
| PCCU | postcoronary care unit | PCI | percutaneous coronary intervention |
| PCD | pacer-cardioverter-defibrillator | | pneumatosis cystoides intestinalis |
| | paroxysmal cerebral dysrhythmia | | prophylactic cranial irradiation |
| | plasma cell dyscrasias | PCINA | patient-controlled intranasal analgesia |
| | postmortem cesarean delivery | PCIOL | posterior chamber intraocular lens |
| | primary ciliary dyskinesia | PC-IRV | pressure-controlled inverse-ratio ventilation |
| | programmed cell death | PCKD | polycystic kidney disease |
| PCDAI | Pediatric Crohn Disease Activity Index | PCL | pacing cycle length |
| PCE | physical capacities evaluation | | plasma cell leukemia |
| | | | posterior chamber lens |
| | potentially compensable event | | posterior cruciate ligament |
| | | | proximal collateral ligament |
| | pseudophakic corneal edema | PCLD | polycystic liver disease |
| PCE® | erythromycin particles in tablets | PCLI | plasma cell labeling index |
| | | PCLN | psychiatric consultation liaison nurse |
| PCEA | patient-controlled epidural analgesia | | |
| | | PCLR | paid claims loss ratio |
| PCEC | purified chick embryo cell (culture) | PCM | primary cutaneous melanoma |
| PCEAO | postcarotid endarterectomy airway obstruction | | protein-calorie malnutrition |
| | | | pubococcygeal muscle |
| PCF | pharyngeal conjunctival fever | PC-MRI | phase-contrast magnetic resonance imaging |
| PCFL | primary cutaneous follicular lymphoma | PCMX | chloroxylenol |
| | | PCN | penicillin |
| PCFT | platelet complement fixation test | | percutaneous nephrostomy |
| | | | primary care nursing |
| PCG | phonocardiogram | PCNA | proliferating cell nuclear antigen |
| | primary congenital glaucoma | | |
| | | PCNL | percutaneous nephrostolithotomy |
| | pubococcygeus (muscle) | | |
| PCGG | percutaneous coagulation of gasserian ganglion | PCNs | posterior cervical nodes |
| | | PCNSL | primary central nervous system lymphoma |
| PCGLV | poorly contractile globular left ventricle | | |
| | | PCNT | percutaneous nephrostomy tube |
| PCH | paroxysmal cold hemoglobinuria | PCO | patient complains of |
| | | | polycystic ovary |
| | periocular capillary hemangioma | | posterior capsular opacification |
| | personal care home | | |
| PCHI | permanent childhood hearing impairment | $PCO_2$ | partial pressure (tension) of carbon dioxide, artery |
| PCHL | permanent childhood hearing loss | PCOD | polycystic ovarian disease |

PCOE    prescriber (physician) computer order entry

P COMM A    posterior communicating artery

PCOS    polycystic ovary syndrome

PCP    Palliative Care Program
patient care plan
phencyclidine (phenylcyclohexyl piperidine)
*Pneumocystis carinii* pneumonia
primary care person
primary care physician
primary care provider
prochlorperazine (Compazine)
pulmonary capillary pressure

PCR    patient care report
percutaneous coronary revascularization
polymerase chain reaction
protein catabolic rate

PCr    plasma creatinine

PCRA    pure red-cell aplasia

PCR/PSA    polymerase chain reaction analysis of prostate-specific antigen

PCS    patient care system
patient-controlled sedation
personal care service
physical component summary
portable cervical spine
portacaval shunt
postconcussion syndrome

P c/s    primary cesarean section

PC-SPES    an herbal refined powder preparation of eight medicinal plants

PCT    percent
poker chip tool (for rating pain)
porphyria cutanea tarda
postcoital test
posterior chest tube
primary chemotherapy
progesterone challenge test

PCTA    percutaneous transluminal angioplasty

PCU    palliative care unit
primary care unit
progressive care unit
protective care unit

PCV    packed cell volume
polycythemia vera
pressure-controlled ventilation
procarbazine, lomustine (CCNU [Cee Nu]), and vincristine

PCV 7    pneumococcal 7-valent conjugate vaccine (Prevnar)

PCV 23    pneumococcal vaccine polyvalent (Pneumovax 23; Pnu-Imune 23)

PCVC    percutaneous central venous catheter

PCWP    pulmonary capillary wedge pressure

PCX    paracervical

PCXR    portable chest radiograph

PCZ    procarbazine (Matulane)
prochlorperazine (Compazine)

PD    interpupillary distance
Paget disease
pancreaticoduodenectomy
panic disorder
Parkinson disease
percutaneous drain
peritoneal dialysis
personality disorder
pharmacodynamics
pocket depth (dental)
poorly differentiated
postural drainage
pressure dressing
prism diopter
progressive disease
pupillary distance

P/D    packs per day (cigarettes)

2PD    two point discriminatory test

$^{103}$Pd    palladium 103

PDA    parenteral drug abuser
patent ductus arteriosus
personal digital assistant
poorly differentiated adenocarcinoma

| | |
|---|---|
| | posterior descending (coronary) artery |
| | property damage accident |
| PDAF | platelet-derived angiogenesis factor |
| PDAP | peritoneal dialysis-associated peritonitis |
| PDB | preperitoneal distention balloon |
| PDC | patient denies complaints |
| | poorly differentiated carcinoma |
| | private diagnostic clinic |
| | property damage collision (crash) |
| | pyruvate dehydogenase complex |
| PD&C | postural drainage and clapping |
| PDCA | Plan-Do-Check-Act (process improvement) |
| PDD | cisplatin |
| | pervasive developmental disorder |
| | premenstrual dysphoric disorder |
| | primary degenerative dementia |
| PDE | paroxysmal dyspnea on exertion |
| | pulsed Doppler echocardiography |
| PDE 5 | phosphodiesterase type 5 |
| PDEGF | platelet-derived epidermal growth factor |
| PDF | Portable Document Format |
| PDFC | premature dead female child |
| PDGF | platelet-derived growth factor |
| PDGXT | predischarge graded exercise test |
| PDH | past dental history |
| | pyruvate dehydrogenase |
| PDI | Pain Disability Index |
| | phasic detrusor instability |
| | psychomotor developmental index |
| PDIGC | patient dismissed in good condition |
| PDL | periodontal ligament |
| | poorly differentiated lymphocytic |

| | |
|---|---|
| | postures of daily living |
| | progressively diffused leukoencephalopathy |
| | pulsed-dye laser |
| PDL-D | poorly differentiated lymphocytic-diffuse |
| PDL-N | poorly differentiated lymphocytic-nodular |
| PDMC | premature dead male child |
| PDN | Paget disease of the nipple |
| | prednisone |
| | private duty nurse |
| | prosthetic disk nucleus |
| PDNE | poorly differentiated neuroendocrine (carcinoma) |
| PDOX | pegylated doxorubicin |
| PDP | pachydermoperiostosis |
| | peak diastolic pressure |
| PD & P | postural drainage and percussion |
| PDPH | postdural puncture headache |
| PDQ | pretty damn quick (at once) |
| PDR | patients' dining room |
| | *Physicians' Desk Reference* |
| | point of decreasing response |
| | postdelivery room |
| | proliferative diabetic retinopathy |
| | prospective drug review |
| PDRcVII | proliferative diabetic retinopathy with vitreous hemorrhage |
| PDRP | proliferative diabetic retinopathy |
| PDS | pain dysfunction syndrome |
| | persistent developmental stuttering |
| | polydioxanone suture |
| | Progressive Deterioration Scale |
| PDSA | Plan, Do, Study, and Act |
| PDT | percutaneous dilatational tracheostomy |
| | photodynamic therapy |
| | postdisaster trauma |

| PDTC | pyrrolidine dithiocarbamate |
| PDU | pulsed Doppler ultrasonography |
| PDUFA | Prescription Drug User Fee Act (1992) |
| PDUR | postdialysis urea rebound |
| | prospective drug utilization review |
| PDW | platelet distribution width |
| PDWHF | platelet-derived wound healing factors |
| PDx | principal diagnosis |
| pDXA | peripheral dual energy x-ray absorptiometry |
| PE | cisplatin (Platinol AQ) and etoposide |
| | pedal edema |
| | pelvic examination |
| | pharyngoesophageal |
| | phenytoin equivalent (150 mg of fosphenytoin sodium is equivalent to 100 mg of phenytoin sodium) |
| | physical education (gym) |
| | physical examination |
| | physical exercise |
| | plasma exchange |
| | pleural effusion |
| | pneumatic equalization |
| | polyethylene |
| | preeclampsia |
| | premature ejaculation |
| | pressure equalization |
| | pulmonary edema |
| | pulmonary embolism |
| P₁E₁® | epinephrine 1%, pilocarpine 1% ophthalmic solution |
| P&E | prep and enema |
| PE24 | Preemie Enfamil 24 |
| PEA | pelvic examination under anesthesia |
| | pre-emptive analgesia |
| | pulseless electrical activity |
| PEARL | physiologic endometrial ablation/resection loop |
| | pupils equal accommodation, reactive to light |
| | pupils equal and reactive to light |

| PEARLA | pupils equal and react to light and accommodation |
| PEB | cisplatin, etoposide, and bleomycin |
| PEC | pectoralis |
| | pulmonary ejection click |
| PECCE | planned extracapsular cataract extraction |
| PECHO | prostatic echogram |
| PECHR | peripheral exudative choroidal hemorrhagic retinopathy |
| PECO₂ | mixed expired carbon dioxide tension |
| PED | paroxysmal exertion-induced dyskinesia |
| | pediatrics |
| | pigment epithelial detachments |
| PEDD | proton-electron dipole-dipole |
| PEDI | pediatric evaluation of disability inventory |
| PEDI-DEG | pediatric deglycerolized red blood cells |
| Peds | pediatrics |
| PEE | punctate epithelial erosion |
| PEEP | positive end-expiratory pressure |
| PEF | cisplatin (Platinol AQ), epirubicin, and fluorouracil |
| | peak expiratory flow |
| PEFR | peak expiratory flow rate |
| PEFSR | partial expiratory flow static recoil curve |
| PEG | pegylated |
| | percutaneous endoscopic gastrostomy |
| | pneumoencephalogram |
| | polyethylene glycol |
| PEG-ELS | polyethylene glycol and iso-osmolar electrolyte solution |
| PEGG | Parent Education and Guidance Group |
| PEG-J | percutaneous endoscopic gastrojejunostomy |
| PEG-JET | percutaneous endoscopic gastrostomy with jejunal extension tube |

| | | | |
|---|---|---|---|
| PEG-SOD | polyethylene glycol-conjugated superoxide dismutase (pegorgotein) | | pertussis (whooping cough) vaccine, antigens not otherwise unspecified |
| PEI | cisplatin (Platinol AQ), etoposide, and ifosfamide | | protein efficiency ratio |
| | | PER$_a$ | pertussis, acellular antigen(s), vaccine |
| | percutaneous ethanol injection | PERC | perceptual |
| | phosphate excretion index | | percutaneous |
| | physical efficiency index | PERF | perfect |
| | polyethylenimine | | perforation |
| PEJ | percutaneous endoscopic jejunostomy | Peri Care | perineum care |
| | | PERIO | periodontal disease |
| PEK | punctate epithelial keratopathy | | periodontitis |
| | | peri-pads | perineal pads |
| PEL | permissible exposure limits | PERL | pupils equal, reactive to light |
| | primary effusion lymphomas | PERLA | pupils equally reactive to light and accommodation |
| PELD | percutaneous endoscopic lumbar diskectomy | per os | by mouth (this is a dangerous abbreviation as it is read as left eye) |
| PELV | pelvimetry | | |
| PEM | prescription event monitoring | PERR | pattern evoked retinal response |
| | protein-energy malnutrition | | |
| PEMA | phenylethylmalonamide | PERRL | pupils equal, round, and reactive to light |
| PEMS | physical, emotional, mental, and safety | PERRLA | pupils equal, round, reactive to light and accommodation |
| | post-exercise muscle soreness | | |
| PEN | parenteral and enteral nutrition | PERR-LADC | pupils equal, round, reactive to light and accommodation directly and consensually |
| | Pharmacy Equivalent Name | | |
| PENS | percutaneous electrical nerve stimulation | PERRRLA | pupils equal, round, regular, react to light and accommodation |
| | percutaneous epidural nerve stimulator | PERT | pancreatic enzyme replacement therapy |
| PEO | progressive external ophthalmoplegia | | program evaluation and review technique |
| PEP | patient education program | | |
| | pharmacologic erection program | PERV | porcine endogenous retroviruses |
| | postexposure prophylaxis | PER$_w$ | pertussis, whole-cell antigens, vaccine |
| | preejection period | | |
| | protein electrophoresis | PES | polyethersulfone |
| PEP/ET | pre-ejection period/ejection time | | preexcitation syndrome |
| | | | programmed electrical stimulation |
| PEPI | preejection period index | | |
| PEPP | payment error prevention program | | pseudoexfoliation syndrome |
| PER | by | peSPL | peak equivalent sound pressure level |
| | pediatric emergency room | | |

P

255

| | | | |
|---|---|---|---|
| PET | poor exercise tolerance | PFHx | positive family history |
| | positron-emission tomography | PFI | pill-free intervals progression-free interval |
| | preeclamptic toxemia | PFJ | patellofemoral joint |
| | pressure equalizing tubes | PFJS | patellofemoral joint syndrome |
| | problem elicitation technique | PFL | cisplatin (Platinol AQ), fluorouracil, and leucovorin |
| PETN | pentaerythritol tetranitrate | | |
| PEX | pseudoexfoliation (glaucoma) | PFL+IFN | cisplatin (Platinol AQ), fluorouracil, leucovorin, and interferon alfa 2b |
| PEx | physical examination | | |
| PEX# 3 | plasma exchange number three | PFM | porcelain fused to metal primary fibromyalgia |
| PF | patellofemoral | PFME | pelvic floor muscle exercise |
| | peak flow | | |
| | peripheral fields | PFO | patent foramen ovale |
| | plantar flexion | PFP | progression free probability |
| | Pontiac fever | | |
| | power factor | | proinsulin fusion protein |
| | preservative free | PFPC | Pall filtered packed cells |
| | prostatic fluid | PFPS | patellofemoral pain syndrome |
| | pulmonary fibrosis | | |
| | push fluids | PFR | parotid flow rate |
| Pf | *Plasmodium falciparum* | | peak flow rate |
| PF3 | platelet factor 3 | PFRC | plasma-free red cells |
| PF4 | platelet factor 4 | PFROM | pain-free range of motion |
| 16PF | The Sixteen Personality Factors test | PFS | patellar femoral syndrome patient financial services |
| PFA | foscarnet (phosphonoformatic acid) (Foscavir) | | prefilled syringe preservative-free solution (system) |
| | patellofemoral arthritis | | primary fibromyalgia syndrome |
| | platelet function analysis | | |
| | psychological first aid | | progression-free survival |
| | pure free acid | | pulmonary function studies (study) |
| PFB | potential for breakdown | | |
| | pseudofolliculitis barbae | | |
| PFC | patient-focused care | PFSH | past, family, and social history (histories) |
| | perfluorochemical | | |
| | permanent flexure contracture | PFT | parafascicular thalamotomy |
| | persistent fetal circulation | | pulmonary function test |
| | prolonged febrile convulsions | PFTC | primary fallopian tube carcinoma |
| P̄ FEEDS | after feedings | PFU | plaque-forming unit |
| PFFD | proximal femoral focal deficiency (defect) | PFW | pHisoHex® face wash |
| | | PFWB | Pall filtered whole blood |
| PFFFP | Pall filtered fresh frozen plasma | | Psychological General Well-Being (index) |
| PFGE | pulsed field gel electrophoresis | PG | paged in hospital paregoric |
| PfHRP-2 | *Plasmodium falciparum* histidine-rich protein 2 | | performance goal (short-term goal) |

P

| | | | |
|---|---|---|---|
| | phosphatidylglycerol | P±GTC | partial seizures with or without generalized tonic-clonic seizures |
| | picogram (pg) ($10^{-12}$ gram) | | |
| | placental grade (biophysical profile) | pGTD | persistent gestational trophoblastic disease |
| | polygalacturonate | PG-TXL | poly (L-glutamic acid)-paclitaxel |
| | practice guidelines | | |
| | pregnant | PGU | postgonococcal urethritis |
| | prostaglandin | PGW | person gametocyte week |
| | pyoderma gangrenosum | PGY-1 | postgraduate year one (first year resident) |
| PGA | prostaglandin A | | |
| | **p**rothrombin time, **g**amma-glutamyl transpeptidase activity, and serum **a**polipoprotein AI concentration | pH | hydrogen ion concentration |
| | | PH | past history |
| | | | personal history |
| | | | pinhole |
| | | | poor health |
| PGCH | postinfantile giant cell hepatitis | | pubic hair |
| | | | public health |
| PGCs | primordial germ cells | | pulmonary hypertension |
| PGD | preimplantation genetic diagnosis | P&H | physical and history |
| | | Ph[1] | Philadelphia chromosome |
| PGE | posterior gastroenterostomy | PHA | arterial pH |
| | | | passive hemagglutinating |
| | proximal gastric exclusion | | peripheral hyperalimentation |
| PGE$_1$ | alprostadil (prostaglandin E$_1$) | | phenylalanine |
| PGE$_2$ | dinoprostone (prostaglandin E$_2$) | | phytohemagglutinin antigen |
| PGF | paternal grandfather | | postoperative holding area |
| PGF$_{2\alpha}$ | dinoprost (prostaglandin F$_{2\alpha}$) | PHACO | phacoemulsification |
| PGGF | paternal great-grandfather | PHACO OD | phacoemulsification of the right eye |
| PGGM | paternal great-grandmother | PHACO OS | phacoemulsification of the left eye |
| PGH | pituitary growth hormones | PHAL | peripheral hyperalimentation |
| PGI | potassium, glucose, and insulin | PHAR | pharmacist |
| | | | pharmacy |
| PGI$_2$ | epoprostenol (Prostacyclin) | | pharynx |
| PGL | persistent generalized lymphadenopathy | Pharm | Pharmacy |
| | | PharmD | Doctor of Pharmacy |
| | primary gastric lymphoma | PHb | pyridoxylated hemoglobin |
| PGM | paternal grandmother | PHC | posthospital care |
| | phosphoglucomutase | | primary health care |
| PGP | paternal grandparent | | primary hepatocellular carcinoma |
| Pgp | P-glycoprotein | | |
| PGR | pulse-generated runoff | PHCA | profound hypothermic cardiac arrest |
| PgR | progesterone receptor | | |
| P-graph | penile plethysmograph | PHD | paroxysmal hypnogenic dyskinesia |
| PGS | Persian Gulf syndrome | | |
| PGT | play-group therapy | | Public Health Department |

P

| | | | |
|---|---|---|---|
| PhD | Doctor of Philosophy | | pseudohypoparathyroidism |
| PHE | periodic health examination | | pyridoxalated hemoglobin polyoxyethylene conjugate |
| PHEN-FEN | phentermine and fenfluramine | | |
| PHEO | pheochromocytoma | PHPT | primary hyperparathyroidism |
| PHEP | progressive home exercise program | PHPV | persistent hyperplastic primary vitreous |
| PHF | paired helical filament | PHR | peak heart rate |
| PHG | portal hypertensive gastropathy | | personal health record |
| PHH | paraesophageal hiatus hernia | PhRMA | Pharmaceutical Research and Manufacturers of America (Formerly the Pharmaceutical Manufacturers Association) |
| | posthemorrhagic hydrocephalus | | |
| PHHI | persistent hyperinsulinemic hypoglycemia of infancy | PHS | partial hospitalization program |
| PHI | phosphohexose isomerase | | US Public Health Service |
| | prehospital index | PHT | phenytoin (Dilantin) |
| | protected health information | | portal hypertension |
| PHIS | posthead injury syndrome | | posterior hyaloidal traction |
| PHL | permanent hearing loss | | postmenopausal hormone therapy |
| | Philadelphia (chromosome) | | primary hyperthyroidism |
| PHLIS | Public Health Laboratory Information System | | pulmonary hypertension |
| PHLS | Public Health Laboratory Service (United Kingdom) | PHTC | pulmonary hypertensive crises |
| | | PHV | peak height velocity |
| PHM | partial hydatidiform mole | PHVA | pinhole visual acuity |
| | preventative health maintenance | pHVA | plasma homovanillic acid |
| PHMB | polyhexamethylene biguanine | PHVD | posthemorrhagic ventricular dilatation |
| PHMD | polyhexamethylene (Baquacil, a pool cleaner) | PHx | past history |
| | | Phx | pharynx |
| | | PHY | physician |
| PHN | postherpetic neuralgia | PhyO | physician's orders |
| | public health nurse | PI | package insert |
| | Puritan® heated nebulizer | | pallidal index |
| | | | pancreatic insufficiency |
| PHNC | public health nurse coordinator | | Pearl Index |
| | | | performance improvement |
| PHNI | pinhole no improvement | | peripheral iridectomy |
| PHO | Physician/Hospital Organization | | persistent illness |
| | | | physically impaired |
| PHOB | phobic anxiety | | poison ivy |
| PHP | pooled human plasma | | postincident |
| | postheparin plasma | | postinjury |
| | prepaid health plan | | premature infant |
| | | | present illness |
| | | | principal investigator |

| | protease inhibitor | PIE | pulmonary infiltration |
|---|---|---|---|
| | pulmonary infarction | | with eosinophilia |
| | pulmonic insufficiency | | pulmonary interstitial |
| PI-3 | parainfluenza 3 virus | | emphysema |
| P & I | probe and irrigation | PIEE | pulsed irrigation for |
| PIA | personal injury | | enhanced evacuation |
| | accident | PIF | peak inspiratory flow |
| PIAT | Peabody Individual | PIFG | poor intrauterine fetal |
| | Achievement Test | | growth |
| PIB | professional information | PIG | pertussis immune |
| | brochure | | globulin |
| PIBD | paucity of interlobular | PIGI | pregnancy-induced |
| | bile ducts | | glucose intolerance |
| PIBF | progesterone-induced | PIGN | postinfectious |
| | blocking factor | | glomerulonephritis |
| PIC | penicillin-inhibitor | PIH | pregnancy-induced |
| | combinations | | hypertension |
| | peripherally inserted | | preventricular |
| | catheter | | intraventricular |
| | personal injury collision | | hemorrhage |
| | (crash) | | prolactin-inhibiting |
| | polysaccharide-iron | | hormone |
| | complex | PIIID | peripheral indwelling |
| | postintercourse | | intermediate infusion |
| PICA | Porch Index of | | device |
| | Communicative Ability | PIIIP | aminoterminal type three |
| | posterior inferior | | procollagen propeptide |
| | cerebellar artery | PIIS | posterior inferior iliac |
| | posterior inferior | | spine |
| | communicating artery | PIL | patient information |
| PICC | peripherally inserted | | leaflet |
| | central catheter | PILO | pilocarpine |
| PICHI | pulse-inversion contrast | PIM | Program Integrity Manual |
| | harmonic imaging | | pulse-inversion mode |
| PICT | pancreatic islet cell | | (ultrasound) |
| | transplantation | PIMIA | potentiometric ionophore |
| PICU | pediatric intensive care | | mediated immunoassay |
| | unit | PIMS | programmable implantable |
| | psychiatric intensive care | | medication system |
| | unit | PIN | pain in the neck (no place |
| PICVA | percutaneous *in situ* | | for such a term in a |
| | coronary venous | | written document) |
| | arterialization | | personal identification |
| PICVC | peripherally inserted | | number |
| | central venous catheter | | posterior interosseous |
| PID | pelvic inflammatory | | nerve |
| | disease | | prostatic intraepithelial |
| | primary | | neoplasia |
| | immunodeficiency | | provider identification |
| | prolapsed intervertebral | | number |
| | disk | PIND | progressive intellectual |
| | proportional-integral- | | and neurological |
| | derivative (controller) | | deterioration |

P

| | | | |
|---|---|---|---|
| PINS | persons in need of supervision | PIVD | protruded intervertebral disk |
| PIO | pemoline (Cylert) | PIVH | periventricular-intraventricular hemorrhage |
| PIO$_2$ | partial pressure of inspired oxygen | | |
| PIOK | poikilocytosis | PIVKA | proteins induced in vitamin K absence |
| PIP | peak inspiratory pressure | | |
| | postictal psychosis | PIWT | partially impacted wisdom teeth |
| | postinfusion phlebitis | | |
| | proximal interphalangeal (joint) | PIXI | Peripheral Instantaneous X-ray Imaging (dual-energy x-ray absorptiometry system) |
| | pulmonary immaturity of prematurity | | |
| | pulmonary insufficiency of the premature | PJ | procelin jacket (crown) |
| PIPB | performance index phonetic balance | PJB | premature junctional beat |
| | | PJC | premature junctional contractions |
| PI-PB | performance intensity-phonemically balanced | PJI | prosthetic joint infection |
| | | PJRT | permanent form of junctional reciprocating tachycardia |
| PIPIDA | N-para-isopropyl-acetanilide-iminodiacetic acid | | |
| | | PJS | peritoneojugular shunt |
| | | | Peutz-Jeghers syndrome |
| PIPJ | proximal interphalangeal joint | PJT | paroxysmal junctional tachycardia |
| PIPP | Premature Infant Pain Profile | PJVT | paroxysmal junctional-ventricular tachycardia |
| PIP/TZ | piperacillin-tazobactam (Zosyn) | PK | penetrating keratoplasty |
| | | | pharmacokinetics |
| PIQ | Performance Intelligence Quotient (part of Wechsler tests) | | plasma potassium |
| | | | pyruvate kinase |
| | | PKB | prone knee bend |
| PIR | pirarubicin | PKC | protein kinase C |
| PIS | pregnancy interruption service | PKD | paroxysmal kinesigenic dyskinesia |
| PISA | phase invariant signature algorithm | | polycystic kidney disease |
| | | PKI | public key infrastructure |
| | proximal isovelocity surface area | PKND | paroxysmal nonkinesigenic dyskinesia |
| PIT | patellar inhibition test | | |
| | peak isometric torque | PKP | penetrating keratoplasty |
| | Pitocin (oxytocin) | PK/PD | pharmacokinetic/pharmacodynamic |
| | Pitressin (vasopressin) (this is a dangerous abbreviation) | PKR | phased knee rehabilitation |
| | | PK Test | Prausnitz-Küstner transfer test |
| | pituitary | | |
| | pulsed-inotrope therapy | PKU | phenylketonuria |
| PITP | pseudo-idiopathic thrombocytopenic purpura | pk yrs | pack-years (smoking one pack of cigarettes a day for one year is termed 1 pack-year of smoking, thus 2 packs a day for 20 years would be 40 |
| PITR | plasma iron turnover rate | | |
| PIV | peripheral intravenous | | |
| PIV-3 | parainfluenza virus type 3 | | |

P

|        |                                         |        | child                         |
|--------|-----------------------------------------|--------|-------------------------------|
| PL     | light perception                        | PLG    | plague (*Yersinia pestis*)    |
|        | palmaris longus                         |        | (*la Peste*) vaccine          |
|        | pharyngolaryngectomy                    | PLH    | paroxysmal localized          |
|        | place                                   |        | hyperhidrosis                 |
|        | placebo                                 | PLIF   | posterior lumbar              |
|        | plantar                                 |        | interbody fusion              |
|        | plethoric (infant color)                | PLL    | posterior longitudinal        |
|        | transpulmonary pressure                 |        | ligament                      |
| PLA    | placebo                                 |        | prolymphocytic leukemia       |
|        | Plasma-Lyte A                           | PLLA   | poly-l-lactic acid            |
|        | posterolateral (coronary)               | PLM    | partial lateral               |
|        | artery                                  |        | meniscectomy                  |
|        | potentially lethal                      |        | periodic leg movement         |
|        | arrhythmia                              |        | Plasma-Lyte M                 |
|        | Product License                         |        | polarized-light microscope    |
|        | Application                             |        | precise lesion measuring      |
|        | pulpolinguoaxial                        |        | (device)                      |
| PLAD   | proximal left anterior                  |        | product-line manager          |
|        | descending (artery)                     | PLMC   | premature living male         |
| Plan B® | levonorgestrel (a                      |        | child                         |
|        | progestogen emergency                   | PLMD   | periodic limb movement        |
|        | contraceptive)                          |        | disorder                      |
| PLAP   | placental alkaline                      | PLMS   | periodic limb movements       |
|        | phosphatase                             |        | during sleep                  |
| PLAT C | platelet concentration                  | PLN    | pelvic lymph node             |
| PLAT P | platelet pheresis                       |        | popliteal lymph node          |
| PLAX   | parasternal long axis                   | PLND   | pelvic lymph node             |
| PLB    | phospholamban                           |        | dissection                    |
|        | placebo                                 | PLO    | pluronic lecithin             |
|        | posterolateral branch                   |        | organogels                    |
| PLBO   | placebo                                 | PLOF   | previous level of             |
| PLC    | peripheral lymphocyte                   |        | functioning                   |
|        | count                                   | PLOSA  | physiologic low stress        |
|        | pityriasis lichenoides                  |        | angioplasty                   |
|        | chronica                                | PLP    | partial                       |
| PLD    | partial lower denture                   |        | laryngopharyngectomy          |
|        | pegylated liposomal                     |        | phantom limb pain             |
|        | doxorubicin                             |        | protolipid protein            |
|        | percutaneous laser                      | PLPH   | postlumbar puncture           |
|        | diskectomy                              |        | headache                      |
| PLDD   | percutaneous laser disk                 | PLR    | pupillary light reflex        |
|        | decompression                           | PLS    | Papillon-Lefèvre              |
| PLE    | polymorphic light                       |        | syndrome                      |
|        | eruption                                |        | plastic surgery               |
|        | protein-losing                          |        | point locator stimulator      |
|        | enteropathy                             |        | Preschool Language Scale      |
| PLED   | periodic lateralizing                   |        | primary lateral sclerosis     |
|        | epileptiform discharge                  | PLs    | premalignant lesions          |
| PLEVA  | pityriasis lichenoides et               | PLSO   | posterior leafspring          |
|        | varioliformis acuta                     |        | orthosis                      |
| PLF    | prior level of function                 | PLST   | progressively lowered         |
| PLFC   | premature living female                 |        | stress threshold              |

| | | | |
|---|---|---|---|
| PLSURG | plastic surgery | PMCT | perinatal mortality counseling team |
| PLT | platelet | | |
| PLT EST | platelet estimate | PMD | perceptual motor development |
| PLTF | plaintiff | | |
| PLTS | platelets | | primary myocardial disease |
| PLUG | plug the lung until it grows | | primidone (Mysoline) |
| | | | private medical doctor |
| PLV | posterior left ventricular | | progressive muscular dystrophy |
| PLX | plexus | | |
| PLYO | plyometric | | |
| PLZF | promyelocytic leukemia zinc finger | PMDD | premenstrual dysphoric disorder |
| | | pMDI | pressurized metered-dose inhaler |
| PM | afternoon | | |
| | evening | PM/DM | polymyositis and dermatomyositis |
| | pacemaker | | |
| | paraspinal mapping | PME | pelvic muscle exercise |
| | particulate matter | | phosphomonoester(s) |
| | petit mal | | polymorphonuclear esosinophil (leukocytes) |
| | physical medicine | | |
| | pneumomediastinum | | postmenopausal estrogen |
| | poliomyelitis | | progressive myoclonus epilepsy |
| | polymyositis | | |
| | poor metabolizers | PMEALS | after meals |
| | postmenopausal | PMEC | pseudomembranous enterocolitis |
| | postmortem | | |
| | presents mainly | PMF | progressive massive fibrosis |
| | pretibial myxedema | | |
| | primary motivation | | pupils mid-position, fixed |
| | prostatic massage | PMH | past medical history |
| | pulpomesial | PMHx | past medical history |
| Pm | *Plasmodium malariae* | PMI | Pain Management Index |
| PM$_{10}$ | particulate matter less than 10 micrometers diameter | | past medical illness |
| | | | patient medication instructions |
| PMA | positive mental attitude | | plea of mental incompetence |
| | premarket approval (application) (for medical devices) | | point of maximal impulse |
| | | | posterior myocardial infarction |
| | premenstrual asthma | | |
| | Prinzmetal angina | PMID | PubMed Unique Identifier (National Library of Medicine) |
| | progress myoclonic ataxia | | |
| PMAA | Premarket Approval Application (medical devices) | PML | polymorphonuclear leukocytes |
| | | | posterior mitral leaflet |
| PMB | polymorphonuclear basophil (leukocytes) | | premature labor |
| | | | progressive multifocal leukoencephalopathy |
| | polymyxin B | | |
| | postmenopausal bleeding | | promyelocytic leukemia |
| PMC | premature mitral closure | PMLCL | primary mediastinal large-cell lymphoma |
| | pseudomembranous colitis | | |
| PMCP | para-monochlorophenol | PMMA | polymethyl methacrylate |
| | perinatal mortality counseling program | | |

| | | | |
|---|---|---|---|
| PMMF | pectoralis major myocutaneous flap | PMTS | premenstrual tension syndrome |
| PMN | polymodal nociceptors | PMV | percutaneous mitral (balloon) valvuloplasty |
| | polymorphonuclear leukocyte | | prolapse of mitral valve |
| | Premarket Notification (medical devices) | PMW | pacemaker wires |
| PMNL | polymorphonuclear leukocyte | PMZ | postmenopausal zest |
| | | PN | parenteral nutrition |
| PMNN | polymorphonuclear neutrophil | | percussion note |
| | | | percutaneous nephrosonogram |
| PMNS | postmalarial neurological syndrome | | percutaneous nucleotomy |
| | | | periarteritis nodosa |
| PMO | postmenopausal osteoporosis | | peripheral neuropathy |
| | | | pneumonia |
| pmol | picomole | | polyarteritis nodosa |
| PMP | pain management program | | poorly nourished |
| | | | positional nystagmus |
| | previous menstrual period | | postnasal |
| | psychotropic medication plan | | postnatal |
| | | | practical nurse |
| PMPA | tenofovir | | premie nipple |
| PMPM | per member, per month | | primary nurse |
| PMPO | postmenopausal palpable ovary | | progress note |
| | | | pyelonephritis |
| PMPY | per member, per year | P & N | pins and needles |
| PMR | pacemaker rhythm | | psychiatry and neurology |
| | percutaneous revascularization | PN$_2$ | partial pressure of nitrogen |
| | polymorphic reticulosis | PNA | Pediatric Nurse Associate |
| | polymyalgia rheumatica | | pneumonia |
| | premedication regimen | | polynitroxyl albumin |
| | prior medical record | PNa | plasma sodium |
| | progressive muscle relaxation | PNAB | percutaneous needle aspiration biopsy |
| | proportional mortality ratios | PNAC | parenteral nutrition associated cholestasis |
| PM&R | physical medicine and rehabilitation | PNAR | perennial nonallergic rhinitis |
| PMS | performance measurement system | PNAS | prudent no added salt |
| | periodic movements of sleep | PNB | percutaneous needle biopsy |
| | poor miserable soul | | popliteal nerve block |
| | postmarketing surveillance | | premature newborn |
| | postmenopausal syndrome | | premature nodal beat |
| | premenstrual syndrome | | prostate needle biopsy |
| | pulse, motor, and sensory | PNC | penicillin |
| PMT | pacemaker-mediated tachycardia | | peripheral nerve conduction |
| | point of maximum tenderness | | premature nodal contraction |
| | premenstrual tension | | prenatal care |

| | | | |
|---|---|---|---|
| | prenatal course | | peripheral nerve stimulator |
| | Psychiatric Nurse Clinician | | peripheral nervous system |
| PNCV7 | pneumococcal 7-valent | | practical nursing student |
| | conjugate vaccine | PNSP | penicillin-nonsusceptible |
| | (Prevnar) | | *S. pneumoniae* |
| PND | paroxysmal nocturnal dyspnea | PNT | percutaneous nephrostomy tube |
| | pelvic node dissection | | percutaneous |
| | postnasal drip | | neuromodulatory |
| | pregnancy, not delivered | | therapy |
| PNDS | Perioperative Nursing | pnthx | pneumothorax |
| | Data Set | PNTML | pudendal-nerve terminal |
| | postnasal drip syndrome | | motor latency |
| PNE | peripheral | PNU | pneumococcal |
| | neuroepithelioma | | (*Streptococcus* |
| | primary nocturnal enuresis | | *pneumoniae*) vaccine, |
| PNET | primitive neuroectodermal | | not otherwise specified |
| | tumors | | protein nitrogen units |
| PNET-MB | primitive neuroectodermal | PNUcn-7 | pneumococcal |
| | tumors-medulloblastoma | | (*Streptococcus* |
| PNEUMO | pneumothorax | | *pneumoniae*) conjugate |
| PNF | primary nonfunction | | vaccine, 7-valent |
| | proprioceptive | | vaccine (Prevnar) |
| | neuromuscular | PNUps23 | pneumococcal |
| | fasciculation (reaction) | | (*Streptococcus* |
| PNH | paroxysmal nocturnal | | *pneumoniae*) |
| | hemoglobinuria | | polysaccharide, |
| | polynitroxyl-hemoglobin | | 23-valent vaccine |
| PNI | peripheral nerve injury | | (Pneumovax-23; |
| | Prognostic Nutrition Index | | Pnu-Imune-23) |
| PNKD | paroxysmal nonkinesigenic | PNV | postoperative nausea and |
| | dyskinesia | | vomiting |
| PNL | percutaneous | | prenatal vitamins |
| | nephrolithotomy | Pnx | pneumonectomy |
| PNMG | persistent neonatal | | pneumothorax |
| | myasthenia gravis | *PO* | by mouth |
| PNMT | phenylethanolamine-N- | | phone order |
| | methyltransferase | | postoperative |
| PNNP | Perinatal Nurse | Po | *Plasmodium ovale* |
| | Practitioner | P&O | parasites and ova |
| PNP | peak negative pressure | | prosthetics and orthotics |
| | Pediatric Nurse | $P_{O2}$ | partial pressure (tension) |
| | Practitioner | | of oxygen, artery |
| | progressive nuclear palsy | $PO_4$ | phosphate |
| | purine nucleoside | POA | pancreatic oncofetal |
| | phosphorylase | | antigen |
| PNR | physician's nutritional | | power of attorney |
| | recommendation | | present on arrival |
| PNRB | partial non-rebreather | | primary optic atrophy |
| | (oxygen mask) | POACH | prednisone, vincristine |
| PNS | partial nonprogressing | | (Oncovin), doxorubicin |
| | stroke | | (Adriamycin), |

|         | cyclophosphamide, and cytarabine | POHI | physically or otherwise health impaired |
| POAG | primary open-angle glaucoma | POHS | presumed ocular histoplasmosis syndrome |
| POB | phenoxybenzamine (Dibenzyline) place of birth | POI | Personal Orientation Inventory postoperative instructions |
| POBC | primary operable breast cancer | POIB | place outpatient in inpatient bed |
| POC | plans of care point-of-care position of comfort postoperative care product of conception | POIK | poikilocytosis |
|  |  | POL | physician's office laboratory poliovirus vaccine, not otherwise specified premature onset of labor |
| POCT | point-of-care testing (test) point-of-care therapy |  |  |
| POD | pacing on demand place of death Podiatry polycystic ovarian disease | POLS | postoperative length of stay |
|  |  | POLY | polychromic erythrocytes polymorphonuclear leukocyte |
| POD 1 | postoperative day one |  |  |
| PODx | preoperative diagnosis | POLY-CHR | polychromatophilia |
| POE | patient-oriented evidence point (portal, port) of entry position of ease provider order entry | POM | pain on motion polyoxymethylene prescription-only medication |
| POEM | Patient-Oriented Evidence That Matters | POMA | Performance-Oriented Mobility Assessment |
| POEMS | plasma cell dyscrasia with polyneuropathy, organomegaly, endocrinopathy, monoclonal protein (M-protein), and skin changes | POMC | pro-opiomelanocortin |
|  |  | POMP | prednisone, vincristine (Oncovin), methotrexate, and mercaptopurine (Purinthol) |
|  |  | POMR | problem-oriented medical record |
| POEx | postoperative exercise | POMS | Profile of Mood States |
| POF | physician's order form position of function premature ovarian failure | POMS-FI | Fatigue-Inertia Subscale of the Profile of Mood States |
| P of I | proof of illness | PON | postoperative note |
| POG | Pediatric Oncology Group Penthrane,® oxygen, and gas (nitrous oxide) products of gestation | PONI | postoperative narcotic infusion |
|  |  | PONV | postoperative nausea and vomiting |
| POGO | percentage of glottic opening | POOH | postoperative open heart (surgery) |
| POH | perillyl alcohol personal oral hygiene presumed ocular histoplasmosis progressive osseous heteroplasia | POOL | premature onset of labor |
|  |  | POP | pain on palpation persistent occipitoposterior persistent organic pollutants |
| POHA | preoperative holding area |  |  |

P

|         | plaster of paris |
|         | popiliteal |
|         | posterior oral pharynx |
| POp | postoperative |
| POPC | Pediatric Overall Performance Category (scale) |
| poplit | popliteal |
| POPs | persistent organic pollutants |
|         | progesterone-only pills |
| POR | physician of record |
|         | problem-oriented record |
| PORP | partial ossicular replacement prosthesis |
| PORR | postoperative recovery room |
| PORT | perioperative respiratory therapy |
|         | portable |
|         | postoperative radiotherapy |
|         | postoperative respiratory therapy |
| POS | parosteal osteosarcoma |
|         | physician's order sheet |
|         | point-of-service |
|         | positive |
| POSHPATE | problem, onset, associated symptoms, previous history, precipitating factors, alleviating/ aggravation factors, timing, an etiology (prompts for taking history and chief complaint) |
| poss | possible |
| post | posterior |
|         | postmortem examination (autopsy) |
| PostC | posterior chamber |
| PostCap | posterior capsule |
| Post-M | urine specimen after prostate massage |
| post op | postoperative |
| Post Sag D | posterior sagittal diameter |
| post tib | posterial tibial |
| PostVD | posterior vitreous detachment |
| POSYC | Pain Observation Scale for Young Children |
| POT | peak occupancy time |
|         | plans of treatment |

|         | potassium |
|         | potential |
| POTS | postural tachycardia syndrome |
| POU | placenta, ovaries, and uterus |
| POV | privately owned vehicle |
| POW | Powassan (virus) |
|         | prisoner of war |
| POWSBP | pulse oximetry waveform systolic blood pressure |
| POX | pulse oximeter (reading) |
| PP | near point of accommodation |
|         | paradoxical pulse |
|         | partial upper and lower dentures |
|         | pedal pulse |
|         | per protocol |
|         | periodontal pockets |
|         | peripheral pulses |
|         | pin prick |
|         | pink puffer (emphysema) |
|         | Planned Parenthood |
|         | plasmapheresis |
|         | plaster of paris |
|         | poor person |
|         | posterior pituitary |
|         | postpartum |
|         | postprandial |
|         | presenting part |
|         | private patient |
|         | prophylactics |
|         | protoporphyria |
|         | proximal phalanx |
|         | pulse pressure |
|         | push pills |
| P-P | probability-probability (plots) |
| P&P | pins and plaster |
|         | policy and procedure |
| PIIIP | aminoterminal type three protocollegan propeptide |
| PPIX | protoporphyrin nine |
| PPA | palpation, percussion, and auscultation |
|         | phenylpropanolamine |
|         | phenylpyruvic acid |
|         | postpartum amenorrhea |
|         | primary progressive aphasia |

| | | | |
|---|---|---|---|
| PP&A | palpation, percussion, and auscultation | | pedal pulses equal and strong |
| PPAR$_g$ | peroxisome-proliferator-activated receptor gamma | PPF | pellagra preventive factor plasma protein fraction |
| PPARs | peroxisome proliferator-activated receptors | PPG | photoplethysmography postprandial glucose |
| PPAS | postpolio atrophy syndrome | | pylorus-preserving gastrectomy |
| PPB | parts per billion pleuropulmonary blastoma | PPGI | psychophysiologic gastrointestinal (reaction) |
| | positive pressure breathing | PPH | postpartum hemorrhage |
| | prostate puncture biopsy | | primary postpartum |
| PPBE | postpartum breast engorgment | | hemorrhage primary pulmonary |
| PPBS | postprandial blood sugar | | hypertension |
| PPBTL | postpartum bilateral tubal ligation | PPHN | persistent pulmonary hypertension of the |
| PPC | plaster of paris cast | | newborn |
| | progressive patient care | PPHx | previous psychiatric |
| PPCD | posterior polymorphous corneal dystrophy | | history |
| PPCF | plasma prothrombin conversion factor | PPIX | protoporphyrin nine |
| PPD | packs per day | PPI | patient package insert permanent pacemaker |
| | posterior polymorphous dystrophy | | insertion prepulse inhibition |
| | postpartum day | | Present Pain Intensity |
| | probing pocket depth (dental) | | proton-pump inhibitor Psychopathic Personality |
| | purified protein derivative (of tuberculin) | | Inventory |
| | pylorus-sparing | PPIVMs | passive physiological intervertebral |
| | pancreaticoduodenectomy | | movements |
| P & PD | percussion & postural drainage | PPJ | pure pancreatic juice |
| PPD-B | purified protein | PPK | population pharmacokinetics |
| | derivative, Battey | PPL | pars plana lensectomy |
| PPDR | preproliferative diabetic retinopathy | Ppl | pleural pressure |
| | | PPLO | pleuropneumonia-like organisms |
| PPD-S | purified protein derivative, standard | PPLOV | painless progressive loss of vision |
| PPE | palmar-plantar erythrodysesthesia (syndrome) | PPM | parts per million permanent pacemaker persistent pupillary |
| | personal protective equipment | | membrane physician practice |
| | professional performance evaluation | | management |
| | pruritic papular eruption | PPMA | postpoliomyelitis muscular atrophy |
| PPES | palmar-plantar erythrodysesthesia syndrome | PPMS | psychophysiologic musculoskeletal (reaction) |

| | | | |
|---|---|---|---|
| PPN | peripheral parenteral nutrition | | postperfusion syndrome |
| PPNAD | primary pigmented nodular adrenocortical disease | | postpoliomyelitis syndrome |
| | | | postpump syndrome |
| PPNG | penicillinase producing *Neisseria gonorrhoeae* | | prospective payment system |
| PPO | permanent punctal occlusion | | pulses per second |
| | | PPSS | peripheral protein sparing solution |
| | preferred provider organization | PPT | parts-per-trillion |
| | pump-prime only | | person, place, and time |
| PPOB | postpartum obstetrics | | Physical Performance Test |
| PPP | patient prepped and positioned | | posterior pelvic tilt |
| | | PPTg | pedunculopontine tegmental nucleus |
| | pearly penile papules | PPTL | postpartum tubal ligation |
| | pedal pulse present | PPU | perforated peptic ulcer |
| | peripheral pulses palpable (present) | PPV | pars plana vitrectomy |
| | platelet-poor plasma | | patent processus vaginalum |
| | postpartum psychosis | | pneumococcal polysaccharide vaccine |
| | preferred practice patterns | | |
| | proportional pulse pressure (SBP minus DBP)/SBP | | positive predictive value |
| | | | positive-pressure ventilation |
| | protamine paracoagulation phenomenon | PPVT | Peabody Picture Vocabulary Test |
| PPPBL | peripheral pulses palpable both legs | PPW | plantar puncture wound |
| | | PPY | packs per year (cigarettes) |
| PPPD | pylorus-preserving pancreatoduodenectomy | PQ | pronator quadratus |
| PPPG | postprandial plasma glucose | pQCT | peripheral quantitative computed tomography |
| PPPM | Parents' Postoperative Pain Measure | PQOCN | Psychiatric Questionnaire Obsessive-Compulsive Neurosis |
| | per patient, per month | | |
| PPPY | per patient, per year | PQRI | Product Quality Research Initiative |
| PPQ | Postoperative Pain Questionnaire | PR | far point of accommodation |
| PPR | patient progress record | | pack removal |
| PPr | periodontal prophylactics | | partial remission |
| PPRC | Physician Payment Review Commission | | partial response |
| | | | patient relations |
| PPROM | prolonged premature rupture of membranes | | perennial rhinitis |
| pPROM | premature rupture of the membranes before 37 weeks gestation | | per rectum |
| | | | pityriasis rosea |
| | | | premature |
| PPS | pentosan polysulfate (Elmiron) | | profile |
| | | | progressive resistance |
| | peripheral pulmonary stenosis | | prolonged remission |
| | | | prone |
| | postpartum sterilization | | Protestant |

|  | Puerto Rican | | preretinal hemorrhage |
|  | pulmonic regurgitation | PRI | Pain Rating Index |
|  | pulse rate | | Patient Review Instrument |
| P=R | pupils equal in size and | prim | primary |
|  | reaction | PRIMIP | primipara (1st pregnancy) |
| P & R | pelvic and rectal | PR | part of the electrocardio- |
|  | pulse and respiration | interval | graphic cycle from |
| PR-2 | Bennett pressure | | onset of atrial |
|  | ventilator | | depolarization on onset |
| PRA | panel reactive antibodies | | of ventricular |
|  | (organ transplants) | | depolarization |
|  | percent reactive | PRISM | Pediatric Risk of |
|  | antibody | | Mortality Score |
|  | plasma renin activity | PRIT® | pretargeted |
| PRAFO | pressure relief ankle-foot | | radioimmunotherapy |
|  | orthosis | PRK | photorefractive |
| PRAT | platelet radioactive | | keratectomy |
|  | antiglobulin test | PRL | prolactin |
| PRBC | packed red blood cells | PRLA | pupils react to light and |
| PRC | packed red cells | | accommodation |
|  | peer review committee | PRM | partial rebreathing mask |
| PRCA | pure red cell aplasia | | passive range of motion |
| PrCa | prostate cancer | | phosphoribomutase |
| PRD | polycystic renal disease | | photoreceptor membrane |
| PRE | passive resistance | | prematurely ruptured |
|  | exercises | | membrane |
|  | progressive resistive | | primidone |
|  | exercise | PRMF | preretinal macular fibrosis |
|  | proton relaxation | PRM-SDX | pyrimethamine; |
|  | enhancement | | sulfadoxine (Fansidar) |
| Pred | prednisone | p.r.n. | as occasion requires |
| PREG | Pregestimil® (infant | PRO | Professional Review |
|  | formula) | | Organization |
| Pre-M | urine specimen before | | proline |
|  | prostate massage | | pronation |
| PREMIE | premature infant | | protein |
| pre-op | before surgery | | prothrombin |
| prep | prepare for surgery | prob | probable |
|  | preposition | PROCTO | procotoscopic |
| PRERLA | pupils round, equal, react | | proctology |
|  | to light and | PROG | prognathism |
|  | accommodation | | prognosis |
| prev | prevent | | program |
|  | previous | | progressive |
| PRFD | percutaneous radio- | PROM | passive range of motion |
|  | frequency denervation | | premature rupture of |
| PRFNB | percutaneous radio- | | membranes |
|  | frequency facet nerve | ProMACE | prednisone, methotrexate, |
|  | block | | calcium leucovorin, |
| PRG | phleborheogram | | doxorubicin |
| PRH | past relevant history | | (Adriamycin), |
|  | postocclusive reactive | | cyclophosphamide, and |
|  | hyperemia | | etoposide |

P

| | | | |
|---|---|---|---|
| PROMM | passive range of motion machine | PRSs | positive rolandic spikes |
| Promy | promyelocyte | PRST | Blood Pressure, Heart Rate, Sweating, and Tears (scale to assess analgesic needs) |
| PRO MYELO | promyelocytes | | |
| PRON | pronation | PRT | pelvic radiation therapy |
| PROS | prostate | | protamine response test |
| | prosthesis | PRTCA | percutaneous rotational transluminal coronary angioplasty |
| PROT REL | protrusive relationship | | |
| prov | provisional | PRTH-C | prothrombin time control |
| PROVIMI | proteins, vitamins, and minerals | PRV | polycythemia rubra vera |
| | | PRVEP | pattern reversal visual evoked potentials |
| PROX | proximal | | |
| PRP | panretinal photocoagulation | PRW | past relevant work |
| | | | polymerized ragweed |
| | patient recovery plan | PRX | panoramic facial x-ray |
| | penicllinase-resistant penicillin | PRZF | pyrazofurin |
| | | PS | paradoxic sleep |
| | penicillin-resistant pneumococci | | paranoid schizophrenia |
| | | | pathologic stage |
| | pityriasis rubra pilaris | | patient's serum |
| | platelet rich plasma | | performance status |
| | polyribose ribitol phosphate | | peripheral smear |
| | | | physical status |
| | poor progression of R wave in precordial leads | | plastic surgery (surgeon) |
| | | | polysulfone (filter) |
| | | | posterior synechiae |
| | | | posterior synechiotomy |
| | progressive rubella panencephalitis | | pressure sore |
| | | | pressure support |
| PrP | prion protein | | protective services |
| PRP-D | *Haemophilus influenzae,* type b diphtheria conjugate vaccine | | Proteus syndrome |
| | | | pulmonary stenosis |
| | | | pyloric stenosis |
| PRPP | 5-phosphoribosyl-1-pyrophosphate | | pyrimethamine; sulfadoxine (Fansidar) |
| PRP-T | polysaccharide tetanus conjugate vaccine | | serum from pregnant women |
| PRRE | pupils round, regular, and equal | P/S | polyunsaturated to saturated fatty acids ratio |
| PRRERLA | pupils round, regular, equal; react to light and accommodation | P & S | pain and suffering |
| | | | paracentesis and suction |
| | | | permanent and stationary |
| PRS | photon radiosurgery system | PS I | healthy patient with localized pathological process |
| | postradiation sarcoma | | |
| | prolonged respiratory support | | |
| PRSL | potential renal solute load | PS II | a patient with mild to moderate systemic disease |
| PRSP | penicillinase-resistant synthetic penicillins | | |
| | penicillin-resistant *Streptococcus pneumoniae* | PS III | a patient with severe systemic disease |

|  |  |
|---|---|
|  | limiting activity but not incapacitating |
| PS IV | a patient with incapacitating systemic disease |
| PS V | moribund patient not expected to live |
|  | (These are American Society of Anesthesiologists' physical status patient classifications. Emergency operations are designated by "E" after the classification.) |
| PSA | polysubstance abuse |
|  | power spectral analysis |
|  | product selection allowed |
|  | prostate-specific antigen |
|  | *Pseudomonas aeruginosa* |
| PsA | psoriatic arthritis |
| PSAB | pretreatment prostate-specific antigen |
| PSAD | prostate-specific antigen density |
| PSADT | prostate-specific antigen doubling time |
| PSAG | *Pseudomonas aeruginosa* |
| PSAV | prostate-specific antigen velocity |
| PSBO | partial small bowel obstruction |
| PSC | Pediatric Symptom Checklist |
|  | percutaneous suprapubic cystostomy |
|  | posterior semicircular canal |
|  | posterior subcapsular cataract |
|  | primary sclerosing cholangitis |
|  | pronation spring control |
|  | pubosacrococcygeal (diameter) |
| PSCA | prostate stem cell antigen |
| PSCC | posterior subcapsular cataract |
| PSC Cat | posterior subcapsular cataract |
| PSCH | peripheral stem cell harvest |

| PSCP | papillary serous carcinoma of the peritoneum |
|---|---|
|  | posterior subcapsular precipitates |
| PSCT | peripheral stem cell transplant |
| PSCU | pediatric special care unit |
| PSD | pilonidal sinus disease |
|  | poststroke depression |
|  | power spectral density |
|  | psychosomatic disease |
| PSDA | Patient Self-Determination Act |
| PSDS | palmar surface desensitization |
| PSE | portal systemic encephalopathy |
|  | pseudoephedrine |
| PSF | posterior spinal fusion |
| PSG | peak systolic gradient |
|  | polysomnogram |
|  | portosystemic gradient |
| PSGN | poststreptococcal glomerulonephritis |
| PSH | past surgical history |
|  | postspinal headache |
| PSHx | past surgical history |
| PSI | passenger space intrusion (motor vehicle accident) |
|  | Physiologic Stability Index |
|  | pounds per square inch |
|  | prostate seed implant |
|  | punctate subepithelial infiltrate |
| PSIC | pediatric surgical intensive care |
| PSIG | pounds per square inch gauge |
| PSIS | posterior superior iliac spine |
| PSM | patient self-management |
|  | presystolic murmur |
| PSMA | personal self-maintenance activities |
|  | progressive spinal muscular atrophy |
|  | prostate-specific membrane antigen |
| PSMF | protein-sparing modified fasting (Blackburn diet) |

271

| | | | |
|---|---|---|---|
| PSM-R | Optimism-Pessimism Scale, revised | PSTT | placental site trophoblastic tumor |
| PSMS | Physical Self Maintenance Scale | PSU | pseudomonas (*P. aeruginosa*) vaccine |
| PSNP | progressive supranuclear palsy | PSUD | psychoactive substance use disorder |
| PSO | pelvic stabilization orthosis | PSUR | periodic safety update reporting |
| | physician supplemental order | PSV | peak systolic velocity |
| | Polysporin ointment | | persistent sciatic vein(s) |
| | proximal subungual onychomycosis | | pressure supported ventilation |
| pSO$_2$ | arterial oxygen saturation | PSVT | paroxysmal supraventricular tachycardia |
| PSOC | Puget Sound Oncology Consortium | | |
| P/sore | pressure sore | PSW | psychiatric social worker |
| PSP | pancreatic spasmolytic peptide | PSWF | positive sharp wave fibrillations (electromyograph) |
| | phenolsulfonphthalein | PSY | presexual youth |
| | photostimulable phosphor | PSZ | pseudoseizures |
| | progressive supranuclear palsy | PT | cisplatin (Platinol AQ) |
| | | | parathormone |
| | | | parathyroid |
| PSPDV | posterior superior pancreaticoduodenal vein | | paroxysmal tachycardia |
| | | | patient |
| | | | phacotrabeculectomy |
| PSR | Psychiatric Status Rating (scale) | | phage type |
| PSRA | pressure sore risk assessment | | phenytoin (Dilantin) |
| | | | phototoxicity |
| PSRBOW | premature spontaneous rupture of bag of waters | | physical therapy |
| | | | pine tar |
| PSReA | poststreptococcal reactive arthritis | | pint |
| | | | posterior tibial |
| PSRT | photostress recovery test | | preterm |
| PSS | painful shoulder syndrome | | pronator teres |
| | pediatric surgical service | Pt | prothrombin time |
| | physiologic saline solution (0.9% sodium chloride) | P/T | platinum |
| | | | pain and tenderness |
| | primary Sjögren syndrome | | piperacillin/tazobactam (Zosyn®) |
| | progressive systemic sclerosis | P1/2T | pressure one-half time |
| PSSP | penicillin-sensitive *Streptococcus pneumoniae* | P&T | pain and tenderness |
| | | | paracentesis and tubing (of ears) |
| PST | paroxysmal supraventricular tachycardia | | peak and trough |
| | | | permanent and total |
| | patient self-testing | | Pharmacy and Therapeutics (Committee) |
| | Patient Service Technician | PTA | patellar tendon autograft |
| | platelet survival time | | percutaneous transluminal angioplasty |
| | postural stress test | | |

|          | Physical Therapy Assistant | PTCRA | percutaneous transluminal coronary rotational atherectomy |
|          | plasma thromboplastin antecedent | PTD | percutaneous transpedicular diskectomy |
|          | posterior tibial artery |  | period to discharge |
|          | post-traumatic amnesia |  | permanent and total disability |
|          | pretreatment anxiety |  |  |
|          | prior to admission |  | persistent trophoblastic disease |
|          | pure-tone average |  |  |
| PTAB     | popliteal-tibial artery bypass |  | pharmacy to dose |
|          |  |  | pharyngotracheal duct |
| PTAS     | percutaneous transluminal angioplasty with stent placement |  | preterm delivery |
|          |  |  | prior to delivery |
| PTB      | patellar tendon bearing | PTDM | post-transplant diabetes mellitus |
|          | prior to birth |  |  |
|          | pulmonary tuberculosis | PTDP | permanent transvenous demand pacemaker |
| PTBA     | percutaneous transluminal balloon angioplasty |  |  |
| PTBD     | percutaneous transhepatic biliary drain (drainage) | PTE | pretibial edema |
|          |  |  | proximal tibial epiphysis |
| PTBD-EF  | percutaneous transhepatic biliary drainage—enteric feeding |  | pulmonary thromboembolectomy |
|          |  |  | pulmonary thromboembolism |
| PTBS     | post-traumatic brain syndrome | PTE-4® | trace metal elements injection (there is also a #5 and #6) |
| PTB-SC-SP | patellar tendon bearing-supracondylar-suprapatellar |  |  |
|          |  | PTED | pulmonary thromboembolic disease |
| PTC      | patient to call | PTER | percutaneous transluminal endomyocardial revascularization |
|          | percutaneous transhepatic cholangiography |  |  |
|          | plasma thromboplastin components | PTF | patient transfer form |
|          | post-tetanic count |  | Patient Treatment File |
|          | premature tricuspid closure |  | pentoxifylline (Trental) |
|          |  |  | post-tetanic facilitation |
|          | prior to conception | PTFE | polytetrafluoroethylene |
|          | pseudotumor cerebri | PTG | parathyroid gland |
| PT-C     | prothrombin time control |  | photoplethysmogram |
| PTCA     | percutaneous transluminal coronary angioplasty | PTGBD | percutaneous transhepatic gallbladder drainage |
| PTCDLF   | pregnancy, term, complicated delivered, living female | PTH | parathyroid hormone |
|          |  |  | post-transfusion hepatitis |
|          |  |  | prior to hospitalization |
| PTCDLM   | pregnancy, term, complicated delivered, living male | PTHC | percutaneous transhepatic cholangiography |
|          |  | PTHrP | parathyroid hormone-related protein |
| PTCL     | peripheral T-cell lymphoma | PTHS | post-traumatic hyperirritability syndrome |
| PTCR     | percutaneous transluminal coronary recanalization |  |  |

| | | | |
|---|---|---|---|
| PTI | pressure-time integral | | prior to surgery |
| PTJV | percutaneous transtracheal jet ventilation | PTSD | post-traumatic stress disorder |
| PTK | phototherapeutic keratectomy | PTT | partial thromboplastin time |
| PTL | preterm labor | | pharyngeal transit time |
| | pudding-thick liquid (diet consistency) | | platelet transfusion therapy |
| | Sodium Pentothal | | protein truncation testing |
| PTLD | post-transplantation lymphoproliferative disorder (disease) | | pulse transit time |
| | | PTT-C | partial thromboplastin time control |
| PTLR | percutaneous transmyocardial laser revascularization | PTTG | pituitary tumor transforming gene |
| | | PTTW | patient tolerated traction well |
| PTM | patient monitored | PTU | pain treatment unit |
| | posterior trabecular meshwork | | pregnancy, term, uncomplicated |
| PTMC | percutaneous transvenous mitral commissurotomy | | propylthiouracil |
| PTMDF | pupils, tension, media, disk, and fundus | PTUCA | percutaneous transluminal ultrasonic coronary angioplasty |
| PTMR | percutaneous transmyocardial revascularization | PTUDLF | pregnancy, term, uncomplicated delivered, living female |
| PT-NANB | post-transfusion non-A, non-B (hepatitis C) | PTUDLM | pregnancy, term, uncomplicated delivered, living male |
| PTNB | preterm newborn | | |
| pTNM | postsurgical resection-pathologic staging of cancer | PTV | patient-triggered ventilation |
| | | | posterior tibial vein |
| PTO | part-time occlusion (eye patch) | PTWTKG | patient's weight in kilograms |
| | please turn over | PTX | paclitaxel (Taxol) |
| | proximal tubal obstruction | | parathyroidectomy |
| PTP | posterior tibial pulse | | pelvic traction |
| | post-transfusion purpura | | pentoxifylline (Trental) |
| PTPM | post-traumatic progressive myelopathy | | phototherapy |
| PTPN | peripheral (vein) total parenteral nutrition | | pneumothorax |
| | | PTZ | pentylenetetrazol |
| P to P | point to point | | phenothiazine |
| PTR | paratesticular rhabdomyosarcoma | PU | pelvic-ureteric |
| | | | pelviureteral |
| | patella tendon reflex | | peptic ulcer |
| | patient to return | | pregnancy urine |
| | prothrombin time ratio | P & U | Pharmacia & Upjohn Company |
| PT-R | prothrombin time ratio | | |
| PTRA | percutaneous transluminal renal angioplasty | PUA | pelvic (examination) under anesthesia |
| PTS | patellar tendon suspension | PUB | pubic |
| | Pediatric Trauma Score | PUBS | percutaneous umbilical blood sampling |
| | permanent threshold shift | | |

| | | | |
|---|---|---|---|
| PUC | pediatric urine collector | | polycythemia vera |
| | | | popliteal vein |
| PUD | partial upper denture | | portal vein |
| | peptic ulcer disease | | postvoiding |
| | percutaneous ureteral dilatation | | prenatal vitamins |
| | | | projectile vomiting |
| PUE | pyrexia of unknown etiology | | pulmonary vein |
| | | Pv | *Plasmodium vivax* |
| PUF | pure ultrafiltration | P & V | peak and valley (this is a dangerous abbreviation, use peak and trough) |
| PUFA | polyunsaturated fatty acids | | |
| PUFFA | polyunsaturated free fatty acids | | pyloroplasty and vagotomy |
| pul. | pulmonary | PVA | polyvinyl alcohol |
| PULP | pulpotomy | | Prinzmetal variant angina |
| Pulse A | pulse apical | PVAD | prolonged venous access devices |
| PULSE OX | pulse oximetry | | |
| | | PVAM | potential visual acuity meter |
| Pulse R | pulse radial | | |
| PULSES | (physical profile) **p**hysical condition, **u**pper limb functions, **l**ower limb functions, **s**ensory components, **e**xcretory functions, and **s**upport factors | PVAR | pulmonary vein atrial reversal |
| | | PVB | cisplatin, (Platinol AQ) vinblastine, and bleomycin |
| | | | paravertebral block |
| | | | porcelain veneer bridge |
| PUN | plasma urea nitrogen | | premature ventricular beat |
| PUND | pregnancy, uterine, not delivered | PVC | paclitaxel, vinblastine, and cisplatin |
| PUNL | percutaneous ultrasonic nephrolithotripsy | | polyethylene vacuum cup |
| | | | polyvinyl chloride |
| PUO | pyrexia of unknown origin | | porcelain veneer crown |
| PUP | percutaneous ultrasonic pyelolithotomy | | postvoiding cystogram |
| | | | premature ventricular contraction |
| | previously untreated patient | | pulmonary venous congestion |
| PU/PL | partial upper and lower dentures | Pvco₂ | partial pressure (tension) of carbon dioxide, vein |
| PUPPP | pruritic urticarial papules and plaque of pregnancy | PVD | patient very disturbed |
| | | | peripheral vascular disease |
| PUS | percutaneous ureteral stent | | posterior vitreous detachment |
| | preoperative ultrasound | | |
| PUU | Puumala hantavirus | | premature ventricular depolarization |
| PUV | posterior urethral valves | | |
| PUVA | psoralen-ultraviolet-light (treatment) | PVDA | prednisone, vincristine, daunorubicin, and asparaginase |
| PUW | pick-up walker | | |
| PV | papillomavirus | PVDF | polyvinylidene difluoride |
| | Parvovirus | PVE | perivenous encephalomyelitis |
| | per vagina | | |
| | plasma volume | | premature ventricular extrasystole |
| | polio vaccine | | |

P

| | | | |
|---|---|---|---|
| | prosthetic value endocarditis | P-VP-B | posteroventral pallidotomy cisplatin (Platinol AQ), etoposide (VP-16), and bleomycin |
| P vera | polycythemia vera | | |
| PVF | peripheral visual field | | |
| PVFS | postviral fatigue syndrome | PVR | peripheral vascular resistance |
| PVGM | perifoveolar vitreoglial membrane | | perspective volume rendering |
| PVH | periventricular hemorrhage | | postvoiding residual proliferative vitreoretinopathy pulmonary vascular resistance pulse-volume recording |
| | periventricular hyperintensity | | |
| | pulmonary vascular hypertension | | |
| PVI | pelvic venous incompetence | PVRI | pulmonary vascular resistance index |
| | peripheral vascular insufficiency | PVS | percussion, vibration and suction |
| | portal-vein infusion protracted venous infusion | | peripheral vascular surgery |
| PVK | penicillin V potassium | | peritoneovenous shunt |
| PVL | Panton-Valentine leukocidin | | persistent vegetative state |
| | peripheral vascular laboratory | | Plummer-Vinson syndrome |
| | periventricular leukomalacia | | pulmonic valve stenosis |
| PVM | paraverteabral muscle | PVT | paroxysmal ventricular tachycardia |
| | proteins, vitamins, and minerals | | previous trouble |
| PVMS | paravertebral muscle spasms | | private proximal vein thrombosis |
| PVN | peripheral venous nutrition | PVTT | tumor thrombus in the portal vein |
| PVNS | pigmented villonodular synovitis | PVV | persistent varicose veins |
| PVO | peripheral vascular occlusion | PW | pacing wires |
| | | | patient waiting |
| | portal vein occlusion | | plantar wart |
| | pulmonary venous occlusion | | posterior wall |
| PVo | pulmonary valve opening | | pulse width |
| | | | puncture wound |
| Pvo$_2$ | partial pressure (tension) of oxygen, vein | P&W | pressures and waves |
| | | PWA | persons with AIDS |
| | peripheral vascular occlusive disease | | P-wave axis |
| | | PWACR | Prader-Willi/Angelman critical region |
| PVOD | pulmonary vascular obstructive disease | P wave | part of the electrocardiographic cycle representing atrial depolarization |
| PVP | cisplatin (Platinol AQ) and etoposide (Ve Pesid) | | |
| | penicillin V potassium | PWB | partial weight bearing |
| | peripheral venous pressure | | Positive Well-being (scale) |
| | polyvinylpyrrolidone | | psychological well-being |

| | |
|---|---|
| PWBL | partial weight bearing, left |
| PWBR | partial weight bearing, right |
| PWCA | personal watercraft accident |
| PWD | patients with diabetes |
| | person(s) with a disability |
| | powder |
| PWE | people with epilepsy |
| PWI | pediatric walk-in clinic |
| | perfusion-weighted (magnetic resonance) imaging |
| | posterior wall infarct |
| PWLV | posterior wall of left ventricle |
| PWM | pokeweed mitogens |
| PWMI | posterior wall myocardial infarction |
| PWO | persistent withdrawal occlusion |
| PWP | pulmonary wedge pressure |
| PWS | port-wine stain |
| | Prader-Willi syndrome |
| PWT | posterior wall thickness |
| PWTd | posterior wall thickness at end-diastole |
| PWV | polistes wasp venom |
| | pulse-wave velocity |
| Px | physical exam |
| | pneumothorax |
| | prognosis |
| | prophylaxis |
| PXAT | paroxysmal atrial tachycardia |
| PXE | pseudoxanthoma elasticum |
| PXF | pseudoexfoliation |
| PXL | paclitaxel (Taxol) |
| PXS | dental prophylaxis (cleaning) |
| PY | pack-years (see pk yrs) |
| PYE | person-years of exposure |
| PYHx | packs per year history |
| PYLL | potential years of life lost |
| PYP | pyrophosphate |
| PYP® | technetium Tc 99m pyrophosphate kit |
| PZ | peripheral zone |
| PZA | pyrazinamide |
| | pyrazoloacridine (a drug class of sidatine/hyponotics) |
| PZD | partial zona drilling |
| | partial zonal dissection |
| PZI | protamine zinc insulin |

P

# Q

Q every
 quadriceps
QA quality assurance
QAC before every meal (this is a dangerous abbreviation)
QALE quality-adjusted life expectancy
QALYs quality-adjusted life years
QAM every morning (this is a dangerous abbreviation because the Q can be read as a 9)
QAS quality-adjusted survival
QATTP quality-adjusted time to progression
QB blood flow
QC quad cane
 quality control
 quick catheter
QCA quantitative coronary angiography
Q compound Chinese cucumber
QCSW Qualified Clinical Social Worker
QCT quantitative computed tomography
QD dialysate flow
 every day (this is a dangerous abbreviation as it is read as four times daily-QID; use "once daily")
QDAM once daily in the morning
QDNs quantum dot nanocrystals
QDPM once daily in the evening
QDS United Kingdom abbreviation for four times a day
QE quinidine effect
QED every even day (this is a dangerous abbreviation as it will be read as four times daily-QID)
 quick and early diagnosis
QEE quadriceps extension exercise

QFB Químico Farmacéutico Biólogo (Chemist Pharmacist Biologist; Pharmacist in Mexico)
QF-PCR quantitative fluorescence polymerase chain reaction
QFV Q fever (*Coxiella burnetii*) vaccine
QGS quantitative gate SPECT (single photon emission computed tomography)
q4h every four hours
*q.h.* every hour
qhs every night (this is a dangerous abbreviation as it is read as every hour-QHR and four times daily-QID)
QIAD Quantitative Inventory of Alcohol Disorders
*q.i.d.* four times daily
QIDM four times daily with meals and at bedtime
QIG quantitative immunoglobulins
QIMT quantitative intima media thickness
QIW four times a week (this is a dangerous abbreviation)
QJ quadriceps jerk
QKD interval Korotkoff sounds
QL quality of life
QLI Quality of Life Index
QLS quality of life score
QM every morning (this is a dangerous abbreviation as it will not be understood)
QMB qualified Medicare beneficiary
QMI Q-wave myocardial infarction
QMRP qualified mental retardation professional
QMT quantitative muscle testing
*q.n.* every night (this is a dangerous abbreviation as it is read as every hour)

| | | | |
|---|---|---|---|
| q.n.s. | quantity not sufficient | Qs/Qt | intrapulmonary shunt fraction |
| qod | every other day (this is a dangerous abbreviation as it is read as every day or four times a day-QID) | QSP | physiological shunt fraction |
| | | QT | the time between the beginning of the QRS complex and the end of the T-wave |
| qoh | every other hour (this is a dangerous abbreviation as it is read as every day or four times a day-QID) | qt | quart |
| | | QTB | quadriceps tendon bearing |
| | | QTC | quantitative tip cultures |
| qohs | every other night (this is a dangerous abbreviation as it is not recognized) | QTc | the QTc interval is the length of time it takes the electrical system in the heart to repolarize, adjusted for heart rate (normal 350-440 milliseconds) |
| QOL | quality of life | | |
| QOLIE-31 | quality of life in epilepsy | | |
| QOM | quality of motion | | |
| QON | every other night (this is a dangerous abbreviation) | QTL | quantitative trait locus |
| QPCR | quantitative polymerase chain reaction | QTP | quetiapine fumarate (Seroquel) |
| qpm | every evening (this is a dangerous abbreviation) | Q-TWiST | quality-adjusted time without symptoms (of disease) and toxicity |
| QPOS | Quality Point of Service | | |
| QP/QS | ratio of pulmonary blood to systemic blood flow | QUAD | quadrant quadriceps quadriplegic |
| qqh | every four hours (United Kingdom) | QU | quiet |
| qqs | every four hours (United Kingdom) | QUART | quadrantectomy, axillary dissection, and radiotherapy |
| QR | quiet room | | |
| QRC | qualitative radiocardiography | QUEST | Quality of Upper Extremity Skills Test |
| QRDR | quinolone resistance-determining region(s) | QUS | quantitative (bone) ultrasound |
| QRE | quality-related event | QW | every week (this is a dangerous abbreviation) |
| QRNG | quinolone-resistant N. gonorrhoeae | q4w | every 4 weeks (this is a dangerous abbreviation) |
| QRS | part of electrocardio-graphic wave representing ventricular depolarization | QWB | Quality of Well-Being (scale) |
| | | QWE | every weekend (this is a dangerous abbreviation) |
| QS | every shift quadriceps set quadrilateral socket Quality Services (Department) sufficient quantity | QWK | once a week (this is a dangerous abbreviation) |
| | | Q4wk | every four weeks (this is a dangerous abbreviation) |
| qs ad | a sufficient quantity to make | QWMI | Q-wave myocardial infarction |
| QS&L | quarters, subsistence, and laundry | | |

Q

# R

| | |
|---|---|
| R | radial |
| | rate |
| | ratio |
| | reacting |
| | rectal |
| | rectum |
| | regular |
| | regular insulin |
| | resistant |
| | respiration |
| | reticulocyte |
| | retinoscopy |
| | right |
| | Ritalin (methylphenidate) as in vitamin R |
| | roentgen |
| | rub |
| r | recombinant |
| ® | registered trademark |
| | right |
| −R | Rinne test, negative |
| +R | Rinne test, positive |
| RA | radial artery |
| | radiographic absorptiometry |
| | rales |
| | readmission |
| | renal artery |
| | repeat action |
| | retinoic acid |
| | rheumatoid arthritis |
| | right arm |
| | right atrium |
| | right auricle |
| | room air |
| | rotational atherectomy |
| RAA | renin-angiotensin-aldosterone |
| | right atrial abnormality |
| | right atrial appendage |
| RAAS | renin-angiotensin-aldosterone system |
| RAB | rabies vaccine, not otherwise specified |
| | rice (rice cereal), applesauce, and banana (diet) |
| RAB_DEV | rabies vaccine, duck embryo culture |
| RAB_FRhL-2 | rabies vaccine, diploid fetal-rhesus-lung-2 cell line |
| RABG | room air blood gas |
| RAB_HDCV | rabies vaccine, human diploid cell culture |
| RABig | rabies immune globulin |
| RAB_PCEC | rabies vaccine, purified chick embryo cell culture |
| RAC | Recombinant DNA Advisory Committee |
| | right antecubital |
| | right atrial catheter |
| RACCO | right anterior caudocranial oblique |
| RACT | recalcified whole-blood activated clotting time |
| RACZ | a procedure of dissolving lumbar scar tissue (epidurolysis) |
| RAD | ionizing radiation unit |
| | radical |
| | radiology |
| | reactive airway disease |
| | reactive attachment disorder |
| | right axis deviation |
| RADCA | right anterior descending coronary artery |
| RADISH | rheumatoid arthritis diffuse idiopathic skeletal hyperostosis |
| RADS | ionizing radiation units |
| | rapid assay delivery systems |
| | reactive airway disease syndrome |
| RAE | right atrial enlargement |
| RAEB | refractory anemia, erythroblastic |
| RAEB-T | refractory anemia with excess blasts in transition |
| RAF | rapid atrial fibrillation |
| RAFF | rectus abdominis free flap |
| RAFT | Rehabilitative Addicted Family Treatment |
| RAG | room air gas |
| RAH | right atrial hypertrophy |
| RAHB | right anterior hemiblock |
| rAHF | antihemophilic factor (recombinant) |

| | | | |
|---|---|---|---|
| RAI | radioactive iodine | RAU | recurrent aphthous ulcers |
| | Resident Assessment Instrument | RAVLT | Rey Auditory Verbal Learning Test |
| RAID | radioimmunodetection | R(AW) | airway resistance |
| RAIT | radioimmunotherapy | RB | relieved by |
| RAIU | radioactive iodine uptake | | retinoblastoma |
| RALT | routine admission laboratory tests | | retrobulbar |
| | | | right breast |
| RAM | radioactive material | | right buttock |
| | rapid alternating movements | R & B | right and below |
| | | RBA | right basilar artery |
| | rectus abdominis myocutaneous | | right brachial artery |
| | | | risks, benefits, and alternatives (discussion with patient) |
| RAN | resident's admission notes | | |
| R₂AN | second year resident's admission notes | | |
| | | RBB | right breast biopsy |
| RANTES | regulated upon activation, normal T cell expressed and secreted | RBBB | right bundle branch block |
| | | RBBX | right breast biopsy examination |
| RAO | right anterior oblique | RBC | ranitidine bismuth citrate |
| rAOM | recurrent acute otitis media | | red blood cell (count) |
| | | RBCD | right border cardiac dullness |
| RAP | request for advance payment | | |
| | | RBCM | red blood cell mass |
| | right abdominal pain | RBC s/f | red blood cells spun filtration |
| | right atrial pressure | | |
| RAPA | radial artery pseudoaneurysm | RBCV | red blood cell volume |
| | | RBD | REM (rapid eye movement sleep) behavior disorder |
| RAQ | right anterior quadrant | | |
| RAP | recurrent abdominal pain | | |
| | Resident Assessment Protocol | | right border of dullness |
| | | RBE | relative biologic effectiveness |
| RAPD | random amplified polymorphic DNA | | |
| | | RBF | renal blood flow |
| | relative afferent pupillary defect | RBG | random blood glucose |
| | | RBILD | respiratory bronchiolitis-associated interstitial lung disease |
| RAPs | Resident Assessment Protocols | | |
| | | RBL | Roche Biomedical Laboratory |
| RAR | right arm, reclining | | |
| RARs | retinoic acid receptors | RBON | retrobulbar optic neuritis |
| RAS | recurrent aphthous stomatitis | RBOW | rupture bag of water |
| | | RBP | retinol-binding protein |
| | renal artery stenosis | RBRVS | Medicare resource-based relative-value scale |
| | renin-angiotensin system | | |
| | reticular activating system | RBS | random blood sugar |
| | right arm, sitting | RBT | rational behavior therapy |
| RASE | rapid-acquisition spin echo | | |
| RAST | radioallergosorbent test | RBV | right brachial vein |
| RAT | right anterior thigh | RBVO | right brachial vein occlusion |
| RA test | test for rheumatoid factor | | |
| RATG | rabbit antithymocyte globulin | RC | race |
| | | | radiocarpal (joint) |
| RATx | radiation therapy | | Red Cross |

R

| | report called | RCM | radiographic contrast media |
| | retrograde cystogram | | restricted cardiomyopathy |
| | retruded contact (position) | | retinal capillary microaneurysm |
| | right coronary | | right costal margin |
| | Roman Catholic | RCN | radiocontrast-agent-induced nephrotoxicity |
| | root canal | | |
| | rotator cuff | RCOG | Royal College of Obstetricians and Gynaecologists |
| R/C | reclining chair | | |
| R & C | reasonable and customary | | |
| RCA | radiographic contrast agent | RCP | respiratory care plan |
| | radionuclide cerebral angiogram | | retrograde cerebral perfusion |
| | right carotid artery | | Royal College of Physicians |
| | right coronary artery | | |
| | root cause analysis | RCPM | raven-colored progressive matrices |
| RC/AL | residential care, assisted living | | |
| RCBF | regional cerebral blood flow | RCPT | Registered Cardiopulmonary Technician |
| RCC | rape crisis center | | |
| | renal cell carcinoma | RCR | replication-competent retrovirus (assay) |
| | Roman Catholic Church | | rotator cuff repair |
| RCCA | right common carotid artery | RCS | repeat cesarean section |
| RCCT | randomized controlled clinical trial | | reticulum cell sarcoma |
| | | | Royal College of Surgeons |
| RCD | relative cardiac dullness | RCT | randomized clinical trial |
| RCE | right carotid endarterectomy | | Registered Care Technologist |
| RCF | Reiter complement fixation | | root canal therapy |
| RCF® | enteral nutrition product | | Rorschach Content Test |
| RCFA | right common femoral angioplasty | | rotator cuff tear |
| | right common femoral artery | RCU | respiratory care unit |
| RCFE | residential care facility for the elderly | RCV | red cell volume |
| | | | right colic vein |
| RCH | residential care home | RCX | ramus circumflexus |
| RCHF | right-sided congestive heart failure | RD | radial deviation |
| | | | Raynaud disease |
| R-CHOP | rituximab, cyclophosphamide, doxorubicin (hydroxydaunorubicin), vincristine (Oncovin), and prednisone | | reaction of degeneration |
| | | | reflex decay |
| | | | Registered Dietitian |
| | | | renal disease |
| | | | respiratory disease |
| RCIN | radiographic-contrast-media-induced nephropathy | | respiratory distress |
| | | | restricted duty |
| | | | retinal detachment |
| RCIP | rape crisis intervention program | | Reye disease |
| | | | rhabdomyosarcoma |
| RCL | range of comfortable loudness | | right deltoid |
| | | | ruptured disk |

| | | | |
|---|---|---|---|
| RDA | recommended daily allowance | | reflux esophagitis |
| | | | regarding |
| | Registered Dental Assistant | | regional enteritis |
| | | | reticuloendothelial |
| | representational difference analysis | | retinol equivalents |
| | | | right ear |
| RDB | randomized double-blind (trial) | | right eye |
| | | | rowing ergometer |
| RDCS | Registered Diagnostic Cardiac Sonographer | $^{186}$Re | rhenium 186 |
| | | R & E | rest and exercise |
| RDD | renal dose dopamine | | round and equal |
| RDE | remote data entry | R ↑ E | right upper extremity |
| RDEA | right deviation of electrical axis | R ↓ E | right lower extremity |
| | | RE✓ | recheck |
| RDG | right dorsogluteal | READM | readmission |
| RDH | Registered Dental Hygienist | REAL | Revised European American Lymphoma (classification) |
| RDI | respiratory disturbance (distress) index | | |
| | | REALM | Rapid Estimation of Adult Literacy in Medicine |
| RDIH | right direct inguinal hernia | | |
| | | REC | gingival recession |
| RDLBBB | rate-dependent left bundle branch block | | rear end collision |
| | | | recommend |
| | | | record |
| RDM | right deltoid muscle | | recovery |
| RDMS | Registered Diagnostic Medical Sonographer | | recreation |
| | | | recur |
| RDMs | reactive drug metabolites | RECA | right external carotid artery |
| RDOD | retinal detachment, right eye | | |
| | | RECT | rectum |
| RDOS | retinal detachment, left eye | REDA | Registered Eating Disorders Associate |
| RDP | random donor platelets | | |
| | right dorsoposterior | REDs | reproductive endocrine diseases |
| RDPE | reticular degeneration of the pigment epithelium | | |
| | | RED SUBS | reducing substances |
| RDS | research diagnostic criteria | REE | resting energy expenditure |
| | | RE-ED | re-education |
| | respiratory distress syndrome | R-EEG | resting electroencephalogram |
| RDT | regular dialysis (hemodialysis) treatment | | |
| | | REEGT | Registered Electroencephalogram Technologist |
| RDTD | referral, diagnosis, treatment, and discharge | | |
| | | REF | referred |
| | | | refused |
| | | | renal erythropoietic factor |
| RDU | recreational drug use | ref→ | refer to |
| RDVT | recurrent deep vein thrombosis | REG | radioencephalogram |
| | | | regression analysis |
| RDW | red (cell) distribution width | Reg block | regional block anesthesia |
| | | regurg | regurgitation |
| RE | concerning | rehab | rehabilitation |
| | Rasmussen encephalitis | REL | relative |
| | rectal examination | | religion |

RELE  resistive exercise, lower extremities
REM  rapid eye movement
recent event memory
remarried
remission
roentgen equivalent unit
REMS  rapid eye movement sleep
REO  respiratory and enteric orphan (viruses)
REP  rapid electrophoresis
repair
repeat
report
REP CK  rapid electrophoresis creatine kinase
REPL  recurrent early pregnancy loss
repol  repolarization
REPS  repetitions
REPT  Registered Evoked Potential Technologist
RER  renal excretion rate
RER+  replication error positive
RES  recurrent erosion syndrome
resection
resident
reticuloendothelial system
RESC  resuscitation
RESP  respirations
respiratory
REST  restoration
restriction of environmental stimulation therapy
RET  retention
reticulocyte
retina
retired
return
right esotropia
ret detach  retinal detachment
retic  reticulocyte
RETRO  retrograde
RETRX  retractions
REUE  resistive exercise, upper extremities
REV  reverse
review
revolutions
RF  radiofrequency
reduction fixation
refill; refilled (prescriptions)
renal failure
respiratory failure
restricted fluids
rheumatic fever
rheumatoid factor
right foot
risk factor
radiofrequency
R/F  retroflexed
R&F  radiographic and fluoroscopic
RF6  rejection-free survival at 6 months
RFA  radiofrequency ablation
right femoral artery
right forearm
right frontoanterior
RFB  retained foreign body
radial flow chromatography
residual functional capacity
RFC  reduced folate carrier
RFCA  radiofrequency catheter ablation
RFD  residue-free diet
RFDT  Reach in Four Directions Test
RFE  return flow enema
RFFIT  rapid fluorescent focus inhibition test
rFVIII FS  antihemophilic factor (recombinant), formulated with sucrose (Kogenate)
RFg  visual fields by Goldmann-type perimeter
rFGF-2  recombinant fibroblast growth factor-2
RFIPC  Rating Form of IBD (inflammatory bowel disease) Patient Concerns
RFL  radionuclide functional lymphoscintigraphy
right frontolateral
RFLF  retained fetal lung fluid
RFLP  restriction fragment length polymorphism (patterns)

R

| RFM | rifampin (Rifadin) |
| RFP | Renal function panel (see page 362) |
| | request for payment |
| | request for proposal |
| | right frontoposterior |
| RFS | rapid frozen section |
| | refeeding syndrome |
| | relapse-free survival |
| RFT | respiratory function test |
| | right frontotransverse |
| | routine fever therapy |
| RFTA | radiofrequency thermal ablation |
| RFTC | radiofrequency thermocoagulation |
| RFUT | radioactive fibrinogen uptake |
| RFV | reason for visit |
| | right femoral vein |
| RG | regurgitated (infant feeding) |
| | right (upper outer) gluteus |
| R/G | red/green |
| RGA | right gastroepiploic artery |
| RGM | recurrent glioblastoma multiforme |
| | right gluteus medius |
| RGO | reciprocating gait orthosis |
| RGP | rigid gas-permeable (contact lens) |
| Rh | Rhesus factor in blood |
| RH | reduced haloperidol |
| | relative humidity |
| | rest home |
| | retinal hemorrhage |
| | right hand |
| | right hemisphere |
| | right hyperphoria |
| | room humidifier |
| Rh+ | Rhesus positive |
| Rh− | Rhesus negative |
| RHA | rheumatoid arthritis (therapeutic) vaccine |
| | right hepatic artery |
| rHA | recombinant human albumin |
| rhAPC | recombinant human activated protein C |
| RHB | raise head of bed |
| | right heart border |

| RH/BSO | radial hysterectomy and bilateral salpingo-oophorectomy |
| RHC | respiration has ceased |
| | right heart catheterization |
| | right hemicolectomy |
| | routine health care |
| | rural health clinic |
| RHD | radial head dislocation |
| | relative hepatic dullness |
| | rheumatic heart disease |
| | right-hand dominant |
| rh-DNase | dornase alfa (Pulmozyme) |
| RHF | rheumatic fever vaccine |
| | right heart failure |
| RHG | right-hand grip |
| r-hGH(m) | mammalian-cell–derived recombinant human growth hormone (Serostim) |
| RHH | right homonymous hemianopsia |
| RHIA | Registered Health Information Administrator |
| RHINO | rhinoplasty |
| RHIT | Registered Health Information Technician |
| RHL | right hemisphere lesions |
| | right heptic lobe |
| rhm | roentgens per hour at one meter |
| RHO | right heel off |
| Rho(D) | immune globulin to an Rh-negative woman |
| RhoGAM® | Rho (D) immune globulin |
| RHP | resting head pressure |
| rhPDGF | recombinant human platelet-derived growth factor |
| RHR | resting heart rate |
| RHS | right-hand side |
| RHT | regional hyperthermia |
| | right hypertropia |
| rHuEPO | recombinant human erythropoietin |
| RHV | right hepatic vein |
| RHW | radiant heat warmer |
| RI | ramus intermedius (coronary artery) |
| | refractive index |
| | regular insulin |

|  | relapse incidence | RIO | right inferior oblique (muscle) |
|  | renal insufficiency |  |  |
|  | respiratory illness | RIOJ | recurrent intrahepatic obstructive jaundice |
|  | rooming in |  |  |
| RIA | radioimmunoassay | R-IOL | remove intraocular lens |
|  | reversible ischemic attack | RIP | radioimmunoprecipitin test |
| RIAT | radioimmune antiglobulin test |  | rapid infusion pump |
| RIBA | recombinant immunoblot assay |  | respiratory inductance plethysmograph |
| RIC | right iliac crest |  | rhythmic inhibitory pattern |
|  | right internal carotid (artery) | RIPA | ristocetin-induced platelet agglutination |
| RICA | right internal carotid artery | RIR | right inferior rectus |
| RICE | rest, ice, compression, and elevation | RIS | responding to internal stimuli |
| RICM | right intercostal margin |  | risperidone (Risperdal) |
| RICS | right intercostal space | RISA | radioactive iodinated serum albumin |
| RICU | respiratory intensive care unit | RIST | radioimmunosorbent test |
| RID | radial immunodiffusion | RIT | radioimmunotherapy |
|  |  |  | ritonavir (Norvir) |
|  | ruptured intervertebral disk |  | Rorschach Inkblot Test |
| RIE | radiation induced emesis | RITA | right internal thoracic artery |
|  | reactive ion etching |  |  |
|  | rocket immunoelectrophoresis | RIVD | ruptured intervertebral disk |
| RIF | rifampin | RIX | radiation-induced xerostomia |
|  | right iliac fossa | RJ | radial jerk (reflex) |
|  | right index finger |  | right jugular |
|  | rigid internal fixation | RK | radial keratotomy |
| RIG | rabies immune globulin |  | right kidney |
| RIGS | radioimmunoguided surgery | RKS | renal kidney stone |
|  |  | RKT | Registered Kinesiotherapist |
| RIH | right inguinal hernia | RL | right lateral |
| RIHP | renal interstitial hydrostatic pressure |  | right leg |
| RIJ | right internal jugular |  | right lower |
| RIMA | reversible inhibitor of monoamine oxidase-type A |  | right lung |
|  |  |  | Ringer lactate |
|  |  |  | rotation left |
|  | right internal mammary anastamosis | R → L | right to left |
|  |  | RLA | right lower arm |
|  | right internal mammary artery | RLB | right lateral bending |
|  |  |  | right lateral border |
| RIN | radiocontrast-induced nephropathy | RLBCD | right lower border of cardiac dullness |
| RIND | reversible ischemic neurologic defect | RLC | residual lung capacity |
|  |  | RLD | related living donor |
| RINV | radiation-induced nausea and vomiting |  | right lateral decubitus |
|  |  |  | ruptured lumbar disk |

| RLDP | right lateral decubital position | | Rivermead motor assessment |
|------|--------------------------|--------|------------------------|
| RLE | right lower extremity | RMB | right main bronchus |
| RLF | retrolental fibroplasia | RMBPC | Revise Memory and |
| | right lateral femoral | | Behavior Problems |
| RLFP | Remaining Lifetime | | Checklist |
| | Fracture Probability | RMCA | right main coronary artery |
| RLG | right lateral gaze | | right middle cerebral |
| RLGS | restriction landmark | | artery |
| | genomic scanning | RMCAT | right middle cerebral |
| RLH | reactive lymphoid | | artery thrombosis |
| | hyperplasia | RMCL | right midclavicular line |
| RLL | right liver lobe | RMD | rippling muscle disease |
| | right lower lid | RME | reasonable maximum |
| | right lower lobe | | exposure |
| RLN | recurrent laryngeal nerve | | resting metabolic |
| | regional lymph node(s) | | expenditure |
| RLND | regional lymph node | | right mediolateral |
| | dissection | | episiotomy |
| RLQ | right lower quadrant | RMEE | right middle ear |
| RLQD | right lower quadrant | | exploration |
| | defect | rMET | recombinant |
| RLR | right lateral rectus | | methioninase |
| RLRTD | recurrent lower respiratory | RMF | right middle finger |
| | tract disease | RMK #1 | remark number 1 |
| RLS | restless legs syndrome | RML | right mediolateral |
| | Ringer lactate solution | | right middle lobe |
| | stammerer who has | RMLE | right mediolateral |
| | difficulty in enunciating | | episiotomy |
| | R, L, and S | RMO | responsible medical |
| RLSB | right lower scapular | | officer |
| | border | rMOG | recombinant myelin |
| | right lower sternal border | | oligodendrocyte |
| RLT | right lateral thigh | | glycoprotein |
| RLTCS | repeat low transverse | RMP | right mentoposterior |
| | cesarean section | | risk management |
| RLUs | relative light units | | program |
| RLWD | routine laboratory work | RMR | resting metabolic rate |
| | done | | right medial rectus |
| RLX | right lower extremity | | root mean square residue |
| RM | radical mastectomy | RMRM | right modified radical |
| | repetitions maximum | | mastectomy |
| | respiratory movement | RMS | red-man syndrome |
| | risk manager | | Rehabilitation Medicine |
| | (management) | | Service |
| | risk model | | repetitive motion |
| | room | | syndrome |
| R&M | routine and microscopic | | rhabdomyosarcoma |
| 1-RM | single repetition | | Rocky Mountain spotted |
| | maximum lift | | fever vaccine |
| RMA | Registered Medical | | root-mean-square |
| | Assistant | RMS® | rectal morphine sulfate |
| | right mentoanterior | | (suppository) |

| RMSB | right middle sternal border | RNUD | recurrent nonulcer dyspepsia |
| RMSE | root-mean-square error | RO | reality orientation |
| RMSF | Rocky Mountain spotted fever | | relative odds |
| | | | report of |
| RMT | Registered Music Therapist | | reverse osmosis |
| | | | routine order(s) |
| | right mentotransverse | | Russian Orthodox |
| RMV | respiratory minute volume | R/O | rule out |
| RN | Registered Nurse | ROA | right occiput anterior |
| | right nostril (nare) | ROAC | repeated oral doses of activated charcoal |
| Rn | radon | | |
| R/N | renew | ROAD | reversible obstructive airway disease |
| RNA | radionuclide angiography | | |
| | Restorative Nursing Assistant | ROBE | routine operative breast endoscopy |
| | ribonucleic acid | ROC | receiver operating characteristic |
| | routine nursing assistance | | |
| RNC | Registered Nurse, Certified | | record of contact |
| | | | resident on call |
| RNCD | Registered Nurse, Chemical Dependency | | residual organic carbon |
| | | ROCF | Rey-Osterrieth complex figure |
| RNCNA | Registered Nurse Certified in Nursing Administration | | |
| | | ROD | rapid opioid detoxification |
| RNCNAA | Registered Nurse Certified in Nursing Administration Advanced | RODA | rapid opiate detoxification under anesthesia |
| | | ROE | report of event |
| | | | right otitis externa |
| RNCS | Registered Nurse Certified Specialist | ROF | review of outside films |
| | | ROG | rogletimide |
| RND | radical neck dissection | ROH | rubbing alcohol |
| RNEF | resting (radio-) nuclide ejection fraction | ROI | region of interest (radiology) |
| RNF | regular nursing floor | | release of information |
| RNFL | retinal nerve fiber layer | ROIDS | hemorrhoids |
| RNFLT | retinal nerve fiber layer thickness | ROIH | right oblique inguinal hernia |
| RNI | reactive nitrogen intermediates | ROJM | range of joint motion |
| | | ROL | right occipitolateral |
| | rubella nonimmune | ROLC | roentgenologically occult lung cancer |
| RNLP | Registered Nurse, license pending | | |
| | | ROM | range of motion |
| RNP | Registered Nurse Practitioner | | rifampicin 600 mg, ofloxacin 400 mg, and minocycline 100 mg |
| | restorative nursing program | | |
| | | | right otitis media |
| | ribonucleoprotein | | rupture of membranes |
| RNS | recurrent nephrotic syndrome | Romb | Romberg |
| | | ROMCP | range of motion complete and painfree |
| | replacement normal saline (0.9% sodium chloride) | | |
| | | ROMI | rule out myocardial infarction |
| RNST | reactive nonstress test | | |

R

| | | |
|---|---|---|
| ROMSA | right otitis media, suppurative, acute | |
| ROMSC | right otitis media, suppurative, chronic | |
| ROMWNL | range of motion within normal limits | |
| RONTD | risk of neural tube defect | |
| ROP | retinopathy of prematurity | |
| | right occiput posterior | |
| ROPS | roll-over protection structures | |
| ROR | the French acronym for measles-mumps-rubella vaccine | |
| | reporting odds ratio | |
| R or L | right or left | |
| RoRx | radiation therapy | |
| ROS | review of systems | |
| | rod outer segments | |
| | rule out sepsis | |
| ROSA | rank-order stability analysis | |
| ROSC | restoration of spontaneous circulation | |
| ROSS | review of signs and symptoms | |
| ROT | remedial occupational therapy | |
| | right occipital transverse | |
| | rotator | |
| ROU | recurrent oral ulcer | |
| ROUL | rouleaux (rouleau) | |
| ROW | rest of (the) week | |
| RP | radial pulse | |
| | radical prostatectomy | |
| | radiopharmaceutical | |
| | Raynaud phenomenon | |
| | responsible party | |
| | resting position | |
| | restorative proctocolectomy | |
| | retinitis pigmentosa | |
| | retrograde pyelogram | |
| | retropubic prostatectomy | |
| | root plane | |
| RPA | radial photon absorptiometry | |
| | recursive partitioning analysis | |
| | Registered Physician's Assistant | |
| | restenosis postangioplasty | |

| | |
|---|---|
| | ribonuclease protection assay |
| | right pulmonary artery |
| RPAC | Registered Physician's Assistant Certified |
| RPC | root planing and curettage |
| RPCDBM | randomized, placebo-controlled, double-blind, multinational (study) |
| RPCF | Reiter protein complement fixation |
| RPD | removable partial denture |
| RPE | rating of perceived exertion |
| | retinal pigment epithelium |
| RPED | retinal pigment epithelium detachment |
| RPEP | rabies postexposure prophylaxis |
| | right pre-ejection period |
| RPF | relaxed pelvic floor |
| | renal plasma flow |
| | retroperitoneal fibrosis |
| RPFT | Registered Pulmonary Function Technologist |
| RPG | retrograde percutaneous gastrostomy |
| | retrograde pyelogram |
| RPGN | rapidly progressive glomerulonephritis |
| RPH | retroperitoneal hemorrhage |
| RPh | Registered Pharmacist |
| RPHA | reverse passive hemagglutination |
| RPI | resting pressure index |
| | reticulocyte production index |
| RPICA | right posterior internal carotid artery |
| RPICCE | round pupil intracapsular cataract extraction |
| RPL | retroperitoneal lymphadenectomy |
| RPLC | reversed-phase liquid chromatography |
| RPLND | retroperitoneal lymph node dissection |
| RPLS | reversible posterior leukoencephalopathy syndrome |

R

| | | | |
|---|---|---|---|
| RPN | renal papillary necrosis | RRC | cohort relative risk |
| | resident's progress notes | RRCT, | regular rate, clear tones, |
| R₂PN | second year resident's | no(m) | no murmurs |
| | progress notes | RRD | rhegmatogenous retinal |
| RPO | right posterior oblique | | detachment |
| RPP | radical perineal | RRE | round, regular, and equal |
| | prostatectomy | | (pupils) |
| | rate-pressure product | RRED® | Rapid Rare Event |
| | retropubic prostatectomy | | Detection |
| RPPS | retropatellar pain | RREF | resting radionuclide |
| | syndrome | | ejection fraction |
| RPR | rapid plasma reagin (test | RRI | renal resistive index |
| | for syphilis) | RR-IOL | remove and replace |
| | Reiter protein reagin | | intraocular lens |
| RPSGT | Registered | RRM | reduced renal mass |
| | Polysomnography | | right radial mastectomy |
| | Technician | | risk-reducing mastectomy |
| RPT | Registered Physical | RRMS | relapsing-remitting |
| | Therapist | | multiple sclerosis |
| RPTA | Registered Physical | RRNA | Resident Registered Nurse |
| | Therapist Assistant | | Anesthetist |
| RPU | retropubic urethropexy | rRNA | ribosomal ribonucleic acid |
| RPV | right portal vein | RRND | right radical neck |
| | right pulmonary vein | | dissection |
| RQ | respiratory quotient | RROM | resistive range of motion |
| RQLQ | Respiratory Quality of | R rot | right rotation |
| | Life Questionnaire | RRP | radical retropubic |
| RR | recovery room | | prostatectomy |
| | regular rate | RRR | recovery room routine |
| | regular respirations | | regular rhythm and rate |
| | relative risk | | relative risk reduction |
| | respiratory rate | RRRN | round, regular, and react |
| | response rate | | normally |
| | retinal reflex | RRRsM | regular rate and rhythm |
| | rotation right | | without murmur |
| R/R | rales-rhonchi | RRSO | risk-reducing salpingo- |
| R&R | rate and rhythm | | oophorectomy |
| | recent and remote | RRT | Registered Respiratory |
| | recession and | | Therapist |
| | resection | RRU | rapid reintegration unit |
| | resect and recess (muscle | RRVO | repair relaxed vaginal |
| | surgery) | | outlet |
| | rest and recuperation | RRVS | recovery room vital |
| | remove and replace | | signs |
| RRA | radioreceptor assay | RRV-TV | rhesus rotavirus |
| | Registered Record | | tetravalent (vaccine) |
| | Administrator (for | RRW | rales, rhonchi or wheezes |
| | newer title, see RHIA) | RS | Raynaud syndrome |
| | right radial artery | | rectal swab |
| | right renal artery | | recurrent seizures |
| RRAM | rapid rhythmic | | Reed-Sternberg (cell) |
| | alternating | | Reiter syndrome |
| | movements | | reschedule |

|  | restart | RSLR | reverse straight leg raise |
|  | Reye syndrome | RSM | remote study monitoring |
|  | rhythm strip | RSNI | round spermatid nuclear injection |
|  | right side |  |  |
|  | Ringer solution | RSO | right salpingooophorectomy |
|  | rumination syndrome |  |  |
| R/S | reschedule |  | right superior oblique |
|  | rest stress | rS$_{02}$ | regional oxygen saturation |
|  | rupture spontaneous | RSOC | regular source of care |
| R & S | restraint and seclusion | RSOP | right superior oblique palsy |
| R/S I | resuscitation status one (full resuscitative effort) | RSP | rapid straight pacing |
|  |  |  | right sacroposterior |
| R/S II | resuscitation status two (no code, therapeutic measures only) | RSR | regular sinus rhythm |
|  |  |  | relative survival rate |
|  |  |  | right superior rectus |
| R/S III | resuscitation status three (no code, comfort measures only) | RSRI | renal:systemic renin index |
|  |  | RSS | reduced space symbologies |
| RSA | right sacrum anterior |  | representative sample |
|  | right subclavian artery |  | sectioned |
| RSAPE | remitting seronegative arthritis with pitting edema |  | Russell-Silver syndrome |
|  |  | RSSE | Russian spring-summer encephalitis |
| RSB | right sternal border | RST | rapid simple tests |
| RSBI | rapid shallow breathing index |  | right sacrum transverse |
|  |  | RSTs | Rodney Smith tubes |
| RSC | right subclavian (artery) (vein) | RSV | respiratory syncytial virus |
|  |  |  | right subclavian vein |
| RScA | right scapuloanterior | RSVC | right superior vena cava |
| RSCL | Rotterdam Symptom Check List | RSV$_{IGIV}$ | respiratory syncytial virus immune globulin, intravenous |
| RScP | right scapuloposterior |  |  |
| RSCS | respiratory system compliance score | RSV$_{mab}$ | respiratory syncytial virus monoclonal antibody, intramuscular (palivizumab; Synagis) |
| rscu-PA | recombinant, single-chain, urokinase-type plasminogen activator |  |  |
|  |  | RSW | right-sided weakness |
|  |  | RT | radiation therapy |
| RSD | reflex sympathetic dystrophy |  | Radiologic Technologist |
|  |  |  | recreational therapy |
| RSDS | reflex-sympathetic dystrophy syndrome |  | rectal temperature |
|  |  |  | renal transplant |
| RSE | reactive subdural effusion |  | repetition time |
|  | refractory status epilepticus |  | Respiratory Therapist |
|  |  |  | reverse transcriptase |
|  | right sternal edge |  | right |
| RSI | rapid sequence intubation |  | right thigh |
|  | repetitive strain (stress) injury |  | room temperature |
|  |  | R/t | related to |
| R-SICU | respiratory-surgical intensive care unit | RTA | ready to administer |
|  |  |  | renal tubular acidosis |
| RSL | renal solute load |  | road traffic accident |

R

| | | | |
|---|---|---|---|
| t-RA | tretinoin (*trans*-retinoic acid) | RTRR | return to recovery room |
| RTAE | right atrial enlargement | RTS | radial tunnel syndrome |
| RTAH | right anterior hemiblock | | raised toilet seat |
| RTAT | right anterior thigh | | real-time scan |
| RTB | return to baseline | | Resolve Through Sharing |
| RTC | Readiness to Change (questionnaire) | | return to school |
| | | | return to sender |
| | return to clinic | | Revised Trauma Score |
| | round the clock | | Rothmund-Thomson syndrome |
| RTCA | ribavirin | | Rubinstein-Taybi syndrome |
| RTER | return to emergency room | RTT | Respiratory Therapy Technician |
| rt.↑ext. | right upper extremity | | |
| RTF | ready-to-feed | $RT_3U$ | resin triiodothyronine uptake |
| | return to flow | | |
| RTFS | return to flying status | RTUS | realtime ultrasound |
| RTH | right total hip (arthroplasty) | RTV | ritonavir (Norvir) |
| | | | rotavirus vaccine, not otherwise specified |
| RTI | respiratory tract infection | | |
| | reverse transcriptase inhibitor | $RTV_{rr}$ | rotavirus vaccine, rhesus reassortant |
| RTK | rhabdoid tumor of the kidney | RTW | return to ward |
| | | | return to work |
| | right total knee (arthroplasty) | | Richard Turner Warwick (urethroplasty) |
| RTL | reactive to light | RTWD | return to work determination |
| RTLF | respiratory-tract lining fluids | RTX | resiniferatoxin |
| RTM | regression to the mean | RTx | radiation therapy |
| | routine medical care | | renal transplantation |
| RTMD | right mid-deltoid | RU | residual urine |
| rTMS | repetitive transcranial magnetic stimulation | | resin uptake |
| | | | retrograde ureterogram |
| RTN | renal tubular necrosis | | right upper |
| RTNM | retreatment staging of cancer | | routine urinalysis |
| | | RU 486 | mifepristone (Mifeprex) |
| RTO | return to office | RUA | right upper arm |
| RTOG | Radiation Therapy Oncology Group | | routine urine analysis |
| | | RUB | rubella virus vaccine |
| RTP | renal transplant patient | RUE | right upper extremity |
| | return to pharmacy | RUG | resource utilization group |
| rtPA | alteplase (recombinant tissue-type plasminogen activator) (Activase) | | retrograde urethrogram |
| | | RUI | recurring urinary infections |
| RT-PCR | reverse transcription polymerase chain reaction | RUL | right upper lid |
| | | | right upper lobe |
| RTR | renal transplant recipient(s) | RUOQ | right upper outer quadrant |
| | | rupt. | ruptured |
| | return to room | RUQ | right upper quadrant |
| RT (R) | Radiologic Technologist (Registered) | RUQD | right upper quadrant defect |

| | | | |
|---|---|---|---|
| RURTI | recurrent upper respiratory tract infection | RVL | right vastus lateralis |
| | | RVO | relaxed vaginal outlet |
| | | | retinal vein occlusion |
| RUSB | right upper scapular border | | right ventricular outflow |
| | | | right ventricular overactivity |
| | right upper sternal border | RVOT | right ventricular outflow tract |
| RUT | rapid urease test | | |
| RUTI | recurring urinary tract infections | RVOTH | right ventricular outflow tract hypertrophy |
| RUV | residual urine volume | RVP | right ventricular pressure |
| RUX | right upper extremity | RVR | rapid ventricular response |
| RV | rectovaginal | | renal vascular resistance |
| | residual volume | | right ventricular rhythm |
| | respiratory volume | RVSP | right ventricular systolic pressure |
| | retinal vasculitis | | |
| | return visit | RVSW | right ventricular stroke work |
| | right ventricle | | |
| | rubella vaccine | RVSWI | right ventricular stroke work index |
| RVA | rabies vaccine, adsorbed | | |
| | right ventricular apex | RVT | recurrent ventricular tachycardia |
| | right vertebral artery | | |
| RVAD | right ventricular assist device | | renal vein thrombosis |
| | | RV/TLC | residual volume to total lung capacity ratio |
| RVCD | right ventricular conduction deficit | | |
| | | RVU | relative-value units |
| RVD | relative vertebral density | RVV | rubella vaccine virus |
| | renal vascular disease | RVVT | Russell viper venom time |
| RVDP | right ventricular diastolic pressure | RW | radiant warmer |
| | | | ragweed |
| RVE | right ventricular enlargement | | red welt |
| | | | rolling walker |
| RVEDP | right ventricular end-diastolic pressure | R/W | return to work |
| | | RWM | regional wall motion |
| RVEDV | right ventricular end-diastolic volume | RWMA | regional wall motion abnormalities |
| | | RWP | ragweed pollen |
| RVEF | right ventricular ejection fraction | RWS | ragweed sensitivity |
| | | RWT | relative wall thickness |
| RVET | right ventricular ejection time | Rx | drug |
| | | | medication |
| RVF | Rift Valley fever | | pharmacy |
| | right ventricular function | | prescription |
| | right visual field | | radiotherapy |
| RVG | radionuclide ventriculography | | take |
| | | | therapy |
| | Radio VisioGraphy | | treatment |
| | right ventrogluteal | RXN | reaction |
| RVH | renovascular hypertension | RXRs | retinoid X receptors |
| | right ventricular hypertrophy | RXT | radiation therapy |
| | | | right exotropia |
| RVHT | renovascular hypertension | | |
| RVI | right ventricle infarction | | |
| RVIDd | right ventricle internal dimension diastole | | |

R

# S

| | | | |
|---|---|---|---|
| S | sacral | | suicide attempt |
| | second (s) | | surface area |
| | sensitive | | surgical assistant |
| | serum | | sustained action |
| | single | S/A | same as |
| | sister | | sugar and acetone |
| | son | S&A | sugar and acetone |
| | South (as in the location | SAA | same as above |
| | 2S would be second | | serum amyloid A |
| | floor, South wing) | | Stokes-Adams attacks |
| | sponge | | synthetic amino acids |
| | *Staphylococcus* | SAAG | serum-ascites albumin |
| | subjective findings | | gradient |
| | suicide | SAANDs | selective apoptotic |
| | suction | | antineoplastic drugs |
| | sulfur | SAARDs | slow-acting antirheumatic |
| | supervision | | drugs |
| | surgery | SAB | serum albumin |
| | susceptible | | sinoatrial block |
| /S/ | signature | | Spanish American Black |
| $\bar{s}$ | without (this is a | | spontaneous abortion |
| | dangerous abbreviation) | | subarachnoid bleed |
| S′ | shoulder | | subarachnoid block |
| $S_1$ | first heart sound | SABR | screening auditory |
| $S^{-1}...S^{-4}$ | suicide risk classifications | | brainstem response |
| $S_2$ | second heart sound | SAC | segmental antigen |
| $S_3$ | third heart sound | | challenge |
| | (ventricular filling | | serum aminoglycoside |
| | gallop) | | concentration |
| $S_4$ | fourth heart sound (atrial | | short arm cast |
| | gallop) | | substance abuse counselor |
| $S_1...S_5$ | sacral vertebra or nerves | SACC | short arm cylinder cast |
| | 1 through 5 | SACD | subacute combined |
| SI..SIV | symbols for the first to | | degeneration |
| | fourth heart sounds | SACH | solid ankle, cushioned |
| SA | sacroanterior | | heel |
| | salicylic acid | SACT | sinoatrial conduction time |
| | semen analysis | SAD | seasonal affective disorder |
| | Sexoholics Anonymous | | Self-Assessment |
| | sinoatrial | | Depression (scale) |
| | sleep apnea | | social anxiety disorder |
| | slow acetylator | | source-axis distance |
| | Spanish American | | subacromial |
| | spinal anesthesia | | decompression |
| | *Staphylococcus aureus* | | subacute dialysis |
| | subarachnoid | | sugar and acetone |
| | substance abuse | | determination |
| | suicide alert | | superior axis deviation |
| | | SADBE | squaric acid dibutyl ester |
| | | SADD | Students Against Drunk |
| | | | Driving |
| | | SADL | simulated activities of |
| | | | daily living |

| | | | |
|---|---|---|---|
| SADR | suspected adverse drug reaction | | and metaproterenol (Metaprel) |
| SADS | Schedule for Affective Disorders and Schizophrenia | | selective antimicrobial modulation |
| SADs | severe autoimmune diseases | | self-administered medication |
| SADS-C | Schedule for Affective Disorders And Schizophrenia – Change Version | | short arc motion |
| | | | sleep apnea monitor |
| | | | Spanish-American male |
| | | | systolic anterior motion |
| | | SAMe | S-adenosylmethionine (ademetionine) |
| SAE | serious adverse event | | |
| | short above elbow (cast) | SAMHSA | Substance Abuse and Mental Health Services Administration |
| SAEG | signal averaging electrocardiogram | | |
| SAEKG | signaled average electrocardiogram | SAMPLE | symptoms/signs, allergies, medications, past medical history, last oral intake, and events prior to arrival (an EMT mnemonic used in initial patient questioning) |
| SAESU | Substance Abuse valuating Screen Unit | | |
| SAF | Self-Analysis Form | | |
| | self-articulating femoral | | |
| | Spanish American female | | |
| | subcutaneous abdominal fat | SAN | side-arm nebulizer |
| | | | sinoatrial node |
| | | | slept all night |
| SAFHS | sonic accelerated fracture healing system | SANC | short arm navicular cast |
| SAG | sodium antimony gluconate | sang | sanguinous |
| Sag D | sagittal diameter | SANS | Schedule (Scale) for the Assessment of Negative Symptoms |
| SAGE | serial analysis of gene expression | | |
| SAH | subarachnoid hemorrhage | | sympathetic autonomic nervous system |
| | systemic arterial hypertension | SAO | small airway obstruction |
| | | | Southeast Asian ovalocytosis |
| SAHA | suberoylanilide hydroxamic acid | | |
| SAHS | sleep apnea/hypopnea (hypersomnolence) syndrome | $SaO_2$ | arterial oxygen percent saturation |
| SAI | Sodium Amytal® interview | SAP | serum alkaline phosphate |
| | | | serum amyloid P |
| SAL | salicylate | | sporadic adenomatous polyps |
| | Salmonella | | |
| | sensory acuity level | SAPD | self-administration of psychotropic drugs |
| | sterility assurance level | | |
| SAL 12 | sequential analysis of 12 chemistry constituents (see page 362) | SAPH | saphenous |
| | | SAPHO | synovitis, acne, pustulosis, hyperostosis, and osteomyelitis (syndrome) |
| SALK | surgical arthroscopy, left knee | | |
| SAM | methylprednisolone sodium succinate (Solu-Medrol), aminophylline, | SAPS | Scale for the Assessment of Positive Symptoms |

| | | | |
|---|---|---|---|
| | short arm plaster splint | SASP | sulfasalazine (salicylazo-sulfapyridine; Azulfidine) |
| | Simplified Acute Physiology Score | | |
| SAPS II | Simplified Acute Physiology Score version II | SASS | Social Adaptation Self-Evaluation Scale |
| SAQ | saquinavir (Invirase) | SAT | methylprednisolone sodium succinate (Solu-Medrol), aminophylline, and terbutaline |
| | Sexual Adjustment Questionnaire | | |
| | short-arc quadriceps | | |
| SAR | seasonal allergic rhinitis | | saturated |
| | Senior Assistant Resident | | saturation |
| | sexual attitudes reassessment | | Saturday |
| | | | self-administered therapy |
| | structural activity relationships | | Senior Apperception Test |
| | | | speech awareness threshold |
| SARA | sexually acquired reactive arthritis | | subacute thyroiditis |
| | SQUID (superconducting quantum interference device) array for reproductive assessment | SATC | substance abuse treatment clinic |
| | | SATL | surgical Achilles tendon lengthening |
| | system for anesthetic and respiratory administration analysis | SATP | substance abuse treatment program |
| | | SATS | refers to oxygen saturation levels |
| SARAN | senior admitting resident's admission note | SATU | substance abuse treatment unit |
| SARC | seasonal allergic rhinoconjunctivitis | SAVD | spontaneous assisted vaginal delivery |
| SARK | surgical arthroscopy, right knee | SB | safety belt |
| | | | sandbag |
| S Arrh | sinus arrhythmia | | scleral buckling |
| SART | standard acid reflux test | | seat belt |
| SAS | saline, agent, and saline | | seen by |
| | scalenus anticus syndrome | | Sengstaken-Blakemore (tube) |
| | Sedation-Agitation Scale | | sick boy |
| | see assessment sheet | | side bend |
| | Self-rating Anxiety Scale | | side bending |
| | short arm splint | | sinus bradycardia |
| | sleep apnea syndrome | | slide board |
| | Social Adjustment Scale | | small bowel |
| | Specific Activity Scale | | spina bifida |
| | statistical applications software | | sponge bath |
| | | | stand-by |
| | subarachnoid space | | Stanford-Binet (test) |
| | subaxial subluxation | | sternal border |
| | sulfasalazine (Azulfidine) | | stillbirth |
| | synthetic absorbable sutures | | stillborn |
| | | | stone basketing |
| SASA | Sex Abuse Survivors Anonymous | Sb | antimony |
| SASH | saline, agent, saline, and heparin | SB+ | wearing seat belt |

| | | | |
|---|---|---|---|
| SB− | not wearing seat belt | SBOS | scleral buckle, left eye |
| SBA | serum bactericidal activity | SBP | school breakfast program |
| | standby angioplasty | | scleral buckling procedure |
| | standby assistant (assistance) | | small bowel phytobezoars |
| | Summary Basis of Approval | | spontaneous bacterial peritonitis |
| | | | systolic blood pressure |
| SBAC | small bowel adenocarcinoma | SBQC | small based quad cane |
| | | SBR | sluggish blood return |
| SBB | stereotactic breast biopsy | | strict bed rest |
| SBBO | small-bowel bacterial overgrowth | SBRN | sensory branch of the radial nerve |
| SBC | sensory binocular cooperation | SBS | serum blood sugar |
| | | | shaken baby syndrome |
| | single base cane | | short (small) bowel syndrome |
| | standard bicarbonate | | sick-building syndrome |
| | strict bed confinement | | side-by-side |
| | superficial bladder cancer | | small bowel series |
| | | SBT | serum bactericidal titers |
| SBD | straight bag drainage | | special baby Travesol |
| SBE | saturated base excess | | spontaneous breathing trial |
| | self-breast examination | | |
| | short below-elbow (cast) | SBTB | sinus breakthrough beat |
| | shortness of breath on exertion | SBTT | small bowel transit time |
| | subacute bacterial endocarditis | SBV | single binocular vision |
| | | SBW | seat belts worn |
| SBFT | small bowel follow through | SBX | symphysis, buttocks, and xiphoid |
| SBG | stand-by guard | SC | schizophrenia |
| SBGM | self blood-glucose monitoring | | Schwann cell |
| | | | self-care |
| SBH | State Board of Health | | serum creatinine |
| SBI | silicone (gel-containing) breast implants | | service connected |
| | | | sick call |
| | systemic bacterial infection | | sickle cell |
| SBJ | skin, bones, and joints | | small (blood pressure) cuff |
| SBK | spinnbarkeit | | Snellen chart |
| SBL | sponge blood loss | | spinal cord |
| sBLA | supplemental Biologic License Application | | sport cord |
| | | | sternoclavicular |
| SB-LM | Stanford-Binet Intelligence Test-Form LM | | subclavian |
| | | | subclavian catheter |
| | | | subcutaneous |
| SBO | small bowel obstruction | | succinylcholine |
| | specified bovine offals | | sugar-coated (tablets) |
| SBOD | scleral buckle, right eye | | sulfur colloid |
| SBOE | surgical blood order equation | | surveillance cultures |
| | | s̄c | without correction (without glasses) |
| SBOH | State Board of Health | | |
| SBOM | soybean oil meal | S&C | sclerae and conjunctivae |

S

| SCA | sickle cell anemia | | subacute combined |
| | spinocerebellar ataxia | | degeneration |
| | subclavian artery | | sudden cardiac death |
| | subcutaneous abdominal | ScDA | scapulodextra anterior |
| | (block) | SCDM | soybean-casein digest |
| | sudden cardiac arrest | | medium |
| | superior cerebellar artery | ScDP | scapulodextra posterior |
| SCa | serum calcium | SCE | sister chromatid |
| SCAD | short chain acyl-coenzyme | | exchange |
| | A dehydrogenase | | soft cooked egg |
| SCAN | suspected child abuse and | | specialized columnar |
| | neglect | | epithelium |
| SCAP | scapula; scapulae; | SCEMIA | self-contained enzymatic |
| | scapular | | membrane |
| | stem cell apheresis | | immunoassay |
| SCARMD | severe childhood | SCEP | somatosensory cortical |
| | autosomal recessive | | evoked potential |
| | muscular dystrophy | SCF | special care formula |
| SCAT | sheep cell agglutination | | stem cell factor |
| | titer | SCFA | short-chain fatty acid |
| | sickle cell anemia test | SCFE | slipped capital femoral |
| SCB | strictly confined to bed | | epiphysis |
| SCBC | small cell bronchogenic | SCFGT | Southern California |
| | carcinoma | | Figure Ground Test |
| SCBE | single-contrast barium | SCG | seismocardiography |
| | enema | | serum Chemogram |
| SCBF | spinal cord blood flow | | sodium cromoglycate |
| SCC | short course | SCH | schistosomiasis |
| | chemotherapy (for | | (*Schistosoma* sp.) |
| | tuberculosis) | | vaccine |
| | sickle cell crisis | | subclinical |
| | small cell carcinoma | | hypothyroidism |
| | spinal cord compression | SCh | succinylcholine chloride |
| | squamous cell carcinoma | SCHISTO | schistocytes |
| SCCA | semi-closed circle | SCHIZ | schizocytes |
| | absorber | | schizophrenia |
| | squamous cell carcinoma | SCHLP | supracricord |
| | antigen | | hemilaryngopharyngec- |
| SCCa | squamous cell carcinoma | | tomy |
| SCCB | small cell cancer of the | SCHNC | squamous cell head and |
| | bladder | | neck cancer |
| SCCE | squamous cell carcinoma | SCI | silent cerebral infarct |
| | of the esophagus | | specific COX-2 inhibitor |
| SCCHN | squamous cell carcinoma | | spinal cord injury |
| | of the head and neck | | subcoma insulin |
| SCCI | subcutaneous continuous | SCID | severe combined |
| | infusion | | immunodeficiency |
| SCD | sequential compression | | disorders (disease) |
| | device | | structured clinical |
| | service connected | | interview for |
| | disability | | DSM-III-R |
| | sickle cell disease | SCII | Strong-Campbell Interest |
| | spinal cord disease | | Inventory |

| | | | |
|---|---|---|---|
| SCIP | Screening and Crisis Intervention Program | S-CPK | serum creatine phosphokinase |
| SCIPP | sacrococcygeal to inferior pubic point | SCPP | spinal cord perfusion pressure |
| SCIT | single-chain immunotoxin | SCR | special care room (seclusion room) |
| SCIU | spinal cord injury unit | | spondylitic caudal radioculopathy |
| SCIV | subclavian intravenous | | standard care regimen |
| SCI-WORA | spinal cord injury without radiographic abnormalities | | stem cell rescue |
| SCJ | sternoclavicular joint | SCr | serum creatinine |
| SCL | skin conductance level | sCR | soluble complement receptor |
| | symptom checklist | SCRIPT | prescription |
| SCL-90 | Symptoms Checklist—90 items | SC/RP | scaling and root planing |
| ScLA | scapulolaeva anterior | SC-RNV | subcutaneous radionuclide venography |
| SCLAX | subcostal long axis | | |
| SCLC | small cell lung cancer | SCS | spinal cord stimulation |
| SCLD | sickle cell lung disease | | splatter control shield |
| SCLE | subacute cutaneous lupus erythematosis | | stem cell support |
| | | | suspected catheter sepsis |
| ScLP | scapulolaeva posterior | | |
| SCLs | soft contact lenses | SCSAX | subcostal short axis |
| | synthetic combinatorial libraries | SCSIT | Southern California Sensory Integration Tests |
| SCM | scalene muscle | | |
| | sensation, circulation, and motion | SCSVT | Southern California Space Visualization Test |
| | spondylitic caudal myelopathy | SCT | Sertoli cell tumor |
| | sternocleidomastoid | | sex chromatin test |
| | supraclavicular muscle | | sickle cell trait |
| SCMD | senile choroidal macular degeneration | | stem cell transplant |
| | | | sugar-coated tablet |
| SCMV | serogroup C meningococcal vaccine | SCTX | static cervical traction |
| | | SCU | self-care unit |
| SCN | severe congenital neutropenia | | special care unit |
| | special care nursery | SCUCP | small cell undifferentiated carcinoma of the prostate |
| | suprachiasmatic nucleus (nuclei) | | |
| SCNT | somatic-cell nuclear transfer | SCUF | slow continuous ultrafiltration |
| SCOB | Schedule-Controlled Operant Behavior | SCUT | schizophrenia, chronic undifferentiated type |
| SCOP | scopolamine | SCV | subclavian vein |
| SCOPE | arthroscopy | | subcutaneous vaginal (block) |
| SCP | secondary care provider | SCY | scytonemin |
| | sodium cellulose phosphate | SD | scleroderma |
| | standardized care plan | | senile dementia |
| SCPF | stem cell proliferation factor | | sensory deficit |
| | | | severe deficit |
| | | | septal defect |

severely disabled

shallow distance (aquatic therapy)

shoulder disarticulation

single dose

skin dose

sleep deprived

solvent-detergent

somatic dysfunction

spasmodic dysphonia

speech discrimination

spontaneous delivery

stable disease

standard deviation

standard diet

step-down

sterile dressing

straight drainage

streptozocin and doxorubicin

sudden death

surgical drain

**S & D**  seen and discussed

stomach and duodenum

**S/D**  sharp/dull

systolic-diastolic ratio

**SDA**  sacrodextra anterior

same day admission

serotonin/dopamine antagonist

Seventh-Day Adventist

steroid-dependent asthmatic

**SDAT**  senile dementia of Alzheimer type

**SDB**  Sabouraud dextrose broth

self-destructive behavior

sleep disordered breathing

**SDBP**  seated diastolic blood pressure

standing diastolic blood pressure

supine diastolic blood pressure

**SDC**  serum digoxin concentration

serum drug concentration

Sleep Disorders Center

sodium deoxycholate

**SD&C**  suction, dilation, and curettage

**SDD**  selective digestive (tract) decontamination

sterile dry dressing

subantimicrobial dose doxycycline (dental; Periostat)

**SDDT**  selective decontamination of the digestive tract

**SDE**  subdural empyema

**SDES**  symptomatic diffuse esophageal spasm

**SDF**  sexual dysfunction

stromal-cell-derived factor

**SDH**  spinal detrusor hyperreflexia

subdural hematoma

**SDHD**  succinate dehydrogenase complex subunit D

**SDI**  Sandimmune (cyclosporine)

State Disability Insurance

**SDII**  sudden death in infancy

**SDL**  serum digoxin level

serum drug level

speech discrimination loss

**SDLE**  sex-difference in life expectancy

somatic dysfunction lower extremity

**SDM**  soft drusen maculopathy

standard deviation of the mean

**S/D/M**  systolic, diastolic, mean

**SDMC**  safety and data monitoring committee

**SD/N**  signal-difference-to-noise ratio

**SDNN**  standard deviation of normal-to-normal beats

**SDO**  surgical diagnostic oncology

**SDP**  sacrodextra posterior

single donor platelets

solvent-detergent plasma

stomach, duodenum, and pancreas

**SDPTG**  second derivative of photoplethysmogram

**SDR**  selective dorsal rhizotomy

short-duration response

**SDS**  same day surgery

Self-Rating Depression Scale

S

| | | | |
|---|---|---|---|
| | sodium dodecyl sulfate | SECG | scalp electrocardiogram |
| | somatropin deficiency syndrome | SECL | seclusion |
| | | SECPR | standard external cardiopulmonary resuscitation |
| | Speech Discrimination Score | | |
| | standard deviation score | SE-CPT | single-electrode current perception threshold |
| | sudden death syndrome | | |
| | Symptom Distress Scale | SED | sedimentation |
| SDSO | same day surgery overnight | | skin erythema dose |
| | | | socially and emotionally disturbed |
| SDS-PAGE | sodium dodecyl sulfate – polyacrylamide gel electrophoresis | | spondyloepiphyseal dysplasia |
| | | SeDBP | seated diastolic blood pressure |
| SDT | sacrodextra transversa | | |
| | speech detection threshold | SEDDS | self-emulsifying drug-delivery system |
| SDU | step-down unit | | |
| SDUE | somatic dysfunction upper extremity | SED-NET | severely emotional disturbed - network |
| SDV | single-dose vial | sed rt | sedimentation rate |
| SE | saline enema (0.9% sodium chloride) | SEER | Surveillance, Epidemiology, and End Results (program) |
| | self-examination | | |
| | side effect | | |
| | soft exudates | SEG | segment |
| | spin echo | | sonoencephalogram |
| | staff escort | segs | segmented neutrophils |
| | standard error | SEH | spinal epidural hematomas |
| | Starr-Edwards (valve, pacemaker) | | |
| | | | subependymal hemorrhage |
| | status epilepticus | | |
| Se | selenium | SEI | subepithelial (comeal) infiltrate |
| S/E | suicidal and eloper | | |
| S & E | seen and examined | SELDI | surface enhanced laser desorption/ionization |
| SEA | sheep erythrocyte agglutination (test) | | |
| | | SELFVD | sterile elective low forceps vaginal delivery |
| | side-entry (venous) access | | |
| | Southeast Asia | SEM | scanning electron microscopy |
| | subdural electrode array | | |
| | synaptic electronic activation | | semen |
| | | | slow eye movement |
| SEAR | Southeast Asia refugee | | standard error of mean |
| SEB | Staphylococcus enterotoxin B | | systolic ejection murmur |
| | | SEMI | subendocardial myocardial infarction |
| | surrogate end-point biomarker | | |
| | | SEN | spray each nostril |
| SEC | second | SENS | sensitivity |
| | secondary | | sensorium |
| | secretary | SEOC | serous epithelial ovarian carcinoma |
| | size exclusion chromatography | | |
| | | SEP | multiple sclerosis (French) |
| | steric exclusion chromatography | | |
| | | | separate |

| | | | |
|---|---|---|---|
| | serum electrophoresis | | skull fracture |
| | somatosensory evoked potential | | soft feces |
| | | | sound field |
| | syringe exchange program | | spinal fluid |
| | | | starch-free |
| | systolic ejection period | | sugar-free |
| SEPS | subfascial endoscopic perforator surgery | | symptom-free |
| | | | synovial fluid |
| SEQ | sequela | S&F | slip and fall |
| SER | scanning equalization radiography | | soft and flat |
| | sertraline (Zoloft) | SF-6 | sulfahexafluoride |
| | side effects records | SF 36 | 36-item short form health survey |
| | signal enhancement ratio | SFA | saturated fatty acids |
| SERA-TEK | technetium-99m hexametazime | | superficial femoral artery |
| | | SFB | single frequency bioimpedance |
| SERF | Severity of Exacerbation and Risk Factors | SFC | spinal fluid count |
| Serial 7's | a mental status examination (starting with a 100, count backward by 7's) | | subarachnoid fluid collection |
| | | SFD | scaphoid fossa depression |
| | | | small for dates |
| SER-IV | supination external rotation, type 4 fracture | SFE | supercritical fluid extraction |
| SERM | selective estrogen-receptor modulator | SFEMG | single-fiber electromyography |
| SERO-SANG | serosanguineous | SFH | schizophrenia family history |
| SERP-ACWA | Skin Exposure Reduction Paste Against Chemical Warfare Agents | SFJ | saphenofemoral junction |
| | | SFM | scanning force microscopy |
| SERs | somatosensory evoked responses | SFNM | subfoveal neovascular membranes |
| SES | sick euthyroid syndrome | SFP | simulated fluorescence process |
| | socioeconomic status | | |
| | standard electrolyte solution | | simultaneous foveal perception |
| SeSBP | seated systolic blood pressure | | spinal fluid pressure |
| | | SFPT | standard fixation preference test |
| SET | signal extraction technology | SFS | split function studies |
| | skin end-point titration | SFTR | sagittal, frontal, transverse, rotation |
| | social environmental therapy | SFUP | surgical follow-up |
| | systolic ejection time | SFV | simian foamy viruses |
| SEV | sevoflurane (Ultane) | | superficial femoral vein |
| SEWHO | shoulder-elbow-wrist-hand orthosis | SFW | shell fragment wound |
| | | SFWB | social/family well-being |
| SF | salt-free | SFWD | symptom-free walking distance |
| | saturated fat | | |
| | scarlet fever | SG | salivary gland |
| | seizure frequency | | scrotography |
| | seminal fluid | | serum glucose |

| | | | |
|---|---|---|---|
| | side glide | S&H | speech and hearing |
| | skin graft | | suicidal and homicidal |
| | specific gravity | S/H | suicidal/homicidal |
| | Swan-Ganz (catheter) | | ideation |
| S/G | swallow/gag | SH2 | sarc homology region 2 |
| SGA | small for gestational age | SHA | super-heated aerosol |
| | subjective global | SHAL | standard |
| | assessment (dietary | | hyperalimentation |
| | history and physical | SHAS | supravalvular |
| | examination) | | hypertrophic aortic |
| | substantial gainful activity | | stenosis |
| | (employment) | S Hb | sickle hemoglobin screen |
| SGAs | second-generation | SHBG | sex hormone-binding |
| | antihistamines | | globulin |
| SGB | Swiss gym ball | sHBO$_2$T | systemic hyperbaric |
| SGC | Swan-Ganz catheter | | oxygen therapy |
| SGCNB | stereotactic guided core-needle biopsy | SHC | subsequent hospital care |
| SGD | straight gravity drainage | SHEENT | skin, head, eyes, ears, |
| SGE | significant glandular | | nose, and throat |
| | enlargement | SHG | shigellosis (*Shigella* sp.) |
| SGHL | superior glenohumeral | | vaccine |
| | ligament | SHGT | somatic-cell human gene |
| s̄ gl | without correction | | therapy |
| | (without glasses) | SHI | standard heparin |
| SGM | serum glucose | | infusion |
| | monitoring | Shig | *Shigella* |
| SGOT | serum glutamic oxalo-acetic transaminase | SHIV | simian-human immunodeficiency virus |
| | (same as AST) | SHL | sudden hearing loss |
| SGP | Schering-Plough | | supraglottic horizontal |
| | Corporation | | laryngectomy |
| SGPT | serum glutamate pyruvate | SHO | Senior House Officer |
| | transaminase (same as | SHP | secondary hypertension, |
| | ALT) | | pulmonary |
| SGRQ-A | St. George's Respiratory | SHR | scapulohumeral rhythm |
| | Questionnaire translated | SHRC | shortened, held, resisted |
| | into American English | | contraction |
| SGS | second-generation | SHS | student health service |
| | sulfonylurea | SHV | short hepatic vein |
| | subglottic stenosis | | sulfhydryl variant |
| sGS | surgical Gleason score | SHx | social history |
| SGTCS | secondarily generalized | SI | International System of |
| | tonic-clonic seizures | | Units |
| SH | serum hepatitis | | sacroiliac |
| | sexual harassment | | sagittal index |
| | short | | sector iridectomy |
| | shoulder | | self-inflicted |
| | shower | | sensory integration |
| | social history | | seriously ill |
| | sulfhydryl (group) | | sexual intercourse |
| | surgical history | | signal intensity |
| | systemic hypertension | | small intestine |

S

303

| | | | |
|---|---|---|---|
| | strict isolation | SIG | let it be marked (appears on prescription before directions for patient) |
| | stress incontinence | | |
| | stroke index | | |
| | suicidal ideation | | sigmoidoscopy |
| Si | silicon | Signal 99 | patient in cardiac or respiratory distress |
| S & I | suction and irrigation | | |
| | support and interpretation | SIJ | sacroiliac joint |
| SIA | small intestinal atresia | SIJS | sacroiliac joint syndrome |
| SIDAM | structured interview for the diagnosis of dementia of Alzheimer type | SIL | seriously ill list |
| | | | sister-in-law |
| | | | squamous intraepithelial lesion |
| SIDAM-A | structured interview for the diagnosis of dementia of the Alzheimer type, multi-infarct dementia, and dementias of other etiology according to ICD-10 and DSM-III-R | SILFVD | sterile indicated low forceps vaginal delivery |
| | | SILV | simultaneous independent lung ventilation |
| | | SIM | selective ion monitoring |
| | | | Similac® |
| | | | surface-induced mineralization |
| SIADH | syndrome of inappropriate antidiuretic hormone secretion | SIMCU | surgical intermediate care unit |
| SIAT | supervised intermittent ambulatory treatment | Sim c̄ Fe | Similac with iron® |
| | | SIMV | synchronized intermittent mandatory ventilation |
| SIB | self-inflating bulb | | |
| | self-injurious behavior | SIN | salpingitis isthmica nodose |
| SIBC | serum iron-binding capacity | | |
| | | SIOD | Schimke immuno-osseous dysplasia |
| sibs | siblings | | |
| SIC | self-intermittent catherization | SIP | Sickness Impact Profile |
| | | | stroke in progression |
| | squamous intraepithelial cells | | sympathetically independent pain |
| | Standard Industrial Classification | SIQ | sick in quarters |
| | | SIQ-JR | Suicidal Ideation Questionnaire-Junior |
| SICD | sudden infant crib death | | |
| SICT | selective intracoronary thrombolysis | SIR | standardized incidence rate (ratio) |
| SICU | surgical intensive care unit | SIRS | systemic inflammatory response syndrome |
| SID | once daily (used in veterinary medicine) | | |
| | | SIS | sister |
| SIDA | French and Spanish abbreviation for AIDS | | Surgical Infection Stratification (system) |
| SIDD | syndrome of isolated diastolic dysfunction | SISI | Short Increment Sensitivity Index |
| SIDERO | siderocyte | SISS | severe invasion streptococcal syndrome |
| SIDFF | superimposed dorsiflexion of foot | SIT | serum inhibitory titers |
| SIDS | sudden infant death syndrome | | silicon-intensified target |
| | | | Slossen Intelligence Test |
| SIEP | serum immunoelectrophoresis | | specific immunotherapy (allergy) |

| | sperm immobilization test | | side-lying |
|---|---|---|---|
| | structured interrupted therapy | | staging laparoscopy |
| | | | slight |
| | supraspinatus, infraspinatus, teres (insertions) | | sublingual |
| | | S/L | slit lamp (examination) |
| | | SLA | sacrolaeva anterior |
| | surgical intensive therapy | | sex and love addictions |
| SITA | standard infertility treatment algorithm | | slide latex agglutination |
| | | | The Satisfaction with Life Areas |
| SIT BAL | sitting balance | | |
| SIT TOL | sitting tolerance | SLAA | Sex and Love Addicts Anonymous |
| SIV | simian immunodeficiency virus | | |
| | | SLAC | scapholunate advanced collapse |
| SIVP | slow intravenous push | | |
| SIW | self-inflicted wound | SLAM | Systemic Lupus Activity Measure |
| SJC | swollen joint count | | |
| SJCRH | St. Jude Children's Research Hospital | SLAP | serum leucine amino-peptidase |
| SJM | St. Jude Medical (heart valve prosthesis) | | superior labral anteroposterior (shoulder lesion) |
| S-JRA | systemic juvenile rheumatoid arthritis | | |
| | | SLB | short leg brace |
| SJS | Schwartz-Jampel syndrome | SLC | short leg cast |
| | | SLCC | short leg cylinder cast |
| | Stevens-Johnson syndrome | SLCG | sulfolithocholyglycine |
| | | SLCT | Sertoli-Leydig cell tumor |
| | Swyer-James syndrome | SLD | specific language disorder |
| $S_{jvO2}$ | jugular venous oxygen saturation | | stealth liposomal doxorubicin |
| SK | seborrheic keratosis | SLE | slit-lamp examination |
| | senile keratosis | | St. Louis encephalitis |
| | SmithKline | | systemic lupus erythematosus |
| | solar keratosis | | |
| | streptokinase | SLEDAI | Systemic Lupus Erythematosus Disease Activity Index |
| S & K | single and keeping (baby) | | |
| SKAO | supracondylar knee-ankle orthosis | SLEX | slit-lamp examination (biomicroscopy) |
| SKB | SmithKline Beecham | SLFVD | sterile low forceps vaginal delivery |
| SKC | single knee to chest | | |
| SKINT | skinfold thickness | SLGXT | symptom-limited graded exercise test |
| SK-SD | streptokinase streptodornase | | |
| SKU | stock keeping unit (related to product identification) | SLI | specific language impairment |
| | | SLK | superior limbic keratoconjunctivitis |
| SKY | spectral karyotyping | SLL | second-look laparotomy |
| SL | scapholunate | | small lymphocytic lymphoma |
| | secondary leukemia | | |
| | sensation level | SLMFVD | sterile low midforceps vaginal delivery |
| | sentinel lymphadenectomy | | |
| | serious list | SLMMS | slightly more marked |
| | shortleg | | since |

S

| | | | |
|---|---|---|---|
| SLMP | since last menstrual period | sl. tr. | slight trace |
| | | SLUD | salivation, lacrimation, urination, and defecation |
| SLN | sentinel lymph node(s) superior laryngeal nerve | | |
| SLND | sentinel lymph node detection | SLUDGE | salivation, lacrimation, urination, diarrhea, gastrointestinal upset, and emesis (signs and symptoms of cholinergic excess) |
| SLNM | sentinel lymph node mapping | | |
| SLNTG | sublingual nitroglycerin | | |
| SLNWBC | short leg nonweight-bearing cast | | |
| | | SLV | since last visit |
| SLNWC | short leg nonwalking cast | SLWB | severely low birth weight |
| SLO | scanning laser ophthalmoscope | SLWC | short leg walking cast |
| | | SM | sadomasochism |
| | second-look operation | | service mark (such as The Pause that Refreshes) |
| | shark liver oil | | |
| | Smith-Lemli-Opitz (syndrome) | | skim milk |
| | | | small |
| | streptolysin O | | sports medicine |
| SLOA | short leave of absence | | Stairmaster® |
| SLP | single-limb progression | | streptomycin |
| | Speech Language Pathologist | | systolic motion |
| | | | systolic murmur |
| | speech language pathology | $^{153}$Sm | samarium 153 |
| SLPI | secretory leukocyte protease inhibitor | SMA | smallpox vaccine, not otherwise specified |
| SLPMS | short-leg posterior-molded splint | | smooth muscle antibody |
| | | | spinal muscular atrophy |
| SLR | straight-leg raising | | superior mesenteric artery |
| SLRT | straight-leg raising tenderness | SMA-6 | simultaneous multichannel autoanalyzer (page 358) |
| | straight-leg raising test | SMA-7 | See page 362 |
| SLS | second-look sonography | SMA-12 | See page 362 |
| | short leg splint | SMA-18 | See page 362 |
| | shrinking lungs syndrome | SMA-23 | See page 362 |
| | single limb support | SMAO | superior mesenteric artery occlusion |
| SLT | sacrolaeva transversa | | |
| | scanning laser tomography | SMAR | self-medication administration record |
| | single lung transplantation | SMAS | superficial musculoaponeurotic system (graft; flat) |
| | Speech Language Therapist | | |
| | spontaneous labor at term | | superior mesenteric artery syndrome |
| | swing light test | SMAST | Short Michigan Alcohol-ism Screening Test |
| SLT-I | Shiga-like toxin I | | |
| SLTA | severe life-threatening asthma | SMAvac | smallpox (vaccinia virus) vaccine |
| | standard language test for aphasia | SMB | simulated moving bed (chromatography) |
| SLTEC | Shiga-like toxin-producing *Escherichia coli* | SMBG | self-monitoring blood glucose |

| | | | |
|---|---|---|---|
| SMC | skeletal myxoid chondrosarcoma | | odds ratios |
| | special mouth care | SMP | self-management program |
| SMCA | sorbitol MacConkey agar | | sympathetic maintained plan |
| SMCD | senile macular chorio-retinal degeneration | SmPC | Summary of Product Characteristics (European Union) |
| SMCs | smooth muscle cells | | |
| SMD | senile macular degeneration | SMPN | sensorimotor polyneuropathy |
| | standardized mean difference | SMR | senior medical resident |
| | | | skeletal muscle relaxant |
| SMDA | Safe Medical Defice Act | | standardized mortality ratio |
| SME | significant medical event | | submucous resection |
| SMF | streptozocin, mitomycin, and fluorouracil | SMRR | submucous resection and rhinoplasty |
| SMFA | sodium monofluoroacetate | SMS | scalded mouth syndrome |
| SMFVD | sterile midforceps vaginal delivery | | senior medical student |
| | | | Smith-Magenis syndrome |
| SMG | submandibular gland | | somatostatin (Zecnil) |
| SMH | state mental hospital | | stiff-man syndrome |
| SMI | sensory motor integration (group) | SMSA | standard metropolitan statistical area |
| | severely mentally impaired | SMT | smooth muscle tumors |
| | service mix index | SMV | stentless mitral valve |
| | small volume infusion | | submentovertical |
| | suggested minimum increment | | superior mesenteric vein |
| | sustained maximal inspiration | SMVT | sustained monomorphic ventricular tachycardia |
| SMIDS | suppertime mixed insulin and daytime sulfonylureas | SMX-TMP | sulfamethoxazole and trimethoprim (SMZ-TMP) |
| SMILE | safety, monitoring, intervention, length of stay and evaluation | SN | sciatic notch |
| | | | sinus node |
| | | | staff nurse |
| | | | student nurse |
| | sustained maximal inspiratory lung exercises | | suprasternal notch |
| | | | superior nasal |
| | | Sn | tin |
| SMIT | standard mycological identification techniques | S/N | signal to noise ratio |
| | | SNA | specimen not available |
| | | | Student Nursing Assistant |
| SMMVT | sustained monomorphic ventricular tachycardia | SNa | serum sodium |
| SMN | second malignant neoplasia | SNAP | scheduled nursing activities program |
| SMO | Senior Medical Officer | | Score for Neonatal Acute Physiology |
| | site management organization(s) | | sensory nerve action potential |
| | slip made out | | Swanson, Nolan, and Pelham (rating scale) |
| SMON | subacute myelo-opticoneuropathy | SNAP-PE | Score for Neonatal Acute Physiology-Perinatal Extension |
| SMORs | standardized mortality | | |

S

| | | | |
|---|---|---|---|
| SNaRI | serotonin noradrenergic reuptake inhibitor | | Medicine, Reference Terminology |
| SNASA | Salford Needs Assessment Schedule for Adolescents | SNOOP | Systematic Nursing Observation of Psychopathology |
| SNAT | suspected nonaccidental trauma | SNOs | S-nitrosothiols |
| | | SNP | simple neonatal procedure |
| SNB | scalene node biopsy | | sodium nitroprusside |
| | sentinel (lymph) node biopsy | SNP-LP | single nucleotide polymorphisms – linkage disequilibrium |
| SNC | skilled nursing care | | |
| SNc | substantia nigra compacta | SNPs | single nucleotide polymorphisms |
| SNCV | sensory nerve conduction velocity | SNR | signal-to-noise ratio (radiology) |
| SND | single needle device | SNr | substantia nigra reticularis |
| | sinus node dysfunction | SNRB | selective nerve root block |
| SNDA | Supplemental New Drug Application | SNRI | selective noradrenergic reuptake inhibitor |
| SNE | subacute necrotizing encephalomyelopathy | | serotonin norepinephrine reuptake inhibitor |
| SNEP | student nurse extern program | SNRT | sinus node recovery time |
| | | SNS | sterile normal saline (0.9% sodium chloride, sterile) |
| SnET2 | tin ethyl etiopurpurin | | |
| SNF | Simon nitinol filter | | |
| | skilled nursing facility | | sympathetic nervous system |
| SnF$_2$ | stannous fluoride | | |
| SNF/MR | skilled nursing facility for the mentally retarded | SNT | sinuses, nose, and throat |
| | | | suppan nail technique |
| SNGFR | single nephron glomerular filtration rate | SNV | Sin Nombre virus |
| | | | skilled nursing visit |
| SNGP | supranuclear gaze palsy | | spleen necrosis virus |
| SNHL | sensorineural hearing loss | SO | second opinion |
| | | | sex offender |
| SNIP | silver nitrate immunoperoxidase | | shoulder orthosis |
| | | | significant other |
| | strict no information in paper | | special observation |
| | | | sphincter of Oddi |
| SNM | sentinel (lymph) node mapping | | standing orders |
| | | | suboccipital |
| | serotoninergic neuroenteric modulators | | suggestive of |
| | | | superior oblique |
| | student nurse midwife | | supraoptic |
| SnMp | tin-mesoporphyrin | | supraorbital |
| SNOMED | Systematized Nomenclature of Medicine | | sutures out |
| | | | sympathetic ophthalmia |
| | | S/O | suggestive of |
| SNOMED CT | Systemized Nomenclature of Medicine, Clinical Terms | S-O | salpingo-oophorectomy |
| | | S&O | salpingo-oophorectomy |
| | | SO$_3$ | sulfite |
| | | SO$_4$ | sulfate |
| SNOMED RT | Systemized Nomenclature of | SOA | serum opsonic activity |
| | | | shortness of air |

S

|  |  |  |  |
|---|---|---|---|
|  | spinal opioid analgesia | SOH | sexually oriented |
|  | supraorbital artery |  | hallucinations |
|  | swelling of ankles | SoHx | social history |
| SOAA | signed out against advice | SOI | slipped on ice |
| SOAM | sutures out in the morning |  | sudden overwhelming |
| SOAMA | signed out against |  | infection |
|  | medical advice |  | surgical orthotopic |
| SOAP | subjective, objective, |  | implantation (implant) |
|  | assessment, and plans |  | syrup of ipecac |
| SOAPIE | subjective, objective, | SOL | solution |
|  | assessment, plan, |  | space occupying lesion |
|  | implementation, | SOL I | special observations level |
|  | (intervention), and |  | one (there are also SOL |
|  | evaluation |  | II and SOL III) |
| SOB | see order book | SOM | secretory otitis media |
|  | shortness of breath (this |  | serous otitis media |
|  | abbreviation has |  | somatization |
|  | caused problems) | SOMI | sterno-occipital |
|  | side of bed |  | mandibular immobilizer |
| SOBE | short of breath on | Sono | sonogram |
|  | exertion | SONP | solid organs not palpable |
| SOBOE | short of breath on | SOOL | spontaneous onset of |
|  | exertion |  | labor |
| SOC | see old chart | SOP | standard operating |
|  | socialization |  | procedure |
|  | stages of change | SOPM | sutures out in afternoon |
|  | standard of care |  | (or evening) |
|  | start of care | SOR | sign own release |
|  | state of consciousness | SOS | if there is need |
|  | system organ class |  | may be repeated once if |
| S & OC | signed and on chart (e.g. |  | urgently required |
|  | permit) |  | (Latin: *si opus sit*) |
| SOD | sinovenous occlusive |  | self-obtained smear |
|  | disease |  | suicidal observation status |
|  | sphincter of Oddi | SOSOB | sit on side of bed |
|  | dysfunction | SOT | solid organ transplant |
|  | superoxide dismutase |  | something other than |
|  | surgical officer of the day |  | stream of thought |
| SODA | Severity of Dyspepsia | SOTP | Sex Offender Treatment |
|  | Assessment |  | Provider |
| SODAS | spheriodal oral drug | SP | sacrum to pubis |
|  | absorption system |  | sequential pulse |
| SOE | source of embolism |  | serum protein |
| SOFA | sepsis-related organ |  | shoulder press |
|  | failure assessment |  | silent period (related to |
|  | Sequential Organ Failure |  | electromyographic |
|  | Assessment (score) |  | responses) |
| SOFAS | Social and Occupational |  | spastic dysphonia |
|  | Functioning Assessment |  | speech |
|  | Scale |  | Speech Pathologist |
| SOG | suggestive of good |  | spinal |
| SOGS | South Oaks Gambling |  | spouse |
|  | Screen |  | stand and pivot |

S

|  |  |  |  |
|---|---|---|---|
|  | stand pivot | SPCT | simultaneous prism and cover test |
|  | status post |  |  |
|  | *Streptococcus pneumoniae* | SPD | subcorneal pustular dermatosis |
|  | systolic pressure |  |  |
| sp | species |  | Supply, Processing, and Distribution (department) |
| S/P | status post |  |  |
|  | suprapubic |  |  |
| SP 1 | suicide precautions number 1 |  | suprapubic drainage |
|  |  | SPE | saw palmetto extract |
| SP 2 | suicide precautions number 2 |  | serum protein electrophoresis |
| SPA | albumin human (formerly known as salt-poor albumin) |  | solid-phase extraction |
|  |  |  | superficial punctate erosions |
|  | scintillation proximity assay | SPEB | streptococcal pyrogenic exotoxins B |
|  | serum prothrombin activity | SPEC | specimen |
|  |  |  | streptococcal pyrogenic exotoxins C |
|  | sheep pulmonary adenomatosis | Spec Ed | special education |
|  | single photon absorptiometry | SPECT | single-photon emission computed tomography |
|  | Speech Pathology and Audiology | SPEEP | spontaneous positive end-expiratory pressure |
|  | stimulation produced analgesia | SPEP | serum protein electrophoresis |
|  | student physician's assistant | SPET | single-photon emission tomography |
|  | subperiosteal abscess | SPF | semipermeable film |
|  | suprapubic aspiration |  | S-phase fraction |
| SpA | spondyloarthropathy |  | split products of fibrin |
| SP-A | surfactant-specific protein A |  | sun protective factor |
| SPAC | satisfactory postanesthesia course | sp fl | spinal fluid |
| SPAG | small-particle aerosol generator | SPG | scrotopenogram |
|  |  |  | sphenopalatine ganglion |
| SPAMM | spatial modulation of magnetization | SpG | specific gravity |
| SPBE | saw palmetto berry extract | SPH | severely and profoundly handicapped |
| SPBI | serum protein bound iodine |  | sighs per hour |
| SPBT | suprapubic bladder tap |  | spherocytes |
| SPC | saturated phosphatidylcholine | SPHERO | spherocytes |
|  | sclerosing pancreatocholangitis | SPI | speech processor interface |
|  |  |  | surgical peripheral iridectomy |
|  | statistical process control | SPIA | solid phase immunoabsorbent assay |
|  | Summary of Product Characteristics | SPIF | spontaneous peak inspiratory force |
|  | suprapubic catheter |  |  |
| SPCA | serum prothrombin conversion accelerator (factor VII) | SPIFE | serum protein and immunofixation electrophoresis (system) |

| | | | |
|---|---|---|---|
| S-PIN | Steinmann pin | SP-RIA | solid-phase radioimmunoassay |
| SPK | simultaneous pancreas-kidney (transplant) | SPROM | spontaneous premature rupture of membrane |
| | single parent keeping (baby) | SPS | shoulder pain and stiffness |
| | superficial punctate keratitis | | simple partial seizure |
| SPL | sound pressure level | | sodium polyethanol sulfonate |
| | superior parietal lobule | | sodium polystyrene sulfonate (Kayexalate; SPS®) |
| SPL® | Staphylococcal Phage Lysate | | status post surgery |
| SPLATTT | split anterior tibial tendon transfer | | systemic progressive sclerosis |
| SPM | scanning probe microscopy | SPT | second primary tumors |
| | second primary malignancy | | skin prick test |
| | | | standing pivot transfer |
| SPM96 | statistical parametric mapping 96 | | supportive periodontal therapy |
| SPMA | spinal progressive muscle atrophy | | suprapubic tenderness |
| | | SP TAP | spinal tap |
| SPMD | scapuloperoneal muscular dystrophy | SPTL | spontaneous preterm labor |
| SPMDs | semipermeable membrane devices | SPTs | second primary tumors |
| | | | single-patient trials |
| SPME | solid-phase microextraction | SP TUBE | suprapubic tube |
| SPMI | severely and persistently mentally ill | SPTX | static pelvic traction |
| | | SPU | short procedure unit |
| SPMSQ | Short Portable Mental Status Questionnaire | SPVR | systemic peripheral vascular resistance |
| SPN | solitary pulmonary nodule | SPX | smallpox vaccine, not otherwise specified |
| | student practical nurse | $SPX_v$ | smallpox vaccine (vaccinia virus) |
| SPNK | single parent not keeping (baby) | SQ | status quo |
| SPO | status postoperative | | subcutaneous (this is a dangerous abbreviation, use subcut) |
| $SpO_2$ | oxygen saturation by pulse oximeter | | |
| spont | spontaneous | Sq CCa | squamous cell carcinoma |
| SponVe | spontaneous ventilation | SQE | subcutaneous emphysema |
| SPP | Sexuality Preference Profile | SQM | square meter(s) |
| | single presentation phenotype | SQUID | superconducting quantum interference device |
| | species (specus) | SQV | saquinavir (Fortovose; Invirase) |
| | super packed platelets | SR | screen |
| | suprapubic prostatectomy | | sedimentation rate |
| SPQ | Schizotypal Personality Questionnaire | | see report |
| | | | senior resident |
| SPR | surface plasmon resonance | | service record |
| | | | side rails |
| SPRAS | Sheehan Patient Rated Anxiety Scale | | sinus rhythm |
| | | | slow release |

|  |  |  |  |
|---|---|---|---|
|  | smooth-rough | SRMs | specified risk materials |
|  | social recreation | SR/NE | sinus rhythm, no ectopy |
|  | stretch reflex | SRNV | subretinal |
|  | superior rectus |  | neovascularization |
|  | sustained release | SRNVM | subretinal neovascular |
|  | sustained response |  | membrane |
|  | suture removal | SRO | sagittal ramus osteotomy |
|  | system review |  | single room occupancy |
| S/R | strong/regular (pulse) |  | smallest region of overlap |
| S&R | seclusion and restraint |  | sustained-release oral |
|  | smooth and rough | SROA | sports-related |
| $^{89}$Sr | strontium 89 |  | osteoarthritis |
| SRA | serotonin release assay | SROCPI | Self-Rating Obsessive- |
|  | steroid-resistant asthma |  | Compulsive Personality |
| SRAN | surgical resident |  | Inventory |
|  | admission note | SROM | spontaneous rupture of |
| SRBC | sheep red blood cells |  | membrane |
|  | sickle red blood cells | SRP | scaling and root planing |
| SRBOW | spontaneous rupture of |  | (dental) |
|  | bag of waters |  | septorhinoplasty |
| SRC | sclerodermal renal crisis |  | stapes replacement |
| SRCC | sarcomatoid renal cell |  | prosthesis |
|  | carcinoma | SRR | surgical recovery room |
| SRCS | Division of Surveillance, | SRS | Silver-Russell syndrome |
|  | Research, and |  | somatostatin receptor |
|  | Communication |  | scintigraphy |
|  | Support (FDA) | $\overline{s}$RS | without redness or |
| SRD | service-related disability |  | swelling |
|  | smallest real difference | SRS-A | slow-reacting substance of |
|  | sodium-restricted diet |  | anaphylaxis |
| SRE | skeletal related event | SRSV | small round structured |
| SRF | somatotropin releasing |  | viruses |
|  | factor | SRT | sedimentation rate test |
|  | subretinal fluid |  | sleep-related tumescence |
| SRF-A | slow-releasing factor of |  | speech reception threshold |
|  | anaphylaxis |  | speech recognition |
| SRGVHD | steroid-resistant graft- |  | threshold |
|  | versus-host disease |  | surfactant replacement |
| SRH | signs of recent |  | therapy |
|  | hemorrhage |  | sustained release |
| SRI | serotonin reuptake |  | theophylline |
|  | inhibitor | SRU | side rails up |
| SRICU | surgical respiratory | SRUS | solitary rectal ulcer |
|  | intensive care unit |  | syndrome |
| SRIF | somatotropin-release | SRVC | subcutaneous reservoir |
|  | inhibiting factor |  | and ventricular |
|  | (somatostatin; Zecnil) |  | catheter |
| SRK | smooth-rod Kaneda | SR ↑ X2 | both siderails up |
|  | (implant) | SS | half |
| SRMD | stress-related mucosal |  | sacral sulcus |
|  | damage |  | sacrosciatic |
| SRMS | sustained-release |  | saline soak (sodium |
|  | morphine sulfate |  | chloride 0.9%) |

saline solution (0.9% sodium chloride)
saliva sample
salt sensitivity (sensitive)
salt substitute
serotonin syndrome
serum sickness
sickle cell
single-session (treatment)
single-strength (as compared to double-strength)
Sjögren syndrome
sliding scale
slip sent
Social Security
social service
somatostatin (Zecnil)
stainless steel
steady state
step stool
subaortic stenosis
susceptible
suprasciatic (notch)
symmetrical strength

**S/S** Saturday and Sunday
**SS#** Social Security number
**S & S** shower and shampoo
signs and symptoms
sitting and supine
sling and swathe
soft and smooth (prostate)
support and stimulation
swish and spit
swish and swallow
**SSA** sagittal split advancement
salicylsalicylic acid (salsalate)
Sjögren syndrome antigen A
Social Security Administration
Subjective Symptoms Assessment (profile)
sulfasalicylic acid (test)
**SSAs** standard sedative agents
**SSBP** sitting systolic blood pressure
**SSC** sign symptom complex
silver sulfadiazine and chlorhexidine
Similac® and special care

Special Services for Children
stainless steel crown
standard straight cane
**SSc** systemic sclerosis (scleroderma)
**SSCA** single shoulder contrast arthrography
**SSCP** single-stranded conformational polymorphism
substernal chest pain
**SSCr** stainless steel crown
**SSCU** surgical special care unit
**SSCVD** sterile spontaneous controlled vaginal delivery
**SSD** serosanguineous drainage
sickle cell disease
silver sulfadiazine
Social Security disability
source to skin distance
**SSDI** Social Security disability income
**ss DNA** single-stranded desoxyribonucleic acid
**SSE** saline solution enema (0.9% sodium chloride)
skin self-examination
soapsuds enema
subacute spongiform encephalopathy
systemic side effects
**SSEH** spontaneous spinal epidural hematoma
**SSEPs** somatosensory evoked potentials
**SSF** subscapular skinfold
**SSG** sodium stibogluconate
sublabial salivary gland
**SSI** sliding scale insulin
Social Skills Inventory
sub-shock insulin
superior sector iridectomy
Supplemental Security Income
surgical site infection
**SSKI** saturated solution of potassium iodide
**SSL** second stage of labor
subtotal supraglottic laryngectomy

S

| | |
|---|---|
| SSLF | sacrospinous ligament fixation |
| SSLR | seated straight leg raise |
| SSM | short stay medical |
| | skin-sparing mastectomy |
| | skin surface microscopy |
| | superficial spreading melanoma |
| SSN | severely subnormal |
| | Social Security number |
| SSO | second surgical opinion |
| | sequence-specific oligonucleotide |
| | short stay observation (unit) |
| | Spanish speaking only |
| SSOP | Second Surgical Opinion Program |
| | sequence-specific oligonucleotide probe |
| SSP | sequence-specific primer |
| | short stay procedure (unit) |
| | superior spermatic plexus |
| | supragingival scaling and prophylaxis (dental) |
| SSPA | staphylococcal-slime polysaccharide antigens |
| SSPE | subacute sclerosing panencephalitis |
| SSPG | steady-state plasma glucose |
| SSPL | saturation sound pressure level |
| SSPU | surgical short procedure unit |
| SSQ | Staring Speel Questionnaire |
| SSR | Sleep Self-Reporting |
| | substernal retractions |
| | sympathetic skin response |
| SSRFC | surrounding subretinal fluid cuff |
| SSRI | selective serotonin reuptake inhibitor |
| SSRP | subgingival scaling and root planing (dental) |
| SSRs | simple sequence repeats |
| SSS | layer upon layer |
| | scalded skin syndrome |
| | Scandinavian Stroke Scale |
| | Sepsis Severity Score |
| | Severity Scoring System (Dart Snakebite) |
| | short stay service (unit) |
| | sick sinus syndrome |
| | skin and skin structures |
| | Spanish-speaking sometimes |
| | sphincter-saving surgery |
| | sterile saline soak |
| SSSB | sagittal split setback |
| SSSDW | significant sharp, spike, or delta waves |
| SSSE | self-sustained status epilepticus |
| SSSIs | skin and skin structure infections |
| SSSS | staphylococcal scalded skin syndrome |
| SSSs | small short spikes (encephalography) |
| SST | sagittal sinus thrombosis |
| | somatostatin (Zecnil) |
| SSTI | skin and skin structure infections |
| SSU | short stay unit |
| SSX | sulfisoxazole acetyl |
| S/SX | signs/symptoms |
| ST | esotropic |
| | sacrum transverse |
| | Schiotz tonometry |
| | shock therapy |
| | sinus tachycardia |
| | skin tear |
| | skin test |
| | slight trace |
| | slow-twitch |
| | smokeless tobacco |
| | sore throat |
| | spasmodic torticollis |
| | speech therapist |
| | speech therapy |
| | sphincter tone |
| | split thickness |
| | spondee threshold |
| | station (obstetrics) |
| | stomach |
| | straight |
| | strength training |
| | stress testing |
| | stretcher |
| | subtotal |
| | Surgical Technologist |
| | survival time |
| | synapse time |

S

| | | | |
|---|---|---|---|
| S & T | sulfamethoxazole and trimethoprim (SMZ-TMP or SMX-TMP) | STD TF | standard tube feeding |
| STA | second trimester abortion | STE | ST-segment elevation |
| | staphylococcus vaccine, not otherwise specified | STEAM | stimulated-echo acquisition mode |
| | superficial temporal artery | STEC | shiga toxin-producing *Escherichia coli* |
| STA_aur | *Staphylococcus aureus* vaccine | STEM | scanning transmission electron microscopic |
| stab. | polymorphonuclear leukocytes (white blood cells, in nonmature form) | STEMI | ST-segment elevation myocardial infarction |
| | | Stereo | steropsis |
| STAI | State-Trait Anxiety Inventory | STEPS | The System for Thalidomide Educating and Prescribing Safety |
| STAI-I | State-Trait-Anxiety Index—I | STET | single photon emission tomography |
| STA-MCA | superficial temporary artery-middle cerebral artery (anastomosis; bypass) | | submaximal treadmill exercise test |
| | | STETH | stethoscope |
| STAPES | stapedectomy | STF | special tube feeding |
| staph | *Staphylococcus aureus* | | standard tube feeding |
| STA_SPL | staphylococcus vaccine, bacteriophage lysate | STG | short-term goals |
| | | | split-thickness graft |
| STAT | immediately | | superior temporal gyri |
| | signal transducers and activators of transcription | STH | soft tissue hemorrhage |
| | | | somatotrophic hormone |
| | | | subtotal hysterectomy |
| STATINS | HMG-CoA reductase inhibitors | | supplemental thyroid hormone |
| | | STHB | said to have been |
| STAXI | State-Trait Anger Expression Inventory | STI | sexually transmitted infection |
| STB | stillborn | | signal transduction inhibitor((s) |
| STBAL | standing balance | | soft tissue injury |
| ST BY | stand by | | structured treatment interruption(s) |
| STC | serum theophylline concentration | | sum total impression |
| | soft tissue calcification | | systolic time interval |
| | special treatment center | STI-571 | imatinib mesylate (Gleevec) |
| | stimulate to cry | STILLB | stillborn |
| | stroke treatment center | STIR | short TI (tau) inversion recovery |
| | subtotal colectomy | STIs | sexually transmitted infections |
| | sugar tongue cast | | |
| ST CLK | station clerk | | systolic time intervals |
| STD | sexually transmitted disease(s) | STJ | scapulothoracic joint |
| | | | subtalar joint |
| | short-term disability | STK | streptokinase |
| | skin test dose | STL | sent to laboratory |
| | skin to tumor distance | | serum theophylline level |
| | sodium tetradecyl sulfate | | |

S

| | | | |
|---|---|---|---|
| STLE | St. Louis encephalitis | Str Post | strictly posterior |
| STLI | subtotal lymphoid irradiation | MI | myocardial infarction |
| | | STS | serologic test for syphilis |
| STLOM | swelling, tenderness, and limitation of motion | | short-term survivors slide thin slab |
| STLV | simian T-lymphotrophic viruses | | sodium tetradecyl sulfate sodium thiosulfate |
| STM | scanning tunneling microscope | | soft tissue sarcoma soft tissue swelling |
| | short-term memory | | somatostatin (Zecnil) |
| | soft tissue mobilization | | staurosporine |
| | streptomycin | | Surgical Technology |
| | supra (significant) | | Student |
| | threshold shift | STSG | split thickness skin graft |
| | (audiology) | STSS | streptococcal-induced |
| STMT | Seat Movement | | toxic shock syndrome |
| STN | subtalar neutral | STS-SPT | simple two-step |
| | subthalamic nucleus | | swallowing |
| STNI | subtotal nodal irradiation | | provocation test |
| STNM | surgical evaluative staging of cancer | STT | scaphoid, trapezium trapezoid |
| STNR | symmetrical tonic neck | | serial thrombin time |
| | reflex | | skin temperature test |
| S to | sensitive to | | soft tissue tumor |
| STOP | sensitive, timely, and | STT#1 | Schirmer tear test one |
| | organized programs | STT#2 | Schirmer tear test two |
| | (battered spouses) | STTb | basal Schirmer tear test |
| STORCH | syphilis, toxoplasmosis, | STTOL | standing tolerance |
| | other agents, rubella, | STU | shock trauma unit |
| | cytomegalovirus, and | | surgical trauma unit |
| | herpes (maternal | STV | short-term variability |
| | infections) | STV+ | short-term variability- |
| STP | short-term plans | | present |
| | sodium thiopental | STV 0 | short-term variability- |
| | step training | | absent |
| | progression | STV inter | short-term variability- |
| STPD | standard temperature and | | intermittent |
| | pressure—dry | STX | stricture |
| STPI | State-Trait Personality | STZ | streptozocin (Zanosar) |
| | Inventory | SU | sensory urgency |
| STPS | Short-Term Performance | | Somogyi units |
| | Status | | stasis ulcer |
| STR | scotopic threshold | | stroke unit |
| | response | | sulfonylurea |
| | short tandem repeat | | supine |
| | sister | S/U | shoulder/umbilicus |
| | small tandem repeat | S&U | supine and upright |
| | stretcher | SUA | serum uric acid |
| Strab | strabismus | | single umbilical artery |
| strep | streptococcus | SUB | Skene urethra and |
| | streptomycin | | Bartholin glands |
| STRICU | shock/trauma/respiratory | Subcu | subcutaneous |
| | intensive care unit | SUBCUT | subcutaneous |

S

316

| | | | |
|---|---|---|---|
| Subepi M Inj | subepicardial myocardial injury | SUV | standard uptake variable |
| SUBL | sublingual | SUVs | standard uptake values |
| SUB-MAND | submandibular | SUX | succinylcholine |
| | | | suction |
| sub q | subcutaneous (this is a dangerous abbreviation since the q is mistaken for every, when a number follows) | SUZI | subzonal insertion |
| | | SV | seminal vesical |
| | | | severe |
| | | | sigmoid volvulus |
| | | | single ventricle |
| | | | single vessel |
| SUCC | succinylcholine | | snake venom |
| SUCT | suction | | stock volume |
| SUD | sudden unexpected death | | subclavian vein |
| | | Sv | sievert (radiation unit) |
| SuDBP | supine diastolic blood pressure | SV40 | simian virus 40 |
| | | SVA | small volume admixture |
| SUDEP | sudden unexpected (unexplained) death in epilepsy | SVAS | supravalvular aortic stenosis |
| SUDS | Subjective Unit of Distress (Disturbance) (Discomfort) Scale | SVB | saphenous vein bypass |
| | | SVBG | saphenous vein bypass graft |
| | sudden unexplained death syndrome | SVC | slow vital capacity |
| | | | subclavian vein compression |
| SUF | symptomatic uterine fibroids | | superior vena cava |
| SUI | stress urinary incontinence | SVCO | superior vena cava obstruction |
| | suicide | | |
| SUID | sudden unexplained infant death | SVC-RPA | superior vena cava and right pulmonary artery (shunt) |
| SULF-PRIM | sulfamethoxazole and trimethoprim | SVCS | superior vena cava syndrome |
| SUN | serum urea nitrogen | SVD | singular value decomposition (analysis) |
| SUNDS | sudden unexplained nocturnal death syndrome | | |
| | | SVD | single-vessel disease |
| SUO | syncope of unknown origin | | spontaneous vaginal delivery |
| SUP | stress ulcer prophylaxis | | structural valve deterioration (dysfunction) |
| | superior | | |
| | supination | | |
| | supinator | SVE | sterile vaginal examination |
| | symptomatic uterine prolapse | | |
| SUPAC | Scale-Up and Post Approval Change | | *Streptococcus viridans* endocarditis |
| supp | suppository | | subcortical vascular encephalopathy |
| SUR | suramin (Metaret) | SV&E | suicidal, violent, and eloper |
| | surgery | | |
| | surgical | SVG | saphenous vein graft |
| Surgi | Surgigator | SVH | subjective visual horizontal (test) |
| SUUD | sudden unexpected, unexplained death | | |

| | | | |
|---|---|---|---|
| SVI | seminal vesicle invasion | | abnormalities |
| | stroke volume index | SWO | superficial white |
| S VISC | serum viscosity | | onychomycosis |
| SVL | severe visual loss | SWOG | Southwest Oncology |
| SVN | small volume nebulizer | | Group |
| SVO | small vessel occlusion | SWOT | strengths, weaknesses, |
| SVO$_2$ | mixed venous oxygen | | opportunities, threats |
| | saturation | | (analysis) |
| SVP | spontaneous venous pulse | SWP | small whirlpool |
| SVPB | supraventricular | SWR | surface wrinkling |
| | premature beat | | retinopathy |
| SVPC | supraventricular premature | | surgical waiting room |
| | contraction | SWS | sheltered workshop |
| SV/PP | stroke volume/pulse | | slow wave sleep |
| | pressure | | social work service |
| SVR | supraventricular rhythm | | student ward secretary |
| | sustained virological | | Sturge-Weber syndrome |
| | response | SWT | stab wound of the throat |
| | systemic vascular | | shuttle-walk test |
| | resistance | SWU | septic work-up |
| SVRI | systemic vascular | SWW | static wall walk (aquatic |
| | resistance index | | therapy) |
| SVT | superficial vein | Sx | signs |
| | thrombosis | | surgery |
| | supraventricular | | symptom |
| | tachycardia | SXA | single-energy x-ray |
| | symptom validity | | absorptiometry |
| | test(s) | SXR | skull x-ray |
| SVVD | spontaneous vertex | SYN | synovial |
| | vaginal delivery | SYN Fl | synovial fluid |
| SW | sandwich | SYPH | syphilis |
| | sea water | SYR | syrup |
| | seriously wounded | SYS BP | systolic blood pressure |
| | shallow walk (aquatic | SZ | schizophrenic |
| | therapy) | | seizure |
| | short wave | | suction |
| | Social Worker | SZN | streptozocin (Zanosar) |
| | stab wound | | |
| | sterile water | | |
| | swallowing reflex | | |
| S&W | soap and water | | |
| S/W | somewhat | | |
| SWA | Social Work Associate | | |
| SWAP | short-wavelength | | |
| | automated perimetry | | |
| SWD | short wave diathermy | | |
| SWFI | sterile water for injection | | |
| SWG | standard wire gauge | | |
| SWI | sterile water for injection | | |
| | surgical wound infection | | |
| S&WI | skin and wound isolation | | |
| SWL | shock wave lithotripsy | | |
| SWMA | segmental wall-motion | | |

# T

T    inverted T wave
     tablespoon (15 mL)
        (this is a dangerous
        abbreviation)
     temperature
     tender
     tension
     tesla (unit of magnetic
        flux density in
        radiology)
     testicles
     testosterone
     thoracic
     thymine
     trace
     transcribed
t    teaspoon (5 mL) (this is
        a dangerous
        abbreviation)
T+   increase intraocular
        tension
T−   decreased intraocular
        tension
2,4,5-T   2,4,5-
        trichlorophenoxyacetic
        acid
T°   temperature
$T_{1/2}$   half-life
$T_1$   tricuspid first sound
$T_2$   tricuspid second sound
T-2   dactinomycin,
        doxorubicin,
        vincristine, and
        cyclophosphamide
$T_3$   triiodothyronine
        (liothyronine)
T3   transurethral thermo-
        ablation therapy
        (Targis)
     Tylenol with codeine 30
        mg (this is a dangerous
        abbreviation)
$T_{3/4}$ind   triiodothyronine to
        thyroxine index
$T_4$   levothyroxine
     thyroxine
T4   CD4 (helper-inducer
        cells)

T-7   free thyroxine factor
T-10   methotrexate, calcium
        leucovorin rescue,
        doxorubicin, cisplatin,
        bleomycin,
        cyclophosphamide,
        and dactinomycin
$T_1...T_{12}$   thoracic nerve 1
        through 12
     thoracic vertebra
        1 through 12
TA   Takayasu arteritis
     temperature axillary
     temporal arteritis
     tendon Achilles
     therapeutic abortion
     tracheal aspirate
     traffic accident
     tricuspid atresia
     truncus arteriosus
Ta   tonometry applanation
T&A   tonsillectomy and
        adenoidectomy
     tonsils and adenoids
T(A)   axillary temperature
TA1   thymosin alpha-1
TA-55   stapling device
TAA   Therapeutic Activities
        Aide
     thoracic aortic aneurysm
     total ankle arthroplasty
     transverse aortic arch
     triamcinolone acetonide
     tumor-associated antigen
        (antibodies)
TAAA   thoracoabdominal aortic
        aneursym
TAB   tablet
     therapeutic abortion
     total androgen blockade
     triple antibiotic
        (bacitracin, neomycin,
        and polymyxin—this is
        a dangerous
        abbreviation)
TAC   docetaxel (Taxotere),
        doxorubicin
        (Adriamycin), and
        cyclophosphamide
     tetracaine, Adrenalin®
        and cocaine
     total arterial compliance
     tibial artery catheter

| | | |
|---|---|---|
| | total abdominal colectomy | **TANI** total axial (lymph) node irradiation |
| | total allergen content | |
| | triamcinolone cream | **TAO** thromboangitis obliterans |
| **TACC** | thoracic aortic cross-clamping | troleandomycin |
| | | **TAP** tone and positioning |
| **TACE** | transarterial chemoembolization | tonometry by applanation |
| | | transabdominal preperitoneal (laparoscopic hernia repair) |
| **TACI** | total anterior cerebral infarct | |
| **TAD** | thoracic asphyxiant dystrophy | transesophageal atrial paced |
| | transverse abdominal diameter | trypsinogen activation peptide |
| **TADAC** | therapeutic abortion, dilation, aspiration, and curettage | tumor-activated prodrug |
| | | **TAPP** transabdominal preperitoneal polypropylene (mesh-plasty) |
| **TADC** | tumor-associated dendritic cells | |
| **TAE** | transcatheter arterial embolization | **T APPL** applanation tonometry |
| | | **TAPVC** total anomalous pulmonary venous connection |
| **TAF** | tissue angiogenesis factor | |
| **TAG** | triacylglycerol | **TAPVD** total anomalous pulmonary venous drainage |
| | tumor-associated glycoprotein | |
| **TA-GVHD** | transfusion-associated graft-versus-host disease | **TAPVR** total anomalous pulmonary venous return |
| **TAH** | total abdominal hysterectomy | **TAR** thrombocytopenia with absent radius |
| | total artificial heart | total ankle replacement |
| **TAHBSO** | total abdominal hysterectomy, bilateral salpingo-oophorectomy | total anorectal reconstruction |
| | | treatment administration record |
| **TAHL** | thick ascending limb of Henle loop | treatment authorization request |
| **T Air** | air puff tonometry | **TARA** total articular replacement arthroplasty |
| **TAL** | tendon Achilles lengthening | |
| | total arm length | **TART** tenderness, asymmetry, restricted motion, and tissue texture changes |
| **T ALCON** | Alcon® tonometry | |
| **TALP** | total alkaline phosphatase | tumorectomy and radiotherapy |
| **TAML** | therapy-related acute myelogenous leukemia | **TAS** therapeutic activities specialist |
| **t-AML** | therapy-related acute myeloid leukemia | Thrombolytic Assessment System |
| **TAM** | tamoxifen | turning against self |
| | teenage mother | typical absence seizures |
| | total active motion | **TAT** tandem autotransplants |
| | tumor-associated macrophages | tell a tale |
| **TAN** | treatment-as-needed | |
| | Treatment Authorization Number | |
| | tropical ataxic neuropathy | |

T

|  | tetanus antitoxin | | eastern encephalitis, Russian spring-summer e., Taiga e.) vaccine |
|  | thematic apperception test | | |
|  | thrombin-antithrombin III complex | T-berg | Trendelenburg (position) |
|  | 'til all taken | TBEV | tick-borne encephalitis virus |
|  | total adipose tissue | | |
|  | transactivator of transcription | TBE_w | tick-bone encephalitis, western subtype (Central European encephalitis) vaccine |
|  | transplant-associated thrombocytopenia | | |
|  | turnaround time | TBF | total-body fat |
|  | tyrosine aminotransferase | TBG | thyroxine-binding globulin |
| TAUC | target area under the curve | | |
|  | time-averaged urea concentration | TBI | toothbrushing instruction total-body irradiation traumatic brain injury |
| TAUSA | thrombolysis and angioplasty in unstable angina | T bili | total bilirubin |
|  | | TBK | total-body potassium |
| TAX | cefotaxime (Claforan) | tbl | tablespoon (15 mL) |
|  | paclitaxel (Taxol) | TBLB | transbronchial lung biopsy |
| TB | Tapes for the Blind | TBLC | term birth, living child |
|  | terrible burning | TBLF | term birth, living female |
|  | thought broadcasting | TBLI | term birth, living infant |
|  | toothbrush | TBLM | term birth, living male |
|  | total base | TBM | tracheobronchomalacia tuberculous meningitis tubule basement membrane |
|  | total bilirubin | | |
|  | total body | | |
|  | tuberculosis | | |
| TBA | to be absorbed | TBMg | total-body magnesium |
|  | to be added | TBN | total-body nitrogen |
|  | to be administered | TBNA | transbronchial needle aspiration treated but not admitted |
|  | to be admitted | | |
|  | to be announced | | |
|  | to be arranged | TBNa | total-body sodium |
|  | to be assessed | TBOCS | Tale-Brown Obsessive-Compulsive Scale |
|  | total body (surface) area | | |
| TBAGA | term birth appropriate for gestational age | TBP | thyroxine-binding protein toe blood pressure total-body phosphorus total-body protein tuberculous peritonitis |
| T-bar | tracheotomy bar (a device used in respiratory therapy) | | |
| TBARS | thiobarbituric acid reactive substances | TBPA | thyroxine-binding prealbumin |
| TBB | transbronchial biopsy | TBR | total-bed rest |
| TBC | to be cancelled total-blood cholesterol total-body clearance tuberculosis | TBS | tablespoon (15ml)(this is a dangerous abbreviation) The Bethesda System (reporting cervical and vagina cytology) total-serum bilirubin |
| TBD | to be determined | | |
| TBE | tick-borne encephalitis to be evaluated | | |
| TBE_e | tick-borne encephalitis, eastern subtype (Far | TBSA | total-body surface area total-burn surface area |

T

| | | | |
|---|---|---|---|
| tbsp | tablespoon (15 mL) | | tumor chemosensitivity assay |
| TBT | tolbutamide test | | tumor clonogenic assays |
| | tracheal bronchial toilet | TCABG | triple coronary artery bypass graft |
| | transbronchoscopic balloon tipped | TCAD | transplant-related coronary-artery disease |
| TBV | thiotepa, bleomycin, and vinblastine | | tricyclic antidepressant |
| | total-blood volume | TCAR | tiazofurin |
| | transluminal balloon valvuloplasty | TCB | to call back |
| | | | tumor cell burden |
| TBW | total-body water | TCBS agar | thiosulfate-citrate-bile salt-sucrose agar |
| TBZ | thiabendazole (Mintezol) | TCC | transitional cell carcinoma |
| TC | paclitaxel (Taxol) and cisplatin | $TcCO_2$ | transcutaneous carbon dioxide |
| | team conference | TCD | transcerebellar diameter |
| | telephone call | | transcranial Doppler (ultrasonography) |
| | terminal cancer | | |
| | testicular cancer | | transverse cardiac diameter |
| | thioguanine and cytarabine | TCCB | transitional cell carcinoma of bladder |
| | thoracic circumference | | |
| | throat culture | TC/CL | ticarcillin-clavulanate (Timentin) |
| | tissue culture | | |
| | tolonium chloride | TCD | transcystic duct |
| | tonic-clonic | TCDB | turn, cough, and deep breath |
| | tonsillar coblation | | |
| | total cholesterol | TCDD | tetrachlorodibenzo-p-dioxin (dioxin) |
| | total communication | | |
| | to (the) chest | $^{99m}Tc$ DTPA | technetium Tc 99m pentetate |
| | tracheal collar | | |
| | trauma center | TCE | tetrachloroethylene |
| | true conjugate | | total-colon examination |
| | tubocurarine | | transcatheter embolotherapy |
| Tc | technetium | | |
| T/C | telephone call | T cell | small lymphocyte |
| | ticarcillin-clavulanic acid (Timentin) | TCES | transcranial electrical stimulation |
| | to consider | $^{99m}TcGHA$ | technetium Tc 99m gluceptate |
| 3TC | lamivudine (Epivir) | | |
| TC7 | Interceed® | TCH | turn, cough, hyperventilate |
| T&C | turn and cough | | |
| | type and crossmatch | $^{99m}Tc$-HAS | technetium Tc 99m-labeled human serum albumin |
| T&C#3 | Tylenol with 30 mg codeine | | |
| TCA | thioguanine and cytarabine | TCHRs | traditional Chinese herbal remedies |
| | | TCI | target-control infusion |
| | tissue concentrations of antibiotic(s) | | to come in |
| | | TCID | tissue culture infective dose |
| | trichloroacetic acid | | |
| | tricuspid atresia | TCIE | transient cerebral |
| | tricyclic antidepressant | | |

|  |  |  |  |
|---|---|---|---|
|  | ischemic episode | TCU | transitional care unit |
| TCL | tibial collateral ligament | TCVA | thromboembolic cerebral |
|  | transverse carpal |  | vascular accident |
|  | ligament | TD | Takayasu disease |
| TCM | tissue culture media |  | tardive dyskinesia |
|  | traditional Chinese |  | temporary disability |
|  | medicine |  | terminal device |
|  | transcutaneous (oxygen) |  | test dose |
|  | monitor |  | tetanus-diphtheria toxoids |
| $^{99m}$Tc-MAA | technetium Tc 99m albumin microaggregated |  | (pediatric use) |
|  |  |  | tidal volume |
|  |  |  | tolerance dose |
| TCMH | tumor-direct cell-mediated |  | tone decay |
|  | hypersensitivity |  | total disability |
| TCMS | transcranial cortical |  | transverse diameter |
|  | magnetic stimulation |  | travelers' diarrhea |
| TCMZ | trichlormethiazide |  | treatment discontinued |
| TCN | tetracycline | Td | tetanus-diphtheria toxoids |
|  | triciribine phosphate |  | (adult type) |
|  | (tricyclic nucleoside) | TDAC | tumor-derived activated |
| TCNS | transcutaneous nerve |  | cell (cultures) |
|  | stimulator | TDD | telephone device for the |
| TCNU | tauromustine |  | deaf |
| TcO$_2$ | transcutaneous oxygen |  | thoracic duct drainage |
|  | pressure |  | total daily dose |
| TcO$_4^-$ | pertechnetate | TDE | total daily energy |
| TCOM | transcutaneous oxygen |  | (requirement) |
|  | monitor | TDF | tenofovir disoproxil |
| T Con | temporary conservatorship |  | fumarate (Virend) |
| TCP | thrombocytopenia |  | testis determining factor |
|  | transcutaneous pacing |  | total-dietary fiber |
|  | tranylcypromine (Parnate) |  | tumor dose fractionation |
|  | tumor control probability | TDI | tolerable daily intake |
| TCPC | total cavopulmonary |  | toluene diisocyanate |
|  | connection | TDK | tardive diskinesia |
| TcPCO$_2$ | transcutaneous carbon | TDL | thoracic duct lymph |
|  | dioxide | TDLN | tumor-draining lymph |
| TcPO$_2$ | transcutaneous oxygen |  | nodes |
| $^{99m}$TcPYP | technetium Tc 99m | TDM | therapeutic drug |
|  | pyrophosphate |  | monitoring |
| TCR | T-cell receptor | TDMAC | tridodecylmethyl |
| TCRE | transcervical resection of |  | ammonium chloride |
|  | the endometrium | TDN | totally digestible nutrients |
| TCS | tonic-clonic seizure |  | transdermal nitroglycerin |
| $^{99m}$TcSC | technetium Tc 99m sulfur | TDNTG | transdermal nitroglycerin |
|  | colloid | TDNWB | touchdown |
| TCT | thyrocalcitonin |  | nonweightbearing |
|  | tincture | TdP | torsades de pointes |
|  | transcatheter therapy | TDPDS | temporomandibular |
|  | triple combination tablet |  | disorder pain |
|  | (abacavir, lamivudine, |  | dysfunction syndrome |
|  | and zidovudine) | TDPWB | touchdown partial |
|  | (Trizivir) |  | weight-bearing |

T

| | | | |
|---|---|---|---|
| TdR | thymidine | TeBG | testeosterone binding globulin |
| TDS | traveler's diarrhea syndrome | TeBIDA | technetium 99m trimethyl 1-bromo-imono diacetic acid |
| *TDS* | three times a day (United Kingdom) | | |
| TDT | tentative discharge tomorrow | TEC | thromboembolic complication |
| | transmission disequilibrium test | | total eosinophil count |
| | | | toxic *Escherichia coli* |
| | Trieger Dot Test | | transient erythroblastopenia of childhood |
| | tumor doubling time | | |
| TdT | terminal deoxynucleotidyl transferase | | transluminal extraction-endarterectomy catheter |
| TDW | target dry weight | | |
| TDWB | touch down weight bearing | | triethyl citrate |
| TDx® | fluorescence polarization immunoassay | T&EC | trauma and emergency center |
| TE | echo time | TECA | titrated extract of *Centella asiatica* |
| | tennis elbow | | |
| | terminal extension | TECAB | totally endoscopic (off-pump) coronary artery bypass grafting |
| | tooth extraction | | |
| | toxoplasmic encephalitis | | |
| | trace elements (chromium, copper, iodine, manganese, selenium, molybdenum and zinc) | TED | thromboembolic disease |
| | | | thyroid eye disease |
| | | TEDS | thromboembolic disease stockings |
| | | | transesophageal echo-Doppler system |
| | tracheoesophageal | | |
| | transesophageal echocardiography | | Treatment Episode Data Set |
| | transrectal electroejaculation | TEE | total energy expended |
| *t*E | total expiratory time | | transnasal endoscopic ethmoidectomy |
| T/E | testosterone to epitestosterone ratio | | transesophageal echocardiography |
| T&E | testing and evaluation | TEF | tracheoesophageal fistula |
| | training and evaluation | TEG | thromboelastogram (thromboelastography) |
| | trial and error | | |
| TEA | thromboendarterectomy | TEH | theophylline, ephedrine, and hydroxyzine |
| | Time and Extent Application (FDA) | | |
| | total elbow arthroplasty | TEI | therapeutic equivalence interchange |
| | transluminal extraction atherectomy | | total episode of illness |
| | | | transesophageal imaging |
| TEAE | treatment-emergent adverse event | TEL | telemetry |
| | | | telephone |
| TEAP | transesophageal atrial pacing | tele | telemetry |
| | | TEM | temozolomide (Temodar) |
| TEB | thoracic electrical bioimpedance | | transanal endoscopic microsurgery |
| TEBG | testosterone-estradiol binding globulin | | transmission electron microscopy |

| | | | |
|---|---|---|---|
| TEMI | transient episodes of myocardial ischemia | TET | transcranial electrostimulation therapy |
| TEMP | temperature | | treadmill exercise test |
| | temporal | TETE | too early to evaluate |
| | temporary | TETig | tetanus immune globulin |
| TEN | tension (intraocular pressure) | TEU | token economy unit |
| | | TEV | talipes equinovarus (deformity) |
| | toxic epidermal necrolysis | | |
| TEN® | Total Enteral Nutrition | TEVAP | transurethral electrovaporization of the prostate |
| TENS | transcutaneous electrical nerve stimulation | | |
| TEOAE | transient evoked otoacoustic emission (test) | TF | tactile fremitus |
| | | | tail flick (reflex) |
| | | | tetralogy of Fallot |
| TEP | total endoprosthesis | | tibiofemoral |
| | total extraperitoneal (laparoscopic hernia repair) | | to follow |
| | | | tube feeding |
| | | TFA | topical fluoride application |
| | tracheoesophageal puncture | | trans fatty acids |
| | | | trifluoroacetic acid |
| | tubal ectopic pregnancy | TFB | trifascicular block |
| TEQ | toxic equivalents | TFBC | The Family Birthing Center |
| TER | terlipressin | | |
| | total elbow replacement | TFC | thoracic fluid content |
| | total energy requirement | | time to following commands |
| | transurethral electroresection | | |
| TERB | terbutaline | TFCC | triangular fibrocartilage complex |
| TERC | Test of Early Reading Comprehension | | |
| | | TFF | tangential flow filtration |
| TERM | full-term | TF-Fe | transferrin-bound iron |
| | terminal | TFL | tensor fasciae latae |
| TERT | human telomerase reverse transcriptase (also hTRT) | | trimetrexate, fluorouracil, and leucovorin |
| | | TFM | transverse friction massage |
| | tertiary | | |
| | total end-range time | TFO | triplex-forming oligonucleotide |
| TES | therapeutic electrical stimulation | | |
| | | TFOs | triplex-forming oligonucleotides |
| | thoracic endometriosis syndrome | | |
| | | TFPI | tissue-factor pathway inhibitor |
| | thoracic endoscopic sympathectomy | | |
| | | TFR | total fertility rate |
| | treatment emergent symptoms | TFT | thumb-finding test |
| | | | trifluridine (trifluorothymidine) |
| TESE | testicular sperm extraction | | |
| TESI | thoracic epidural steroid injection | TFTs | thyroid function tests |
| TESS | Toronto Extremity Salvage Score | TG | total gym |
| | | | triglycerides |
| | Treatment Emergent Symptom Scale | Tg | thyroglobulin |
| | | 6-TG | thioguanine |

T

325

| | | | |
|---|---|---|---|
| TGA | Therapeutic Goods Administration (Australia) | THBI | thyroid hormone binding index |
| | third-generation antidepressant | THBR | thyroid hormone-binding ratio |
| | transient global amnesia | THAM® | tromethamine |
| | transposition of the great arteries | THBO₂ | topical hyperbaric oxygen |
| TGAR | total graft area rejected | THC | tetrahydrocannabinol (dronabinol) |
| TGB | tiagabine (Gabatril) | | thigh circumference |
| TGCT | testicular germ cell tumor(s) | | transhepatic cholangiogram |
| TGD | thyroglossal duct | THCT | triple-phase helical computer tomography |
| | tumor growth delay | TH-CULT | throat culture |
| TGE | transmissible gastroenteritis | tHcy | total homocysteine |
| TGFA | triglyceride fatty acid | THE | total-head excursion |
| TGF | transforming growth factor | | transhepatic embolization |
| | | Ther Ex | therapeutic exercise |
| TGF-β | transforming growth factor-beta | THF | thymic humoral factor |
| | | THI | transient hypogamma-globinemia of infancy |
| TGGE | temperature-gradient gel electrophoresis | THKAFO | trunk-hip-knee-ankle-foot orthosis |
| TGR | tenderness, guarding, and rigidity | THL | transvaginal hydrolaparoscopy |
| TGS | tincture of green soap | THLAA | tubular hypoplasia left aortic arch |
| TGs | triglycerides | | |
| TGT | thromboplastin generation test | THP | take home packs |
| | | | total hip prosthesis |
| TGTL | total glottic transverse laryngectomy | | transhepatic portography |
| | | | trihexyphenidyl (Artane) |
| TGV | thoracic gas volume | THR | target heart rate |
| | transposition of great vessels | | thrombin receptor |
| | | | total hip replacement |
| TGXT | thallium-graded exercise test | | training heart rate |
| | | THRL | total hip replacement, left |
| TGZ | troglitazone (Rezulin) | | |
| TH | thrill | THRR | total hip replacement, right |
| | thyroid hormone | | |
| | total hysterectomy | THS | Tolosa-Hunt syndrome |
| T&H | type and hold | THTV | therapeutic home trial visit |
| THA | tacrine (tetrahydroacridine; Cognex) | THV | therapeutic home visit |
| | | TI | terminal ileus |
| | total hip arthroplasty | | thought insertion |
| | transient hemispheric attack | | time following inversion pulse (radiology) |
| THAA | thyroid hormone autoantibodies | | transischial |
| | tubular hypoplasia aortic arch | | transverse diameter of inlet |
| | | | tricuspid incompetence |
| THAL | thalassemia | | tricuspid insufficiency |
| | thalidomide (Thalomid) | TIA | transient ischemic attack |

| | | | |
|---|---|---|---|
| TIB | tibia | TIPSS | transjugular intrahepatic portosystemic shunt (stent) |
| TIBC | total iron-binding capacity | | |
| TIC | paclitaxel (Taxol), ifosfamide, and cisplain | TIRFM | total-internal reflection microscopy |
| | trypsin-inhibitor capacity | TIS | tumor *in situ* |
| TICOSMO | trauma, infection, chemical/drug exposure, organ systems, stress, musculoskeletal, and other (prompts used during history taking for possible etiologies of problems) | TISS | Therapeutic Intervention Scoring System |
| | | TIT | *Treponema* (*pallidum*) immobilization test |
| | | | triiodothyronine (liothyronine) |
| | | TIUP | term intrauterine pregnancy |
| TICS | diverticulosis | TIVA | total intravenous anethesia |
| TICU | thoracic intensive care unit | TIVC | thoracic inferior vena cava |
| | transplant intensive care unit | +tive | positive |
| | | TIW | three times a week (this is a dangerous abbreviation) |
| | trauma intensive care unit | | |
| *t.i.d.* | three times a day | | |
| TIDM | three times daily with meals | TJ | tendon jerk |
| | | | triceps jerk |
| TIE | transient ischemic episode | TJA | total joint arthroplasty |
| TIF | tracheal intubation fiberscope | TJC | tender joint count |
| | | TJN | tongue jaw neck (dissection) |
| TIG | tetanus immune globulin | | |
| TIH | tumor-inducing hypercalcemia | | twin-jet nebulizer |
| | | TJR | total joint replacement |
| TIL | tumor-infiltrating lymphocytes | TK | thymidine kinase |
| | | | toxicokinetics |
| %tile | percentile | TKA | total knee arthroplasty |
| TIMI | Thrombolysis in Myocardial Infarction (studies) | | tyrosine kinase activity |
| | | TKD | tokodynamometer |
| | | TKE | terminal knee extension |
| TIMP | tissue inhibitor of metalloproteinase | TKIC | true knot in cord |
| | | TKNO | to keep needle open |
| TIN | three times a night (this is a dangerous abbreviation) | TKP | thermokeratoplasty |
| | | | total knee prosthesis |
| | | TKO | to keep open |
| | tubulointerstitial nephritis | TKR | total knee replacement |
| tinct | tincture | TKRL | total knee replacement, left |
| TIND | Treatment Investigational New Drug (application) | TKRR | total knee replacement, right |
| TINEM | there is no evidence of malignancy | TKVO | to keep vein open |
| TIP | toxic interstitial pneumonitis | TL | team leader |
| | | | thoracolumbar |
| | tubularized incised plate (urethroplasty) | | total laryngectomy |
| | | | transverse line |
| TIPS | transjugular intrahepatic portosystemic shunt (stent-shunt) | | trial leave |
| | | | tubal ligation |
| | | T/L | terminal latency |

**327**

| Tl | thallium | TMA | thrombotic microangiopathy |
| TLA | translumbar arteriogram (aortogram) | | trained medication aid |
| | transverse ligament of atlas | | transcription mediated amplification |
| TLAC | triple lumen Arrow catheter | | transmetatarsal amputation |
| | | | trimethylamine |
| TL BLT | tubal ligation, bilateral | T/MA | tracheostomy mask |
| TLC | tender loving care | TMAS | Taylor Manifest Anxiety Scale |
| | therapeutic lifestyle changes | TMA-uria | trimethylaminuria |
| | thin layer chromatography | $T_{max}$ | temperature maximum |
| | titanium linear cutter | $t_{max}$ | time of occurrence for maximum (peak) drug concentration |
| | T-lymphocyte choriocarcinoma | | |
| | total lung capacity | TMB | tetramethylberizidine |
| | total lymphocyte count | | transient monocular blindness |
| | triple lumen catheter | | trimethoxybenzoates |
| TLD | thermoluminescent dosimeter | TMC | transmural colitis |
| | | | triamcinolone |
| TLE | temporal lobe epilepsy | TMCA | trimethylcolchicinic acid |
| TLFB | timeline follow back (interview) | | |
| TLI | total lymphoid irradiation | TMCN | triamcinolone |
| | translaryngeal intubation | TMD | temporomandibular dysfunction (disorder) |
| TLK | thermal laser keratoplasty | | treating physician |
| TLM | torn lateral meniscus | | |
| TLNB | term living newborn | t-MDS | therapy-related myelodysplastic syndrome |
| TLOA | temporary leave of absence | | |
| TLP | transitional living program | TME | thermolysin-like metalloendopeptidase |
| TLR | target lesion reintervention | | |
| | tonic labyrinthine reflex | | total mesorectal excision |
| TLS | tumor lysis syndrome | TMET | treadmill exercise test |
| TLSO | thoracic lumbar sacral orthosis | TMEV | Theiler murine encephalomyelitis virus |
| TLSSO | thoracolumbosacral spinal orthosis | TMH | trainable mentally handicapped |
| TLT | tonsillectomy | TMI | threatened myocardial infarction |
| TLV | threshold limit value | | |
| | total lung volume | | transmandibular implant |
| TM | temperature by mouth | | transmural infarct |
| | thalassemia major | T>MIC | time above minimum inhibitory concentration |
| | Thayer-Martin (culture) | | |
| | Tibetan Medicine | TMJ | temporomandibular joint |
| | trabecular meshwork | TMJD | temporomandibular joint dysfunction |
| | trademark (unregistered) | | |
| | transcendental meditation | TMJS | temporomandibular joint syndrome |
| | treadmill | | |
| | tropical medicine | TML | tongue midline |
| | tumor | | treadmill |
| | tympanic membrane | TMLR | transmyocardial laser revascularization |
| T & M | type and crossmatch | | |

| | | | |
|---|---|---|---|
| TMM | torn medial meniscus | TND | term, normal delivery |
| | total muscle mass | TNDM | transient neonatal diabetes |
| Tmm | McKay-Marg tension | | mellitus |
| TMNG | toxic multinodular goiter | TNF | tumor necrosis factor |
| TMO | transcaruncular medial | TNF-bp | tumor necrosis factor |
| | orbitotomy | | binding protein |
| TMP | thallium myocardial | TNG | nitroglycerin |
| | perfusion | | toxic nodular goiter |
| | transmembrane pressure | TNI | total nodal irradiation |
| | trimethoprim | TnI | troponin I |
| TMP/SMZ | trimethoprim and | TNKase® | tenecteplase |
| | sulfamethoxazole | TNM | primary tumor, regional |
| | (correct name is | | lymph nodes, and |
| | sulfamethoxazole and | | distant metastasis (used |
| | trimethoprin; SMZ- | | with subscripts for the |
| | TMP) | | staging of cancer) |
| TMR | trainable mentally | t-NNT | threshold number needed |
| | retarded | | to treat |
| | transmyocardial | TNR | tonic neck reflex |
| | revascularization | TNS | transcutaneous nerve |
| TMS | transcranial magnetic | | stimulation (stimulator) |
| | stimulation | | transient neurologic |
| TMSI | Task Management | | symptoms |
| | Strategy Index | | Tullie-Niebörg syndrome |
| TMST | treadmill stress test | TNT | thiotepa, mitoxantrone |
| TMT | tarsometatarsal | | (Novantrone), and |
| | teratoma with malignant | | paclitaxel (Taxol) |
| | transformation | | triamcinolone and |
| | treadmill test | | nystatin |
| | tympanic membrane | TnT | troponin T |
| | thermometer | TNTC | too numerous to count |
| TMTC | too many to count | TNU | tobacco nonuser |
| TMTX | trimetrexate (Neutrexin) | TNY | trichomonas and yeast |
| TMUGS | Tumor Marker Utility | TO | old tuberculin |
| | Grading Scale | | telephone order |
| TMX | tamoxifen | | time off |
| TMZ | temazepam (Restoril) | | tincture of opium |
| | temozolomide (Temodar) | | (warning: this is NOT |
| TN | normal intraocular tension | | paregoric) |
| | team nursing | | total obstruction |
| | temperature normal | | transfer out |
| | trigeminal neuralgia | T(O) | oral temperature |
| T&N | tension and nervousness | T/O | time out |
| | tingling and numbness | T&O | tubes and ovaries |
| TNA | total nutrient admixture | TOA | time of arrival |
| TNAB | transthoracic needle biopsy | | tubo-ovarian abscess |
| TNB | term newborn | TOAA | to affected areas |
| | transnasal butorphanol | TOB | tobacco |
| | transrectal needle biopsy | | tobramycin |
| | (of the prostate) | TOC | table of contents |
| | Tru-Cut® needle biopsy | | test-of-cure (post-therapy |
| TNBP | transurethral needle | | visit) |
| | biopsy of prostate | | total organic carbon |

**T**

| | | | |
|---|---|---|---|
| TOCE | transcatheter oily chemoembolization | TORP | total ossicular replacement prosthesis |
| TOCO | tocodynamometer | TOS | intraocular pressure of the left eye |
| TOD | intraocular pressure of the right eye | | thoracic outlet syndrome |
| | target organ damage | TOT BILI | total bilirubin |
| | target-organ disease | TOTM | trioctyltrimellitate |
| | time of death | TOV | trial of void |
| | time of departure | TOWL | Test of Written Language |
| | tubal occlusion device | TOX | toxoplasmosis |
| TOF | tetralogy of Fallot | | *(Toxoplasma gondii)* |
| | time of flight (radiology) | | vaccine |
| | total of four | TOXO | toxoplasmosis |
| | train-of-four | TP | temperature and pressure |
| TOFMS | time-of-flight mass spectrometry | | temporoparietal |
| | | | tender point |
| TOGV | transposition of the great vessels | | therapeutic pass |
| | | | ThinPrep Pap (test) |
| TOH | throughout hospitalization | | thought process |
| TOI | Trial Outcome Index | | thrombophlebitis |
| TOL | tolerate | | thymidine phosphorylase |
| | trial of labor | | time to progression |
| TOLD | Test of Language Development | | Todd paralysis |
| | | | toe pressure |
| TOM | therapeutic outcomes monitoring | | toilet paper |
| | | | total protein |
| | tomorrow | | "T" piece |
| | transcutaneous oxygen monitor | | treating physician |
| | | | trigger point |
| Tomo | tomography | T:P | trough-to-peak ratio |
| TON | tonight | T & P | temperature and pulse |
| TOP | termination of pregnancy | | turn and position |
| | Topografov (virus) | TPA | alteplase, recombinant (tissue plasminogen activator) (Activase) |
| | topotecan (Hycamtin) | | |
| TOP-8 | Treatment Outcome PTSD (post-traumatic stress disorder) (scale) | | temporary portacaval anastomosis |
| | | | third-party administrator |
| TOPO | topotecan (Hycamtin) | | tissue polypeptide antigen |
| TOPO 1 | topoisermerase | | |
| TOPS | Take Off Pounds Sensibly | | total parenteral alimentation |
| TOPV | trivalent oral polio vaccine | TPAL | term infant(s), premature infant(s), abortion(s), living children |
| TOR | toremifene (Faneston) | | |
| TORC | Test of Reading Comprehension | TPC | target plasma concentration |
| TORCH | toxoplasmosis, others (other viruses known to attack the fetus), rubella, cytomegalovirus, and herpes simplex (maternal viral infections) | | total patient care |
| | | TPD | tropical pancreatic diabetes |
| | | | typhoid vaccine, not otherwise specified |

| | | | |
|---|---|---|---|
| TPD<sub>a</sub> | typhoid vaccine, attenuated live (oral Ty21a strain) | TPPV | trans pars plana vitrectomy |
| TPD<sub>AKD</sub> | typhoid vaccine, acetone-killed and dried (U.S. military) | TPR | temperature temperature, pulse, and respiration total peripheral resistance |
| TPD<sub>HP</sub> | typhoid vaccine, heat and phenol inactivated, dried | TPRI | total peripheral resistance index |
| TPD<sub>VI</sub> | typhoid vaccine, *Vi* capsular polysaccharide | T PROT TPS | total protein tender point score typhus (*rickettsiae* sp.) vaccine |
| TPE | therapeutic plasma exchange total placental estrogens total protective environment | TPT | time to peak tension topotecan (Hycamtin) transpyloric tube treadmill performance test |
| T-penia | thrombocytopenia | | |
| TPF | trained participating father | *t*PTEF | time to peak tidal expiratory flow |
| TPH | thromboembolic pulmonary hypertension | TPU | tropical phagedenic ulcer |
| | trained participating husband | T-putty TPVA | Theraputty tibioperoneal vessel angioplasty |
| TPHA | *Treponema pallidum* hemagglutination | TPVR | total peripheral vascular resistance |
| T PHOS | triple phosphate crystals | | |
| TPI | *Treponema pallidum* immobilization triose phosphate isomerase | TPZ TQM TR | tirapazamine total quality management therapeutic recreation time to repeat |
| TPIT | trigger point injection therapy | | time to repetition (radiology) |
| t<sub>pk</sub> | time to peak | | tincture |
| TPL | thromboplastin | | to return |
| T plasty | tympanoplasty | | trace |
| TPLSM | two-photon laser-scanning microscope | | transfusion reaction transplant recipients |
| TPM | temporary pacemaker topiramate (Topamax) | | treatment tremor |
| TPMT | thiopurine methyltransferase | | tricuspid regurgitation tumor registry |
| TPN | total parenteral nutrition | T(R) | rectal temperature |
| TPO | thrombopoietin thyroid peroxidase trial prescription order | T & R | tenderness and rebound treated and released turn and reposition |
| TPP | thiamine pyrophosphate | TRA | therapeutic recreation associate |
| TpP | thrombus precursor protein | | to run at |
| TP & P | time, place, and person | | tumor regression antigen |
| TPPN | total peripheral parenteral nutrition | TRAb | thyrotropin-receptor antibody |
| TPPS | Toddler-Preschooler Postoperative Pain Scale | TRAC TRACH | traction tracheal tracheostomy |

| | | | |
|---|---|---|---|
| TRAFO | tone-reducing ankle/foot orthosis | TRH | protirelin (thyrotropin-releasing hormone) (Relefact TRH®; Thypinone®) |
| TRAIL | tumor-necrosis-factor-related apoptosis-inducing ligand | | |
| TRALI | transfusion-associated lung injury | TRI | transient radicular irritation |
| TRAM | transverse rectus abdominis myocutaneous (flap) | T₃RIA | trimester |
| | | $T_3RIA$ | triiodothyronine level by radioimmunoassay |
| | transverse rectus abdominum muscle | TRIAC | triiodothyroacetic acid |
| | Treatment Response Assessment Method | TRIC | trachoma inclusion conjunctivitis |
| TRAMP | transversus and rectus abdominis musculo-peritoneal (flap) | TRICH | *Trichomonas* |
| | | TRICKS | time-resolved imaging contrast kinetics |
| TRANCE | tumor necrosis factor–related activation-induced cytokine | TRIG | triglycerides |
| | | TRISS | Trauma Related Injury Severity Score |
| | | TR-LSC | time-resolved liquid scintillation counting |
| TRANS | transfers | TRM | transplant-related mortality |
| Trans D | transverse diameter | | treatment-related mortality |
| TRANS Rx | transfusion reaction | TRM-SMX | trimethoprim-sulfamethoxazole (correct name is sulfamethoxazole and trimethoprim; SMZ-TMP; SMX-TMP) |
| TRAP | tartrate-resistant (leukocyte) acid phophatase | | |
| | Telomeric Repeat Amplification Protocol | | |
| | thrombospondin-related anonymous protein | tRNA | transfer ribonucleic acid |
| | | TRNBP | transrectal needle biopsy prostate |
| | total radical-trapping antioxidant parameter | TRND | Trendelenburg (position) |
| | trapezium | TRNG | tetracycline-resistant *Neisseria gonorrhoeae* |
| | trapezius muscle | | |
| TRAS | transplant renal artery stenosis | TRO | to return to office |
| | | TROFO | trofosfamide |
| TRB | return to baseline | TROM | torque range of motion |
| TRBC | total red blood cells | | total range of motion |
| TRC | tanned red cells | TRP | tubular reabsorption of phosphate |
| TRD | tongue-retaining device | | |
| | total-retinal detachment | TRP-1 | tyrosine-related protein-1 |
| | traction retinal detachment | TrPs | trigger points |
| | | TRPT | transplant |
| | treatment-related death | TRS | Therapeutic Recreation Specialist |
| | treatment-resistant depression | | the real symptom |
| TRDN | transient respiratory distress of the newborn | TRT | tangential radiation therapy |
| | | | thermoradiotherapy |
| TREC | T-cell receptor-rearrangement excision circles | | thoracic radiation therapy |
| Tren | Trendelenburg | | treatment-related toxicity |

| | | | |
|---|---|---|---|
| TR/TE | time to repetition and time to echo in spin (echo sequence of magnetic resonance imaging) | TSB | total serum bilirubin trypticase soy broth |
| T₃RU | triiodothyronine resin uptake | TSBB | transtracheal selective bronchial brushing |
| TRUS | transrectal ultrasonography | TSC | technetium sulfur colloid theophylline serum concentration total symptom complex tuberous sclerosis complex |
| TRUSP | transrectal ultrasonography of the prostate | | |
| TRUST | toluidine red unheated serum test | T-score | number of standard deviations from the average bone mineral density (BMD) of a 25-30 year old woman |
| TRZ | triazolam (Halcion) | | |
| TS | Tay-Sachs (disease) telomerase temperature sensitive test solution thoracic spine throat swab thymidylate synthase toe signs Tourette syndrome transsexual Trauma Score tricuspid stenosis triple strength tuberous sclerosis Turner syndrome | TSD | target to skin distance Tay-Sachs disease total sleep deprivation T-(tumor) stage downstaging |
| | | TSDP | tapered steroid dosing package |
| | | TSE | targeted systemic exposure testicular self-examination total skin examination transmissible spongiform encephalopathy |
| | | TSEBT | total skin electron beam therapy |
| T/S | trimethoprim/ sulfamethoxazole (correct name is sulfamethoxazole and trimethoprin) | T set | tracheotomy set |
| | | TSF | tricep skin fold (thickness) |
| | | TSGs | tumor suppressor genes |
| T&S | type and screen | TSH | thyroid-stimulating hormone |
| Ts | Schiotz tension T suppressor cell | TSH-RH | thyrotropin-releasing hormone |
| TSAb | thyroid stimulating antibodies | TSI | thyroid stimulating immunoglobulin tobramycin solution for inhalation (TOBI®) |
| TSA | toluenesulfonic acid total shoulder arthroplasty tryptone soya (blood) agar tumor-specific antigen type-specific antibody tyramine signal amplification | | |
| | | TSIs | thymidylate synthase inhibitors |
| | | T-SKULL | trauma skull |
| | | tsp | teaspoon (5 mL) |
| | | TSP | thrombospondin total serum protein tropical spastic paraparesis |
| TSAR® | tape surrounded Appli-rulers | | |
| TSAS | Total Severity Assessment Score | TSPA | thiotepa |
| | | T-SPINE | thoracic spine |
| TSAT | transferrin saturation | TSR | total shoulder replacement |

**T**

| | | | |
|---|---|---|---|
| TSS | total serum solids | TTE | transthoracic echocardiography |
| | toxic shock syndrome | | |
| | tumor score system | *t* test | Student's *t*-test |
| TSST | toxic shock syndrome toxin | TTF | time-to-treatment failure |
| | | TTGE | timed-temperature gradient electrophoresis |
| TST | titmus stereocuity test | | |
| | trans-scrotal testosterone | | |
| | treadmill stress test | TTI | Teflon tube insertion |
| | tuberculin skin test(s) | | total time to intubate |
| TSTA | tumor-specific transplantation antigens | | transfer to intermediate |
| | | TTII | thyrotropin-binding inhibitory immunoglobulins |
| TSTM | too small to measure | | |
| TT | testicular torsion | | |
| | Test Tape® | TTJV | transtracheal jet ventilation |
| | tetanus toxoid | | |
| | thiotepa (Thioplex) | TTM | total tumor mass |
| | thoracostomy tube | | transtelephonic monitoring |
| | thrombin time | | trichotillomania |
| | thrombolytic therapy | TTN | time to normalization |
| | thymol turbidity | | transient tachypnea of the newborn |
| | tilt table | | |
| | tonometry | TTNA | transthoracic needle aspiration |
| | total thyroidectomy | | |
| | transit time | TTNB | transient tachypnea of the newborn |
| | transtracheal | | |
| | tuberculin tested | TTND | time to nondetectable |
| | twitch tension | TTO | tea tree oil |
| | tympanic temperature | | time trade-off |
| T-T | time-to-time | | to take out |
| T/T | trace of ____/ trace of ____ | | transfer to open |
| | | | transtracheal oxygen |
| T&T | tobramycin and ticarcillin | TTOD | tetanus toxoid outdated |
| | | TTOT | transtracheal oxygen therapy |
| | touch and tone | | |
| | tympantomy and tube (insertion) | TTP | tender to palpation |
| | | | tender to pressure |
| TT4 | total thyroxine | | thrombotic thrombocytopenic purpura |
| TTA | total toe arthroplasty | | |
| | transtracheal aspiration | | time to pregnancy |
| TTAT | toe touch as tolerated | | time to tumor progression |
| TTC | transtracheal catheter | | |
| TTD | tarsal tunnel decompression | | time-to-progression |
| | | TTR | time in therapeutic range |
| | temporary total disability | | transthyretin |
| | total tumor dose | | triceps tendon reflex |
| | transverse thoracic diameter | TTS | tarsal tunnel syndrome |
| | | | temporary threshold shift |
| TTDE | transthoracic color Doppler echocardiography | | through the skin |
| | | | transdermal therapeutic system |
| TTDM | thallim threadmill | | |
| TTDP | time-to-disease progression | | transfusion therapy service |

**334**

| | | | |
|---|---|---|---|
| TTT | tilt-table test | TUR | transurethral resection |
| | tolbutamide tolerance test | T₃UR | triiodothyronine uptake ratio |
| | total tourniquet time | | |
| | transpupillary thermotherapy | TURB | transurethral resection of the bladder |
| | turn-to-turn transfusion | | turbidity |
| TTTS | twin-twin transfusion syndrome | TURBN | transurethral resection bladder neck |
| TTUTD | tetanus toxoid up-to-date | TURBT | transurethral resection bladder tumor |
| TTV | total tumor volume | | |
| | transfusion-transmitted virus | TURP | transurethral resection of prostate |
| TTVP | temporary transvenous pacemaker | TURV | transurethral resection valves |
| TTWB | touch-toe weight bearing | TURVN | transurethral resection of vesical neck |
| TTx | thrombolytic therapy | TUTL | transuterine tubal lavage |
| TU | Todd units | TUU | transureteroureterostomy |
| | transrectal ultrasound | TUV | transurethral valve |
| | transurethral | TUVP | transurethral vaporization of the prostate |
| | tuberculin units | | |
| | tumor | TV | television |
| 1-TU | 1 tuberculin unit | | temporary visit |
| 5-TU | 5 tuberculin units | | tidal volume |
| 250-TU | 250 tuberculin units | | tonic vergence |
| TUB | tuberculosis vaccine, not BCG | | transvenous |
| | | | trial visit |
| TUE | transurethral extraction | | *Trichomonas vaginalis* |
| TUF | total ultrafiltration | | tricuspid value |
| TUG | total urinary gonadotropin | | touch-verbal |
| TUIBN | transurethral incision of bladder neck | T/V | |
| | | TVC | triple voiding cystogram |
| TUIP | transurethral incision of the prostate | | true vocal cord |
| | | TVc | tricuspid valve closure |
| TUL | tularemia (*Francisella tularensis*) vaccine | TVD | triple vessel disease |
| | | TVDALV | triple vessel disease with an abnormal left ventricle |
| TULIP® | transurethral ultrasound-guided laser-induced prostatectomy (system) | | |
| | | TVF | tactile vocal fremitus |
| TULIPS | touch-up and loop incorporated primers (an alternative PCR technique) | | true vocal fold |
| | | TVH | total vaginal hysterectomy |
| | | TVI | time velocity integral |
| | | TVN | tonic vibration response |
| TUMT | transurethral microwave thermotherapy | TVP | tensor veli palatini (muscle) |
| | | | transvenous pacemaker |
| TUN | total urinary nitrogen | | transvesicle prostatectomy |
| TUNA | transurethral needle ablation | TVR | tricuspid valve replacement |
| TUNEL | terminal deoxynucleotidyl transferase-mediated dUTP-biotin nick-end labeling | | |
| | | TVRSS | total vasomotor rhinitis symptom score |
| | | TVS | transvaginal sonography |
| TUPR | transurethral prostatic resection | | transvenous system |
| | | | trigemino-vascular system |

T

335

| | | | |
|---|---|---|---|
| TVSC | transvaginal sector scan | | transfuse |
| TVT | transvaginal taping | | transplant |
| | transvaginal tension-free | | transplantation |
| TVU | total volume of urine | | treatment |
| | transvaginal | | tympanostomy |
| | ultrasonography | T & X | type and crossmatch |
| TVUS | transvaginal | TXA$_2$ | thromboxane A$_2$ |
| | ultrasonography | TXB$_2$ | thromboxane B$_2$ |
| TW | talked with | TXE | Timoptic-XE® |
| | tapwater | TXL | paclitaxel (Taxol) (this is |
| | test weight | | a dangerous |
| | thought withdrawal | | abbreviation as it can |
| | *Trophermyma whippleii* | | be read as TXT) |
| TW2 | Tanner-Whitehouse mark | TXM | type and crossmatch |
| | 2 (bone-age assessment) | TXS | type and screen |
| 5TW | five times a week (this is | TXT | docetaxel (Taxotere) (this |
| | a dangerous | | is a dangerous |
| | abbreviation) | | abbreviation as it can |
| TWA | time-weighted average | | be read as TXL) |
| | total wrist arthroplasty | T & Y | trichomonas and yeast |
| | T-wave alternans | TYCO #3 | Tylenol with 30 mg of |
| TWAR | *Chlamydia pneumoniae* | | codeine (#1=7.5 mg, |
| T-wave | part of the | | #2=15 mg and #4=60 |
| | electrocardiographic | | mg of codeine present) |
| | cycle, representing a | Tyl | Tylenol (acetaminophen) |
| | portion of ventricular | | tyloma (callus) |
| | repolarization | TYMP | tympanogram |
| TWB | total weight bearing | TYR | tyrosine |
| TWD | total white and | TZ | temozolomide (Temodar) |
| | differential count | | transition zone |
| TWE | tapwater enema | TZD | thiazolidinedione |
| TWETC | tapwater enema 'til | TZDs | thiazolidinediones |
| | clear | TZM | temozolomide (Temodar) |
| TWG | total weight gain | | |
| TWH | transitional wall | | |
| | hyperplasia | | |
| TWHW ok | toe walking and heel | | |
| | walking all right | | |
| TWI | T-wave inversion | | |
| TWiST | time without symptoms | | |
| | of progression or | | |
| | toxicity | | |
| TWR | total wrist replacement | | |
| TWSTRS | Toronto Western | | |
| | Spasmodic Torticollis | | |
| | Rating Scale | | |
| T1WT | T1 weighted image | | |
| TWWD | tap water wet dressing | | |
| Tx | therapist | | |
| | therapy | | |
| | traction | | |
| | transcription | | |

# U

| | |
|---|---|
| U | Ultralente Insulin® |
| | units (this is the most dangerous abbreviation—spell out "unit") |
| | unknown |
| | upper |
| | urine |
| Ⓤ | Kosher |
| U/1 | 1 finger breadth below umbilicus |
| 1/U | 1 finger over umbilicus |
| U/ | at umbilicus |
| 24U | 24-hour urine (collection) |
| U100 | 100 units per milliliters |
| UA | umbilical artery |
| | unauthorized absence |
| | uncertain about |
| | unstable angina |
| | upper airway |
| | upper arm |
| | uric acid |
| | urinalysis |
| UABD | upper airway bronchodilation |
| UAC | umbilical artery catheter |
| | under active |
| | upper airway congestion |
| UA/C | uric acid to creatinine (ratio) |
| UAD | upper airway disease |
| UADT | upper aerodigestive tract |
| UAE | urinary albumin excretion |
| | uterine artery embolization |
| UACEs | unplanned acute care encounters |
| UAER | urinary albumin excretion rate |
| UAL | umbilical artery line |
| | up *ad lib* |
| UA&M | urinalysis and microscopy |
| UA/ NSTEMI | unstable angina and non-ST-segment elevation myocardial infarction |
| UAO | upper airway obstruction |
| UAP | upper abdominal pain |
| UAPD | Union of American Physicians and Dentists |

| | |
|---|---|
| UAPF | upon arrival patient found |
| UAPs | unlicensed assistive personnel |
| U-ARM | upper arm |
| UARS | upper airway resistance syndrome |
| UAS | upstream activating sequence |
| UASA | upper airway sleep apnea |
| UAT | up as tolerated |
| UAVC | univentricular atrioventricular connection |
| UBC | University of British Columbia (brace) |
| UBD | universal blood donor |
| UBE | upper body ergometer |
| UBF | unknown black female |
| | uterine blood flow |
| UBI | ultraviolet blood irradiation |
| UBM | ultrasound biomicroscopy |
| | unknown black male |
| UBO | unidentified bright object |
| UBT | $^{13}$C-urea breath test |
| | uterine balloon therapy |
| UBW | usual body weight |
| UC | ulcerative colitis |
| | umbilical cord |
| | unchanged |
| | unconscious |
| | Unit clerk |
| | United Church of Christ |
| | urea clearance |
| | urinary catheter |
| | urine culture |
| | usual care |
| | uterine contraction |
| U&C | urethral and cervical |
| | usual and customary |
| UCAD | unstable coronary artery disease |
| UCB | umbilical cord blood |
| | unconjugated bilirubin (indirect) |
| | Unicorn Campbell Boy (orthotics) |
| UCBT | unrelated cord-blood transplant |
| UCD | urine collection device |
| | usual childhood diseases |
| UCE | urea cycle enzymopathy |

U

| | | | |
|---|---|---|---|
| UCG | urinary chorionic gonadotropins | UDS | unconditioned stimulus |
| | | | urine drug screen |
| UCHD | usual childhood diseases | UDT | undescended testicle(s) |
| UCHI | usual childhood illnesses | UE | under elbow |
| UCHS | uncontrolled hemorrhagic shock | | undetermined etiology |
| | | | upper extremity |
| UCI | urethral catheter in | U & E | urea and electrolytes (see page 362) |
| | usual childhood illnesses | | |
| UCL | uncomfortable loudness level | UEC | uterine endometrial carcinoma |
| UCLP | unilateral cleft lip and palate | UEDs | unilateral epileptiform discharges |
| UCN | urocortin | UES | undifferentiated embryonal sarcoma |
| UCN-01 | 7-hydroxystaurosporin | | upper esophageal sphincter |
| UCO | urethral catheter out | | |
| UCP | umbilical cord prolapse | UESEP | upper extremity somatosensory evoked potential |
| | urethral closure pressure | | |
| UCPs | urine collection pads | | |
| UCR | unconditioned reflex | UESP | upper esophageal sphincter pressure |
| | unconditioned response | | |
| | usual, customary, and reasonable (fees) | UF | ultrafiltration |
| | | | until finished |
| UCP-3 | uncoupling protein $-3$ | UFC | urinary free cortisol |
| UCRE | urine creatinine | UFF | unusual facial features |
| UCRP | universal coagulation reference plasma | UFFI | urea formaldehyde foam insulation |
| UCS | unconscious | UFH | unfractionated heparin |
| UC&S | urine culture and sensitivity | UFN | until further notice |
| UCTD | undifferentiated connective tissue disease | UFO | unflagged order |
| | | | unidentified foreign object |
| UCVA | uncorrected visual acuity | UFOV | useful field of view |
| | | UFR | ultrafiltration rate |
| UCX | urine culture | UFT | uracil and tegafur |
| UD | as directed | UFV | ultrafiltration volume |
| | ulnar deviation | UG | until gone |
| | urethral dilatation | | urinary glucose |
| | urethral discharge | | urogenital |
| | urodynamics | UGA | under general anesthesia |
| | uterine distension | | urogenital atrophy |
| u.d. | as directed | UGCR | ultrasound-guided compression repair |
| UDC | uninhibited detrusor (muscle) capacity | | |
| | usual diseases of childhood | UGDP | University Group Diabetes Project |
| UDCA | ursodeoxycholic acid | UGH | uveitis, glaucoma, and hyphema (syndrome) |
| UDN | updraft nebulizer | | |
| UDO | undetermined origin | UGI | upper gastrointestinal series |
| UDP | unassisted diastolic pressure | UGIB | upper gastrointestinal bleeding |
| UDPGT | uridinediphospho-glucuronyl transferase | UGIH | upper gastrointestinal hemorrhage |

U

| | | | |
|---|---|---|---|
| UGIS | upper gastrointestinal series | | upper limb |
| | | | upper lobe |
| UGIT | upper gastrointestinal tract | U/L | upper and lower |
| | | U & L | upper and lower |
| UGI w/SBFT | upper gastrointestinal (series) with small bowel follow through | ULBW | ultra low birth weight (between 501 and 750 g) |
| UGK | urine, glucose, and ketones | ULDT | ultra low-dose therapy |
| | | ULLE | upper lid, left eye |
| UGP | urinary gonadotropin peptide | ULN | upper limits of normal |
| | | ULPA | ultra-low particulate air |
| UGVA | ultrasound-guided vascular access | ULQ | upper left quadrant |
| | | ULRE | upper lid, right eye |
| UH | umbilical hernia unfavorable history University Hospital | ULSB | upper left sternal border |
| | | ULTT1 | upper limb tension test 1 (median nerve) |
| UHBI | upper hemibody irradiation | ULTT2a | upper limb tension test 2a (medial nerve) |
| UHDDS | Uniform Hospital Discharge Data Set | ULTT2b | upper limb tension test 2b (radial nerve) |
| UHDRS | Unified Huntington Disease Rating Scale | ULTT3 | upper limb tension test 3 (ulnar nerve) |
| | | ULYTES | electrolytes, urine |
| UHDs | ulcer-healing drugs | UM | unmarried utilization management |
| UHMWPE | ultra-high molecular weight polyethylene | Umb A Line | umbilical artery line |
| UHP | University Health Plan | | |
| UI | urinary incontinence | Umb V Line | umbilical venous line |
| UIB | Unemployment Insurance Benefits | umb ven | umbilical vein |
| UIBC | unbound iron binding capacity | UMCD | uremic medullary cystic disease |
| | unsaturated iron binding capacity | UMLS | Unified Medical Language System |
| UID | once daily (this is a dangerous abbreviation, spell out "once daily") | UMN | upper motor neuron (disease) |
| | | UN | undernourished urinary nitrogen |
| UIEP | urine (urinary) immunoelectrophoresis | UNA | urinary nitrogen appearance |
| UIP | usual interstitial pneumonitis (pneumonia) | UNa | urine sodium |
| | | unacc | unaccompanied |
| UIQ | upper inner quadrant | UNC | uncrossed |
| UJ | universal joint (syndrome) | UNDEL | undelivered |
| UK | United Kingdom unknown | UNDP | United Nations Development Program |
| | urine potassium | UNG | ointment |
| | urokinase | UNHS | universal newborn hearing screening |
| UK IC | urokinase intracoronary | UNK | unknown |
| UKO | unknown origin | UNL | upper normal levels |
| UL | Unit Leader upper left upper lid | UNOS | United Network for Organ Sharing |

| | | | |
|---|---|---|---|
| UN/P | unpatched eye | URA | unilateral renal agenesis |
| UN/P OD | unpatched right eye | | |
| UN/P OS | unpatched left eye | URAC | Utilization Review Accreditation Commission |
| UNS | unsatisfactory | | |
| UNSAT | unsatisfactory | | |
| UO | under observation | UR AC | uric acid |
| | undetermined origin | URAS | unilateral renal artery stenosis |
| | ureteral orifice | | |
| | urinary output | URD | undifferentiated respiratory disease |
| UONx | unilateral optic nerve transection | | |
| | | | unrelated donor |
| UOP | urinary output | URE | Uniform Rules of Evidence |
| UOQ | upper outer quadrant | | |
| Uosm | urinary osmolality | URG | urgent |
| ✓ up | check up | URI | upper respiratory infection |
| UP | unipolar | URIC A | uric acid |
| | ureteropelvic | url | unrelated |
| U/P | urine to plasma (creatinine) | UR&M | urinalysis, routine and microscopic |
| UPC | unknown primary carcinoma | URO | urology |
| | | UROB | urobilinogen |
| UPD | uniparental disomy | UROD | ultra-rapid opiate detoxification [under anesthesia] |
| UPDRS | Unified Parkinson Disease Rating Scale | | |
| UPEP | urine protein electrophoresis | UROL | Urologist |
| | | | urology |
| UPG | uroporphyrinogen | URQ | upper right quadrant |
| UPIN | unique physician (provided) identification number | URR | urea reduction ratio |
| | | URS | ureterorenoscopy |
| | | URSB | upper right sternal border |
| UPJ | ureteropelvic junction | | |
| UPLIF | unilateral posterior lumbar interbody fusion | URT | upper respiratory tract |
| | | | uterine resting tone |
| UPN | unique patient number | URTI | upper respiratory tract infection |
| UPO | metastatic carcinoma of unknown primary origin | | |
| | | US | ultrasonography |
| | | | unit secretary |
| UPOR | usual place of residence | | United States of America |
| UPP | urethral pressure profile | USA | unit services assistant |
| UPPP | uvulopalatopharyngo-plasty | | United States Army |
| | | | United States of America |
| U/P ratio | urine to plasma ratio | | unstable angina |
| UPS | ubiquitin-proteasome system | USAF | United States Air Force |
| | | USAN | United States Adopted Names |
| UPSC | uterine papillary serous carcinoma | | |
| | | USAP | unstable angina pectoris |
| UPT | uptake | | |
| | urine pregnancy test | USB | upper sternal border |
| UR | unrelated | U-SCOPE | ureteroscopy |
| | upper respiratory | USCVD | unsterile controlled vaginal delivery |
| | upper right | | |
| | urinary retention | USDA | United States Department of Agriculture |
| | utilization review | | |

| | | |
|---|---|---|
| USED-CARP | **u**reterosigmoidostomy, **s**mall bowel fistula, **e**xtra chloride, **d**iarrhea, **c**arbonic anhydrase inhibitors, **a**drenal insufficiency, **r**enal tubular acidosis, and **p**ancreatic fistula (common causes of nonanion gap metabolic acidosis) | |

UTR — untranslated region
UTS — ulnar tunnel syndrome — ultrasound
U/U− — uterine fundus at umbilicus (usually modified as number of finger breadths below)
U/U+ — uterine fundus at umbilicus (usually modified as number of finger breadths above)

USG — ultrasonography
USH — United Services for Handicapped — usual state of health
USI — urinary stress incontinence
USM — ultrasonic mist
USMC — United States Marine Corps
USN — ultrasonic nebulizer — United States Navy
USO — unilateral salpingo-oophorectomy
USOGH — usual state of good health
USOH — usual state of health
USP — unassisted systolic pressure — United States Pharmacopeia
USPHS — United States Public Health Service
USUCVD — unsterile uncontrolled vaginal delivery
USVMD — urine specimen volume measuring device
UT — upper thoracic
UTA — urinary tract anomaly
UTD — unable to determine — up to date
*ut dict* — as directed
UTF — usual throat flora
UTI — urinary tract infection
UTL — unable to locate
UTM — urinary-tract malformations
UTMDACC — University of Texas M.D. Anderson Cancer Center
UTO — unable to obtain — upper tibial osteotomy
UTP — uridine triphosphate

UUD — uncontrolled unsterile delivery
UUN — urinary urea nitrogen
UUTI — uncomplicated urinary tract infections
UV — ultraviolet — ureterovesical — urine volume
UVA — ultraviolet A light — ureterovesical angle
UVB — ultraviolet B light
UVC — umbilical vein catheter — ultraviolet C light
UVEB — unifocal ventricular ectopic beat
UVH — univentricular heart
UVJ — ureterovesical junction
UVL — ultraviolet light — umbilical venous line
UVR — ultraviolet radiation
UVT — unsustained ventricular tachycardia
U/WB — unit of whole blood
UW — unilateral weakness
UWF — unknown white female
UWM — unknown white male — unwed mother

U

# V

| | | | |
|---|---|---|---|
| | | | vincristine, dactinomycin (actinomycin D), and cyclophosphamide |
| | | | vincristine, doxorubicin (Adriamycin), and cyclophosphamide |
| V | five | | |
| | gas volume | VA cc | distance visual acuity with correction |
| | minute volume | | |
| | vaccinated | VA ccl | near visual acuity with correction |
| | vagina | | |
| | vein | VACE | *Vitex agnus-castus* extract (Chaste tree berry extract) |
| | ventricular | | |
| | verb | | |
| | verbal | VAC EXT | vacuum extractor |
| | vertebral | $VAC_{ig}$ | vaccinia immune globulin |
| | very | VACO | Veterans Administration Central Office |
| | Viagra (sildenafil citrate) as in "vitamin V" | | |
| | viral | VACTERL | vertebral, **a**nal, **c**ardiac, **t**racheal, **e**sophageal, **r**enal, and **l**imb anomalies |
| | vision | | |
| | vitamin | | |
| | vomiting | VAD | vascular (venous) access device |
| $\dot{V}$ | ventilation (L/min) | | |
| +V | positive vertical divergence | | ventricular assist device |
| V1 | fifth cranial nerve, ophthalmic division | | vertebral artery dissection |
| | | | Veterans Administration Domiciliary |
| V2 | fifth cranial nerve, maxillary division | | vincristine, doxorubicin (Adriamycin), and dexamethasone |
| V3 | fifth cranial nerve, mandibular division | | |
| $V_1$ to $V_6$ | precordial chest leads | VaD | vascular dementia |
| VA | vacuum aspiration | VADCS | ventricular atrial distal coronary sinus |
| | valproic acid | | |
| | ventriculoatrial | VADRIAC | vincristine, doxorubicin (Adriamycin), and cyclophosphamide |
| | vertebral artery | | |
| | Veterans Administration | | |
| | visual acuity | VAERS | Vaccine Adverse Events Reporting System |
| $V_A$ | alveolar gas volume | | |
| V&A | vagotomy and antrectomy | VAFD | vascular access flush device |
| VAAESS | Vaccine-Associated Adverse Events Surveillance System (Canada) | | |
| | | VAG | vagina |
| | | VAG HYST | vaginal hysterectomy |
| VAB | variable atrial blockage | VAH | Veterans Administration Hospital |
| | vinblastine, dactinomycin (actinomycin D), bleomycin | | |
| | | VAHBE | ventricular atrial His bundle electrocardio-gram |
| VABS | Vineland Adaptive Behavior Scales | | |
| | | VAHRA | ventricular atrial height right atrium |
| VAC | vacuum-assisted closure (dressings) | | |
| | | VAI | vertebral artery injury |
| | ventriculoarterial conduction | VAIN | vaginal intraepithelial neoplasia |

| VALE | visual acuity, left eye |
| VAMC | Veterans Affairs Medical Center |
| VAMP® | venous-arterial management protection system |
| VAMS | Visual Analogue Mood Scale |
| VANCO/P | vancomycin-peak |
| VANCO/T | vancomycin-trough |
| VAOD | visual acuity, right eye |
| VAOS | visual acuity, left eye |
| VA OS LP with P | visual acuity, left eye, left perception with projection |
| VAP | venous access port |
| | ventilator-associated pneumonia |
| | vincristine, asparaginase, and prednisone |
| VAPCS | ventricular atrial proximal coronary sinus |
| VAPP | vaccine-associated paralytic poliomyelitis |
| VAR | variant |
| | varicella (chickenpox) (*varicella zoster* virus) vaccine |
| VARE | visual acuity, right eye |
| VARig | varicella-zoster immune globulin |
| VAS | vasectomy |
| | vascular |
| | Visual Analogue Scale (Score) |
| VASC | Visual-Auditory Screen Test for Children |
| VA sc | distance visual acuity without correction |
| VA scl | near visual acuity without correction |
| VASPI | Visual Analogue Self Assessment Scales For Pain Intensity |
| VAS RAD | vascular radiology |
| VAT | ventilatory anaerobic threshold |
| | vertebral artery test |
| | video-assist thoracoscopy |
| | visceral adipose tissue |
| VATER | vertebral, anal, tracheal, esophageal, and renal anomalies |

| VATH | vinblastine, doxorubicin (Adriamycin), thiotepa, and fluoxymesterone (Halotestin) |
| VATS | video assisted thoracic surgery |
| VAX-D | vertebral axial decompression |
| VB | Van Buren (catheter) |
| | venous blood |
| | vinblastine |
| | vinblastine and bleomycin |
| | virtual bronchoscopy |
| VB$_1$ | first voided bladder specimen |
| VB$_2$ | second midstream bladder specimen |
| VB$_3$ | third voided urine specimen |
| VBAC | vaginal birth after cesarean |
| VBAI | vertebrobasilar artery insufficiency |
| VBAP | vincristine, carmustine (BiCNU), doxorubicin (Adriamycin), and prednisone |
| VBC | vinblastine, bleomycin, and cisplatin |
| VBG | venous blood gas |
| | vertical banded gastroplasty |
| VBGP | vertical banded gastroplasty |
| VBI | vertebrobasilar insufficiency |
| VBL | vinblastine |
| VBM | vinblastine, bleomycin, and methotrexate |
| VBP | vinblastine, bleomycin, and cisplatin |
| VBR | ventricular brain ratio |
| VBS | vertebral-basilar system |
| | videofluoroscopic barium swallow (evaluation) |
| VC | color vision |
| | etoposide (VePesid) and carboplatin |
| | pulmonary capillary blood volume |
| | vena cava |
| | verbal cues |

V

|  |  |  |  |
|---|---|---|---|
|  | vincristine | VDC | vincristine, doxorubicin, |
|  | vital capacity |  | and cyclophosphamide |
|  | vocal cords | VDD | atrial synchronous |
| V&C | vertical and centric (a bite) |  | ventricular inhibited |
| VCA | vasoconstrictor assay |  | pacing |
| VCAM | vascular cell adhesion | VDDR I | vitamin D dependency |
|  | molecule |  | rickets type I |
| VCAP | vincristine, cyclophospha- | VDDR II | vitamin D dependency |
|  | mide, doxorubicin |  | rickets type II |
|  | (Adriamycin), and | VDE | vasodilatory edema |
|  | prednisone | VDEPT | virus-directed enzyme |
| Vcc | vision with correction |  | prodrug therapy |
| VCCA | velocity common carotid | VDG | venereal disease– |
|  | artery |  | gonorrhea |
| VCD | vocal cord dysfunction | Vdg | voiding |
| VCDR | vertical cup-to-disk ratio | VDH | valvular disease of the |
| VCE | vaginal cervical |  | heart |
|  | endocervical (smear) | VDJ | variable diversity joining |
| VCF | Vaginal Contraception | VDL | vasodepressor lipid |
|  | Film™ |  | visual detection level |
| VCFS | velo-cardio-facial | VDO | varus derotational |
|  | syndrome |  | osteotomy |
| VCG | vectorcardiography | VD or M | venous distention or |
|  | voiding cystogram |  | masses |
| vCJD | variant Creutzfeldt-Jakob | VDP | vinblastine, dacarbazine, |
|  | disease |  | and cisplatin |
| VCO | ventilator CPAP oxyhood |  | (Platinol AQ) |
| Vco$_2$ | carbon dioxide output | VDPCA | variable-dose patient- |
| VCR | video cassette recorder |  | controlled analgesia |
|  | vincristine sulfate | VDR | vitamin D receptor (gene) |
| VCT | venous clotting time | VDRF | ventilator dependent |
|  | voluntary counselling and |  | respiratory failure |
|  | testing | VDRL | Venereal Disease |
| VCTS | vitreal corneal touch |  | Research Laboratory |
|  | syndrome |  | (test for syphilis) |
| VCU | voiding cystourethrogram | VDRR | vitamin D-resistant rickets |
| VCUG | vesicoureterogram | VDRS | Verdun Depression Rating |
|  | voiding cystourethrogram |  | Scale |
| VCV | volume-control ventilation | VDS | vasodepressor syncope |
| VD | venereal disease |  | venereal disease—syphilis |
|  | vessel disease |  | vindesine (Eldisine) |
|  | viral diarrhea | VDT | video display terminal |
|  | voided | VD/VT | dead space to tidal |
|  | volume of distribution |  | volume ratio |
| V$_D$ | deadspace volume | VE | vaginal examination |
| V$_d$ | volume of distribution |  | vertex |
| V&D | vomiting and diarrhea |  | Vietnam era |
| 1-VD | one-vessel disease |  | virtual endoscopy |
| VDA | venous digital angiogram |  | visual examination |
|  | visual discriminatory |  | vitamin E |
|  | acuity |  | vocational evaluation |
| VDAC | vaginal delivery after | V$_E$ | minute volume (expired) |
|  | cesarean | V/E | violence and eloper |

| VEA | ventricular ectopic activity | VFC | Vaccines for Children (program) |
| | viscoelastic agent | | |
| VEB | ventricular ectopic beat | VFCB | vertical flow clean bench |
| VEC | vecuronium (Norcuron) | VFD | ventilator-free days |
| | velocity-encoded cine | | visual fields |
| VECG | vector electrocardiogram | VFFC | visual fields full to confrontation |
| VED | vacuum erection device | | |
| | vacuum extraction delivery | VFI | visual fields intact |
| | ventricular ectopic depolarization | | Visual Functioning index |
| | | V. Fib | ventricular fibrillation |
| VEE | Venezuelan equine encephalitis | VFL | vinflunine |
| | | VFP | vertical float progression (aquatic therapy) |
| VEE$_a$ | Venezuelan equine encephalitis vaccine, attenuated live | | vitreous fluorophotometry |
| | | | vocal fold paralysis |
| VEE$_I$ | Venezuelan equine encephalitis vaccine, inactivated | VFPN | Volu-feed premie nipple |
| | | VFR | visiting friends and relatives (possible contacts for communicable diseases) |
| VEF | visually evoked field | | |
| VEG | vegetation (bacterial) | | |
| VEGF | vascular endothelial growth factor | VFRN | Volu-feed regular nipple |
| | | VFSS | videofluoroscopic swallowing study |
| VeIP | vinblastine (Velban), ifosfamide, and cisplatin (Platinol AQ) | | |
| | | VFT | venous filling time |
| | | | ventricular fibrillation threshold |
| VENC | velocity encoding value (radiology) | VG | vein graft |
| | | | ventricular gallop |
| VENT | ventilation | | ventrogluteal |
| | ventilator | | very good |
| | ventral | V&G | vagotomy and gastroenterotomy |
| | ventricular | | |
| VEP | visual evoked potential | VGAD | vein of Galen aneurysmal dilatation |
| VER | ventricular escape rhythm | | |
| | visual evoked responses | VGAM | vein of Galen aneurysmal malformation |
| VERDICT | Veterans Evidence-based Research Dissemination Implementation Center | | |
| | | VGB | vigabatrin (Sabril) |
| | | VGE | viral gastroenteritis |
| VERP | ventricular effective refractory period | VGH | very good health |
| | | VGM | vein graft myringoplasty |
| VERT | velocity-enhanced resistance training | VGPO | volume-guaranteed pressure option |
| | | VH | vaginal hysterectomy |
| VES | ventricular extrasystoles | | Veterans Hospital |
| | video-endoscopic surgery | | viral hepatitis |
| | vitamin E succinate | | visual hallucinations |
| VET | veteran | | vitreous hemorrhage |
| | Veterinarian | | von Herrick (grading system) |
| | veterinary | | |
| VF | left leg (electrode) | VH I | very narrow anterior chamber angles |
| | ventricular fibrillation | | |
| | vertical float (aquatic therapy) | VH II | moderately narrow anterior chamber angles |
| | visual field | | |
| | vocal fremitus | | |

V

| | | | |
|---|---|---|---|
| VH III | moderately wide open anterior chamber angles | | Visual Impairment Service |
| VH IV | wide open anterior chamber angles | VISA | vancomycin-intermediate-resistant *Staphylococcus aureus* |
| VHD | valvular heart disease vascular hemostatis device | VISC | vitreous infusion suction cutter |
| VHF | viral hemorrhagic fever | VISI | Vaccine Identification |
| VHI | Voice Handicap Index | | Standards Initiative |
| VHL | von Hippel-Lindau disease (complex) | | volar intercalated segmental instability |
| VI | six | VISN | Veterans Integrated |
| | velocity index | | Service Networks |
| | volume index | VISs | Vaccine Information |
| *via* | by way of | | Statements |
| vib | vibration | VIT | venom immunotherapy |
| VIBS | Victim's Information Bureau Service | | vital vitamin |
| VICA | velocity internal carotid artery | | vitreous |
| VICP | Vaccine Injury Compensation Program | Vitamin | see individual letters such as R, V, etc. |
| Vi CPs | typhoid Vi (capsular) | VIT CAP | vital capacity |
| | polysaccharide vaccine (Typhim Vi) | VIU | visual internal urethrotomy |
| VID | videodensitometry | *VIZ* | namely |
| VIG | vaccinia immune globulin | V-J | ventriculo-jugular (shunt) |
| | vinblastine, ifosfamide, and gallium nitrate | VKC | vernal keratoconjunctivitis |
| VIH | human immunodeficiency virus (Spanish and French abbreviation) | VKDB | vitamin K deficiency bleeding |
| | | VKH | Vogt-Koyanagi-Harada disease |
| VIN | vulvar intraepithelial neoplasm | VL | left arm (electrode) vial |
| VIP | etopside (VePesid), ifosfamide, and cisplatin (Platinol AQ) | | viral load |
| | | VLA | very-late antigen |
| | vasoactive intestinal peptide | VLAD | variable life-adjusted display |
| | vasoactive intracorporeal pharmacotherapy | VLAP | vaporization laser ablation of the prostate |
| | very important patient | VLBW | very low birth weight (less than 1500 g) |
| | vinblastine, ifosfamide, and cisplatin (Platinol) | VLBWPN | very low birth weight preterm neonate |
| | voluntary interruption of pregnancy | VLCAD | very-long-chain acyl coenzyme A dehydrogenase |
| VIPomas | vasoactive intestinal peptide-secreting tumors | VLCD | very low calorie diet |
| | | VLCFA | very-long-chain fatty acids |
| VIQ | Verbal Intelligence Quotient (part of Wechsler tests) | VLDL | very-low-density lipoprotein |
| | | VLE | vision left eye |
| VIS | Vaccine Information Statement | VLH | ventrolateral nucleus of the hypothalamus |

V

| | | | |
|---|---|---|---|
| VLM | visceral larva migrans | VOL | volume |
| VLP | virus-like particle | | voluntary |
| VLR | vastus lateralis release | VOM | vomited |
| VM | venous malformation | VOO | continuous ventricular |
| | ventilated mask | | asynchronous pacing |
| | ventimask | VOR | vestibular ocular reflex |
| | Venturi mask | VOS | vision left eye |
| | vestibular membrane | VOSS | visual observation |
| VM 26 | teniposide (Vumon) | | shivering score |
| VMA | vanillylmandelic acid | VOT | Visual Organization Test |
| VMATs | Veterinary Medical | VOU | vision both eyes |
| | Assistance Teams | VP | etoposide (VePesid) and |
| VMCP | vincristine, melphalan, | | cisplatin (Platinol AQ) |
| | cyclophosphamide, and | | vagal paraganglioma |
| | prednisone | | variegate porphyria |
| VMD | Doctor of Veterinary | | venipuncture |
| | Medicine (DVM) | | venous pressure |
| | vertical maxillary | | ventriculoperitoneal |
| | deficiency | | visual perception |
| VME | vertical maxillary excess | | voiding pressure |
| VMH | ventromedial | V & P | vagotomy and |
| | hypothalamus | | pyloroplasty |
| VMI | vendor-managed inventory | | ventilation and perfusion |
| | visual motor integration | VP-16 | etoposide |
| VMO | vaccinia melanoma | VPA | valproic acid |
| | oncolysate | | ventricular premature |
| | vastus medialis oblique | | activation |
| VMR | vasomotor rhinitis | | vigorous physical activity |
| VMS | vanilla milkshake | V-Pad | sanitary napkin |
| VN | visiting nurse | VPB | ventricular premature beat |
| VNA | Visiting Nurses' | VPC | ventricular premature |
| | Association | | contractions |
| VNB | vinorelbine (Navelbine) | VPD | ventricular premature |
| VNC | vesicle neck contracture | | depolarization |
| VNS | vagal nerve stimulation | VPDC | ventricular premature |
| VNTR | variable number of | | depolarization |
| | tandem repeats | | contraction |
| VO | verbal order | VPDF | vegetable protein diet plus |
| VO$_2$ | oxygen consumption | | fiber |
| VOCAB | vocabulary | VPDs | ventricular premature |
| VOCOR | vaso-occlusive crisis | | depolarizations |
| | void on-call to operating | VPI | velopharyngeal |
| | room | | incompetence |
| VOCs | volatile organic | | velopharyngeal |
| | compounds | | insufficiency |
| VOCTOR | void on-call to operating | VPL | ventro-posterolateral |
| | room | VPLN | vaccine-primed lymph |
| VOD | veno-occlusive disease | | node (cells) |
| | vision right eye | VPLS | ventilation-perfusion lung |
| VOE | vascular occlusive | | scan |
| | episode | VPM | venous pressure module |
| VO$_2$I | oxygen consumption | VPR | virtual patient record |
| | index | | volume pressure response |

V

347

| | | | |
|---|---|---|---|
| VPS | valvular pulmonic stenosis | | vital signs (temperature, pulse, and respiration) |
| | ventriculoperitoneal shunt | VSADP | vocational skills assessment and development program |
| VPT | vascularized patellar tendon | | |
| | vibration perception threshold | VSBE | very short below elbow (cast) |
| VQ | ventilation perfusion | VSD | ventricular septal defect |
| VR | right arm (electrode) | | vesicosphincter dyssynergia |
| | valve replacement | | |
| | venous resistance | VSI | visual motor integration |
| | ventricular rhythm | VSMC | vascular smooth muscle cell |
| | verbal reprimand | | |
| | vocational rehabilitation | VSN | vital signs normal |
| V₃R··V₆R | right sided precordial leads | VSO | vertical subcondylar oblique |
| VRA | visual reinforcement audiometry | VSOK | vital signs normal |
| | | VSP | vertical stabilization program |
| | visual response audiometry | VSQOL | Vital Signs Quality of Life |
| VRB | vinorelbine (Navelbine) | | |
| VRC | vocational rehabilitation counselor | VSR | venous stasis retinopathy |
| | | | ventricular septal rupture |
| VRE | vancomycin-resistant enterococci | VSS | variable spot scanning |
| | | | vital signs stable |
| | vision right eye | V_SS | apparent volume of distribution |
| VREF | vancomycin-resistant *Enterococcus faecium* | | |
| | | VSSAF | vital signs stable, afebrile |
| VRI | viral respiratory infection | VST | visual search task |
| VRL | ventral root, lumbar | VSULA | vaccination scar, upper left arm |
| | vinorelbine (Navelbine) | | |
| VRP | vocational rehabilitation program | VSV | vesicular stomatitis virus |
| | | VT | validation therapy |
| VRS | viral rhinosinusitis | | ventricular tachycardia |
| VRSA | vancomycin-resistant *Staphylococcus aureus* | V_t | tidal volume |
| | | VTA | ventral tegmentum area |
| VRT | variance of resident time | VTBI | volume to be infused |
| | ventral root, thoracic | v. tach. | ventricular tachycardia |
| | vertical radiation topography | VTE | venous thromboembolism |
| | | VTEC | verotoxin-producing *Escherichia coli* |
| | Visual Retention Test | | |
| | vocational rehabilitation therapy | VTED | venous thromboembolic disease |
| VRTA | Vocational Rehabilitation Therapy Assistant | VT-NS | ventricular tachycardia nonsustained |
| VRU | ventilator rehabilitation unit | VTOP | voluntary termination of pregnancy |
| VS | vagal stimulation | VTP | voluntary termination of pregnancy |
| | vegetative state | | |
| | versus *(vs)* | VTS | Volunteer Transport Service |
| | very sensitive | | |
| | visit | VT-S | ventricular tachycardia sustained |
| | visited | | |

| | | | |
|---|---|---|---|
| VTSRS | Verdun Target Symptom Rating Scale | VY | surgical replacement flap |
| | | VZ | varicella zoster |
| VT/VF | ventricular tachycardia/fibrillation | VZIG | varicella zoster immune globulin |
| VTX | vertex | VZV | varicella zoster virus |
| VU | venous ulcer vesicoureteral (reflux) | | |
| V/U | verbalize understanding | | |
| VUD-BMT | volunteer unrelated-donor bone marrow transplantation | | |
| VUJ | vesico ureteral junction | | |
| VUR | vesicoureteric reflux | | |
| VV | vaccina virus varicose veins | | |
| V-V | ventriculovenous (shunt) | | |
| V&V | vulva and vagina | | |
| V/V | volume to volume ratio | | |
| VVB | venovenous bypass | | |
| VVC | vulvovaginal candidiasis | | |
| VVD | vaginal vertex delivery | | |
| VVETP | Vietnam Veterans Evaluation and Treatment Program | | |
| VVFR | vesicovaginal fistula repair | | |
| V/VI | grade 5 on a 6 grade basis | | |
| VVI | ventricular demand pacing | | |
| VVIR | ventricular demand inhibited pacemaker (V = chamber paced-ventricle, V = chamber sensed-ventricle, I = response to sensing-inhibited, R = programmability–rate modulation) | | |
| VVL | varicose veins ligation verruca vulgaris of the larynx | | |
| VVOR | visual-vestibulo-ocular-reflex | | |
| VVR | ventricular response rate | | |
| VVT | ventricular synchronous pacing | | |
| VW | vessel wall | | |
| VWD | ventral wall defect | | |
| vWD | von Willebrand disease | | |
| vWF | von Willebrand factor | | |
| VWM | ventricular wall motion | | |
| $V_x$ | vitrectomy | | |
| V-XT | V-pattern exotropia | | |

V

# W

| | |
|---|---|
| W | wash |
| | watts |
| | wearing glasses |
| | week |
| | weight |
| | well |
| | West (as in the location e.g. 2W, is second floor, West wing) |
| | white |
| | widowed |
| | wife |
| | with |
| | work |
| W-1 | insignificant (allergies) |
| W-3 | minimal (allergies) |
| W-5 | moderate (allergies) |
| W-7 | moderate-severe (allergies) |
| W-9 | severe (allergies) |
| WA | when awake |
| | while awake |
| | White American |
| | wide awake |
| | with assistance |
| W-A | Wyeth-Ayerst Laboratories |
| W & A | weakness and atrophy |
| W or A | weakness or atrophy |
| WACH | wedge adjustable cushioned heel |
| WAF | weakness, atrophy, and fasciculation |
| | white adult female |
| WAGR | Wilm tumor, aniridia, genitourinary malformations, and mental retardation (syndrome) |
| WAIS | Wechsler Adult Intelligence Scale |
| WAIS-R | Wechsler Adult Intelligence Scale-Revised |
| WAL | Wyeth-Ayerst Laboratories |
| WALK | weight-activated locking knee (prosthesis) |
| WAM | white adult male |
| WAP | wandering atrial pacemaker |
| WARI | wheezing associated respiratory infection |
| WAS | whiplash-associated disorders |
| | Wiskott-Aldrich syndrome |
| WASO | wakefulness after sleep onset |
| WASP | Wiskott-Aldrich syndrome protein |
| WASS | Wasserman test |
| WAT | word association test |
| WB | waist belt |
| | weight bearing |
| | well baby |
| | Western blot |
| | whole blood |
| WBACT | whole-blood activated clotting time |
| WBAT | weight bearing as tolerated |
| WBC | weight bearing with crutches |
| | well baby clinic |
| | white blood cell (count) |
| WBCT | whole-blood clotting time |
| WBD | weeks by dates (for gestational age) |
| WBE | weeks by examination (for gestational age) |
| WBGD | whole-body glucose disposal |
| WBH | weight-based heparin (dosing) |
| | whole-body hyperthermia |
| WBI | whole-bowel irrigation |
| W Bld | whole blood |
| WBN | wellborn nursery |
| WBNAA | whole-brain N-acetylaspartate |
| WBOS | wide base of support |
| WBPTT | whole-blood partial thromboplastin time |
| WBQC | wide-base quad cane |
| WBR | whole-body radiation |
| WBRT | whole-brain radiotherapy |
| WBS | weeks by size (for gestational age) |
| | whole body scan |
| | Williams-Beuren syndrome |

W

| | | | |
|---|---|---|---|
| WBTF | Waring Blender tube feeding | WDM | white divorced male |
| WBTT | weight bearing to tolerance | WDS | word discrimination score |
| WBUS | weeks by ultrasound | WDTC | well-differentiated thyroid cancer |
| WBV | whole blood volume | | |
| WC | ward clerk | WDWG | well dressed, well groomed |
| | ward confinement | | |
| | warm compress | WDWN-AAF | well-developed, well-nourished African-American female |
| | wet compresses | | |
| | wheelchair | | |
| | when called | WDWN-BM | well-developed, well-nourished black male |
| | white count | | |
| | whooping cough | | |
| | will call | WDWN-WF | well-developed, well-nourished white female |
| | workers' compensation | | |
| WCA | work capacity assessment | | |
| WCC | well-child care | WDXRF | wavelength-dispersive x-ray fluorescence |
| | white cell count | | |
| WCE | white coat effect | WE | weekend |
| | work capacity evaluation | | wide excision |
| WCH | white coat hypertension | W/E | weekend |
| WC/LC | warm compresses and lid scrubs | WEBINO | wall-eyed bilateral internuclear ophthalmoplegia |
| WCM | whole cow's milk | | |
| WCS | work capacity specialist | WE-D | withdrawal-emergent dyskinesia |
| WCST | Wisconsin Card Sorting Test | | |
| | | WEE | Western equine encephalitis |
| WCT | wide-complex tachycardia | | |
| WD | ward | WEMINO | wall-eyed monocular internuclear ophthalmoplegia |
| | well developed | | |
| | well differentiated | | |
| | wet dressing | WEP | weekend pass |
| | Wilson disease | WESR | Westergren erythrocyte sedimentation rate |
| | word | | |
| | working distance | | Wintrobe erythrocyte sedimentation rate |
| | wound | | |
| W/D | warm and dry | WEUP | willful exposure to unwanted pregnancy |
| | withdrawal | | |
| W → D | wet to dry | WF | well flexed |
| W4D | Worth four-dot (test for fusion) | | wet film |
| | | | white female |
| WDCC | well-developed collateral circulation | W/F | weakness and fatigue |
| | | WFB | wooden foreign body |
| WDF | white divorced female | WFE | Williams flexion exercises |
| WDHA | watery diarrhea, hypokalemia, and achlorhydria | W FEEDS | with feedings |
| | | WFH | white-faced hornet |
| | | WFI | water for injection |
| WDHH | watery diarrhea, hypokalemia, and hypochlorhydria | WFL | within full limits |
| | | | within functional limits |
| | | WFLC | white female living child |
| WDL | within defined limits | WF-O | will follow in office |
| WDLL | well-differentiated lymphocytic lymphoma | WFR | wheel-and-flare reaction |
| | | WG | Wegener granulomatosis |

W

| | | | |
|---|---|---|---|
| WGA | wheat germ agglutinin | WIT | water-induced thermotherapy |
| WH | walking heel (cast) | WK | week |
| | well healed | | work |
| | well hydrated | WKI | Wakefield Inventory |
| WHA | warmed humidified air | WKS | Wernicke-Korsakoff Syndrome |
| WHAS | Women's Health Assessment Scale | WL | waiting list |
| WHIS | War Head-Injury Score | | wave length |
| WHNR | well-healed, no residuals | | weight loss |
| WHNS | well-healed, no sequelae | WLE | wide local excision |
| | well-healed, nonsymptomatic | WLM | working level months |
| | well-healed, no sequelae | WLQ | Work Limitation Questionnaire |
| WHO | World Health Organization | WLS | weight-loss surgery |
| | wrist-hand orthosis | | wet lung syndrome |
| WHOART | World Health Organization Adverse Reaction Terms (Terminology) | WLT | waterload test |
| | | WM | wall motion |
| | | | warm, moist |
| | | | wet mount |
| WHOQOL-100 | World Health Organization Quality of Life 100-Item (instrument) | | white male |
| | | | white matter |
| | | | whole milk |
| | | WMA | wall motion abnormality |
| WHP | whirlpool | WMD | warm moist dressings (sterile) |
| WHPB | whirlpool bath | | |
| WHR | ratio of waist to hip circumference | | weapons of mass destruction |
| | | | weighted mean differences |
| WHV | woodchuck hepatitis virus | | |
| WHVP | wedged hepatic venous pressure | WMF | white married female |
| | | WMFT | Wolf Motor Function Test |
| WH/WD | withholding/withdrawal (of life support) | WMI | wall motion index |
| | | | weighted mean index |
| WHZ | wheezes | WML | white matter lesions (cerebral) |
| WI | ventricular demand pacing | | |
| | walk-in | WMLC | white male living child |
| W/I | within | WMM | white married male |
| W+I | work and interest | WMP | warm moist packs (unsterile) |
| WIA | wounded in action | | |
| WIC | Women, Infants, and Children (program) | | weight management program |
| WID | widow | WMS | Wechsler Memory Scale |
| | widower | | Wilson-Mikity syndrome |
| WIED | walk-in emergency department | WMT | Word Memory Test |
| WIP | work in progess | WMX | whirlpool, massage, and exercise |
| WIS | Ward Incapacity Scale | | |
| | Wister Institute | WN | well nourished |
| WISC | Wechsler Intelligence Scale for Children | WND | wound |
| | | WNE | West Nile encephalitis |
| WISC-R | Wechsler Intelligence Scale for Children-Revised | WNF | well-nourished female |
| | | | West Nile fever |
| | | WNL | within normal limits |

W

| | | | |
|---|---|---|---|
| WNL x 4 | upper and lower extremities within normal limits | WR | Wassermann reaction wrist |
| WNLS | weighted nonlinear least squares | WRA | with-the-rule astigmatism |
| WNM | well-nourished male | WRAIR | Walter Reed Army Institute of Research |
| WNR | within normal range | WRAMC | Walter Reed Army Medical Center |
| $WNt^{50}$ | Wagner-Nelson time 50 hours | WRARU | Walter Reed AFRIMS (Armed Forces Research Institute of Medical Sciences) Research Unit |
| WNV | West Nile virus | | |
| WO | weeks old wide open written order | WRAT | Wide Range Achievement Test |
| W/O | water-in-oil without | WRAT-R | The Wide Range Achievement Test, Revised |
| WOB | work of breathing | WRBC | washed red blood cells |
| WOCN | Wound, Ostomy and Continence Nurses (Society)-formerly known as the International Association for Enterostomal Therapy (IEAT) | WRC | washed red (blood) cells |
| | | WRIOT | Wide Range Interest-Opinion Test (for career planning) |
| | | WRL | World Reference Laboratory for Foot-and-Mouth Disease (Institute for Animal Health, Survey, United Kingdom) |
| WOMAC | Western Ontario and McMaster Universities Osteoarthritis Index | | |
| WOP | without pain | WRT | weekly radiation therapy with respect (regards) to |
| W or A | weakness or atrophy | | |
| WORD | Wechsler objective reading dimensions | WRUED | work-related upper-extremity disorder |
| WORLD/ DLROW | a test used in mental status examinations (patient is asked to spell WORLD backwards) | WS | walking speed ward secretary watt seconds Williams syndrome work simplification work simulation work status |
| WP | whirlpool | | |
| WPBT | whirlpool, body temperature | | |
| WPCs | washed packed cells | W&S | wound and skin |
| WPFM | Wright peak flow meter | WSCP | Williams Syndrome Cognitive Profile |
| WPOA | wearing patch on arrival | WSEP | Williams syndrome, early puberty |
| WPP | Wechsler Preschool and Primary Scale of Intelligence | WSepF | white separated female |
| | | WSepM | white separated male |
| | | WSF | white single female |
| WPPSI | Wechsler Preschool and Primary Scale of Intelligence | WSLP | Williams syndrome, late puberty |
| WPPSI-R | WPPSI revised | WSM | white single male |
| WPR | written progress report | WSO | white superficial onychomycosis |
| WPV | within-person variability | | |
| WPW | Wolff-Parkinson-White (syndrome) | | |

**W**

| | | | |
|---|---|---|---|
| WSOC | water-soluble organic compounds | | **X** |
| WSP | wearable speech processor | | |
| WT | walking tank | | |
| | walking training | | |
| | weight (wt) | X | break |
| | wild type | | cross |
| | Wilms tumor | | crossmatch |
| | wisdom teeth | | exophoria for distance |
| 0WT | zero work tolerance | | extra |
| W-T-D | wet to dry | | female sex chromosome |
| WTP | willingness to pay | | start of anesthesia |
| WTS | whole tomography slice | | ten |
| W/U | work-up | | times |
| WV | whispered voice | | xylocaine |
| W/V | weight-to-volume ratio | $\bar{x}$ | except |
| WW | Weight Watchers | | mean |
| | wheeled walker | X' | exophoria at 33 cm |
| WWI | World War One | $X^2$ | chi-square |
| WWII | World War Two | X+# | xyphoid plus number of fingerbreadths |
| W/W | weight-to-weight ratio | | |
| W → W | wet-to-wet | X3 | orientation as to time, place and person |
| WWAC | walk with aid of cane | | |
| WW Brd | whole wheat bread | X-ALD | X-linked adrenoleukodystrophy |
| WWidF | white widowed female | | |
| WWidM | white widowed male | XBT | xylose breath test |
| WWTP | wastewater treatment plant | XC | excretory cystogram |
| WWW | World Wide Web | XCF | aortic cross clamp off |
| WYOU | women years of usage | | |
| | | XCO | aortic cross clamp on |
| | | XD | times daily |
| | | X&D | examination and diagnosis |
| | | X2d | times two days |
| | | XDP | xeroderma pigmentosum |
| | | Xe | xenon |
| | | $^{133}$Xe | xenon, isotope of mass 133 |
| | | XeCl | xenon chloride |
| | | XeCT | xenon-enhanced computed tomography |
| | | X-ed | crossed |
| | | XEM | xonics electron mammography |
| | | XES | x-ray energy spectrometer |
| | | XFER | transfer |
| | | XGP | xanthogranulomatous pyelonephritis |
| | | XI | eleven |
| | | XII | twelve |
| | | XIP | x-ray in plaster |
| | | XKO | not knocked out |

W

| | | | |
|---|---|---|---|
| XL | extended release (once a day oral solid dosage form) | XX | normal female sex chromosome type twenty |
| | extra large | XX/XY | sex karyotypes |
| | forty | XXX | thirty |
| XLA | X-linked infantile agammaglobulinemia | XY | normal male sex chromosome type |
| X-leg | cross leg | XYL | Xylocaine® |
| XLFDP | cross-linked fibrin degradation products | | xylose |
| | | XYLO | Xylocaine® |
| XLH | X-linked hypophos-phatemia | | |
| XLJR | X-linked juvenile retinoschisis | | |
| XLMR | X-linked mental retardation | | |
| XLP | X-linked proliferative (syndrome) | | |
| XLRS | X-linked retinoschisis | | |
| XM | crossmatch | | |
| X-mat. | crossmatch | | |
| XML | extensible markup language | | |
| XMM | xeromammography | | |
| XNA | xenoreactive natural antibodies | | |
| XOM | extraocular movements | | |
| XOP | x-ray out of plaster | | |
| XP | xeroderma pigmentosum | | |
| XR | x-ray | | |
| XRF | x-ray fluorescence | | |
| XRT | radiation therapy | | |
| XS | excessive | | |
| X-SCID | X-linked severe combined immunodeficiency disease | | |
| XS-LIM | exceeds limits of procedure | | |
| XT | exotropia | | |
| | extract | | |
| | extracted | | |
| X(T') | intermittent exotropia at 33 cm | | |
| X(T) | intermittent exotropia | | |
| XTLE | extratemporal-lobe epilepsy | | |
| XU | excretory urogram | | |
| XULN | times upper limit of normal | | |
| XV | fifteen | | |
| 3X/WK | three times a week | | |

X

| | | | |
|---|---|---|---|
| Y | male sex chromosome | Z | impedance |
| | year | ZAP | zoster-associated pain |
| | yellow | ZDV | zidovudine (Retrovir) |
| YAC | yeast artificial chromosome | Z-E | Zollinger-Ellison |
| YACs | yeast artificial chromosomes | | (syndrome) |
| | | ZEEP | zero end-expiratory pressure |
| YACP | young adult chronic patient | | |
| | | ZES | Zollinger-Ellison syndrome |
| YAG | yttrium aluminum garnet (laser) | | |
| | | Z-ESR | zeta erythrocyte sedimentation rate |
| YAS | youth action section (police) | | |
| | | ZIFT | zygote intrafallopian (tube) transfer |
| Yb | ytterbium | | |
| YBOCS | Yale-Brown Obsessive-Compulsive Scale | ZIG | zoster serum immune globulin |
| | | ZIP | zoster immune plasma |
| Yel | yellow | ZMC | zygomatic |
| YF | yellow fever | | zygomatic maxillary compound (complex) |
| YFH | yellow-faced hornet | | |
| YFI | yellow fever immunization | Zn | zinc |
| | | ZnO | zinc oxide |
| YHL | years of healthy life | ZnOE | zinc oxide and eugenol |
| YJV | yellow jacket venom | ZnPc | zinc phthalocyanine |
| Y2K | year 2,000 | ZnPP | zinc protoporphyrin |
| YLC | youngest living child | ZNS | zonisamide (Zonegran) |
| YLD | years of life with disability | ZOI | zone of inhibition |
| YLL | years of life lost | ZOOM | Guarana |
| YMC | young male Caucasian | ZOT | zonula occludens toxin |
| YMRS | Young Mania Rating Scale | ZPC | zero point of charge |
| Y/N | yes/no | | zopiclone |
| YO | years old | z-Plasty | surgical relaxation of contracture |
| YOB | year of birth | | |
| YOD | year of death | ZPO | zinc peroxide |
| YORA | younger-onset rheumatoid arthritis | ZPP | zinc protoporphyrin |
| | | ZPT | zinc pyrithione |
| YPC | YAG (yttrium aluminum garnet) posterior capsulotomy | ZSB | zero stools since birth |
| | | ZSR | zeta sedimentation rate |
| | | ZSRDS | Zung Self-Rating Depression Scale |
| YPLL | years of potential life lost before age 65 | | |
| yr | year | | |
| YSC | yolk sac carcinoma | | |
| YTD | year to date | | |
| YTDY | yesterday | | |

Y

# Chapter 5

# Symbols and Numbers

**Symbols**

| | | | |
|---|---|---|---|
| ↑ | above | | to and from |
| | alive | | unchanging |
| | elevated | ↓↓ | flexor |
| | greater than | | plantar response |
| | high | | (Babinski) |
| | improved | | testes descended |
| | increase | | |
| | rising | ↑↑ | extensor |
| | up | | extensor response |
| | upper | | (positive Babinsky) |
| ↑g | increasing | | testes undescended |
| ↓ | dead | ‖ | parallel |
| | decrease | | parallel bars |
| | depressed | √ | check |
| | diminished | | flexion |
| | down | | |
| | falling | √'d | checked |
| | lower | | |
| | lowered | √'ing | checking |
| | normal plantar | | |
| | reflex | # | fracture |
| | restricted | | number |
| | | | pound |
| ↓g | decreasing | | weight |
| → | causes to | ∴ | therefore |
| | greater than | ∵ | because |
| | progressing | Δ scan | delta scan (computed |
| | results in | | tomography scan) |
| | showed | | |
| | to the right | + | plus |
| | transfer to | | positive |
| | | | present |
| ← | less than | − | absent |
| | resulted from | | minus |
| | to the left | | negative |
| ↔ | same as | / | slash mark signifying per, |
| | stable | | and, over, as a blood |

|  |  |
|---|---|
|  | pressure of 160 over 100, or with (this is a dangerous symbol as it is mistaken for a one) |
| ± | either positive or negative<br>no definite cause<br>plus or minus<br>very slight trace |
| L | right lower quadrant |
| Γ | right upper quadrant |
| ⌐ | left upper quadrant |
| ⌐ | left lower quadrant |
| > | greater than (can be confused with <, use "greater than")<br>left ear-bone conduction threshold |
| ≥ | greater than or equal to |
| < | caused by<br>less than (can be confused with >, use "less than")<br>right ear-bone conduction threshold |
| ≤ | less than or equal to |
| ≮ | not less than |
| ≯ | not more than<br>above<br>diastolic blood pressure<br>increased |
| V | below<br>systolic blood pressure |
| ≠ | not equal to |
| ≅ | approximately equal to |
| = | equal<br>equal to<br>feet |
| ' | minutes (as in 30') |
| " | inches<br>seconds |
| ~ | about<br>approximately<br>difference |
| ≈ | approximately equal to |
| ≡ | identical |

|  |  |
|---|---|
| × | left ear-air conduction threshold<br>ten |
| ] | left ear-masked bone conduction threshold |
| △ | right ear-masked air conduction threshold<br>change |
| [ | right ear-masked bone conduction threshold<br>reversible |
| ○ |  |
| ? | questionable |
| — | not tested |
| Ø | no<br>none<br>without |
| ⊙ | start of an operation |
| ⊗ | end of anesthesia |
| @ | at |
| ☥ | one |
| ☥☥ | two |
| ♂ | male |
| ♀ | female |
| ⚣ | gay |
| ⚢ | lesbian |
| ■ | deceased male |
| ● | deceased female |
| □ | living male<br>left ear-masked air conduction threshold |
| ○ | living female<br>respiration<br>right ear-air conduction threshold |
| ◇ | sex unknown |
| (□) | adopted living male |
| * | birth |
| † | dead<br>death |
| ♀ | standing |
| O—< | recumbent position |
| ♀ | sitting position |
| ♥ | heart |

## Numbers (Arabic and Roman)

| | |
|---|---|
| 1/2 and 1/2 | half Dakin solution and half glycerin |
| 1° | first degree<br>primary |
| 1:1 | one-to-one (individual session with staff) |
| 2° | second degree<br>secondary |
| 2×2 | gauze dressing folded 2″×2″ |
| 3° | tertiary<br>third degree |
| 3× | three times |
| 4×4 | gauze dressing folded 4″×4″ |
| 7+3 | 7 days of cytarabine and 3 days of daunorubicin leukemia therapy |
| Serial 7's | a mental status examination (starting with 100, count backward by 7's) |
| 24° | twenty-four hours (24 hr is safer as the ° is seen as a zero) |
| 777 | Ortho Novum 777® (a triphasic oral contraceptive) |
| 1500 | Health Insurance Claim Form HCFA 1500 |
| 1,000 | one thousand ($1 \times 10^3$) |
| 10,000 | ten thousand ($1 \times 10^4$) |
| 100,000 | one hundred thousand ($1 \times 10^5$) |
| 1,000,000 | one million ($1 \times 10^6$) |
| 10,000,000 | ten million ($1 \times 10^7$) |
| 100,000,000 | one hundred million ($1 \times 10^8$) |
| 1,000,000,000 | one billion ($1 \times 10^9$) |
| i | one (Roman numerals are dangerous expressions and should not be used because they are not universally understood) |
| ii | two |
| iii | three |
| iiii | four |
| iv | four (this is a dangerous abbreviation as it is read as intravenous, use 4) |
| v | five |
| vi | six |
| vii | seven |
| viii | eight |
| ix | nine |
| x | ten |
| xi | eleven |
| xii | twelve |
| XL | forty<br>extended release dosage form |

## Greek Letters

| | |
|---|---|
| A α | alpha |
| β B | beta |
| Γ γ | gamma |
| Δ δ | anion gap<br>change<br>delta<br>delta gap<br>prism diopter<br>temperature<br>trimester |
| E ε | epsilon |
| Z ζ | zeta |
| H η | eta |
| Θ θ | negative<br>theta |
| I ι | iota |
| K κ | kappa |
| Λ λ | lambda |
| M μ | micro<br>mu |
| N ν | nu |
| Ξ ξ | xi |
| O o | omicron |
| Π π | pi |
| P ρ | rho |
| Σ σ | sigma |

|   |   |   |
|---|---|---|
|   |   | sum of |
|   |   | summary |
| # | T τ | tau |
|   | Υ υ | upsilon |
|   | Φ φ | phenyl |
|   |   | phi |
|   |   | thyroid |
|   | X χ | chi |

Ψ ψ  psi
    psychiatric
Ω ω  omega

## Miscellaneous

liver, kidneys, and spleen negative, no masses, or tenderness

# Chapter 6

# Tables and Lists

## Numbers and letters for teeth

Two adult numbering systems and a deciduous system are shown. The adult systems are shown as numbers, whereas deciduous teeth are lettered. The system commonly used in the U.S. is 1 to 32 (shown in bold face type).

| | | |
|---|---|---|
| **1** (18) | upper right 3rd molar | |
| **2** (17) (A) | upper right 2nd molar | |
| **3** (16) (B) | upper right 1st molar | |
| **4** (15) | upper right 2nd bicuspid | |
| **5** (14) | upper right 1st bicuspid | |
| **6** (13) (C) | upper right canine (eyetooth) | |
| **7** (12) (D) | upper right lateral incisor | |
| **8** (11) (E) | upper right central incisor | |
| **9** (21) (F) | upper left central incisor | |
| **10** (22) (G) | upper left lateral incisor | |
| **11** (23) (H) | upper left canine | |
| **12** (24) | upper left 1st bicuspid | |
| **13** (25) | upper left 2nd bicuspid | |
| **14** (26) (I) | upper left 1st molar | |
| **15** (27) (J) | upper left 2nd molar | |
| **16** (28) | upper left 3rd molar | |
| **17** (38) | lower left 3rd molar | |
| **18** (37) (K) | lower left 2nd molar | |
| **19** (36) (L) | lower left 1st molar | |
| **20** (35) | lower left 2nd bicuspid | |
| **21** (34) | lower left 1st bicuspid | |
| **22** (33) (M) | lower left canine | |
| **23** (32) (N) | lower left lateral incisor | |
| **24** (31) (O) | lower left central incisor | |
| **25** (41) (P) | lower right central incisor | |
| **26** (42) (Q) | lower right lateral incisor | |
| **27** (43) (R) | lower right canine | |
| **28** (44) | lower right 1st bicuspid | |
| **29** (45) | lower right 2nd bicuspid | |
| **30** (46) (S) | lower right 1st molar | |
| **31** (47) (T) | lower right 2nd molar | |
| **32** (48) | lower right 3rd molar | |

| UPPER | | | | | | | | | | | | | | | | UPPER |
|---|---|---|---|---|---|---|---|---|---|---|---|---|---|---|---|---|
| | **1** | **2** | **3** | **4** | **5** | **6** | **7** | **8** | **9** | **10** | **11** | **12** | **13** | **14** | **15** | **16** |
| | 18 | 17 | 16 | 15 | 14 | 13 | 12 | 11 | 21 | 22 | 23 | 24 | 25 | 26 | 27 | 28 |
| **Right** | A | B | | | C | D | E | F | G | H | | | I | J | | **Left** |
| | T | S | | | R | Q | P | O | N | M | | | L | K | | |
| | 48 | 47 | 46 | 45 | 44 | 43 | 42 | 41 | 31 | 32 | 33 | 34 | 35 | 36 | 37 | 38 |
| | **32** | **31** | **30** | **29** | **28** | **27** | **26** | **25** | **24** | **23** | **22** | **21** | **20** | **19** | **18** | **17** |
| LOWER | | | | | | | | | | | | | | | | LOWER |

## Laboratory Test Panels*

| | Cl CO₂ K Na | BUN Ca Creat Gluc | Alb Alk P AST(SGOT) ALT(SGPT) T Bili TP | ANA ESR RF Ur Ac | Calc LDL HDL T Chol Trig VLDL | Alb Phos | HAAb, IgM Ab HbcAb, IgM Ab HbsAG HCAb |
|---|---|---|---|---|---|---|---|
| Lytes (electrolyte panel) | X | | | | | | |
| BMP (basic metabolic panel) or MBP, MPB | X | X | | | | | |
| CMP (comprehensive metabolic panel) | X | X | X | | | | |
| HFP (hepatitis function panel) | | | X plus D Bili | | | | |
| AP (arthritis panel) | | | | X | | | |
| LP (lipid Panel) | | | | | X | | |
| RFP (renal function panel) | X | X | | | | X | |
| AHP (acute hepatitis panel) | | | | | | | X |

*These can vary from institution to institution and from year to year

**Abbreviation Key**
Ab–antibody
Alb–albumin
Alk P–alkaline phosphate
ALT (SGPT)–alanine aminotransferase
  (serum glutamate pyruvate)
ANA–antinuclear antibody
AST (SGOT)–aspartate-aminotransferase
  (serum glutamate oxaloacetic transaminase)
BUN–blood urea nitrogen
Ca–calcium
Calc LDL–calculated low-density lipoprotein
LDL–low density lipoprotein

Cl–chloride
CO₂–carbon dioxide
Creat–creatinine
D Bili–direct bilirubin
ESR–erythrocyte sedimentation rate
Gluc–glucose
HAAb–hepatitis A antibody
HBcAb–hepatitis B core antibody
HBsAg–hepatitis B surface antigen
HCAb–hepatitis C antibody
HDL–high-density lipoprotein

IgM–immunoglobulin M
K–potassium
Na–sodium
Phos–phosphate
RF–rheumatoid factor
T Bili–total bilirubin
T Chol–total cholesterol
TP–total protein
Trig–triglycerides
Ur Ac–uric acid
VLDL–very low-density lipoprotein

See text for meaning of the abbreviations shown

## Complete Blood Count

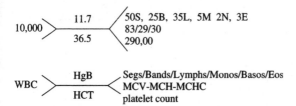

$$10,000 \diagdown \begin{array}{c} 11.7 \\ 36.5 \end{array} \diagup \begin{array}{c} \text{50S, 25B, 35L, 5M 2N, 3E} \\ 83/29/30 \\ 290,00 \end{array}$$

$$\text{WBC} \diagdown \begin{array}{c} \text{HgB} \\ \text{HCT} \end{array} \diagup \begin{array}{c} \text{Segs/Bands/Lymphs/Monos/Basos/Eos} \\ \text{MCV-MCH-MCHC} \\ \text{platelet count} \end{array}$$

## Electrolyte Panel

| 142 | 99 | sodium | chloride |
|---|---|---|---|
| 4.7 | 25 | potassium | carbon dioxide |

## Blood Gases

7.4/80/48/98/25    pH/$PO_2$/$PCO_2$/% $O_2$ saturation/bicarbonate

## Obstetrical shorthand

$$\frac{2 \text{ cm}|80\%}{-2 \text{ Vtx}}$$    2 cm = dilation of cervix

80% = degree of cer-        Vtx = vertex; presen-
vix effacement                    tation of fetus,
                                           (breech = Br)

−2 = station; distance
        above (−) or
        below (+) the
        spine of the ischium measured in cm

## Reflexes

Reflexes are usually graded on a 0 to 4+ scale. The designations +, ++, +++, and ++++ should not be used.

4+   may indicate disease
       often associated with clonus
       very brisk, hyperactive
3+   brisker than average
       possibly but not necessarily indicative of disease
2+   average
       normal
1+   low normal
       somewhat diminished
0    may indicate neuropathy
       no response

## Muscle strength[1]

0—No muscular contraction detected
1—A barely detectable flicker or trace of contraction
2—Active movement of the body part with gravity eliminated
3—Active movement against gravity
4—Active movement against gravity and some resistance
5—Active movement against full resistance without evident fatigue. This is
      normal muscle strength

## Pulse[1]

| | |
|---|---|
| 0 | completely absent |
| +1 | markedly impaired (or 1+) |
| +2 | modererately impaired (or 2+) |
| +3 | slightly impaired (or 3+) |
| +4 | normal (or 4+) |

## Gradation of intensity of heart murmurs[1]

| | |
|---|---|
| 1/6 or I/VI | may not be heard in all positions<br>very faint, heard only after the listener has "tuned in" |
| 2/6 or II/VI | quiet, but heard immediately upon placing the stethoscope on the chest |
| 3/6 or III/VI | moderately loud |
| 4/6 or IV/VI | loud |
| 5/6 orV/VI | very loud, may be heard with a stethoscope partly off the chest (thrills are associated) |
| 6/6 or VI/VI | may be heard with the stethoscope entirely off the chest (thrills are associated) |

## Tonsil Size

| | |
|---|---|
| 0 | no tonsils |
| 1 | less than normal |
| 2 | normal |
| 3 | greater than normal |
| 4 | touching |

## Metric Prefixes and Symbols

| Prefix | Symbol | |
|---|---|---|
| tera- | T | 1,000,000,000,000 or $(10^{12})$ one trillion |
| giga- | G | 1,000,000,000 or $(10^{9})$ one billion |
| mega- | M | 1,000,000 or $(10^{6})$ one million |
| kilo- | k | 1,000 or $(10^{3})$ one thousand |
| hecto- | h | 100 or $(10^{2})$ one hundred |
| deka- | da | 10 or $(10^{1})$ ten |
| deci- | d | 0.1 or $(10^{-1})$ one-tenth |
| centi- | c | 0.01 or $(10^{-2})$ one-hundredth |
| milli- | m | 0.001 or $(10^{-3})$ one-thousandth |
| micro- | μ | 0.000,001 or $(10^{-6})$ one-millionth |
| nano- | n | 0.000,000,001 or $(10^{-9})$ one-billionth |
| pico- | p | 0.000,000,000,000,001 or $(10^{-12})$ one-trillionth |
| femto- | f | 0.000,000,000,000,001 or $(10^{-15})$ one-quadrillionth |
| atto- | a | 0.000,000,000,000,000,001 or $(10^{-18})$ one-quintillionth |

## Apothecary symbols (Should never be used)

The symbols presented below are for informational use. The apothecary system should *not* be used. Only the metric system should be used. The methods of expressing the symbols, the meanings, and the equivalence are not the classic ones, nor are they accurate, but reflect the usual intended meanings when used by some older physicians in writing prescription directions.

|  |  |  |  |
|---|---|---|---|
| ℨ or ℨ𝖎 | dram, teaspoonful, (5 mL) | ℥ or ℥𝖎 | ounce, (30 mL) |
| | | **gr** | grain (approximately 60 mg) |
| ℨ𝖎𝖎 | two drams, 2 teaspoonfuls, (10 mL) | | |
| | | ♏ | minim (approximately 0.06 mL) |
| ℥ss | half ounce, tablespoonful, (15 mL) | **gtt** | drop |

## Reference

1. Adopted from Bates B. Bates guide to physical examinations and history taking, 8th ed. Philadelphia: J.B. Lippincott; 2003.

If you encounter abbreviations which are not in this book or on the web-version, please send them to—

Neil M Davis
1143 Wright Drive
Huntingdon Valley, PA 19006

or E-mail them to med@neilmdavis.com
or fax them to 215 938 1937

---

Have you investigated the web-version of this book? See the Preface for access instructions.

- It is instantaneously searchable for the meanings of abbreviations
- It is reverse searchable (search for all abbreviations containing the word "cardiac")
- Each month, about 100 new entries are added

# Chapter 7

# Cross-Referenced List of Generic and Brand Drug Names

Listed below is a cross-referenced index of generic and brand drug names. Generic names begin with a lower case letter while brand names begin with a capital letter. This partial list consists of frequently prescribed and new drugs.

The meanings of abbreviated and coded drug names can be found in Chapter 4 (Lettered Abbreviations and Acronyms).

Complete indices of United States drug names can be found in current editions of Drug Facts and Comparisons[1], the American Drug Index[2], and Physicians GenRx[3]. A complete list of world-wide names may be found in Martindales.[4] These and other references should be used to determine the equivalence of products, strengths, and dosage forms. Although several products may be listed under one generic name they may differ in strength, dosage form, or concentration available, as is the case with estradiol transdermal (Climara, Estraderm, and Vivelle).

Some products are marketed without a brand name, as in the case of thioguanine. In such cases only the generic name is listed. When a product is often prescribed and/or labeled generically, the generic name is shown in italics.

The following abbreviations are used in this listing:

| | | | |
|---|---|---|---|
| EC | enteric coated | SR | sustained release tablets or capsules |
| HCl | hydrochloride | | (and other forms of extended |
| IM | intramuscular | | release) |
| IV | intravenous | susp | suspension |
| inj | injection | (W) | withdrawn or discontinued from |
| oint | ointment | | US market |
| ophth | ophthalmic | (WA) | withdrawn or discontinued from |
| soln | solution | | US market but available under |
| | | | different name from another |
| | | | manufacturer |

# A

| | |
|---|---|
| abacavir sulfate | Ziagen |
| Abbokinase | urokinase |
| abciximab | ReoPro |
| Abelcet | amphotericin B lipid complex |
| acarbose | Precose |
| Accolate | zafirlukast |
| AccuNeb | albuterol inhalation soln |
| Accupril | quinapril HCl |
| Accuretic | quinapril; hydrochlorothiazide |
| Accutane | isotretinoin |
| Accuzyme | papain; urea oint |
| acebutolol HCl | Sectral |
| Aceon | perindopril erbumine |
| *acetaminophen* | paracetamol Tylenol |
| acetaminophen 300 mg with Codeine Phosphate (15, 30, and 60 mg) | Phenaphen with Codeine (#2, 3, and 4) Tylenol with Codeine (#2, 3, and 4) |
| acetazolamide | Diamox |
| acetohexamide | Dymelor |
| acetohydroxamic acid | Lithostat |
| acetylcholine ophth | Miochol E |
| acetylcysteine | Mucomyst |
| Achromycin (WA) | tetracycline HCl |
| Aciphex | rabeprazole sodium |
| acitretin | Soriatane |
| Acora | argatroban |
| Acthar | corticotropin |
| ActHIB/Tripedia | *Haemophilus b* conjugate vaccine reconstituted with diphtheria and tetanus toxoids and acellular pertussis vaccine adsorbed |
| Acthrel | corticorelin ovine triflutate |
| Actifed | triprolidine HCl; pseudo-ephedrine HCl |
| Actigall | ursodiol |
| Actimmune | interferon gamma 1-b |
| Actiq | fentanyl oral transmucosal |
| Activase | alteplase, recombinant |
| Activella (WA) | norethindrone acetate; estradiol |
| Actonel | risedronate sodium |
| Actos | pioglitazone HCl |
| Acular | ketorolac tromethamine ophth |
| acyclovir | Zovirax |
| Adalat | nifedipine |
| Adalat CC | nifedipine SR |
| adapalene | Differin |
| Adapin | doxepin HCl |
| Adderall | amphetamine; dextroamphetamine mixed salts |
| adefovir dipivoxil | Preveon |
| Adenocard | adenosine |
| adenosine | Adenocard |
| Adrenalin | epinephrine |
| Adriamycin | doxorubicin HCl |
| Advair Diskus | fluticasone propionate; salmeterol inhalation powder |
| Advicor | lovastatin; niacin |
| Advil | ibuprofen |
| AeroBid | flunisolide |
| Afrin nasal spray | oxymetazoline HCl |

| | | | |
|---|---|---|---|
| Agenerase | amprenavir | Alfenta | alfentanil HCl |
| Aggrastat | tirofiban HCl | alfentanil HCl | Alfenta |
| Aggrenox | aspirin; extended-release dipyridamole | alglucerase | Ceredase |
| | | Alimta | pemetrexed disodium |
| Agrylin | anagrelide HCl | alitretinoin | Panretin |
| Akineton | biperiden | Allegra | fexofenadine HCl |
| Alamast | pemirolast potassium ophth soln | Alkeran | melphalan |
| | | allopurinol | Zyloprim |
| alatrofloxacin mesylate IV | Trovan inj | almotriptan malate | Axert |
| albendazole | Albenza | Alocril | nedocromil ophth soln |
| Albenza | albendazole | | |
| albumin human | Albuminar Albutein Buminate Plasbumin Albunex | Alomide | lodoxamide tromethamine ophth soln |
| | | Alora | estradiol transdermal |
| albumin (human), sonicated | Albunex | alosetron | Lotronex |
| | | Alphagan | brimonidine tartrate ophth |
| Albuminar | albumin human | | |
| Albunex | albumin (human), sonicated | alpha$_1$-proteinase inhibitor (human) | Prolastin |
| Albutein | albumin human | alprazolam | Xanax |
| albuterol | AccuNeb Proventil salbutamol Ventolin | alprostadil | Caverject Edex Prostin VR |
| albuterol SR | Proventil Repetabs Volmax | alprostadil urethral suppository | Muse |
| albuterol sulfate inhalation aerosol | Proventil HFA | Alrex | loteprednol etabonate ophth susp |
| Aldactazide | spironolactone; hydrochloro-thiazide | Altace | ramipril |
| | | alteplase, recombinant | Activase |
| Aldactone | spironolactone | alteplase (for catheter occlusions) | Cathflo Activase |
| Aldara | imiquimod cream | | |
| aldesleukin | Proleukin | altretamine | Hexalen |
| Aldomet | methyldopa | aluminum acetate | Domeboro |
| Aldoril | methyldopa; hydrochloro-thiazide | aluminum carbonate | Basaljel |
| alemtuzumab | Campath | aluminum hydroxide | Amphojel |
| alendronate sodium | Fosamax | aluminum hydroxide; magnesium hydroxide | Maalox |
| Alesse | levonorgestrel; ethinyl estradiol | | |

| | | | |
|---|---|---|---|
| Alupent | metaproterenol sulfate | amlodipine besylate | Norvasc |
| Alustra | hydroquinone topical susp | amlodipine besylate; benazepril HCl | Lotrel |
| amantadine HCl | Symmetrel | | |
| Amaryl | glimepiride | | |
| Ambien | zolpidem tartrate | ammonium lactate lotion | AmLactin |
| AmBisome | liposomal amphotericin B | amobarbital sodium | Amytal |
| amcinonide | Cyclocort | amoxapine | Asendin |
| Amerge | naratriptan HCl | *amoxicillin* | Amoxil Trimox Wymox |
| Amicar | aminocaproic acid | amoxicillin; clavulanic acid | Augmentin |
| Amidate | etomidate | | |
| amifostine | Ethyol | Amoxil | amoxicillin |
| amikacin sulfate | Amikin | amphetamine resins (W) | Biphetamine (W) |
| Amikin | amikacin sulfate | | |
| amiloride HCl | Midamor | amphetamine; dextroamphet- amine mixed salts | Adderall |
| amiloride; hydro- chlorothiazide | Moduretic | | |
| amino acid inj | Aminosyn Travasol TrophAmine | Amphojel | aluminum hydroxide |
| amino acid with electrolytes in dextrose with calcium inj (various concentrations) | Clinimix E | Amphotec | amphotericin B cholesteryl sulfate |
| | | amphotericin B | Fungizone |
| | | amphotericin B cholesteryl sulfate | Amphotec |
| aminocaproic acid | Amicar | amphotericin B lipid complex | Abelcet |
| aminocaproic acid gel | Caprogel | *ampicillin* | Principen |
| | | ampicillin sodium; sulbactam sodium | Unasyn |
| aminogluteth- imide | Cytadren | | |
| aminolevulinic acid HCl topical soln | Levulan Kerastick | amprenavir | Agenerase |
| | | amrinone (former name) | inamrinone (new name) |
| aminophylline | aminophylline | | |
| aminosalicylic acid | Paser | amsacrine | Amsidyl |
| Aminosyn | amino acid inj | Amsidyl | amsacrine |
| amiodarone HCl | Cordarone | Amvisc | sodium hyaluronate |
| *amitriptyline HCl* | Elavil Endep | Amytal | amobarbital sodium |
| AmLactin | ammonium lactate lotion | Anadrol-50 | oxymetholone |
| amlexanox oral paste | Aphthasol | Anafranil | clomipramine HCl |

| | | | |
|---|---|---|---|
| anagrelide HCl | Agrylin | Apresoline | hydralazine HCl |
| anakinra | Kineret | aprotinin | Trasylol |
| Anaprox | naproxen sodium | AquaMEPHY-TON | phytonadione |
| anastrozole | Arimidex | Aralen | chloroquine phosphate |
| Anbesol | benzocaine | | |
| Ancef | cefazolin sodium | Aramine | metaraminol bitartrate |
| Ancobon | flucytosine | Aranesp | darbepoetin |
| Androderm | testosterone transdermal system | Arava | leflunomide |
| | | arbutamine HCl | GenEsa |
| | | arcitumomab | CEA-Scan |
| AndroGel | testosterone gel | ardeparin sodium (W) | Normiflo (W) |
| Androgel-DHT | dihydro-testosterone transdermal | Arduan | pipecuronium bromide |
| Anectine | succinylcholine chloride | Aredia | pamidronate disodium |
| Anexsia | hydrocodone bitartrate; acetaminophen | Arestin | minocycline HCl dental microspheres |
| Angiomax | bivalirudin | Arfonad | trimethaphan camsylate |
| Ansaid | flurbiprofen | | |
| Antabuse | disulfiram | argatroban | argatroban |
| Antagon | ganirelix acetate | arginine HCl | R-Gene |
| antihemophilic factor (recombinant) | Kogenate ReFacto | Aricept | donepezil HCl |
| | | Arimidex | anastrozole |
| | | Aristocort | triamcinolone acetonide |
| Antilirium | physostigmine salicylate | Arixtra | fondaparinux sodium |
| antipyrine otic | Auralgan | | |
| antithrombin III (human) | Thrombate III | Aromasin | exemestane |
| | | arsenic trioxide | Trisenox |
| antithymocyte globulin, (rabbit) | Thymoglobulin | Artane (W) | trihexyphenidyl HCl (W) |
| | | Arthrotec | diclofenac; misoprostol |
| Antivert | meclizine | | |
| Antizol | fomepizole | Asacol | mesalamine |
| Anturane | sulfinpyrazone | Asendin | amoxapine |
| Anzemet | dolasetron mesylate | Aslera | prasterone |
| | | asparaginase | Elspar |
| Aphthasol | amlexanox oral paste | aspirin 325 mg with codeine phosphate (30 and 60 mg) | Empirin with codeine #3 and #4 |
| A.P.L. | chorionic gonadotropin | | |
| apligraf | Graftskin | aspirin buffered | Bufferin |
| Aplisol | tuberculin skin test | *aspirin EC* | Ecotrin |
| | | Astelin | azelastine HCl nasal spray |
| apomorphine HCl | Uprima | | |
| Aposyn | exisulind | astemizole (W) | Hismanal (W) |
| Apresazide | hydralazine HCl; hydrochloro-thiazide | Atacand | candesartan cilexetil |
| | | Atarax | hydroxyzine HCl |

| | | | |
|---|---|---|---|
| *atenolol* | Tenormin | Axert | almotriptan |
| atenolol; | Tenoretic | | malate |
| chlorthalidone | | Axid | nizatidine |
| Atgam | lymphocyte | Azactam | aztreonam |
| | immune | azatadine | Optimine |
| | globulin | maleate | |
| articaine; | Septocaine | azathioprine | Imuran |
| epinephrine | | azelaic acid | Azelex |
| aspirin; extended- | Aggrenox | cream | Finevin |
| release | | azelastine HCl | Astelin |
| dipyridamole | | nasal spray | |
| Atacand HCT | candesartan | azelastine HCl | Optivar |
| | cilexetil; | ophth soln | |
| | hydrochloro- | Azelex | azelaic acid |
| | thiazide | | cream |
| Ativan | lorazepam | azithromycin | Zithromax |
| atorvastatin | Lipitor | Azmacort | triamcinolone |
| calcium | | | acetonide |
| atovaquone | Mepron | | aerosol |
| atovaquone; | Malarone | Azopt | brinzolamide |
| proguanil HCl | | | ophth susp |
| atracurium | Tracrium | aztreonam | Azactam |
| besylate | | Azulfidine | sulfasalazine |
| Atridox | doxycycline | | |
| | hyclate gel | | |
| Atromid-S | clofibrate | **B** | |
| atropine sulfate | Sal-Tropine | | |
| tablets | | | |
| Atrovent | ipratropium | | |
| | bromide | Baciguent | bacitracin |
| Augmentin | amoxicillin; | | ointment |
| | clavulanic acid | bacitracin | Baciguent |
| Auralgan | antipyrine otic | ointment | |
| auranofin | Ridaura | baclofen | Lioresal |
| Aurolate | gold sodium | Bactrim | sulfamethoxa- |
| | thiomalate | | zole; trimeth- |
| aurothioglucose | Solganal | | oprim |
| Avalide | irbesartan; | Bactroban | mupirocin nasal |
| | hydrochloro- | | ointment |
| | thiazide | BAL in Oil | dimercaprol |
| Avandia | Rosiglitazone | Basaljel | aluminum |
| | maleate | | carbonate |
| Avanir | docosanol cream | balsalazide | Colazal |
| Avapro | irbesartan | disodium | |
| Avelox | moxifloxacin HCl | basiliximab | Simulect |
| Aventyl | nortriptyline HCl | Baycol (W) | cerivastatin |
| Avinza | morphine sulfate | | sodium (W) |
| | tab SR | BCG intravesical | Pacis TheraCys |
| Avita | tretinoin cream | | TICE BCG |
| | 0.025% | becaplermin gel | Regranex |
| Avitene | collagen | beclomethasone | Beclovent |
| | hemostat | dipropionate | Beconase AQ |
| Avonex | interferon beta-la | | Nasal |

| | |
|---|---|
| | Qvar |
| | Vancenase |
| | Vancenase AQ Nasal |
| | Vanceril |
| Beclovent | beclomethasone dipropionate |
| Beconase AQ Nasal | beclomethasone dipropionate |
| belladonna alkaloids; phenobarbital | Donnatal |
| Bellergal-S | phenobarbital; ergotamine; belladonna |
| Benadryl | diphenhydramine HCl |
| benazepril HCl | Lotensin |
| BeneFix | factor IX, (recombinant) |
| Benemid | probenecid |
| Benicar | olmesartan medoxomil |
| bentoquatam | IvyBlock |
| Bentyl | dicyclomine HCl |
| Benzamycin | erythromycin; benzoyl peroxide topical gel |
| benzocaine | Anbesol |
| | Hurricaine |
| | Orabase |
| | Orajel |
| benzocaine; tetracaine HCl | Cetacaine |
| benztropine mesylate | Cogentin |
| bepridil | Vascor |
| beractant | Survanta |
| Berroca | vitamin B complex; folic acid; vitamin C |
| Betadine | povidone iodine |
| 17β-estradiol; norgestimate | Ortho-Prefest |
| Betagan | levobunolol HCl |
| betaine anhydrous | Cystadane |
| betamethasone | Celestone |
| betamethasone dipropionate | Diprosone |

| | |
|---|---|
| betamethasone; clotrimazole cream | Lotrisone |
| betamethasone valerate (foam) | Luxiq |
| Betapace | sotalol |
| Betaseron | interferon beta-1b |
| betaxolol | Kerlone |
| betaxolol HCl ophth soln | Betoptic |
| betaxolol HCl ophth susp | Betoptic S |
| betaxolol HCl; pilocarpine HCl ophth soln | Betoptic Pilo |
| bethanechol chloride | Urecholine |
| Betoptic | betaxolol HCl ophth soln |
| Betoptic Pilo | betaxolol HCl; pilocarpine HCl, ophth soln |
| Betoptic S | betaxolol HCl ophth suspension |
| bexarotene gel | Targretin |
| Bextra | valdecoxib |
| Bexxar | tositumomab and I-131 tositumomab |
| Biaxin | clarithromycin |
| Biaxin XL | clarithromycin SR |
| bicalutamide | Casodex |
| Bicillin C-R | penicillin G benzathine; penicillin G procaine (for IM use only) |
| Bicillin L-A | penicillin G benzathine (for IM use only) |
| Bicitra | sodium citrate; citric acid |
| BiCNU | carmustine |
| Bilopaque | tyropanoate sodium |
| bimatoprost ophth soln | Lumigan |
| biperiden | Akineton |
| Biphetamine (W) | amphetamine resins (W) |

B
R℞

373

| | |
|---|---|
| bisacodyl | Dulcolax |
| bismuth subsalicylate; metronidazole; tetracycline HCl | Helidac |
| bisoprolol fumarate; hydrochlorothi- azide | Ziac |
| bitolterol mesylate | Tornalate |
| bivalirudin | Angiomax |
| Blenoxane | bleomycin sulfate |
| bleomycin sulfate | Blenoxane |
| Blocadren | timolol maleate |
| bosentan | Tracleer |
| B & O Supprettes | opium; belladonna suppositories |
| Botox | botulinum toxin type A |
| botulinum toxin type A | Botox |
| botulinum toxin type B | Myobloc |
| Bravelle | urofollitropin |
| Brethaire | terbutaline sulfate aerosol |
| Brethine | terbutaline sulfate tablets and inj |
| bretylium tosylate | Bretylol |
| Bretylol | bretylium tosylate |
| Brevibloc | esmolol HCl |
| Brevital Sodium | methohexital sodium |
| Bricanyl | terbutaline sulfate tablets and inj |
| brimonidine tartrate ophth | Alphagan |
| brinzolamide ophth suspension | Azopt |
| bromocriptine mesylate | Parlodel |
| brompheniramine maleate | Dimetane |

| | |
|---|---|
| brompheniramine maleate; phenylpropan- olamime | Dimetapp Extentabs |
| Bronkometer | isoetharine HCl aerosol |
| Bronkosol | isoetharine HCl soln |
| Bucladin-S | buclizine HCl |
| buclizine HCl | Bucladin-S |
| budesonide capsule SR | Entocort EC |
| budesonide inhalation powder | Pulmicort Turbuhaler |
| budesonide nasal inhaler | Rhinocort |
| Bufferin | aspirin buffered |
| bumetanide | Bumex |
| Bumex | bumetanide |
| Buminate | albumin human |
| Buphenyl | phenylbutyrate sodium |
| bupivacaine HCl | Marcaine HCl |
| bupropion HCl | Wellbutrin |
| bupropion HCl SR | Wellbutrin SR Zyban |
| BuSpar | buspirone HCl |
| buspirone HCl | BuSpar |
| busulfan | Myleran |
| busulfan inj | Busulfex |
| Busulfex | busulfan inj |
| butabarbital sodium | Butisol |
| butalbital; acetaminophen; caffeine | Fioricet |
| butalbital; aspirin; caffeine | Fiorinal |
| butenafine HCl | Mentax |
| Butisol | butabarbital sodium |
| butoconazole nitrate vaginal cream | Gynazole |
| butorphanol tartrate inj | Stadol |
| butorphanol tartrate nasal spray | Stadol NS |

# C

| | |
|---|---|
| cabergoline | Dostinex |
| Cafcit | caffeine citrate inj |
| Cafergot | ergotaminetartrate; caffeine |
| caffeine citrate inj | Cafcit |
| Calan SR | verapamil HCl SR |
| Calciferol | ergocalciferol |
| Calcimar | calcitonin |
| calcipotriene cream | Dovonex |
| calcitonin | Calcimar |
| calcitonin-salmon | Miacalcin |
| calcitriol | Rocaltrol |
| calcium carbonate | Os-Cal 500 Tums |
| calcium carbonate; vitamin D and K chewable | Viactiv |
| calfactant intratracheal susp | Infasurf |
| Campath | alemtuzumab |
| camphorated tincture of opium | paregoric |
| Camptosar | irinotecan HCl |
| candesartan cilexetil | Atacand |
| candesartan cilexetil; hydrochlorothiazide | Atacand HCT |
| Cancidas | caspofungin acetate |
| Capastat Sulfate | capreomycin sulfate |
| capecitabine | Xeloda |
| Capital w/ Codeine Suspension | codeine phosphate; acetaminophen suspension |
| Capitrol | chloroxine |
| Capoten | captopril |
| capreomycin sulfate | Capastat Sulfate |
| Caprogel | aminocaproic acid gel |
| capromab pendetide | ProstaScint |
| captopril | Capoten |
| Carafate | sucralfate |
| carbachol | Isopto Carbachol |
| carbamazepine | Tegretol |
| carbamazepine SR | Carbatrol Tegretol-XR |
| carbamide peroxide otic | Debrox |
| Carbatrol | carbamazepine SR |
| carbenicillin | Geocillin |
| Carbex | selegiline |
| Carbocaine | mepivacaine HCl |
| carboplatin | Paraplatin |
| Cardene | nicardipine HCl |
| Cardiolite | technetium Tc99m sestamibi |
| Cardiotec | technetium Tc-99m teboroxime kit |
| Cardizem | diltiazem HCl |
| Cardizem CD | diltiazem HCl SR |
| Cardura | doxazosin mesylate |
| carisoprodol | Soma |
| carmustine | BiCNU |
| carmustine implantable wafer | Gliadel |
| Carnitor | levocarnitine |
| Cartia XR | diltiazem HCl SR |
| carvedilol | Coreg |
| Casodex | bicalutamide |
| caspofungin acetate | Cancidas |
| Cataflam | diclofenac potassium |
| Catapres | clonidine HCl |
| Cathflo Activase | alteplase (for catheter occlusions) |

C
R

| | | | |
|---|---|---|---|
| Caverject | alprostadil | CellCept | mycophenolate mofetil |
| CEA-SCAN | arcitumomab | | |
| Ceclor | cefaclor | Cenestin | synthetic conjugated estrogens, A |
| Cedax | ceftibuten | | |
| CeeNu | lomustine | | |
| cefaclor | Ceclor | Centrum | vitamins; minerals |
| cefadroxil | Duricef | cephalexin | Keflex |
| Cefadyl | cephapirin sodium | cephalexin HCl | Keftab |
| cefamandole nafate | Mandol | cephalothin sodium (W) | Keflin (W) |
| cefazolin sodium | Ancef Kefzol | cephapirin sodium | Cefadyl |
| cefdinir | Omnicef | cephradine | Velosef |
| cefditoren pivoxil | Spectracef | Cephulac | lactulose |
| | | Ceptaz | ceftazidime |
| cefepime HCl | Maxipime | Cerebyx | fosphenytoin sodium |
| cefixime | Suprax | | |
| Cefizox | ceftizoxime sodium | Ceredase | alglucerase |
| | | Cerezyme | imiglucerase |
| Cefobid | cefoperazone sodium | cerivastatin sodium (W) | Baycol (W) |
| cefonicid sodium | Monocid | Cernevit-12 | multivitamins for infusion |
| cefoperazone sodium | Cefobid | | |
| | | Cerubidine | daunorubicin HCl |
| Cefotan | cefotetan | Cervidil | dinoprostone vaginal insert |
| cefotaxime sodium | Claforan | | |
| | | Cetacaine | benzocaine; tetracaine HCl |
| cefotetan | Cefotan | | |
| cefoxitin sodium | Mefoxin | cetirizine HCl | Zyrtec |
| cefpodoxime proxetil | Vantin | cetirizine HCL; pseudoephedrine HCl SR | Zyrtec-D |
| cefprozil | Cefzil | | |
| ceftazidime | Ceptaz Fortaz Tazicef Tazidime | cetrorelix | Cetrotide |
| | | Cetrotide | cetrorelix |
| | | cevimeline HCl | Evoxac |
| | | Chirocaine | levobupivacaine |
| ceftibuten | Cedax | chloral hydrate | chloral hydrate |
| Ceftin | cefuroxime axetil | chlorambucil | Leukeran |
| ceftizoxime sodium | Cefizox | chloramphenicol | Chloromycetin |
| | | chloramphenicol ophth | Chloroptic ophth |
| ceftriaxone sodium | Rocephin | | |
| | | chlordiazepoxide HCl | Librium |
| cefuroxime axetil | Ceftin | | |
| cefuroxime sodium | Kefurox Zinacef | chlordiazepoxide HCl; amitriptyline HCl | Limbitrol |
| Cefzil | cefprozil | | |
| Celebrex | celecoxib | | |
| celecoxib | Celebrex | chlorhexidine gluconate | Hibiclens PerioChip |
| Celestone | betamethasone | | |
| Celexa | citalopram hydrobromide | chlorhexidine gluconate mouth rinse | Peridex |

| | | | |
|---|---|---|---|
| Chloromycetin | chloramphenicol | ciprofloxacin HCl | Cipro |
| chloroprocaine HCl | Nesacaine | ciprofloxacin; hydrocortisone otic | Cipro HC Otic |
| Chloroptic ophth | chloramphenicol ophth | ciprofloxacin ophth soln | Ciloxan |
| chloroquine phosphate | Aralen | Cipro HC Otic | ciprofloxacin; hydrocortisone otic |
| chlorothiazide | Diuril | | |
| chloroxine | Capitrol | cisapride (W) | Propulsid (W) |
| chlorpheniramine maleate | Chlor-Trimeton | cisatracurium besylate | Nimbex |
| chlorpheniramine maleate SR | Teldrin | cisplatin | Platinol AQ |
| chlorpromazine | Thorazine | citalopram hydrobromide | Celexa |
| chlorpropamide | Diabinese | cladribine | Leustatin |
| chlorthalidone | Hygroton | Claforan | cefotaxime sodium |
| chlorthalidone; reserpine | Regroton | | |
| Chlor-Trimeton | chlorpheniramine maleate | Clarinex | desloratadine |
| | | clarithromycin | Biaxin |
| chlorzoxazone 250 mg | Paraflex | clarithromycin SR | Biaxin XL |
| | | Claritin | loratadine |
| chlorzoxazone 500 mg | Parafon Forte DSC | Claritin D | loratadine; pseudoephedrine sulfate |
| Cholebrine | iocetamic acid | | |
| Choledyl | oxtriphylline | | |
| cholestyramine | Questran | clemastine fumarate | Tavist |
| choline chloride inj | Intrachol | Cleocin | clindamycin HCl |
| choline magnesium trisalicylate | Trilisate | clidinium (W) bromide | Quarzan (W) |
| | | clidinium; chlordiazepoxide | Librax |
| Choloxin (W) | dextrothyroxine sodium (W) | | |
| | | Climara | estradiol transdermal |
| chorionic gonadotropin | A.P.L. | clindamycin; benzoyl peroxide gel | BenzaClin |
| choriogonadotropin alfa | Ovidrel | | |
| Chronulac | lactulose | clindamycin HCl | Cleocin |
| Chymodiactin | chymopapain | clindamycin phosphate pledgets | Clindets |
| chymopapain | Chymodiactin | | |
| Cibalith-S | lithium citrate | | |
| ciclopirox cream and lotion | Loprox | Clindets | clindamycin phosphate pledgets |
| ciclopirox soln | Penlac Nail Lacquer | | |
| cidofovir | Vistide | Clinimix E | amino acid with electrolytes in dextrose with calcium inj (various concentrations) |
| cilostazol | Pletal | | |
| Ciloxan | ciprofloxacin ophth soln | | |
| cimetidine HCl | Tagamet | | |
| Cipro | ciprofloxacin HCl | Clinoril | sulindac |

C
R

| | | | |
|---|---|---|---|
| clioquinol | Vioform | colistin sulfate; | Coly-Mycin S |
| clobetasol foam | Olux | hydrocortisone, | |
| clobetasol | Clobevate | and neomycin | |
| propionate | | otic soln | |
| gel | | collagen | Avitene |
| Clobevate | clobetasol | hemostat | |
| | propionate gel | collagenase | Santyl |
| clofibrate | Atromid-S | Collyrium | tetrahydrozoline |
| Clomid | clomiphene citrate | | HCl ophth |
| clomiphene | Clomid | Colomed | short chain fatty |
| citrate | | | acids enema |
| clomipramine | Anafranil | Coly-Mycin M | colistimethate |
| HCl | | | sodium |
| clonazepam | Klonopin | Coly-Mycin S | colistin sulfate; |
| clonidine HCl | Catapres | | hydrocortisone, |
| clonidine HCl inj | Duraclon | | and neomycin |
| clopidogrel | Plavix | | otic soln |
| bisulfate | | CoLyte | polyethylene |
| clorazepate | Tranxene | | glycol- |
| dipotassium | | | electrolyte soln |
| Clorpactin WCS- | oxychlorosene | CombiPatch | norethindrone |
| 90 | sodium | | acetate; |
| clotrimazole | Gyne-Lotrimin | | estradiol |
| | Lotrimin | | transdermal |
| | Mycelex | Combivent | ipratropium |
| clozapine | Clozaril | | bromide; |
| Clozaril | clozapine | | albuterol |
| coagulation | BeneFix | | sulfate |
| factor IX | | Combivir | lamivudine; |
| (recombinant) | | | zidovudine |
| coagulation factor | NovoSeven | Compazine | prochlorperazine |
| VII a | | Comtan | entacapone |
| (recombinant) | | Comvax | *Haemophilus b* |
| coal tar product | Zetar | | conjugate; |
| codeine | Capital w/ | | Hepatitis B |
| phosphate; | Codeine | | vaccine |
| acetaminophen | Suspension | Concerta | methylphenidate |
| suspension | | | HCl SR |
| coenzyme Q10 | UbiQGel | Condylox | podofilox gel |
| Cogentin | benztropine | Copaxone | glatiramer |
| | mesylate | | acetate |
| Cognex | tacrine HCl | Cordarone | amiodarone |
| Colace | docusate sodium | | HCl |
| Colazol | balsalazide | Coreg | carvedilol |
| | disodium | Corgard | nadolol |
| ColBENEMID | probenecid; | Corlopam | fenoldopam |
| (W) | colchicine (W) | | mesylate |
| colchicine | colchicine | Cortef | hydrocortisone |
| colesevelam HCl | Welchol | corticorellin | Acthrel |
| Colestid | colestipol HCl | ovine triflutate | |
| colestipol HCl | Colestid | corticotropin | Acthar |
| colistimethate | Coly-Mycin M | cortisone acetate | Cortone Acetate |
| sodium | | Cortone Acetate | cortisone acetate |

| | | | |
|---|---|---|---|
| Cortrosyn | cosyntropin | Cyclogyl | cyclopentolate HCl |
| Corvert | ibutilide fumarate | | |
| Cosmegen | dactinomycin | cyclopentolate HCl | Cyclogyl |
| Cosopt | dorzolamide HCl; timolol maleate ophth soln | cyclophospha-mide | Cytoxan Neosar Seromycin |
| | | cycloserine | |
| cosyntropin | Cortrosyn | cyclosporine | Sandimmune |
| Cotazym | pancrelipase | cyclosporine capsules (modified) and oral soln | Neoral |
| Cotazym-S | pancrelipase EC | | |
| Cotrim | sulfamethoxa-zole; trimethoprim | cyclosporine capsules, (modified) | Gengraf |
| co-trimoxazole | Bactrim Cotrim Septra sulfamethoxa-zole; trimetho-prim | cyclosporine ophth emulsion | Restasis |
| | | Cycrin | medroxyproges-terone acetate |
| | | Cylert | pemoline |
| Coumadin | warfarin sodium | cyproheptadine HCl | Periactin |
| Covera HS | verapamil HCl SR bedtime formulation | Cystadane | betaine anhydrous |
| Cozaar | losartan potassium | Cystospaz-M | hyoscyamine sulfate SR |
| Crinone | progesterone gel | Cytadren | aminogluteth-imide |
| Crixivan | indinavir | | |
| CroFab | crotalidae polyvalent immune fab (ovine) | cytarabine | Cytosar-U |
| | | cytarabine, liposomal inj | DepoCyt |
| | | Cytomel | liothyronine sodium |
| cromolyn sodium | Gastrocrom Nasalcrom Opticrom | | |
| | | Cytosar-U | cytarabine |
| | | Cytotec | misoprostol |
| crotalidae polyvalent immune fab (ovine) | CroFab | Cytovene | ganciclovir |
| | | Cytoxan | cyclophosphamide |
| crotamiton | Eurax | | |
| Cuprimine | penicillamine | | |
| Curosurf | poractant alpha intratracheal susp | | |

## D

| | | | |
|---|---|---|---|
| Cutivate | fluticasone propionate cream & ointment | dacarbazine | DTIC-Dome |
| | | daclizumab | Zenapax |
| | | dactinomycin | Cosmegen |
| | | Dalmane | flurazepam HCl |
| cyanocobalamin nasal gel | Nascobal | dalteparin sodium | Fragmin |
| cyclobenzaprine HCl | Flexeril | danaparoid sodium | Orgaran |
| | | danazol | Danocrine |
| Cyclocort | amcinonide | Danocrine | danazol |

C
R

379

| | | | |
|---|---|---|---|
| Dantrium | dantrolene sodium | denileukin diftitox | Ontak |
| dantrolene sodium | Dantrium | Depacon | valproate sodium inj |
| dapsone | dapsone | Depakene | valproic acid |
| Daranide | dichlorphenamide | Depakote | divalproex sodium |
| Daraprim | pyrimethamine | Depakote ER | divalproex sodium SR |
| darbepoetin | Aranesp | | |
| Darvocet-N 100 | propoxyphene napsylate; acetaminophen | DepoCyt | cytarabine, liposomal inj |
| Darvon | propoxyphene HCl | Depo-Medrol | methylprednisolone acetate SR |
| Darvon Compound 65 | propoxyphene HCl; aspirin; caffeine | Depo-Provera | medroxyprogesterone acetate SR |
| daunorubicin citrate liposomal | DaunoXome | Depo-Testosterone | testosterone cypionate SR |
| daunorubicin HCl | Cerubidine | Desferal | deferoxamine mesylate |
| DaunoXome | daunorubicin citrate liposomal | desflurane | Suprane |
| | | desipramine HCl | Norpramin |
| Daypro | oxaprozin | desloratadine | Clarinex |
| DDAVP | desmopressin acetate | desmopressin acetate | DDAVP |
| Debrox | carbamide peroxide otic | Desogen | desogestrel; ethinyl estradiol |
| Decadron | dexamethasone | | |
| Deca-Durabolin | nandrolone decanoate | desogestrel; ethinyl estradiol | Desogen |
| Declomycin | demeclocycline HCl | desogestrel and ethinyl estradiol; ethinyl estradiol | Mircette |
| deferoxamine mesylate | Desferal | | |
| delavirdine mesylate | Rescriptor | | |
| | | desonide | Tridesilon |
| Delestrogen | estradiol valerate | desoximetasone | Topicort |
| Deltasone | prednisone | Desoxyn | methamphetamine HCl |
| Demadex | torsemide | | |
| demecarium bromide | Humorsol | Desyrel | trazodone HCl |
| | | Detrol | tolterodine tartrate |
| demeclocycline HCl | Declomycin | Detrol LA | tolterodine tartrate (SR) |
| Demerol | meperidine HCl | dexamethasone | Decadron |
| Demser | metyrosine | | Hexadrol |
| Demulen | ethynodiol diacetate; ethinyl estradiol | dexchlorpheniramine maleate SR | Polaramine Repetabs |
| | | Dexedrine | dextroamphetamine sulfate |
| Denavir | penciclovir cream | | |

| | | | |
|---|---|---|---|
| dexfenfluramine HCl (W) | Redux (W) | diethylcarbamazine citrate | Hetrazan |
| Dexferrum | iron dextran inj | diethylpropion HCl | Tenuate |
| dexmedetomidine HCl inj | Precedex | Differin | adapalene |
| dexmethylphenidate HCl | Focalin | diflorasone diacetate | Florone |
| | | Diflucan | fluconazole |
| dexrazoxane | Zinecard | diflunisal | Dolobid |
| dextroamphetamine sulfate | Dexedrine | Digibind | digoxin immune fab |
| | | digoxin | Lanoxin |
| | | digoxin capsules | Lanoxicaps |
| dextrothyroxine sodium (W) | Choloxin (W) | digoxin immune fab | Digibind |
| D.H.E. 45 | dihydroergotamine mesylate inj | dihydroergotamine mesylate inj | D.H.E. 45 |
| DiaBeta | glyburide | dihydroergotamine mesylate nasal spray | Migranol |
| Diabinese | chlorpropamide | | |
| Diamox | acetazolamide | | |
| Diapid (W) | lypressin (W) | dihydrotestosterone transdermal | Androgel-DHT |
| Diastat | diazepam rectal gel | | |
| diazepam | Valium | Dilacor XR | diltiazem HCl SR |
| diazepam emulsified inj | Dizac | Dilantin | phenytoin |
| | | Dilaudid | hydromorphone HCl |
| diazepam rectal gel | Diastat | diltiazem HCl | Cardizem |
| | | diltiazem HCl SR | Cardizem CD |
| diazoxide | Hyperstat | | Cartia XR |
| Dibenzyline | phenoxybenzamine HCl | | Dilacor XR |
| | | | Tiazac |
| dibucaine | Nupercainal | diltiazem maleate SR | Tiamate |
| dichlorphenamide | Daranide | | |
| diclofenac gel | Solaraze | dimenhydrinate | Dramamine |
| diclofenac potassium | Cataflam | dimercaprol | BAL in Oil |
| | | Dimetane | brompheniramine maleate |
| diclofenac sodium | Voltaren | | |
| diclofenac sodium; misoprostol | Arthrotec | dinoprostone gel | Prepidil |
| | | dinoprostone vaginal insert | Cervidil |
| diclofenac sodium SR | Voltaren-XR | dinoprostone vaginal suppositories | Prostin E2 |
| dicloxacillin sodium | Dynapen | | |
| | | Diovan | valsartan |
| dicyclomine HCl | Bentyl | Diovan HCT | valsartan; hydrochlorothiazide |
| didanosine | Videx | | |
| didanosine SR | Videx EC | Dipentum | olsalazine sodium |
| Didronel | etidronate disodium | | |
| | | diphenhydramine HCl | Benadryl |

**D**
**R**

| | | | |
|---|---|---|---|
| diphenoxylate HCl; atropine sulfate | Lomotil | dorzolamide HCl | Trusopt |
| dipivefrin | Propine | dorzolamide HCl; timolol maleate ophth soln | Cosopt |
| Diprivan | propofol | | |
| Diprosone | betamethasone dipropionate | | |
| dipyridamole | Persantine | Dostinex | cabergoline |
| dirithromycin | Dynabac | Dovonex | calcipotriene cream |
| Disalcid | salsalate | | |
| disopyramide phosphate | Norpace | doxacurium chloride | Nuromax |
| disulfiram | Antabuse | doxapram HCl | Dopram |
| Ditropan | oxybutynin chloride | doxazosin mesylate | Cardura |
| Diulo (WA) | metolazone | doxepin HCl | Adapin Sinequan |
| Diuril | chlorothiazide | | |
| divalproex sodium | Depakote | doxepin HCl cream | Prudoxin |
| divalproex sodium SR | Depakote ER | doxercalciferol | Hectorol |
| Dizac | diazepam emulsified inj | Doxidan | docusate calcium; phenolphthalein |
| dobutamine HCl | Dobutrex | Doxil | doxorubicin, liposomal |
| Dobutrex | dobutamine HCl | doxorubicin HCl | Adriamycin Rubex |
| docetaxel | Taxotere | | |
| docosanol cream | Avanir | doxorubicin, liposomal | Doxil |
| docusate calcium | Surfak | | |
| docusate calcium; phenolphthalein | Doxidan | doxycycline hyclate | Vibramycin |
| docusate sodium | Colace | doxycycline hyclate 20 mg tab & cap | Periostat |
| docusate sodium; casanthranol | Peri-Colace | | |
| dofetilide | Tikosyn | doxycycline hyclate gel | Atridox |
| dolasetron mesylate | Anzemet | Dramamine | dimenhydrinate |
| Dolobid | diflunisal | Drisdol | ergocalciferol |
| Dolophine | methadone HCl | Dristan Long Lasting | oxymetazoline HCl |
| Domeboro | aluminum acetate | Drixoral Syrup | pseudoephedrine HCl; bromphiramine maleate |
| donepezil HCl | Aricept | | |
| Donnatal | belladonna alkaloids; phenobarbital | dronabinol | Marinol |
| | | droperidol | Inapsine |
| dopamine HCl | Intropin | drospirenone; ethinyl estradiol | Yasmin |
| Dopar | levodopa | | |
| Dopram | doxapram HCl | drotrecogin alfa | Xigris |
| | | Droxia | hydroxyurea |
| dornase alpha | Pulmozyme | DTIC-Dome | dacarbazine |

| | | | |
|---|---|---|---|
| Dulcolax | bisacodyl | Elidel | pimecrolimus cream |
| Durabolin (W) | nandrolone phenpropionate (W) | Eligard | leuprolide acetate |
| | | Elitek | rasburicase |
| Duraclon | clonidine HCl inj | Elixophyllin | theophylline |
| | | Ellence | epirubicin HCl |
| Duragesic | fentanyl transdermal | Elmiron | pentosan polysulfate sodium |
| Duramorph | morphine sulfate inj | Elocon | mometasone furoate topical |
| Duranest | etidocaine HCl | | |
| Duricef | cefadroxil | Eloxatin | oxaliplatin |
| Dyazide | triamterene 37.5 mg; hydro-chlorothiazide 25 mg | Elspar | asparaginase |
| | | Emadine | emedastine difumarate opthth soln |
| Dymelor | acetohexamide | Emcyt | estramustine phosphate sodium |
| Dynabac | dirithromycin | | |
| DynaCirc | isradipine | | |
| Dynapen | dicloxacillin sodium | emedastine difumarate opthth soln | Emadine |
| dyphylline | Lufyllin | EMLA Cream | lidocaine; prilocaine cream |
| Dyrenium | triamterene | | |
| | | Empirin with codeine #3 and #4 | aspirin 325 mg with codeine phosphate (30 and 60 mg) |
| **E** | | | |
| | | E-Mycin | erythromycin |
| EchoGen | perflenapent emulsion | enalapril maleate | Vasotec |
| | | enalapril maleate; diltiazem malate | Teczem |
| echothiophate iodide (W) | Phospholine Iodide (W) | | |
| Ecotrin | aspirin EC | enalapril maleate; felodipine SR | Lexxel |
| Edecrin | ethacrynic acid | | |
| edetate disodium | Endrate | | |
| Edex | alprostadil inj | enalapril maleate; hydrochlorothi-azide | Vaseretic |
| edrophonium chloride | Tensilon | | |
| E.E.S. 400 | erythromycin ethylsuccinate | Enbrel | etanercept |
| | | encainide HCl | Enkaid |
| efavirenz | Sustiva | Endep | amitriptyline HCl |
| Effexor | venlafaxine HCl | Endocet | oxycodone HCl; acetaminophen |
| Effexor XR | venlafaxine HCl SR | | |
| | | Endrate | edetate disodium |
| eflornithine HCl cream | Vaniqa | Enduron | methyclothiazide |
| | | enflurane | Ethrane |
| Efudex | fluorouracil cream; soln | Engerix-B | hepatitis B vaccine |
| Elavil | amitriptyline HCl | | |
| Eldepryl | selegiline HCl | | |
| Eldisine | vindesine sulfate | | |

D
R

383

| | |
|---|---|
| Enkaid | encainide HCl |
| enoxaparin sodium | Lovenox |
| entacapone | Comtan |
| Entex LA | phenylpropanol-amine HCl; guaifenesin SR |
| Entocort EC | budesonide capsule SR |
| epinephrine | Adrenalin |
| epinephrine racemic | Vaponefrin |
| epirubicin HCl | Ellence |
| Epivir | lamivudine |
| Epivir HBV | lamivudine |
| eplerenone | Inspra |
| epoetin alfa | Epogen Procrit |
| Epogen | epoetin alfa |
| epoprostenol sodium | Flolan |
| eprosartan mesylate | Teveten |
| eptifibatide | Integrilin |
| Equanil (WA) | meprobamate |
| Ergamisol (W) | levamisole HCl (W) |
| ergocalciferol | Calciferol Drisdol |
| ergoloid mesylates | Hydergine |
| ergotamine tartrate; caffeine | Cafergot |
| ergotamine tartrate | Ergostat |
| Ergotrate | ergonovine maleate |
| ertapenem sodium | Invanz |
| Ery-Tab | erythromycin EC |
| Erythrocin Stearate | erythromycin stearate |
| erythromycin | E-Mycin |
| erythromycin base coated particles | PCE Dispertab |
| erythromycin; benzoyl peroxide topical gel | Benzamycin |

| | |
|---|---|
| erythromycin EC | Ery-Tab |
| erythromycin estolate | Ilosone |
| erythromycin ethylsuccinate | E.E.S. 400 |
| erythromycin ethylsuccinate; sulfisoxazole | Pediazole |
| erythromycin stearate | Erythrocin Stearate |
| escitalopram oxalate | Lexapro |
| Esclim | estradiol transdermal |
| Eserine Sulfate | physostigmine ophth ointment |
| Esidrix | hydrochlorothi-azide |
| Esimil | guanethidine monosulfate; hydrochloro-thiazide |
| Eskalith | lithium carbonate |
| esmolol HCl | Brevibloc |
| esomeprazole magnesium | Nexium |
| estazolam | ProSom |
| Estinyl | ethinyl estradiol |
| Estrace | estradiol |
| Estraderm | estradiol transdermal |
| estradiol | Estrace |
| estradiol hemihydrate vaginal tab | Vagifem |
| estradiol transdermal | Alora Climara Esclim Estraderm FemPatch Vivelle |
| estradiol vaginal ring | Estring |
| estradiol valerate | Delestrogen |
| estramustine phosphate sodium | Emcyt |
| Estratest | estrogens, esterified; methyltestos-terone |

| | | | |
|---|---|---|---|
| Estratest H.S. | estrogens, esterified; methyltestosterone, half strength | etomidate | Amidate |
| | | etonogestrel; ethinyl estradiol vagina ring | NuvaRing |
| Estring | estradiol vaginal ring | Etopophos | etoposide phosphate diethanolate |
| estrogens, conjugated | Premarin | etoposide | VePesid |
| estrogens conjugate, A synthetic | Cenestin | etoposide phosphate diethanolate | Etopophos |
| estrogens, conjugated; medroxyprogesterone acetate | Premphase Prempro | Etrafon | perphenazine; amitriptyline HCl |
| | | Eulexin | flutamide |
| estrogens, esterified; methyltestosterone | Estratest | Eurax | crotamiton |
| | | Euthroid (WA) | liotrix |
| | | Eutonyl | pargyline HCl |
| estrogens, esterified methyltestosterone, half strength | Estratest H.S. | Evista | raloxifene HCl |
| | | Evoxac | cevimeline HCl |
| | | Exelon | rivastigmine tartrate |
| estropipate | Ogen | exemestane | Aromasin |
| Estrostep | norethindrone acetate; ethinyl estradiol | exisulind | Aposyn |
| | | Ex-Lax | sennosides |
| etanercept | Enbrel | | |
| ethacrynic acid | Edecrin | | |
| ethambutol HCl | Myambutol | factor IX, concentrate | BeneFix |
| ethchlorvynol | Placidyl | Factrel | gonadorelin HCl |
| Ethezyme | papain; urea oint | famciclovir | Famvir |
| ethinyl estradiol | Estinyl | famotidine | Pepcid |
| ethionamide | Trecator-SC | famotidine, oral disintegrating tablet | Pepcid RPD |
| Ethmozine | moricizine | | |
| ethopropazine HCl | Parsidol | Famvir | famciclovir |
| ethosuximide | Zarontin | Fansidar | sulfadoxine; pyrimethamine |
| Ethrane | enflurane | | |
| ethyl chloride | ethyl chloride | Fareston | toremifene citrate |
| ethynodiol diacetate; ethinyl estradiol | Demulen | | |
| | | Faslodex | fulvestrant |
| | | Fastin | phentermine HCl |
| Ethyol | amifostine | fat emulsion | Intralipid Liposyn II and III |
| etidocaine HCl | Duranest | | |
| etidronate disodium | Didronel | felbamate | Felbatol |
| etodolac | Lodine | Felbatol | felbamate |
| etodolac SR | Lodine XL | Feldene | piroxicam |

F

| | | | |
|---|---|---|---|
| felodipine | Plendil | Fiorinal | butalbital; aspirin; caffeine |
| Femara | Ietrozole | | |
| Femhrt | norethindrone acetate; ethinyl estradiol | Flagyl | metronidazole |
| | | Flagyl ER | metronidazole SR |
| FemPatch | estradiol transdermal | flavoxate HCl | Urispas |
| fenfluramine HCl (W) | Pondimin (W) | Flaxedil | gallamine triethiodide |
| fenofibrate | Tricor | flecainide acetate | Tambocor |
| fenoldopam mesylate | Corlopam | Flexeril | cyclobenzaprine HCl |
| fenoprofen calcium | Nalfon | Flolan | epoprostenol sodium |
| fentanyl citrate | Sublimaze | Flomax | tamsulosin HCl |
| fentanyl citrate; droperidol | Innovar | Flonase | fluticasone propionate spray |
| Fentanyl Oralet | fentanyl transmucosal | Florinef | fludrocortisone acetate |
| fentanyl transdermal | Duragesic | Florone | diflorasone diacetate |
| fentanyl transmucosal | Actiq | Floropryl | isoflurophate |
| | Fentanyl Oralet | Florotag | synopinine |
| Feosol | ferrous sulfate | Flovent | fluticasone propionate spray |
| Fer-In-Sol | ferrous sulfate | | |
| Fergon | ferrous gluconate | | |
| Feridex | ferumoxide HCl | Floxin | ofloxacin |
| Ferrlecit | sodium ferric gluconate complex in sucrose inj | Floxin Otic | ofloxacin otic soln |
| | | floxuridine | FUDR |
| | | fluconazole | Diflucan |
| ferrous gluconate | Fergon | flucytosine | Ancobon |
| ferrous sulfate | Feosol Fer-In-Sol | Fludara | fludarabine phosphate |
| ferrous sulfate SR | SlowFe | fludarabine phosphate | Fludara |
| Fertinex | urofollitropin for inj | fludrocortisone acetate | Florinef |
| ferumoxetil oral suspension | Gastromark | Flumadine | rimantadine |
| | | flumazenil | Romazicon |
| ferumoxide HCl | Feridex | flunisolide | Aero Bid |
| fexofenadine HCl | Allegra | fluocinolone acetonide | Synalar |
| filgrastim | Neupogen | fluocinonide | Lidex |
| finasteride | Propecia 1 mg tablet | Fluor-I-Strip | fluorescein sodium strips |
| | Proscar 5 mg tablet | fluorescein sodium soln | Fluorescite |
| Finevin | azelaic cream | fluorescein sodium strips | Fluor-I-Strip |
| Fioricet | butalbital; acetamino-phen; caffeine | Fluorescite | fluorescein sodium soln |

| | |
|---|---|
| fluorometholone | FML |
| Fluoroplex | fluorouracil cream; soln |
| *fluorouracil inj* | *fluorouracil inj* |
| fluorouracil cream; soln | Efudex |
| | Fluoroplex |
| Fluothane | halothane |
| fluoxetine HCl | Prozac |
| | Sarafem |
| fluoxymesterone | Halotestin |
| fluphenazine HCl | Permitil |
| | Prolixin |
| flurazepam HCl | Dalmane |
| flurbiprofen | Ansaid |
| flutamide | Eulexin |
| fluticasone propionate spray | Flonase |
| | Flovent |
| fluticasone propionate cream & ointment | Cutivate |
| fluticasone propionate; salmeterol inhalation powder | Advair Diskus |
| fluvastatin sodium | Lescol |
| fluvoxamine maleate | Luvox |
| FML | fluorometholone |
| Focalin | dexmethyl-phenidate HCl |
| Folex PFS | methotrexate inj |
| *folic acid* | Folvite |
| Follistim | follitropin beta |
| follitropin alfa | Gonal-F |
| follitropin beta | Follistim |
| Folvite | folic acid |
| fomepizole | Antizol |
| fomivirsen sodium inj | Vitravene |
| fondaparinux sodium | Arixtra |
| Foradil | formoterol fumarate |
| Forane | isoflurane |
| formoterol fumarate | Foradil |
| Fortaz | ceftazidime |
| Fortovase | saquinavir soft gel capsule |
| Fosamax | alendronate sodium |
| foscarnet | Foscavir |
| Foscavir | foscarnet |
| fosfomycin tromethamine | Monurol |
| fosinopril sodium | Monopril |
| fosphenytoin sodium | Cerebyx |
| Fragmin | dalteparin sodium |
| Frova | frovatriptan succinate |
| frovatriptan succinate | Frova |
| FUDR | floxuridine |
| fulvestrant | Faslodex |
| Fulvicin P/G | griseofulvin |
| Fungizone | amphotericin B |
| Furacin | nitrofurazone |
| *furosemide* | Lasix |

## G

| | |
|---|---|
| gabapentin | Neurontin |
| Gabitril | tiagabine HCl |
| gadoteridol | ProHance |
| gadoversetamide | OptiMark |
| galantamine HBr | Reminyl |
| gallamine triethiodide | Flaxedil |
| gallium nitrate | Ganite |
| Galzin | zinc acetate |
| Gamimune N | immune globulin intravenous |
| Gammagard S/D | immune globulin intravenous |
| ganciclovir | Cytovene |
| ganciclovir ophthalmic implant | Vitrasert |
| ganirelix acetate | Antagon |
| Ganite | gallium nitrate |
| Gantanol (W) | sulfamethoxazole (W) |
| Garamycin | *gentamicin sulfate* |

F
R

| | | | |
|---|---|---|---|
| Gastrocrom | cromolyn sodium | glycopyrrolate | Robinul |
| Gastromark | ferumoxetil oral suspension | Glynase | glyburide micronized |
| gatifloxacin | Tequin | Glyset | miglitol |
| gemcitabine HCl | Gemzar | gold sodium thiomalate | Aurolate |
| gemfibrozil | Lopid | GoLYTELY | polyethylene glycol-electrolyte soln |
| gemtuzumab ozogamicin | Mylotarg | | |
| Gemzar | gemcitabine HCl | gonadorelin HCl | Factrel |
| GenEsa | arbutamine HCl | Gonal-F | follitropin alfa |
| Gengraf | cyclosporine capsules, (modified) | goserelin acetate implant | Zoladex |
| | | graftskin | Apligraf |
| Genotropin | somatropin for inj | granisetron HCl | Kytril |
| | | grepafloxacin HCl (W) | Raxar (W) |
| *gentamicin sulfate* | Garamycin | Grifulvin V | griseofulvin |
| Geocillin | carbenicillin | griseofulvin | Fulvicin P/G |
| Geodon | ziprasidone HCl | | Grifulvin V |
| Geref | sermorelin acetate | guaifenesin | Organidin NR |
| glatiramer acetate | Copaxone | | Robitussin |
| | | guaifenesin; codeine phosphate | Robitussin A-C Tussi-Organidin NR |
| Gleevec | imatinib mesylate | | |
| Gliadel | carmustine implantable wafer | | |
| | | guaifenesin; dextromethor-phan | Robitussin-DM |
| glimepiride | Amaryl | | |
| glipizide | Glucotrol | guanabenz acetate | Wytensin |
| glipizide SR | Glucotrol XL | | |
| GlucaGen | glucagon (rDNA origin) | guanadrel sulfate | Hylorel |
| | | guanethidine monosulfate | Ismelin |
| glucagon | glucagon | | |
| glucagon (rDNA origin) | GlucaGen | guanethidine monosulfate; hydrochlorothi-azide | Esimil |
| Glucophage | metformin HCl | | |
| Glucophage XR | metformin HCl SR | guanfacine HCl | Tenex |
| Glucotrol | glipizide | Gynazole | butoconazole nitrate vaginal cream |
| Glucotrol XL | glipizide SR | | |
| Glucovance | glyburide; metformin HCl | Gyne-Lotrimin | clotrimazole |
| glyburide | DiaBeta Micronase | | |
| glyburide; metformin HCl | Glucovance | **H** | |
| glyburide micronized | Glynase | | |
| glycerin ophth soln | Ophthalgan | Habitrol | nicotine transdermal system |

*Haemophilus b* conjugate vaccine reconstituted with diphtheria and tetanus toxoids and acellular pertussis vaccine adsorbed — ActHIB/Tripedia

*Haemophilus b* conjugate; Hepatitis B vaccine — Comvax

haemophilus b vaccine — Hib-Immune (W)
HibTITER
PedvaxHIB
ProHIBiT

halcinonide — Halog
Halcion — triazolam
Haldol — haloperidol
Halfan — halofantrine HCl
halofantrine HCl — Halfan
Halog — halcinonide
haloperidol — Haldol
haloprogin — Halotex
Halotestin — fluoxymesterone
Halotex — haloprogin
halothane — Fluothane
Havrix — hepatitis A vaccine, inactivated
Healon — sodium hyaluronate
Hectorol — doxercalciferol
Helidac — bismuth subsalicylate; metronidazole; tetracycline HCl
*heparin sodium* — *heparin sodium*
hepatitis A inactivated; hepatitis B (recombinant) vaccine — Twinrix
hepatitis A vaccine, inactivated — Havrix
Vaqta
hepatitis B immune — NABI-HB

globulin (human)
hepatitis B vaccine — Engerix-B
Recombivax HB
Herceptin — trastuzumab
Herplex (W) — idoxuridine (W)
Hespan — hetastarch
hetastarch — Hespan
hetastarch in lactated electrolyte inj — Hextend
Hetrazan — diethylcarbamazine citrate
Hexadrol — dexamethasone
Hexalen — altretamine
Hextend — hetastarch in lactated electrolyte inj
Hib-Immune (WA) — haemophilus b vaccine
Hibiclens — chlorhexidine gluconate
HibTITER — haemophilus b vaccine
Hiprex — methenamine hippurate
Hismanal (W) — astemizole (W)
Hivid — zalcitabine
homatropine hydrobromide ophth — Isopto Homatropine
Humalog — insulin, lispro (human)
Humalog Mix75/25 — insulin lispro protamine susp 75%; insulin lispro inj 25% [rDNA origin]
Humatin — paromomycin sulfate
Humatrope — somatropin
Humorsol — demecarium bromide
Humulin 70/30 — isophane insulin suspension 70%, insulin inj 30% (human)
Humulin L — insulin zinc suspension (Lente) (human)

H
R

| | | | |
|---|---|---|---|
| Humulin N | isophane insulin suspension (NPH) (human) | *hydrocortisone* | Cortef |
| | | | Hydrocortone |
| Humulin R | insulin inj (human) | hydrocortisone buteprate cream | Pandel |
| Humulin U Ultralente | insulin zinc suspension, extended, (human) | hydrocortisone sodium succinate | Solu-Cortef |
| Hurricane | benzocaine | Hydrocortone | hydrocortisone |
| Hyalgan | sodium hyaluronate | HydroDIURIL | hydrochlorothiazide |
| hyaluronidase | Wydase | hydroflumethiazide | Saluron |
| Hycamtin | topotecan HCl | | |
| Hydergine | ergoloid mesylates | *hydromorphone HCl* | Dilaudid |
| hydralazine HCl | Apresoline | hydromorphone HCl SR | Palladone XL |
| hydralazine HCl; hydrochlorothiazide | Apresazide | Hydromox (W) | quinethazone (W) |
| hydralazine; hydrochlorothiazide; reserpine | Ser-Ap-Es | hydroquinone topical susp | Alustra |
| Hydrea | hydroxyurea | hydroquinone; tretinoin; fluocinolone cream | Tri-Luma |
| *hydrochlorothiazide* | Esidrix | hydroxychloroquine sulfate | Plaquenil |
| | HydroDIURIL | hydroxyurea | Droxia |
| | Microzide | | Hydrea |
| | Oretic | hydroxyzine HCl | Atarax |
| hydrocodone bitartrate; acetaminophen | Anexsia 5/500 | hydroxyzine pamoate | Vistaril |
| | Anexsia 7.5/650 | | |
| | Lorcet 10/650 | Hygroton | chlorthalidone |
| | Lorcet-HD (5/500) | hylan G-F 20 | Synvisc |
| | Lorcet plus (7.5/650) | Hylorel | guanadrel sulfate |
| | Lortab 2.5/500; 5/500; 7.5/500; 10/500 | hyoscyamine sulfate orally disintegrating tab | NuLev |
| | Norco | hyoscyamine sulfate SR | Cystospaz-M |
| | Vicodin | | Levbid |
| | Vicodin ES | Hyperab (W) | rabies immune globulin, human |
| | Zydone 5/400, 7.5/400, 10/400 | Hyperstat | diazoxide |
| hydrocodone bitartrate 7.5 mg; ibuprofen 200 mg | Vicoprofen | Hyper-Tet (W) | tetanus immune globulin (human) (W) |
| | | Hytrin | terazosin HCl |
| hydrocodone polistirex; chlorpheniramine | Tussionex | Hyzaar | losartan potassium; hydrochlorothiazide |

# I-J

ibritumomab tiuxetan — Zevalin
*ibuprofen* — Advil
Motrin
Nuprin
ibutilide fumarate — Corvert
Idamycin — idarubicin
idarubicin — Idamycin
idoxuridine (W) — Herplex (W)
IFEX — ifosfamide
ifosfamide — IFEX
Ilosone — erythromycin estolate
Imagent GI — perflubron
imatinib mesylate — Gleevec
imciromab pentetate — Myoscint
Imdur — isosorbide mononitrate SR
imiglucerase — Cerezyme
imipenem-cilastatin sodium — Primaxin
imipramine HCl — Tofranil
imiquimod cream — Aldara
Imitrex — sumatriptan
immune globulin intravenous — Gamimune N
Gammagard S/D
Sandoglobulin
Imodium — loperamide HCl
Imogam — rabies immune globulin, human
Imuran — azathioprine
inamrinone — Inocor
Inapsine — droperidol
indapamide — Lozol
Inderal — propranolol HCl
Inderide — propranolol HCl; hydrochlorothiazide
indinavir — Crixivan
indium In-111 pentetreotide — OctreoScan
Indocin — indomethacin

indomethacin — Indocin
Infasurf — calfactant intratracheal susp
INFeD — iron dextran inj
Infergen — interferon alfacon-1
infliximab — Remicade
Innohep — tinzaparin sodium
Innovar — fentanyl citrate; droperidol
Inocor — inamrinone
INOmax — nitric oxide for inhalation
Inspra — eplerenone
insulin aspart (rDNA origin) — NovoLog
insulin glargine (rDNA origin) — Lantus
insulin inj (human) — Humulin R
Novolin R
Velosulin Human
insulin lispro (human) — Humalog
insulin lispro protamine susp 75%; insulin lispro inj 25% [rDNA origin] — Humalog Mix75/25
insulin zinc suspension (Lente) (human) — Humulin L
Novolin L
insulin zinc suspension, extended (beef) — Ultralente U
insulin zinc suspension, extended, (human) — Humulin U
Ultralente
Integrilin — eptifibatide
interferon alfa-2a — Roferon-A
interferon alfa-2b — Intron A
interferon alfa-n[1] lymphoblastoid — Wellferon
interferon alfa-n3 (human leukocyte derived) — Alferon
interferon alfacon-1 — Infergen
interferon beta-la — Avonex

| | |
|---|---|
| | Rebif |
| interferon beta-1b | Betaseron |
| interferon gamma 1-b | Actimmune |
| Intrachol | choline chloride inj |
| Intralipid | fat emulsion |
| Intron A | interferon alfa-2b |
| Intropin | dopamine HCl |
| Invanz | ertapenem sodium |
| Inversine | mecamylamine HCl |
| Invirase | saquinavir mesylate |
| iocetamic acid | Cholebrine |
| iodamide meglumine | Renovue 65 |
| iodixanol | Visipaque |
| iohexol | Omnipaque |
| Ionamin | phentermine resin |
| iopamidol | Isovue |
| iopanoic acid | Telepaque |
| iopromide | Ultravist |
| iotrolan | Osmovist |
| ioversol | Optiray |
| ioxilan | Oxilan |
| Ipol | poliovirus vaccine inactivated |
| ipratropium bromide | Atrovent |
| ipratropium bromide; albuterol sulfate | Combivent |
| irbesartan | Avapro |
| irbesartan; hydrochlorothiazide | Avalide |
| irinotecan HCl | Camptosar |
| iron dextran inj | INFeD / Dexferrum |
| iron sucrose inj | Venofer |
| Ismelin | guanethidine monosulfate |
| ISMO | isosorbide mononitrate |
| isocarboxazid | Marplan |
| isoetharine HCl aerosol | Bronkometer |
| isoetharine HCl soln | Bronkosol |
| isoflurane | Forane |
| isoflurophate | Floropryl |
| *isoniazid* | Nydrazid |
| isoniazid; rifampin | Rifamate |
| isophane insulin suspension (NPH) (human) | Humulin N / Novolin N |
| isophane insulin suspension (NPH) 70%, insulin inj 30% (human) | Humulin 70/30 / Novolin 70/30 |
| isoproterenol HCl | Isuprel |
| Isoptin | verapamil HCl |
| Isopto Carbachol | carbachol ophth |
| Isopto Carpine | pilocarpine HCl ophth |
| Isopto Homatropine | homatropine hydrobromide ophth |
| Isopto Hyoscine | scopolamine hydrobromide ophth |
| Isordil | isosorbide dinitrate |
| isosorbide dinitrate | Isordil |
| isosorbide mononitrate | ISMO |
| isosorbide mononitrate SR | Imdur |
| isotretinoin | Accutane |
| Isovue | iopamidol |
| isoxsuprine HCl | Vasodilan |
| isradipine | DynaCirc |
| Isuprel | isoproterenol HCl |
| itraconazole | Sporanox |
| ivermectin | Stromectol |
| IvyBlock | bentoquatam |

## K

| | |
|---|---|
| Kadian | morphine sulfate SR |
| Kaletra | lopinavir; ritonavir |

| | | | |
|---|---|---|---|
| kanamycin sulfate | Kantrex | | bicarbonate effervescent |
| Kantrex | kanamycin sulfate | Kogenate | antihemophilic factor (recombinant) |
| Kaon | potassium gluconate | Kolyum | potassium chloride; potassium gluconate |
| Kaon-Cl | potassium chloride SR | | |
| Kayexalate | polystyrene sulfonate sodium | Konsyl-D | psyllium |
| | | Kwell (WA) | lindane |
| K-Dur | potassium chloride SR | Kytril | granisetron HCl |
| Keflex | cephalexin | | |
| Keflin (W) | cephalothin sodium (W) | **L** | |
| Keftab | cephalexin HCl | | |
| Kefurox | cefuroxime sodium | labetalol HCl | Normodyne Trandate |
| Kefzol | cefazolin sodium | Lac-Hydrin | lactic acid; ammonium lactate lotion |
| Kemadrin | procyclidine HCl | | |
| Kenalog | triamcinolone acetonide | | |
| Keppra | levetiracetam | lactic acid; ammonium lactate lotion | Lac-Hydrin |
| Kerlone | betaxolol | | |
| Ketalar | ketamine HCl | | |
| ketamine HCl | Ketalar | lactulose | Cephulac Chronulac |
| ketoconazole | Nizoral | Lamictal | lamotrigine |
| ketoprofen | Orudis | Lamisil | terbinafine HCl |
| ketoprofen SR | Oruvail | lamivudine | Epivir Epivir HBV |
| ketorolac tromethamine | Toradol | | |
| ketorolac tromethamine ophth | Acular | lamivudine; zidovudine | Combivir |
| | | lamivudine; zidovudine; abacavir sulfate | Trizivir |
| ketotifen fumarate ophth soln | Zaditor | | |
| Kineret | anakinra | lamotrigine | Lamictal |
| Klaron | sodium sulfacetamide lotion | Lanoxicaps | digoxin capsules |
| | | Lanoxin | digoxin |
| | | lansoprazole | Prevacid |
| Klonopin | clonazepam | lansoprazole; amoxicillin; clarithromycin | Prevpac |
| Klor-Con 10 | potassium chloride SR | | |
| K-Lyte | potassium bicarbonate; potassium citrate effervescent | Lantus | insulin glargine (rDNA origin) |
| | | Lariam | mefloquine HCl |
| | | Larodopa | levodopa |
| | | Lasix | furosemide |
| K-Lyte/Cl | potassium chloride potassium | latanoprost | Xalatan |
| | | leflunomide | Arava |
| | | lepirudin | Refludan |

393

| | | | |
|---|---|---|---|
| Lescol | fluvastatin sodium | | Tri-Levlen Triphasil |
| letrozole | Femara | levonorgestrel | Norplant (W) |
| *leucovorin* | Wellcovorin | implant (W) | |
| *calcium* | | levonorgestrel- | Mirena |
| Leukeran | chlorambucil | releasing | |
| Leukine | sargramostim | intrauterine | |
| leuprolide | Eligard | system | |
| acetate | Lupron | Levophed | norepinephrine |
| leuprolide | Viadur | | bitartrate |
| acetate | | levorphanol | Levo-Dromoran |
| implant | | tartrate | |
| Leustatin | cladribine | levothyroxine | Levoxyl |
| levalbuterol HCl | Xopenex | sodium | Synthroid |
| inhalation soln | | Levoxyl | levothyroxine |
| levamisole | Ergamisol (W) | | sodium |
| HCl (W) | | Levulan Kerastick | aminolevulinic |
| Levaquin | levofloxacin | | acid HCl |
| Levbid | hyoscyamine | | topical soln |
| | sulfate SR | Lexapro | escitalopram |
| levetiracetam | Keppra | | oxalate |
| Levlite | levonorgestrel; | Lexxel | enalapril maleate; |
| | ethinyl | | felodipine SR |
| | estradiol | Librax | clidinium; |
| levobupivacaine | Chirocaine | | chlordiaz- |
| levocabastine | Livostin | | epoxide |
| HCl ophth | | Librium | chlordiazepoxide |
| susp | | | HCl |
| Levo-Dromoran | levorphanol | Lidex | fluocinonide |
| | tartrate | lidocaine HCl | Xylocaine |
| levobunolol | Betagan | | HCl |
| HCl | | lidocaine patch | Lidoderm |
| levocarnitine | Carnitor | lidocaine; | EMLA Cream |
| levodopa | Dopar | prilocaine | |
| | Larodopa | cream | |
| levodopa; | Sinemet | Lidoderm | lidocaine patch |
| carbidopa | | Limbitrol | chlordiazepoxide |
| levodopa; | Sinemet CR | | HCl; amitrip- |
| carbidopa | | | tyline HCl |
| SR | | Lincocin | lincomycin |
| levofloxacin | Levaquin | | HCl |
| levofloxacin | Quixin | lincomycin HCl | Lincocin |
| ophth soln | | *lindane* | Kwell (WA) |
| levomethadyl | Orlaam | | lindane |
| acetate HCl | | linezolid | Zyvox |
| levonorgestrel | Plan B | Lioresal | baclofen |
| levonorgestrel; | Alesse | liothyronine | Cytomel |
| ethinyl | Levlite | sodium | |
| estradiol | Nordette | liothyronine | Triostat |
| | Preven | sodium inj | |
| | Emergency | liotrix | Thyrolar |
| | Contraceptive | Lipitor | atorvastatin |
| | Kit | | calcium |

394

L
R

| | | | |
|---|---|---|---|
| liposomal amphotericin B | AmBisome | Lorcet (various combinations) | hydrocodone bitartrate; acetaminophen |
| Liposyn II and III | fat emulsion | Lortab (various combinations) | hydrocodone bitartrate; acetaminophen |
| lisinopril | Prinivil Zestril | | |
| lisinopril; hydrochloro-thiazide | Zestoretic | losartan potassium | Cozaar |
| *lithium carbonate* | Eskalith Lithobid | losartan potassium; hydrochlorothi-azide | Hyzaar |
| lithium citrate | Cibalith-S | | |
| Lithobid | lithium carbonate | Lotemax | loteprednol etabonate ophth susp |
| Lithostat | acetohydroxamic acid | Lotensin | benazepril HCl |
| Livostin | levocabastine HCl ophth susp | loteprednol etabonate ophth susp | Alrex Lotemax |
| Lodine | etodolac | | |
| Lodine XL | etodolac SR | Lotrel | amlodipine besylate; benazepril HCl |
| lodoxamide tromethamine ophth soln | Alomide | | |
| | | Lotrimin | clotrimazole |
| Loestrin | norethindrone acetate; ethinyl estradiol | Lotrisone | betamethasone; clotrimazole cream |
| | | Lotronex (W) | alosetron (W) |
| lomefloxacin | Maxaquin | lovastatin | Mevacor |
| Lomotil | diphenoxylate HCl; atropine sulfate | lovastatin; niacin | Advicor |
| | | Lovenox | enoxaparin sodium |
| lomustine | CeeNu | | |
| Loniten | minoxidil tablets | loxapine succinate | Loxitane |
| Lo/Ovral | norgestrel; ethinyl estradiol | | |
| | | Loxitane | loxapine succinate |
| loperamide HCl | Imodium | Lozol | indapamide |
| Lopid | gemfibrozil | Ludiomil (W) | maprotiline HCl (W) |
| lopinavir; ritonavir | Kaletra | Lufyllin | dyphylline |
| Lopressor | metoprolol tartrate | LumenHance | manganese chloride |
| Loprox | ciclopirox cream and lotion | Lunelle | medroxy-progesterone acetate; estradiol cypionate inj |
| Lorabid | loracarbef | | |
| loracarbef | Lorabid | | |
| loratadine | Claritin | Lupron | leuprolide acetate |
| loratadine; pseudoephe-drine sulfate | Claritin D | Luride | sodium fluoride |
| | | Luvox | fluvoxamine maleate |
| lorazepam | Ativan | Luxiq | betamethasone valerate (foam) |

L R

| | | | |
|---|---|---|---|
| Lyme disease vaccine (W) | LYMErix (W) | Maxaquin | lomefloxacin |
| LYMErix (W) | Lyme disease vaccine (W) | Maxipime | cefepime HCl |
| | | Maxzide | triamterene 75 mg; hydro-chlorothiazide 50 mg |
| lymphocyte immune globulin | Atgam | | |
| lypressin (W) | Diapid (W) | Maxzide-25MG | triamterene 37.5 mg; hydro-chlorothiazide 25 mg |
| Lysodren | mitotane | | |
| | | mazindol | Sanorex |
| **M** | | measles, mumps, rubella vaccines, combined | M-M-R II |
| Maalox | aluminum hydroxide; magnesium hydroxide | Mebaral | mephobarbital |
| | | mebendazole | Vermox |
| | | mecamylamine HCl | Inversine |
| Macrobid | nitrofurantoin macrocrystals and mono-hydrate | mechlorethamine HCl | Mustargen |
| | | Meclan | meclocycline sulfosalicylate |
| Macrodantin | nitrofurantoin macrocrystals | meclizine | Antivert |
| magaldrate | Riopan | meclocycline sulfosalicylate | Meclan |
| manganese chloride | LumenHance | meclofenamate sodium | Meclomen |
| magnesium chloride SR | Slow-Mag | Meclomen | meclofenamate sodium |
| magnesium oxide | MAG-OX 400 | Medrol | methylpredniso-lone |
| magnesium sulfate | magnesium sulfate | medroxyproges-terone acetate | Cycrin Provera |
| MAG-OX 400 | magnesium oxide | medroxyproges-terone acetate; estradiol cypionate inj | Lunelle |
| Malarone | atovaquone; proguanil HCl | | |
| Mandol | cefamandole nafate | | |
| mangofodipir trisodium | Teslascan | medroxyproges-terone acetate SR | Depo-Provera |
| maprotiline HCl (W) | Ludiomil (W) | mefenamic acid | Ponstel |
| | | mefloquine HCl | Lariam |
| Marcaine HCl | bupivacaine HCl | Mefoxin | cefoxitin sodium |
| Marinol | dronabinol | Megace | megestrol acetate |
| Marplan | isocarboxazid | megestrol acetate | Megace |
| Matulane | procarbazine HCl | Mellaril | thioridazine HCl |
| Mavik | trandolapril | meloxicam | Mobic |
| Maxalt | rizatriptan benzoate | melphalan | Alkeran |
| | | menadiol sodium diphosphate | Synkayvite |
| Maxalt-MLT | rizatriptan oral disintegrating tablet | menotropins | Pergonal Repronex |

L
R

| | |
|---|---|
| Mentax | butenafine HCl |
| *meperidine HCl* | Demerol |
| mephentermine sulfate | Wyamine |
| mephenytoin | Mesantoin |
| mephobarbital | Mebaral |
| mepivacaine HCl | Carbocaine |
| meprobamate | Equanil (WA) |
| | Miltown |
| Mepron | atovaquone |
| mercaptopurine | Purinethol |
| Meridia | sibutramine HCl monohydrate |
| meropenem | Merrem |
| Merrem | meropenem |
| Meruvax II | rubella virus vaccine live attenuated |
| mesalamine | Asacol |
| | Rowasa |
| Mesantoin | mephenytoin |
| mesna | Mesnex |
| Mesnex | mesna |
| mesoridazine | Serentil |
| Mestinon | pyridostigmine bromide |
| Metadate ER | methylphenidate HCl SR |
| Metamucil | psyllium |
| Metaprel | metaproterenol sulfate |
| metaproterenol sulfate | Alupent |
| | Metaprel |
| metaraminol bitartrate | Aramine |
| Metaret | suramin |
| Metastron | strontium-89 chloride inj |
| metformin HCl | Glucophage |
| metformin HCl SR | Glucophage XR |
| methadone HCl | Dolophine |
| methamphetamine HCl | Desoxyn |
| methazolamide | Neptazane |
| methenamine combination | Urised |
| methenamine hippurate | Hiprex |
| Methergine | methylergonovine maleate |
| methicillin sodium (W) | Staphcillin (W) |

| | |
|---|---|
| methimazole | Tapazole |
| methocarbamol | Robaxin |
| methohexital sodium | Brevital Sodium |
| *methotrexate* | Mexate |
| | Rheumatrex |
| | Trexall |
| methotrexate, preservative-free inj | Folex PFS |
| methoxamine HCl | Vasoxyl |
| methoxsalen | Oxsoralen |
| methoxsalen extracorporeal administration | Uvadex |
| methscopolamine bromide | Pamine |
| methyclothiazide | Enduron |
| methyldopa | Aldomet |
| methyldopa; hydrochlorothiazide | Aldoril |
| methylergonovine maleate | Methergine |
| Methylin | methylphenidate HCl |
| Methylin ER | methylphenidate HCl SR |
| methylphenidate HCl | Methylin |
| | Ritalin |
| methylphenidate SR | Concerta |
| | Metadate ER |
| | Methylin ER |
| | Ritalin SR |
| methylprednisolone | Medrol |
| methylprednisolone acetate SR inj | Depo-Medrol |
| methylprednisolone sodium succinate inj | Solu-Medrol |
| methyltestosterone | *methyltestosterone* |
| methysergide maleate | Sansert |
| Meticorten | prednisone |
| metoclopramide HCl | Reglan |
| metolazone | Mykrox |
| | Zaroxolyn |
| Metopirone | metyrapone |

M
R

| | | | |
|---|---|---|---|
| metoprolol succinate SR | Toprol XL | MiraLax | polyethylene glycol 3350 powder |
| metoprolol tartrate | Lopressor | Mirapex | pramipexole dihydrochloride |
| MetroGel-Vaginal | metronidazole vaginal gel | Mircette | desogestrel; ethinyl estradiol and |
| *metronidazole* | Flagyl | | ethinyl estradiol |
| metronidazole SR | Flagyl ER | | |
| metronidazole vaginal gel | MetroGel-Vaginal | | |
| metyrapone | Metopirone | Mirena | levonorgestrel-releasing intrauterine system |
| metyrosine | Demser | | |
| Mevacor | lovastatin | | |
| Mexate | methotrexate | | |
| mexiletine HCl | Mexitil | mirtazapine | Remeron |
| Mexitil | mexiletine HCl | misoprostol | Cytotec |
| Mezlin | mezlocillin | Mithracin | plicamycin |
| mezlocillin | Mezlin | mitomycin | Mutamycin |
| Miacalcin | calcitonin-salmon | mitotane | Lysodren |
| mibefradil dihydrochloride (W) | Posicor (W) | mitoxantrone HCl | Novantrone |
| | | Mivacron | mivacurium chloride |
| Micardis | telmisartan | | |
| Micro K | potassium chloride SR | mivacurium chloride | Mivacron |
| miconazole nitrate | Monistat | M-M-R II | measles, mumps, rubella vaccines, combined |
| Micronase | glyburide | | |
| Micronor | norethindrone | | |
| Microzide | hydrochloro-thiazide | Moban | molindone HCl |
| | | Mobic | meloxicam |
| Midamor | amiloride HCl | modafinil | Provigil |
| midazolam HCl | Versed | Moduretic | amiloride HCl; hydrochloro-thiazide |
| midodrine HCl | ProAmatine | | |
| Mifeprex | mifepristone | | |
| mifepristone | Mifeprex | moexipril HCl | Univasc |
| miglitol | Glyset | moexipril HCl; hydrochloro-thiazide | Uniretic |
| Migranol | dihydroergota-mine mesylate nasal spray | | |
| | | molindone HCl | Moban |
| milrinone lactate | Primacor | mometasone furoate topical | Elocon |
| Miltown | meprobamate | | |
| Minipress | prazosin HCl | Mometasone furoate monohydrate nasal spray | Nasonex |
| Minocin | minocycline HCl | | |
| minocycline HCl | Minocin | | |
| minocycline HCl dental microspheres | Arestin | | |
| | | Monistat | miconazole nitrate |
| minoxidil tablets | Loniten | Monocid | cefonicid sodium |
| minoxidil topical | Rogaine | Monopril | fosinopril sodium |
| Mintezol | thiabendazole | | |
| Miochol E | acetylcholine ophth | montelukast sodium | Singulair |

M R

| | |
|---|---|
| Monurol | fosfomycin tromethamine |
| moricizine | Ethmozine |
| morphine sulfate | Roxanol |
| morphine sulfate, immediate release concentrated oral soln | Roxanol-T |
| *morphine sulfate inj* | Duramorph |
| *morphine sulfate SR* | Avinza<br>Kadian<br>MS Contin<br>Oramorph SR<br>Roxanol SR |
| Motrin | ibuprofen |
| moxifloxacin HCl | Avelox |
| MS Contin | morphine sulfate SR |
| Mucomyst | acetylcysteine |
| multivitamins for infusion | Cernevit-12<br>Multi-12 (vial 1 and vial 2) |
| mupirocin nasal ointment | Bactroban |
| muromonab-CD3 | Orthoclone OKT3 |
| Muse | alprostadil urethral suppository |
| Mustargen | mechlorethamine HCl |
| Mutamycin | mitomycin |
| M.V.I.-12 | vitamin, multiple inj |
| Myambutol | ethambutol HCl |
| Mycelex | clotrimazole |
| Mycifradin Sulfate | neomycin sulfate oral soln |
| Myciguent | neomycin sulfate ointment and cream |
| Mycolog Cream | nystatin; triamcinolone cream |
| mycophenolate mofetil | CellCept |
| Mycostatin | nystatin |
| Mydriacyl | tropicamide |
| Mykrox | metolazone |
| Myleran | busulfan |
| Mylicon | simethicone |

| | |
|---|---|
| Mylotarg | gemtuzumab ozogamicin |
| Myobloc | botulinum toxin type B |
| Myochrysine (WA) | gold sodium thiomalate |
| Myoscint | imciromab pentetate |
| Mysoline | primidone |

## N

| | |
|---|---|
| NABI-HB | hepatitis B immune globulin (human) |
| nabumetone | Relafen |
| nadolol | Corgard |
| Nafcil (W) | nafcillin sodium |
| nafcillin sodium (W) | Nafcil (W)<br>Unipen (W) |
| nalbuphine HCl | Nubain |
| Nalfon | fenoprofen calcium |
| nalidixic acid | NegGram |
| nalmefene HCl | Revex |
| naloxone HCl | Narcan |
| naltrexone | ReVia |
| nandrolone phenpropionate (W) | Durabolin (W) |
| nandrolone decanoate | Deca-Durabolin |
| naphazoline ophth soln | Vasocon |
| Naprelan | naproxen sodium SR |
| Naprosyn | naproxen |
| naproxen | Naprosyn |
| naproxen sodium | Anaprox |
| naproxen sodium SR | Naprelan |
| naratriptan HCl | Amerge |
| Narcan | naloxone HCl |
| Nardil | phenelzine sulfate |
| Naropin | ropivacaine HCl |
| Nasacort | triamcinolone acetonide nasal inhaler |
| Nasalcrom | cromolyn sodium |

M
R

| | | | |
|---|---|---|---|
| Nascobal | cyanocobalamin nasal gel | nesiritide | Natrecor |
| Nasonex | Mometasone furoate monohydrate nasal spray | netilmicin sulfate | Netromycin |
| | | Netromycin | netilmicin sulfate |
| | | Neulasta | pegfilgrastim |
| | | Neumega | oprelvekin |
| nateglinide | Starlix | Neupogen | filgrastim |
| Natrecor | nesiritide | Neurolite | technetium Tc-99m bicisate kit |
| Navane | thiothixene | | |
| Navelbine | vinorelbine tartrate | Neurontin | gabapentin |
| Nebcin | tobramycin sulfate | Neutrexin | trimetrexate glucuronate |
| NebuPent | pentamidine isethionate aerosol | nevirapine | Viramune |
| | | Nexium | esomeprazole magnesium |
| nedocromil inhalation | Tilade | niacin SR | Niaspan |
| | | Niaspan | Nicobid |
| nedocromil ophth soln | Alocril | | niacin SR |
| | | nicardipine HCl | Cardene |
| nefazodone HCl | Serzone | Niclocide | niclosamide |
| NegGram | nalidixic acid | niclosamide | Niclocide |
| nelfinavir mesylate | Viracept | Nicobid | niacin SR |
| | | Nicorette | nicotine polacrilex |
| Nembutal | pentobarbital sodium | nicotine nasal spray | Nicotrol NS |
| Neo-Synephrine | phenylephrine HCl | nicotine polacrilex | Nicorette |
| neomycin sulfate ointment and cream | Myciguent | nicotine transdermal | Habitrol Nicotrol Prostep |
| neomycin sulfate oral soln | Mycifradin Sulfate | Nicotrol | nicotine transdermal |
| Neoral | cyclosporine capsules (modified) and oral soln | Nicotrol NS | nicotine nasal spray |
| | | nifedipine | Adalat Procardia |
| Neosar | cyclophosphamide | nifedipine SR | Adalat CC Procardia XL |
| Neosporin Cream | polymyxin; neomycin | Nilandron | nilutamide |
| Neosporin Ointment | polymyxin; neomycin; bacitracin | nilutamide | Nilandron |
| | | Nimbex | cisatracurium besylate |
| Neosporin ophth Ointment | polymyxin; neomycin; bacitracin | nimodipine | Nimotop |
| | | Nimotop | nimodipine |
| | | Nipent | pentostatin inj |
| Neosporin ophth soln | polymyxin; neomycin | Nipride | nitroprusside sodium |
| neostigmine methylsulfate | Prostigmin | nisoldipine SR | Sular |
| Neptazane | methazolamide | nitisinone | Orfadin |
| Nesacaine | chloroprocaine HCl | Nitrek | nitroglycerin transdermal |

| | | | |
|---|---|---|---|
| nitric oxide for inhalation | INOmax | norepinephrine bitartrate | Levophed |
| Nitro-Bid | nitroglycerin SR | norethindrone | Micronor |
| Nitro-Dur | nitroglycerin transdermal | norethindrone acetate; ethinyl estradiol | Estrostep Loestrin |
| nitrofurantoin macrocrystals | Macrodantin | | |
| nitrofurantoin macrocrystals and monohydrate | Macrobid | norethindrone; ethinyl estradiol (or mestranol) | Femhrt Ortho-Novum (products) |
| nitrofurazone | Furacin | norethindrone acetate; estradiol transdermal | CombiPatch |
| nitroglycerin transdermal | Transderm-Nitro | | |
| nitroglycerin inj | Tridil | | |
| *nitroglycerin ointment* | Nitrol | Norflex | orphenadrine citrate |
| nitroglycerin SR | Nitro-Bid | norfloxacin | Noroxin |
| *nitroglycerin sublingual tablets* | Nitrostat | Norgesic | orphenadrine citrate; aspirin; caffeine |
| nitroglycerin transdermal | Nitrek Nitro-Dur | norgestimate; ethinyl estradiol | Ortho Tri-Cyclen |
| Nitrol | nitroglycerin ointment | norgestrel; ethinyl estradiol | Lo/Ovral Ovral |
| nitroprusside sodium | Nipride | | |
| Nitrostat | nitroglycerin sublingual tablets | Normiflo (W) | ardeparin sodium (W) |
| | | Normodyne | labetalol HCl |
| Nix | permethrin | Noroxin | norfloxacin |
| nizatidine | Axid | Norpace | disopyramide phosphate |
| Nizoral | ketoconazole | | |
| nofetumomab | Verluna | Norplant (W) | levonorgestrel implant (W) |
| nolatrexed dihydro- chloride | Thymitaq | Norpramin | desipramine HCl |
| | | nortriptyline HCl | Aventyl Pamelor |
| Nolvadex | tamoxifen citrate | | |
| Norco | hydrocodone bitartrate; acetaminophen | Norvasc | amlodipine besylate |
| | | Norvir | ritonavir |
| | | Novantrone | mitoxantrone HCl |
| Norcuron | vecuronium bromide | | |
| | | Novocain HCl | procaine HCl |
| Nordette | levonorgestrel; ethinyl estradiol | Novolin 70/30 | isophane insulin suspension (NPH) 70%, insulin inj 30% (human) |
| Norditropin | somatropin inj | | |
| norelgestromin; ethinyl estradiol transdermal system | Ortho Evra | | |
| | | Novolin L | insulin zinc suspension (Lente) (human) |

| | | | |
|---|---|---|---|
| Novolin N | isophane insulin suspension (NPH) (human) | olanzapine | Zyprexa |
| | | olmesartan medoxomil | Benicar |
| | | olopatadine HCl ophth soln | Patanol |
| Novolin R | insulin inj (human) | olsalazine sodium | Dipentum |
| NovoLog | insulin aspart (rDNA origin) | Olux | clobetasol foam |
| NovoSeven | coagulation factor VII a (recombinant) | omeprazole | Prilosec |
| | | Omnicef | cefdinir |
| | | Omnipaque | iohexol |
| Nubain | nalbuphine HCl | Oncaspar | pegaspargase |
| NuLev | hyoscyamine sulfate orally disintegrating tab | OncoScint | satumomab pendetide |
| | | Oncovin | vincristine sulfate |
| Numorphan | oxymorphone HCl | ondansetron | Zofran |
| | | ondansetron orally disintegrating tab | Zofran ODT |
| Nupercainal | dibucaine | | |
| Nuromax | doxacurium chloride | | |
| Nuprin | ibuprofen | Ontak | denileukin diftitox |
| Nutropin | somatropin for inj | Onxol | paclitaxel inj |
| Nutropin AQ | somatropin inj | Ophthaine (WA) | proparacaine |
| NuvaRing | etonogestrel; ethinyl estradiol vaginal ring | Ophthalgan | glycerin ophth soln |
| | | Ophthetic | proparacaine HCl |
| Nydrazid | isoniazid | opium; belladonna suppositories | B & O Supprettes |
| *nystatin* | Mycostatin | | |
| nystatin topical powder | Nystop | oprelvekin | Neumega |
| | | Opticrom | cromolyn sodium |
| nystatin; triamcinolone cream | Mycolog Cream | OptiMark | gadoversetamide |
| | | Optimine | azatadine maleate |
| Nystop | nystatin topical powder | Optiray | ioversol |
| | | Optivar | azelastine HCl ophth soln |
| | | Orabase | benzocaine |
| **O** | | Orajel | benzocaine |
| | | Oramorph SR | morphine sulfate SR |
| | | Orap | pimozide |
| OctreoScan | indium In-111 pentetreotide | Oretic | hydrochlorothi-azide |
| octreotide acetate | Sandostatin | Orfadin | nitisinone |
| octreotide acetate susp for inj | Sandostatin LAR Depot | Organidin NR | guaifenesin |
| | | Orgaran | danaparoid sodium |
| ofloxacin | Floxin | Orinase | tolbutamide |
| ofloxacin otic soln | Floxin Otic | Orlaam | levomethadyl acetate HCl |
| Ogen | estropipate | | |

| | | | |
|---|---|---|---|
| orlistat | Xenical | Oxistat | oxiconazole nitrate cream |
| Ornade Spansules | phenylpropanolamine HCl; chlorpheniramine maleate SR | Oxsoralen | methoxsalen |
| | | oxtriphylline | Choledyl |
| | | oxybate sodium | Xyrem |
| orphenadrine citrate | Norflex | oxybutynin chloride | Ditropan |
| orphenadrine citrate; aspirin; caffeine | Norgesic | oxychlorosene sodium | Clorpactin WCS-90 |
| | | oxycodone HCl | Percolone Roxicodone |
| Ortho-Cept | desogestrel; ethinyl estradiol | oxycodone HCl SR | OxyContin |
| | | oxycodone HCl; acetaminophen | Percocet 5/325; 7.5/500; 10/650 |
| Orthoclone OKT3 | muromonab-CD3 | | Endocet Roxicet |
| Ortho Evra | norelgestromin; ethinyl estradiol transdermal system | oxycodone HCl; aspirin | Percodan |
| | | OxyContin | oxycodone HCl SR |
| Ortho-Novum (products) | norethindrone; ethinyl estradiol (or mestranol) | oxymetazoline HCl | Afrin nasal spray Dristan Long Lasting |
| | | oxymetholone | Anadrol-50 |
| Ortho-Prefest | 17β-estradiol; norgestimate | oxymorphone HCl | Numorphan |
| Ortho Tri-Cyclen | norgestimate; ethinyl estradiol (combinations) | oxytocin | Pitocin |

**P**

| | | | |
|---|---|---|---|
| Orudis | ketoprofen | | |
| Oruvail | ketoprofen SR | | |
| Os-Cal 500 | calcium carbonate | Pacis | BCG intravesical |
| oseltamivir phosphate | Tamiflu | paclitaxel | Onxol Taxol |
| Osmovist | iotrolan | palivizumab | Synagis |
| Otrivin | xylometazoline | Palladone XL | hydromorphone HCl SR |
| Ovidrel | choriogonadotropin alfa | Pamelor | nortriptyline HCl |
| Ovral | norgestrel; ethinyl estradiol | pamidronate disodium | Aredia |
| | | Pamine | methscopolamine bromide |
| oxaliplatin | Eloxatin | | |
| Oxandrin | oxandrolone | Pancrease | pancrelipase EC |
| oxandrolone | Oxandrin | pancrelipase | Cotazym |
| oxaprozin | Daypro | pancrelipase EC | Cotazym-S Pancrease |
| oxazepam | Serax | | |
| oxcarbazepine | Trileptal | pancuronium bromide | Pavulon |
| oxiconazole nitrate cream | Oxistat | | |
| Oxilan | ioxilan | Pandel | hydrocortisone buteprate cream |

| | |
|---|---|
| Panretin | alitretinoin |
| pantoprazole | Protonix |
| papain; urea oint | Accuzyme |
| | Ethezyme |
| papaverine HCl SR | Pavabid |
| paracetamol | acetaminophen |
| Paradione | paramethadione |
| Paraflex | chlorzoxazone 250 mg |
| Parafon Forte DSC | chlorzoxazone 500 mg |
| paramethadione | Paradione |
| Paraplatin | carboplatin |
| Parathar | teriparatide acetate |
| paregoric | camphorated tincture of opium |
| pargyline HCl | Eutonyl |
| paricalcitol | Zemplar |
| Parlodel | bromocriptine mesylate |
| Parnate | tranylcypromine sulfate |
| paromomycin sulfate | Humatin |
| paroxetine HCl | Paxil |
| Parsidol | ethopropazine HCl |
| Paser | aminosalicylic acid |
| Patanol | olopatadine HCl ophth soln |
| Pavabid | papaverine HCl SR |
| Pavulon | pancuronium bromide |
| Paxil | paroxetine HCl |
| PBZ | tripelennamine HCl |
| PCE Dispertab | erythromycin base coated particles |
| Pediazole | erythromycin ethylsuccinate; sulfisoxazole |
| PedvaxHIB | haemophilus b vaccine |
| pegaspargase | Oncaspar |
| pegfilgrastim | Neulasta |
| peginterferon alfa-2b (recombinant) | PEG-Intron |

| | |
|---|---|
| PEG-Intron | peginterferon alfa-2b (recombinant) |
| pemetrexed disodium | Alimta |
| pemirolast potassium ophth soln | Alamast |
| pemoline | Cylert |
| penicillamine | Cuprimine |
| penciclovir cream | Denavir |
| penicillin G benzathine | Bicillin L-A (for IM use only) Permapen (for IM use only) |
| penicillin G benzathine; penicillin G procaine | Bicillin C-R (for IM use only) |
| penicillin G procaine | Wycillin (for IM use only) |
| *penicillin V potassium* | Pen Vee K |
| Penlac Nail Lacquer | ciclopirox soln |
| pentaerythritol tetranitrate | Peritrate |
| pentagastrin | Peptavlon |
| Pentam 300 | pentamidine isethionate inj |
| pentamidine isethionate aerosol | NebuPent |
| pentamidine isethionate inj | Pentam 300 |
| Pentaspan | pentastarch |
| pentastarch | Pentaspan |
| pentazocine HCl | Talwin |
| pentazocine HCl; naloxone HCl | Talwin Nx |
| pentobarbital sodium | Nembutal |
| pentosan polysulfate sodium | Elmiron |
| pentostatin inj | Nipent |
| Pentothal | thiopental sodium |
| pentoxifylline | Trental |
| Pen Vee K | penicillin V potassium |

| | | | |
|---|---|---|---|
| Pepcid | famotidine | phenelzine sulfate | Nardil |
| Pepcid RPD | famotidine, oral disintegrating tablet | Phenergan | promethazine HCl |
| Peptavlon | pentagastrin | phenobarbital | phenobarbital |
| Percocet 5/325; 7.5/500; 10/650 | oxycodone HCl; acetaminophen | phenobarbital, ergotamine; belladonna | Bellergal-S |
| Percodan | oxycodone HCl; aspirin | phenoxybenza-mine HCl | Dibenzyline |
| Percolone | oxycodone HCl | phentermine HCl | Fastin |
| perflenapent emulsion | EchoGen | phentermine resin | Ionamin |
| perflubron | Imagent GI | phentolamine mesylate | Regitine |
| Pergonal | menotropins | | |
| Periactin | cyproheptadine HCl | phenylbutyrate sodium | Buphenyl |
| Peri-Colace | docusate sodium; casanthranol | phenylephrine HCl | Neo-Synephrine |
| Peridex | chlorhexidine gluconate mouth rinse | phenylpropanol-amine HCl; chlorphenir-amine maleate SR | Ornade |
| perindopril erbumine | Aceon | | |
| PerioChip | chlorhexidine gluconate | phenylpropanol-amine HCl; guaifenesin SR | Entex LA |
| Periostat | doxycycline hyclate 20 mg tab & cap | | |
| Peritrate | pentaerythritol tetranitrate | Phenytek | phenytoin sodium extended |
| Permapen | penicillin G benzathine (for IM use only) | phenytoin | Dilantin |
| | | phenytoin sodium extended | Phenytek |
| permethrin | Nix | | |
| Permitil | fluphenazine HCl | Phospholine Iodide (W) | echothiophate iodide (W) |
| perphenazine | Trilafon | Photofrin | porfimer sodium |
| perphenazine; amitriptyline HCl | Etrafon Triavil | physostigmine ophth ointment | Eserine Sulfate |
| Persantine | dipyridamole | physostigmine salicylate | Antilirium |
| petrolatum, white | Vaseline | phytonadione | AquaMEPHY-TON |
| Phenaphen with Codeine (#2, 3, and 4) | acetaminophen 300 mg with Codeine Phosphate (15, 30, and 60 mg) | pilocarpine HCl ophth | Isopto Carpine |
| | | pilocarpine HCl tablet | Salagen |
| phenazopyridine HCl | Pyridium | pimecrolimus cream | Elidel |
| phendimetrazine tartrate | Plegine | pimozide | Orap |
| | | pindolol | Visken |

405

| | | | |
|---|---|---|---|
| pioglitazone HCl | Actos | poliovirus | Ipol |
| pipecuronium bromide | Arduan | vaccine inactivated | |
| piperacillin sodium | Pipracil | polyethylene glycolelectro- | CoLyte GoLYTELY |
| piperacillin sodium; tazobactam sodium | Zosyn | lyte soln polyethylene glycol 3350 powder | MiraLax |
| Pipracil | piperacillin sodium | polymyxin B sulfate; | Polytrim |
| piroxicam | Feldene | trimethoprim ophth soln | |
| Pitocin | oxytocin | | |
| Pitressin | vasopressin | polymyxin; neomycin | Neosporin Cream |
| Placidyl | ethchlorvynol | | Neosporin ophth |
| Plan B | levonorgestrel | | soln |
| Plaquenil | hydroxychloro- quine sulfate | polymyxin; neomycin; | Neosporin Ointment |
| Plasbumin | albumin human | bacitracin | Neosporin ophth Ointment |
| plasma protein fraction | Plasma-Plex Plasmanate Plasmatein Protenate | polystyrene sulfonate sodium | Kayexalate |
| Plasma-Plex | plasma protein fraction | polythiazide Polytrim | Renese polymyxin B |
| Plasmanate | plasma protein fraction | | sulfate; trimethoprim ophth soln |
| Plasmatein | plasma protein fraction | Pondimin (W) | fenfluramine HCl (W) |
| Platinol AQ | cisplatin | Ponstel | mefenamic acid |
| Plavix | clopidogrel bisulfate | Pontocaine poractant alpha | tetracaine HCl Curosurf |
| Plegine | phendimetrazine tartrate | intratracheal susp | |
| Plendil | felodipine | porfimer sodium | Photofrin |
| Pletal | cilostazol | | |
| Plexion | sulfacetamide sodium and sulfur lotion | Posicor (W) | mibefradil dihydro- chloride (W) |
| plicamycin | Mithracin | potassium bicarbonate; | K-Lyte |
| pneumococcal vaccine | Pneumovax | potassium citrate | |
| pneumococcal 7-valent conjugate vaccine | Prevnar | effervescent potassium chloride; potassium bicarbonate | K-Lyte/Cl |
| Pneumovax | pneumococcal vaccine | effervescent | |
| podofilox gel | Condylox | *potassium* | Kaon-Cl |
| Polaramine Repetabs | dexchlorphenir- amine maleate SR | *chloride SR* | K-Dur Klor-Con 10 |

| | | | |
|---|---|---|---|
| | Slow-K | Priftin | rifapentine |
| | Micro K | Prilosec | omeprazole |
| potassium | Kolyum | Primacor | milrinone lactate |
| chloride; | | Primaxin | imipenem-cila- |
| potassium | | | statin sodium |
| gluconate | | primidone | Mysoline |
| potassium | Urocit-K | Primsol | trimethoprim |
| citrate tab | | Principen | ampicillin |
| potassium | Kaon | Prinivil | lisinopril |
| gluconate | | Priscoline | tolazoline |
| povidone iodine | Betadine | ProAmatine | midodrine HCl |
| pralidoxime | Protopam | Pro-Banthine | propantheline |
| chloride | | | bromide |
| pramipexole | Mirapex | probenecid | Benemid |
| dihydrochloride | | probenecid; | ColBENEMID |
| pramoxine HCl | Tronothane | colchicine | (W) |
| | HCl | procainamide | Pronestyl |
| Prandin | repaglinide | procainamide | Procan SR |
| prasterone | Aslera | HCl SR | Procanbid |
| Pravachol | pravastatin | procaine HCl | Novocain HCl |
| | sodium | Procan SR | procainamide |
| pravastatin | Pravachol | | HCl SR |
| sodium | | Procanbid | procainamide |
| prazosin HCl | Minipress | | HCl SR |
| Precedex | dexmedetomidine | procarbazine | Matulane |
| | HCl inj | HCl | |
| Precose | acarbose | Procardia | nifedipine |
| prednisolone | Prelone | Procardia XL | nifedipine SR |
| syrup | | prochlorperazine | Compazine |
| *prednisone* | Deltasone | Procrit | epoetin alfa |
| | Meticorten | procyclidine HCl | Kemadrin |
| Prelone | prednisolone | progesterone gel | Crinone |
| | syrup | progesterone | Prometrium |
| Premarin | estrogens, | micronized | |
| | conjugated | Prograf | tacrolimus |
| Premphase | estrogens, | ProHance | gadoteridol |
| Prempro | conjugated; | ProHIBiT | haemophilus b |
| | medroxyproges- | | vaccine |
| | terone acetate | Prokine (WA) | sargramostim |
| Prepidil | dinoprostone gel | Prolastin | alpha$_1$-proteinase |
| Preven | levonorgestrel; | | inhibitor |
| Emergency | ethinyl | | (human) |
| Contraceptive | estradiol | Proleukin | aldesleukin |
| Kit | | Prolixin | fluphenazine HCl |
| Prevacid | lansoprazole | Proloid (W) | thyroglobulin (W) |
| Prevnar | pneumococcal | promethazine | Phenergan |
| | 7-valent | HCl | |
| | conjugate | Prometrium | progesterone |
| | vaccine | | micronized |
| Preveon | adefovir dipivoxil | Pronestyl | procainamide |
| Prevpac | lansoprazole; | Propacet-100 | propoxyphene |
| | amoxicillin; | | napsylate; |
| | clarithromycin | | acetaminophen |

| | | | |
|---|---|---|---|
| propafenone HCl | Rythmol | Proventil | albuterol SR |
| propantheline bromide | Pro-Banthine | Repetabs | |
| | | Provera | medroxyproges-terone acetate |
| proparacaine HCl | Ophthaine (WA) | | |
| | Ophthetic | Provigil | modafinil |
| Propecia | finasteride tablets 1 mg | Prozac | fluoxetine HCl |
| | | Prudoxin | doxepin HCl cream |
| Propine | dipivefrin | | |
| propofol | Diprivan | pseudoephedrine HCl | Sudafed |
| propoxyphene HCl | Darvon | | |
| | | pseudoephedrine HCl; bromphiramine maleate | Drixoral Syrup |
| propoxyphene HCl; acetaminophen | Wygesic | | |
| propoxyphene HCl; aspirin; caffeine | Darvon Compound 65 | psyllium | Konsyl-D Metamucil |
| | | Pulmicort Turbuhaler | budesonide inhalation powder |
| propoxyphene napsylate; acetaminophen | Darvocet-N 100 Propacet-100 | | |
| | | Pulmozyme | dornase alfa |
| propranolol HCl | Inderal | Purinethol | mercaptopurine |
| propranolol HCl; hydrochlorothi-azide | Inderide | Pyridium | phenazopyridine HCl |
| | | pyridostigmine bromide | Mestinon |
| Propulsid (W) | cisapride (W) | | |
| Proscar | finasteride tablets 5 mg | pyrimethamine | Daraprim |
| | | pyrimethamine; sulfadoxine | Fansidar |
| ProSom | estazolam | | |
| ProstaScint | capromab pendetide | | |
| | | | |
| Prostep | nicotine transdermal system | **Q** | |
| Prostigmin | neostigmine methylsulfate | Quadramet | samarium SM 153 lexidronam |
| Prostin E$_2$ | dinoprostone vaginal suppositories | | |
| | | Quarzan (W) | clidinium bromide (W) |
| Prostin VR | alprostadil | Questran | cholestyramine |
| protamine sulfate | protamine sulfate | quetiapine fumerate | Seroquel |
| Protenate | plasma protein fraction | | |
| | | Quinaglute | quinidine gluconate SR |
| Protonix | pantoprazole | | |
| Protopam | pralidoxime chloride | quinapril HCl | Accupril |
| | | quinapril; hydrochloro-thiazide | Accuretic |
| Protopic | tacrolimus oint | | |
| protriptyline HCl | Vivactil | | |
| Protropin | somatrem | quinethazone | Hydromox |
| Protropin II | somatropin for inj | Quinidex Extentabs | quinidine sulfate SR |
| Proventil | albuterol | | |
| Proventil HFA | albuterol sulfate inhalation aerosol | quinidine gluconate SR | Quinaglute |

| | |
|---|---|
| quinidine sulfate | quinidine sulfate |
| quinidine sulfate SR | Quinidex Extentabs |
| quinupristin; dalfopristin | Synercid |
| Quixin | levofloxacin ophth soln |
| Qvar | beclomethasone diproprionate inhalation aerosol |

## R

| | |
|---|---|
| RabAvert | rabies vaccine for human use |
| rabeprazole sodium | Aciphex |
| rabies immune globulin, human | Hyperab (W) Imogam |
| rabies vaccine, adsorbed | rabies vaccine, adsorbed |
| rabies vaccine for human use | RabAvert |
| raloxifene HCl | Evista |
| ramipril | Altace |
| ranitidine bismuth citrate | Tritec |
| ranitidine HCl | Zantac |
| rapacuronium bromide (W) | Raplon (W) |
| Rapamune | sirolimus |
| Raplon (W) | rapacuronium bromide (W) |
| rasburicase | Elitek |
| rattlesnake anti-venom | CroFab |
| Raxar (W) | grepafloxacin HCl (W) |
| Rebetol | ribavirin |
| Rebetron | ribavirin; interferon alfa-2b |
| Rebif | interferon beta-1a |
| reboxetine mesylate | Vestra |
| Recombivax HB | hepatitis B vaccine |
| Redux (W) | dexfenfluramine HCl (W) |

| | |
|---|---|
| Refacto | antihemophilic factor (recombinant) |
| Refludan | lepirudin |
| Regitine | phentolamine mesylate |
| Reglan | metoclopramide HCl |
| Regranex | becaplermin gel |
| Regroton | chlorthalidone; reserpine |
| Relafen | nabumetone |
| Relenza | zanamivir for inhalation |
| Remeron | mirtazapine |
| Remicade | infliximab |
| remifentanil HCl | Ultiva |
| Reminyl | galanthamine HBr |
| Remodulin | treprostinil sodium |
| Renagel | sevelamer HCl |
| Renese | polythiazide |
| Renova | tretinion topical |
| Renovue 65 | iodamide meglumine |
| ReoPro | abciximab |
| repaglinide | Prandin |
| Repronex | menotropins |
| Requip | ropinirole HCl |
| Rescriptor | delavirdine mesylate |
| Rescula | unoprostone isopropyl ophth soln |
| *reserpine* | Serpasil |
| RespiGam | respiratory syncytial virus immune globulin intravenous (human) |
| respiratory syncytial virus immune globulin intravenous (human) | RespiGam |
| Restasis | cyclosporine ophth emulsion |
| Restoril | temazepam |
| Retavase | reteplase |
| reteplase | Retavase |

Q
R

| | | | |
|---|---|---|---|
| Retin-A | tretinoin topical | rizatriptan oral | Maxalt-MLT |
| Retin-A Micro | tretinoin gel | disintegrating | |
| Retrovir | zidovudine | tablet | |
| Revex | nalmefene | Robaxin | methocarbamol |
| | HCl | Robinul | glycopyrrolate |
| ReVia | naltrexone | Robitussin | guaifenesin |
| Rezulin (W) | troglitazone (W) | Robitussin A-C | guaifenesin; |
| R-Gene | arginine HCl | | codeine |
| Rheumatrex | methotrexate | | phosphate |
| | tablets | Robitussin-DM | guaifenesin; |
| Rhinocort | budesonide nasal | | dextrometh- |
| | inhaler | | orphan |
| RH$_O$ (D) immune | RhoGAM | Rocaltrol | calcitriol |
| globulin | | Rocephin | ceftriaxone sodium |
| RH$_O$ (D) immune | WinRho SD | rofecoxib | Vioxx |
| globulin IV | | Roferon-A | interferon alfa-2a |
| (human) | | Rogaine | minoxidil topical |
| RhoGAM | RH$_O$ (D) immune | Romazicon | flumazenil |
| | globulin | ropinirole HCl | Requip |
| ribavirin | Rebetol | ropivacaine HCl | Naropin |
| | Virazole | Rosiglitazone | Avandia |
| ribavirin; | Rebetron | maleate | |
| interferon alfa- | | Rotashield (W) | rotavirus (W) |
| 2b | | | vaccine, live, |
| Ridaura | auranofin | | oral, tetravalent |
| Rifadin | rifampin | rotavirus | Rotashield (W) |
| Rifamate | isoniazid; | vaccine, live, | |
| | rifampin | oral, (W) | |
| rifampin | Rifadin | tetravalent | |
| | Rimactane | Rowasa | mesalamine |
| rifapentine | Priftin | Roxanol | morphine sulfate |
| Rilutek | riluzole | Roxanol SR | morphine sulfate |
| riluzole | Rilutek | | SR |
| Rimactane | rifampin | Roxanol-T | morphine sulfate, |
| rimantadine | Flumadine | | immediate |
| rimexolone | Vexol | | release |
| Riopan | magaldrate | | concentrated |
| risedronate | Actonel | | oral soln |
| sodium | | Roxicet | oxycodone HCl; |
| Risperdal | risperidone | | acetaminophen |
| risperidone | Risperdal | Roxicodone | oxycodone HCl |
| Ritalin | methylphenidate | rubella virus | Meruvax II |
| | HCl | vaccine live | |
| Ritalin SR | methylphenidate | attenuated | |
| | SR | Rubex | doxorubicin HCl |
| ritodrine HCl | Yutopar | Rythmol | propafenone HCl |
| ritonavir | Norvir | | |
| Rituxan | rituximab | | |
| rituximab | Rituxan | | |
| rivastigmine | Exelon | | **S** |
| tartrate | | | |
| rizatriptan | Maxalt | sacrosidase | Sucraid |
| benzoate | | Saizen | somatropin |

410

| | | | |
|---|---|---|---|
| Salagen | pilocarpine HCl tablet | sennosides | Ex Lax |
| salbutamol sulfate | albuterol sulfate | sennosides | Senokot |
| salmeterol xinafoate | Serevent | sennosides; docusate sodium | Senokot-S |
| salmeterol xinafoate inhalation powder | Serevent Diskus | Senokot | senna concentrates |
| | | Senokot-S | sennosides; docusate sodium |
| salsalate | Disalcid | | |
| Sal-Tropine | atropine sulfate tablets | Septocaine | articaine; epinephrine |
| Saluron | hydroflume-thiazide | Septra | sulfamethox-azoletrimeth-oprim |
| samarium SM 153 lexidronam | Quadramet | Ser-Ap-Es | hydralazine; hydrochloro-thiazide; reserpine |
| Sandimmune | cyclosporine | | |
| Sandoglobulin | immune globulin intravenous | Serax | oxazepam |
| | | Serentil | mesoridazine |
| Sandostatin | octreotide acetate | Serevent | salmeterol xinafoate |
| Sandostatin LAR Depot | octreotide acetate susp for inj | Serevent Diskus | salmeterol xinafoate inhalation powder |
| Sanorex | mazindol | | |
| Sansert | methysergide maleate | | |
| Santyl | collagenase | Serlect | sertindole |
| saquinavir mesylate | Invirase | sermorelin acetate | Geref |
| saquinavir soft gel capsule | Fortovase | Seromycin | cycloserine |
| | | Seroquel | quetiapine fumerate |
| Sarafem | fluoxetine | | |
| sargramostim | Leukine Prokine (WA) | Serostim | somatropin (rDNA origin) for inj |
| satumomab pendetide | OncoScint | | |
| | | Serpasil | *reserpine* |
| Sclerosol | talc, sterile aerosol | sertindole | Serlect |
| | | sertraline HCl | Zoloft |
| scopolamine hydrobromide ophth | Isopto Hyoscine | Serzone | nefazodone HCl |
| | | sevelamer HCl | Renagel |
| scopolamine transdermal | Transderm Scop | sevoflurane | Ultane |
| Sectral | acebutolol HCl | short chain fatty acids enema | Colomed |
| Seldane (W) | terfenadine (W) | | |
| Seldane D (W) | terfenadine; pseudoephed-rine HCl (W) | sibutramine HCl monohydrate | Meridia |
| | | sildenafil citrate | Viagra |
| selegiline HCl | Carbex Eldepryl | Silvadene | silver sulfadiazine |
| selenium sulfide | Selsun Blue | silver sulfadiazine | Silvadene |
| Selsun Blue | selenium sulfide | simethicone | Mylicon |

| Simulect | basiliximab | somatostatin | Zecnil |
|---|---|---|---|
| simvastatin | Zocor | somatrem | Protropin |
| Sinemet | levodopa; carbidopa | somatropin for inj | Genotropin |
| | | | Humatrope |
| Sinemet CR | levodopa; carbidopa SR | | Norditropin |
| | | | Nutropin |
| Sinequan | doxepin HCl | | Protropin II |
| Singulair | montelukast sodium | | Saizen |
| sirolimus | Rapamune | somatropin inj | Nutropin AQ |
| Skelid | tiludronate disodium | somatropin (rDNA origin) for inj | Serostim |
| Slo-bid | theophylline SR | Sonata | zaleplon |
| Slo-Phyllin | theophylline | Soriatane | acitretin |
| Slow Fe | ferrous sulfate SR | sotalol | Betapace |
| Slow-K | potassium chloride SR | Sotradecol | sodium tetradecyl sulfate |
| Slow-Mag | magnesium chloride SR | sparfloxacin | Zagam |
| | | stavudine | Zerit |
| sodium citrate; citric acid | Bicitra | spectinomycin HCl | Trobicin |
| sodium ferric gluconate complex in sucrose inj | Ferrlecit | Spectracef | cefditoren pivoxil |
| | | spironolactone | Aldactone |
| | | spironolactone; hydrochlorothiazide | Aldactazide |
| sodium fluoride | Luride | Sporanox | itraconazole |
| sodium hyaluronate | Amvisc | Stadol | butorphanol tartrate inj |
| | Healon | | |
| | Hyalgan | Stadol NS | butorphanol tartrate nasal spray |
| sodium oxybate | Xyrem | | |
| sodium phenylbutyrate | Buphenyl | stanozolol | Winstrol |
| sodium phosphate tab | Visicol | Staphcillin | methicillin sodium |
| sodium sulfacetamide lotion | Klaron | Starlix | nateglinide |
| | | Stelazine | trifluoperazine HCl |
| sodium tetradecyl sulfate | Sotradecol | Streptase | streptokinase |
| | | streptokinase | Streptase |
| Solaraze | diclofenac gel | streptomycin sulfate | streptomycin sulfate |
| Solganal | aurothioglucose | streptozocin | Zanosar |
| Solu-Cortef | hydrocortisone sodium succinate | Stromectol | ivermectin |
| | | strontium-89 chloride inj | Metastron |
| Solu-Medrol | methylprednisolone sodium succinate | Sublimaze | fentanyl citrate |
| | | succinylcholine chloride | Anectine |
| Soma | carisoprodol | Sucraid | sacrosidase |

S
Rx

| | | |
|---|---|---|
| sucralfate | Carafate | |
| Sudafed | pseudoephedrine HCl | |
| Sufenta | sufentanil citrate | |
| sufentanil citrate | Sufenta | |
| Sulamyd sodium | sulfacetamide sodium ophth | |
| Sular | Nisoldipine SR | |
| sulfacetamide sodium and sulfur lotion | Plexion | |
| sulfacetamide sodium ophth | Sulamyd sodium | |
| sulfadoxine; pyrimethamine | Fansidar | |
| sulfamethoxazole (W) | Gantanol (W) | |
| sulfamethoxazole-trimethoprim | Bactrim Cotrim co-trimoxazole Septra | |
| sulfasalazine | Azulfidine | |
| sulfinpyrazone | Anturane | |
| sulindac | Clinoril | |
| Sultrin | triple sulfa vaginal cream | |
| sumatriptan | Imitrex | |
| Sumycin | tetracycline HCl | |
| Suprane | desflurane | |
| Suprax | cefixime | |
| suramin | Metaret | |
| Surfak | docusate calcium | |
| Surmontil | trimipramine maleate | |
| Survanta | beractant | |
| Sustiva | Efavirenz | |
| Symmetrel | amantadine HCl | |
| Synagis | palivizumab | |
| Synalar | fluocinolone acetonide | |
| Synercid | quinupristin; dalfopristin | |
| Synkayvite | menadiol sodium diphosphate | |
| synopinine | Florotag | |
| synthetic conjugated estrogens, A | Cenestin | |
| Synthroid | levothyroxine sodium | |
| Synvisc | hylan G-F 20 | |

# T

| | |
|---|---|
| tacrine HCl | Cognex |
| tacrolimus | Prograf |
| tacrolimus oint | Protopic |
| Tagamet | cimetidine HCl |
| talc, sterile aerosol | Sclerosol |
| Talwin | pentazocine HCl |
| Talwin Nx | pentazocine HCl; naloxone HCl |
| Tambocor | flecainide acetate |
| Tamiflu | oseltamivir phosphate |
| tamoxifen citrate | Nolvadex |
| tamsulosin HCl | Flomax |
| Tapazole | methimazole |
| Targretin | bexarotene gel |
| Tarka | trandolapril; verapamil SR |
| tarzarotene gel | Tazorac |
| Tasmar | tolcapone |
| tasosartan | Verdia |
| Tavist | clemastine fumarate |
| Taxol | paclitaxel |
| Taxotere | docetaxel |
| Tazicef | ceftazidime |
| Tazidime | ceftazidime |
| Tazorac | tarzarotene gel |
| technetium Tc-99m bicisate kit | Neurolite |
| technetium Tc-99m red blood cell kit | Ultratag |
| technetium Tc-99m | Cardiotec |
| technetium Tc99m sestamibi teboroxime kit | Cardiolite |
| Teczem | enalapril maleate; diltiazem malate |
| tegaserod maleate | Zelnorm |
| Tegretol | carbamazepine |

| | | | |
|---|---|---|---|
| Teldrin | chlorpheniramine maleate SR | tetrahydrozoline HCl ophth | Collyrium Visine Extra |
| Telepaque | iopanoic acid | Teveten | eprosartan mesylate |
| telmisartan | Micardis | | |
| temazepam | Restoril | thalidomide | Thalomid |
| Temodar | temozolomide | Thalomid | thalidomide |
| temozolomide | Temodar | Tham | tromethamine |
| tenecteplase | TNKase | Theo-Dur | theophylline SR |
| Tenex | guanfacine HCl | theophylline | Elixophyllin |
| teniposide | Vumon | | Slo-Phyllin |
| tenofovir disoproxil fumarate | Viread | theophylline SR | Slo-bid Theo-Dur Uniphyl |
| Tenoretic | atenolol; chlorthalidone | TheraCys | BCG intravesical |
| Tenormin | atenolol | Theragran-M | vitamins; minerals |
| Tensilon | edrophonium chloride | thiabendazole | Mintezol |
| | | thiethylperazine maleate | Torecan |
| Tenuate | diethylpropion HCl | thioguanine | thioguanine |
| Tequin | gatifloxacin | thiopental sodium | Pentothal |
| Terazol | terconazole | | |
| terazosin HCl | Hytrin | Thioplex | thiotepa |
| terbinafine HCl | Lamisil | thioridazine HCl | Mellaril |
| terbutaline sulfate aerosol | Brethaire | thiotepa | Thioplex |
| | | thiothixene | Navane |
| terbutaline sulfate tablets and inj | Brethine Bricanyl | Thorazine | chlorpromazine |
| | | Thrombate III | antithrombin III (human) |
| terconazole | Terazol | thymalfasin | Zadaxin |
| terfenadine (W) | Seldane (W) | Thymitaq | nolatrexed dihydrochloride |
| terfenadine; pseudoephe-drine HCl (W) | Seldane D (W) | Thymoglobulin | anti-thymocyte globulin, (rabbit) |
| teriparatide acetate | Parathar | thyroglobulin (W) | Proloid (W) |
| Teslac | testolactone | thyroid | thyroid |
| Teslascan | mangofodipir trisodium | Thyrogen | thyrotropin alpha |
| Testoderm | testosterone transdermal | Thyrolar | liotrix |
| | | thyrotropin (W) | Thytropar (W) |
| Testoderm TTS | testosterone transdermal | thyrotropin alpha | Thyrogen |
| testolactone | Teslac | Thytropar (W) | thyrotropin (W) |
| testosterone cypionate SR | DEPO-Testosterone | tiagabine HCl | Gabitril |
| testosterone gel | AndroGel | Tiamate | diltiazem maleate SR |
| testosterone transdermal | Androderm Testoderm Testoderm TTS | Tiazac | diltiazem HCl SR |
| | | Ticar | ticarcillin disodium |
| tetracaine HCl | Pontocaine | ticarcillin disodium | Ticar |
| *tetracycline HCl* | Achromycin (WA) Sumycin | ticarcillin; clavulanic acid | Timentin |

414

| | | | |
|---|---|---|---|
| TICE BCG | BCG intravesical | Tobrex | tobramycin sulfate ophth |
| Ticlid | ticlopidine | | |
| ticlopidine | Ticlid | tocainide HCl | Tonocard |
| Tigan | trimethobenz- amide HCl | Tofranil | imipramine HCl |
| Tikosyn | dofetilide | tolazamide | Tolinase |
| Tilade | nedocromil inhalation | tolazoline | Priscoline |
| | | tolbutamide | Orinase |
| tiludronate disodium | Skelid | tolcapone | Tasmar |
| | | Tolectin | tolmetin sodium |
| Timentin | ticarcillin; clavulanic acid | Tolinase | tolazamide |
| timolol maleate ophth soln | Timoptic | tolmetin sodium | Tolectin |
| | | tolnaftate | Tinactin |
| timolol maleate ophth soln, gel forming | Timoptic-XE | tolterodine tartrate | Detrol |
| | | tolterodine tartrate (SR) | Detrol LA |
| timolol maleate | Blocadren | Tonocard | tocainide HCl |
| timolol maleate; dorzolamide HCl | Cosopt | Topamax | topiramate |
| | | Topicort | desoximetasone |
| | | topiramate | Topamax |
| Timoptic-XE | timolol maleate ophth soln, gel forming | topotecan HCl | Hycamtin |
| | | Toprol XL | metoprolol succinate SR |
| Timoptic | timolol maleate ophth soln | Toradol | ketorolac tromethamine |
| Tinactin | tolnaftate | Torecan | thiethylperazine maleate |
| Tine Test Tuberculin Old | tuberculin, old | | |
| | | toremifene citrate | Fareston |
| Tine Test PPD | tuberculin, purified protein derivative | Tornalate | bitolterol mesylate |
| | | torsemide | Demadex |
| tinzaparin sodium | Innohep | tositumomab and I-131 | Bexxar |
| TNKase | tenecteplase | tositumomab | |
| tioconazole | Vagistat-1 | Totacillin-N | ampicillin sodium |
| tirofiban HCl | Aggrastat | Tracleer | bosentan |
| tizanidine HCl | Zanaflex | Tracrium | atracurium besylate |
| TOBI | tobramycin soln for inhalation | | |
| | | tramadol; acetaminophen | Ultracet |
| TobraDex | tobramycin; dexamethasone oint and susp | tramadol HCl | Ultram |
| | | Trandate | labetalol HCl |
| | | trandolapril | Mavik |
| tobramycin sulfate | Nebcin | trandolapril; verapamil SR | Tarka |
| tobramycin sulfate ophth | Tobrex | Transderm Scop | scopolamine transdermal |
| tobramycin; dexamethasone oint and susp | TobraDex | Transderm-Nitro | nitroglycerin transdermal |
| tobramycin soln for inhalation | TOBI | | |

T
R

415

| | | | |
|---|---|---|---|
| Tranxene | clorazepate dipotassium | Tricor | fenofibrate |
| tranylcypromine sulfate | Parnate | Tri-Cyclen | norgestimate; ethinyl estradiol |
| trastuzumab | Herceptin | Tridesilon | desonide |
| Trasylol | aprotinin | Tridil | nitroglycerin inj |
| Travasol | amino acid inj | | |
| Travatan | travoprost ophth soln | Tridione | trimethadione |
| travoprost ophth soln | Travatan | trifluoperazine HCl | Stelazine |
| trazodone HCl | Desyrel | trifluridine | Viroptic |
| Trecator-SC | ethionamide | trihexyphenidyl HCl (W) | Artane (W) |
| Trelstar Depot | triptorelin pamoate | Trileptal | oxcarbazepine |
| | | Trilafon | perphenazine |
| Trelstar LA | triptorelin pamoate (3 month inj) | Tri-Levlen | levonorgestrel; ethinyl estradiol |
| Trental | pentoxifylline | Trilisate | choline magnesium trisalicylate |
| treprostinil sodium | Remodulin | | |
| tretinoin cream 0.025% | Avita | Tri-Luma | hydroquinone; tretinoin; fluocinolone cream |
| tretinoin gel | Retin-A Micro | | |
| tretinion topical | Renova Retin-A | trimethadione | Tridione |
| tretinoin capsules | Vesanoid | trimethaphan camsylate | Arfonad |
| Trexall | methotrexate tablets | trimethobenza- mide HCl | Tigan |
| triamcinolone acetonide | Aristocort Kenalog | trimethoprim | Primsol |
| triamcinolone acetonide aerosol | Azmacort | trimetrexate glucuronate | Neutrexin |
| | | trimipramine maleate | Surmontil |
| triamcinolone acetonide nasal inhaler | Nasacort | Trimox | amoxicillin |
| | | Tri-Nasal | triamcinolone acetonide nasal spray |
| triamcinolone acetonide nasal spray | Tri-Nasal | Triostat | liothyronine sodium inj |
| triamterene | Dyrenium | | |
| triamterene 37.5 mg; hydro- chlorothiazide 25 mg | Maxzide -25MG Dyazide | tripelennamine HCl | PBZ |
| | | Triphasil | levonorgestrel; ethinyl estradiol |
| triamterene 75 mg; hydro- chlorothiazide 50 mg | Maxzide | triple sulfa vaginal cream | Sultrin |
| Triavil | perphenazine; amitriptyline HCl | triprolidine HCl; pseudoephe- drine HCl | Actifed |
| triazolam | Halcion | triptorelin pamoate | Trelstar Depot |

T
R

| | | | |
|---|---|---|---|
| triptorelin pamoate (3 month inj) | Trelstar LA | Tylenol | acetaminophen |
| | | Tylenol with Codeine (#2, 3, and 4) | acetaminophen 300 mg with Codeine Phosphate (15, 30, and 60 mg) |
| Trisenox | arsenic trioxide | | |
| Tritec | ranitidine bismuth citrate | | |
| Tri-Vi-Flor | vitamins A, D, & C; fluoride | Typhim Vi | typhoid Vi polysaccharide vaccine |
| Trizivir | lamivudine; zidovudine; abacavir sulfate | typhoid Vi polysaccharide vaccine | Typhim Vi |
| Trobicin | spectinomycin HCl | tyropanoate sodium | Bilopaque |
| troglitazone (W) | Rezulin (W) | | |
| tromethamine | Tham | | |
| Tronothane HCl | pramoxine HCl | **U** | |
| TrophAmine | amino acid inj | | |
| Tropicacyl | tropicamide | | |
| tropicamide | Mydriacyl Tropicacyl | UbiQGel | coenzyme Q10 |
| trovafloxacin | Trovan tablets | Ultane | sevoflurane |
| Trovan tablet | trovafloxacin mesylate | Ultiva | remifentanil HCl |
| Trovan inj | alatrofloxacin mesylate IV | Ultracet | tramadol HCl; acetaminophen |
| Trusopt | dorzolamide HCl | Ultralente U | insulin zinc suspension, extended (beef) |
| tuberculin, old | Tine Test, Tuberculin Old | | |
| tuberculin, purified protein derivative | Tine Test PPD | Ultram | tramadol HCl |
| | | Ultratag | technetium Tc-99m red blood cell kit |
| tuberculin skin test | Aplisol | Ultravist | iopromide |
| tubocurarine | tubocurarine | Unasyn | ampicillin sodium; sulbactam sodium |
| Tucks | witch hazel pads | | |
| Tums | calcium carbonate | Unipen (W) | nafcillin sodium (W) |
| Tussi-Organidin NR | guaifenesin; codeine phosphate | Uniphyl | theophylline SR |
| | | Uniretic | moexipril HCl; hydrochloro-thiazide |
| Tussionex | hydrocodone polistirex; chlorphenir-amine | | |
| | | Univasc | moexipril HCl |
| | | Urecholine | bethanechol chloride |
| Twinrix | hepatitis A inactivated; hepatitis B (recombinant) vaccine | Urised | methenamine combination |
| | | Urispas | flavoxate HCl |

| | | | |
|---|---|---|---|
| urofollitropin | Bravelle | Vantin | cefpodoxime proxetil |
| urofollitropin for inj | Fertinex | Vaponefrin | epinephrine racemic |
| urokinase | Abbokinase | | |
| unoprostone isopropyl ophth soln | Rescula | Vaqta | hepatitis A vaccine, inactivated |
| Uprima | apomorphine HCl | varicella virus vaccine | Varivax |
| Urocit-K | potassium citrate tab | Varivax | varicella virus vaccine |
| URSO | ursodiol | Vascor | bepridil |
| ursodiol | Actigall | Vaseline | petrolatum, white |
| | URSO | Vaseretic | enalapril maleate; hydrochloro- thiazide |
| Uvadex | methoxsalen extracorporeal administration | | |
| | | Vasocon | naphazoline ophth soln |
| **V** | | Vasodilan | isoxsuprine HCl |
| | | vasopressin | Pitressin |
| | | Vasotec | enalapril maleate |
| | | Vasoxyl | methoxamine HCl |
| Vagifem | estradiol hemihydrate vaginal tab | vecuronium bromide | Norcuron |
| | | Velban | vinblastine sulfate |
| Vagistat-1 | tioconazole | Velosef | cephradine |
| valacyclovir | Valtrex | Velosulin Human | insulin inj (human) |
| Valcyte | valganciclovir | | |
| valdecoxib | Bextra | venlafaxine HCl | Effexor |
| valganciclovir | Valcyte | venlafaxine HCl SR | Effexor XR |
| Valium | diazepam | | |
| valproate sodium inj | Depacon | Venofer | iron sucrose inj |
| | | Ventolin | albuterol |
| valproic acid | Depakene | VePesid | etoposide |
| valrubicin, (for intravesical use) | Valstar | verapamil HCl | Isoptin |
| | | verapamil HCl SR | Calan SR |
| valsartan | Diovan | | Verelan |
| valsartan; hydro- chlorothiazide | Diovan HCT | verapamil HCl SR bedtime formulation | Covera HS Verelan PM |
| Valstar | valrubicin, (for intravesical use) | | |
| | | Verdia | tasosartan |
| Valtrex | valacyclovir | Verelan | verapamil HCl SR |
| Vancenase | beclomethasone dipropionate | Verelan PM | verapamil HCl SR bedtime formulation |
| Vancenase AQ Nasal | beclomethasone dipropionate | | |
| | | Verluna | nofetumomab |
| Vanceril | beclomethasone dipropionate | Vermox | mebendazole |
| | | Versed | midazolam HCl |
| Vancocin | vancomycin HCl | verteporfin inj | Visudyne |
| vancomycin HCl | Vancocin | Vesanoid | tretinoin capsules |
| Vaniqa | eflornithine HCl cream | Vestra | reboxetine mesylate |
| | | Vexol | rimexolone |

U
R

418

| | |
|---|---|
| Vfend | voriconazole |
| Viactiv | calcium carbonate; vitamin D and K chewable |
| Viadur | leuprolide acetate implant |
| Viagra | sildenafil citrate |
| Vibramycin | doxycycline hyclate |
| Vicodin | hydrocodone bitartrate; acetaminophen |
| Vicoprofen | hydrocodone bitartrate 7.5 mg; ibuprofen 200 mg |
| vidarabine monohydrate | Vira-A |
| Videx | didanosine |
| Videx EC | didanosine SR |
| vinblastine sulfate | Velban |
| vincristine sulfate | Oncovin |
| vindesine sulfate | Eldisine |
| vinorelbine tartrate | Navelbine |
| Vioform | clioquinol |
| Vioxx | rofecoxib |
| Vira-A | vidarabine monohydrate |
| Viracept | nelfinavir mesylate |
| Viramune | nevirapine |
| Virazole | ribavirin |
| Viread | tenofovir disoproxil fumarate |
| Viroptic | trifluridine |
| Visicol | sodium phosphate tab |
| Visine Extra | tetrahydrozoline HCl ophth |
| Visipaque | iodixanol |
| Visken | pindolol |
| Vistaril | hydroxyzine pamoate |
| Vistide | cidofovir |
| Visudyne | verteporfin inj |
| Vitravene | fomivirsen sodium inj |

| | |
|---|---|
| Vivelle | estradiol trans-dermal system |
| Volmax | albuterol SR |
| Voltaren | diclofenac sodium |
| Voltaren-XR | diclofenac sodium SR |
| voriconazole | Vfend |
| Vumon | teniposide |

## W

| | |
|---|---|
| warfarin sodium | Coumadin |
| Welchol | colesevelam HCl |
| Wellbutrin | bupropion HCl |
| Wellbutrin SR | bupropion HCl SR |
| Wellcovorin | *leucovorin calcium* |
| Wellferon | interferon ALFA-n[1] lymphoblastoid |
| WinRho SD | $RH_O$ (D) immune globulin IV (human) |
| Winstrol | stanozolol |
| witch hazel pads | Tucks |
| Wyamine | mephentermine sulfate |
| Wycillin (for IM use only) | penicillin G procaine (for IM use only) |
| Wydase | hyaluronidase |
| Wygesic | propoxyphene HCl; acetaminophen |
| Wymox | amoxicillin |
| Wytensin | guanabenz acetate |

## XYZ

| | |
|---|---|
| Xalatan | latanoprost |
| Xanax | alprazolam |
| Xeloda | capecitabine |
| Xenical | orlistat |
| Xigris | drotrecogin alfa |
| Xopenex | levalbuterol HCl inhalation soln |
| Xylocaine HCl | lidocaine HCl |

V
R

**References**

1. Facts and Comparisons. St. Louis: Facts and Comparisons, Inc. (published monthly and online)
2. Billup NF, Billup SM. American drug index. St. Louis: Facts and Comparisons, Inc.yw (published yearly)
3. Physicians GenRx. St. Louis: Mosby. (published yearly)
4. Parfitt K. Ed. Martindale: 33rd edition. The Pharmaceutical Press. London, 2002.

# Chapter 8

## Normal Laboratory Values*

In the following tables, normal reference values for commonly requested laboratory tests are listed in traditional units and in SI units. The tables are a guideline only. Values are method dependent and "normal values" may vary between laboratories.

| Blood, Plasma or Serum | | |
|---|---|---|
| | **Reference Value** | |
| **Determination** | **Conventional Units** | **SI Units** |
| Ammonia ($NH_3$) − diffusion | 20–120 mcg/dl | 12–70 mcmol/L |
| Ammonia Nitrogen | 15–45 mcg/dl | 11–32 µmol/L |
| Amylase | 35–118 IU/L | 0.58–1.97 mckat/L |
| Anion Gap ($Na^+ − [Cl^- + HCO_3^-]$) (P) | 7–16 mEq/L | 7–16 mmol/L |
| Antinuclear antibodies | negative at 1:10 dilution of serum | negative at 1:10 dilution of serum |
| Antithrombin III (AT III) | 80–120 units/dl | 800–1200 units/L |
| Bicarbonate: Arterial  Venous | 21–28 mEq/L  22–29 mEq/L | 21–28 mmol/L  22–29 mmol/L |
| Bilirubin: Conjugated (direct)  Total | ≤0.2 mg/dl  0.1–1 mg/dl | ≤4 mcmol/L  2–18 mcmol/L |
| Calcitonin | <100 pg/mL | <100 ng/L |
| Calcium: Total  Ionized | 8.6–10.3 mg/dl  4.4–5.1 mg/dl | 2.2–2.74 mmol/L  1–1.3 mmol/L |
| Carbon dioxide content (plasma) | 21–32 mmol/L | 21–32 mmol/L |
| Carcinoembryonic antigen | <3 ng/mL | <3 mcg/L |
| Chloride | 95–110 mEq/L | 95–110 mmol/L |
| Coagulation screen:  Bleeding time  Prothrombin time  Partial thromboplastin time (activated)  Protein C  Protein S | 3–9.5 min  10–13 sec  22–37 sec  0.7–1.4 µ/mL  0.7–1.4 µ/mL | 180–570 sec  10–13 sec  22–37 sec  700–1400 units/mL  700–1400 units/mL |
| Copper, total | 70–160 mcg/dl | 11–25 mcmol/L |
| Corticotropin (ACTH adrenocorticotropic hormone) − 0800 hr | <60 pg/mL | <13.2 pmol/L |
| Cortisol: 0800 hr  1800 hr  2000 hr | 5–30 mcg/dl  2–15 mcg/dl  ≤50% of 0800 hr | 138–810 nmol/L  50–410 nmol/L  ≤50% of 0800 hr |
| Creatine kinase: Female  Male | 20–170 IU/L  30–220 IU/L | 0.33–2.83 mckat/L  0.5–3.67 mckat/L |
| Creatine kinase isoenzymes, MB fraction | 0–12 IU/L | 0–0.2 mckat/L |
| Creatinine | 0.5–1.7 mg/dl | 44–150 mcmol/L |
| Fibrinogen (coagulation factor I) | 150–360 mg/dl | 1.5–3.6 g/L |

| Blood, Plasma or Serum (Cont.) | | |
|---|---|---|
| | **Reference Value** | |
| **Determination** | **Conventional Units** | **SI Units** |
| Follicle-stimulating hormone (FSH): | | |
|   Female | 2–13 mIU/mL | 2–13 IU/L |
|   Midcycle | 5–22 mIU/mL | 5–22 IU/L |
|   Male | 1–8 mIU/mL | 1–8 IU/L |
| Glucose, fasting | 65–115 mg/dl | 3.6–6.3 mmol/L |
| Glucose Tolerance Test (Oral) | mg/dL | mmol/L |
| | Normal | Normal |
|   Fasting | 70–105 | 3.9–5.8 |
|   60 min | 120–170 | 6.7–9.4 |
|   90 min | 100–140 | 5.6–7.8 |
|   120 min | 70–120 | 3.9–6.7 |
| | Diabetic | Diabetic |
|   Fasting | >140 | >7.8 |
|   60 min | ≥200 | ≥11.1 |
|   90 min | ≥200 | ≥11.1 |
|   120 min | ≥140 | ≥7.8 |
| (γ) − Glutamyltransferase (GGT): | | |
|   Male | 9–50 units/L | 9–50 units/L |
|   Female | 8–40 units/L | 8–40 units/L |
| Haptoglobin | 44–303 mg/dl | 0.44–3.03 g/L |
| *Hematologic tests:* | | |
|   Fibrinogen | 200–400 mg/dl | 2–4 g/L |
|   Hematocrit (Hct), female | 36%–44.6% | 0.36–0.446 fraction of 1 |
|     male | 40.7%–50.3% | 0.4–0.503 fraction of 1 |
|   Hemoglobin $A_{1c}$ | 5.3%–7.5% of total Hgb | 0.053–0.075 |
|   Hemoglobin (Hb), female | 12.1–15.3 g/dl | 121–153 g/L |
|     male | 13.8–17.5 g/dl | 138–175 g/L |
|   Leukocyte count (WBC) | 3800–9800/mcl | $3.8–9.8 \times 10^9$/L |
|   Erythrocyte count (RBC), female | $3.5–5 \times 10^6$/mcl | $3.5–5 \times 10^{12}$/L |
|     male | $4.3–5.9 \times 10^6$/mcl | $4.3–5.9 \times 10^{12}$/L |
|   Mean corpuscular volume (MCV) | 80–97.6 mcm³ | 80–97.6 fl |
|   Mean corpuscular hemoglobin (MCH) | 27–33 pg/cell | 1.66–2.09 fmol/cell |
|   Mean corpuscular hemoglobin concentrate (MCHC) | 33–36 g/dl | 20.3–22 mmol/L |
|   Erythrocyte sedimentation rate (sedrate, ESR) | ≤30 mm/hr | ≤30 mm/hr |
| Erythrocyte enzymes: | $250–5000$ units/$10^6$ cells | 250–5000 mcunits/cell |
|   Glucose-6-phosphate dehydrogenase (G-6-PD) | | |
| Ferritin | 10–383 ng/mL | 23–862 pmol/L |
| Folic acid: normal | >3.1–12.4 ng/mL | 7–28.1 nmol/L |
| Platelet count | $150–450 \times 10^3$/mcl | $150–450 \times 10^9$/L |
| Reticulocytes | 0.5%–1.5% of erythrocytes | 0.005–0.015 |
| Vitamin $B_{12}$ | 223–1132 pg/mL | 165–835 pmol/L |
| Iron: Female | 30–160 mcg/dl | 5.4–31.3 mcmol/L |
|   Male | 45–160 mcg/dl | 8.1–31.3 mcmol/L |
| Iron binding capacity | 220–420 mcg/dl | 39.4–75.2 mcmol/L |
| Isocitrate Dehydrogenase | 1.2–7 units/L | 1.2–7 units/L |
| Isoenzymes | | |
|   Fraction 1 | 14%–26% of total | 0.14–0.26 fraction of total |
|   Fraction 2 | 29%–39% of total | 0.29–0.39 fraction of total |
|   Fraction 3 | 20%–26% of total | 0.20–0.26 fraction of total |
|   Fraction 4 | 8%–16% of total | 0.08–0.16 fraction of total |
|   Fraction 5 | 6%–16% of total | 0.06–0.16 fraction of total |
| Lactate dehydrogenase | 100–250 IU/L | 1.67–4.17 mckat/L |

# Normal Laboratory Values (Cont.) Blood

| Blood, Plasma or Serum (Cont.) | | |
|---|---|---|
| | **Reference Value** | |
| **Determination** | **Conventional Units** | **SI Units** |
| Lactic acid (lactate) | 6–19 mg/dl | 0.7–2.1 mmol/L |
| Lead | ≤50 mcg/dl | ≤2.41 mcmol/L |
| Lipase | 10–150 units/L | 10–150 units/L |
| *Lipids:*<br>Total Cholesterol<br>  Desirable<br>  Borderline-high<br>  High<br>LDL<br>  Desirable<br>  Borderline-high<br>  High<br>HDL (low)<br>Triglycerides<br>  Desirable<br>  Borderline-high<br>  High<br>  Very high | <br><br><200 mg/dl<br>200–239 mg/dl<br>>239 mg/dl<br><br><130 mg/dl<br>130–159 mg/dl<br>>159 mg/dl<br><35 mg/dl<br><br><200 mg/dl<br>200–400 mg/dl<br>400–1000 mg/dl<br>>1000 mg/dl | <br><br><5.2 mmol/L<br><5.2–6.2 mmol/L<br>>6.2 mmol/L<br><br><3.36 mmol/L<br>3.36–4.11 mmol/L<br>>4.11 mmol/L<br><0.91 mmol/L<br><br><2.26 mmol/L<br>2.26–4.52 mmol/L<br>4.52–11.3 mmol/L<br>>11.3 mmol/L |
| Magnesium | 1.3–2.2 mEq/L | 0.65–1.1 mmol/L |
| Osmolality | 280–300 mOsm/kg | 280–300 mmol/kg |
| Oxygen saturation (arterial) | 94%–100% | 0.94–1 fraction of 1 |
| $PCO_2$, arterial | 35–45 mm Hg | 4.7–6 kPa |
| pH, arterial | 7.35–7.45 | 7.35–7.45 |
| $PO_2$, arterial: Breathing room air[1]<br>On 100% $O_2$ | 80–105 mm Hg<br><500 mm Hg | 10.6–14 kPa |
| Phosphatase (acid), total at 37°C | 0.13–0.63 IU/L | 2.2–10.5 IU/L or<br>2.2–10.5 mckat/L |
| Phosphatase alkaline[2] | 20–130 IU/L | 20–130 IU/L or<br>0.33–2.17 mckat/L |
| Phosphorus, inorganic,[3] (phosphate) | 2.5–5 mg/dl | 0.8–1.6 mmol/L |
| Potassium | 3.5–5 mEq/L | 3.5–5 mmol/L |
| Progesterone<br>Female<br>  Follicular phase<br>  Luteal phase<br>Male | <br>0.1–1.5 ng/mL<br>0.1–1.5 ng/mL<br>2.5–28 ng/mL<br><0.5 ng/mL | <br>0.32–4.8 nmol/L<br>0.32–4.8 nmol/L<br>8–89 nmol/L<br><1.6 nmol/L |
| Prolactin | 1.4–24.2 ng/mL | 1.4–24.2 mcg/L |
| Prostate specific antigen<br>Protein: Total<br>  Albumin<br>  Globulin | 0–4 ng/mL<br>6–8 g/dl<br>3.6–5 g/dl<br>2.3–3.5 g/dl | 0–4 ng/mL<br>60–80 g/L<br>36–50 g/L<br>23–35 g/L |
| Rheumatoid factor | <60 IU/mL | <60 kIU/L |
| Sodium | 135–147 mEq/L | 135–147 mmol/L |
| Testosterone: Female<br>Male | 6–86 ng/dl<br>270–1070 ng/dl | 0.21–3 nmol/L<br>9.3–37 nmol/L |

[1]Age dependent
[2]Infants and adolescents up to 104 IU/L
[3]Infants in the first year up to 6 mg/dl

## Normal Laboratory Values (Cont.) Blood

| Blood, Plasma or Serum (Cont.) | | |
|---|---|---|
| | **Reference Value** | |
| **Determination** | **Conventional Units** | **SI Units** |
| *Thyroid Hormone Function Tests:*<br>Thyroid-stimulating hormone (TSH)<br>Thyroxine-binding globulin capacity<br>Total triiodothyronine ($T_3$)<br>Total thyroxine by RIA ($T_4$)<br>$T_3$ resin uptake | 0.35–6.2 mcU/mL<br>10–26 mcg/dl<br>75–220 ng/dl<br>4–11 mcg/dl<br>25%–38% | 0.35–6.2 mU/L<br>100–260 mcg/L<br>1.2–3.4 nmol/L<br>51–142 nmol/L<br>0.25–0.38 fraction of 1 |
| Transaminase, AST (aspartate aminotransferase, SGOT) | 11–47 IU/L | 0.18–0.78 mckat/L |
| Transaminase, ALT (alanine aminotransferase, SGPT) | 7–53 IU/L | 0.12–0.88 mckat/L |
| Transferrin | 220–400 mg/dL | 2.20–4.00 g/L |
| Urea nitrogen (BUN) | 8–25 mg/dl | 2.9–8.9 mmol/L |
| Uric acid | 3–8 mg/dl | 179–476 mcmol/L |
| Vitamin A (retinol) | 15–60 mcg/dl | 0.52–2.09 mcmol/L |
| Zinc | 50–150 mcg/dl | 7.7–23 mcmol/L |

## Normal Laboratory Values—Urine

| Urine | | |
|---|---|---|
| | **Reference Value** | |
| **Determination** | **Conventional Units** | **SI Units** |
| Calcium[1] | 50–250 mcg/day | 1.25–6.25 mmol/day |
| *Catecholamines:* Epinephrine<br>Norepinephrine | <20 mcg/day<br><100 mcg/day | <109 nmol/day<br><590 nmol/day |
| Catecholamines, 24-hr | <110 mcg | <650 nmol |
| Copper[1] | 15–60 mcg/day | 0.24–0.95 mcmol/day |
| Creatinine: Child<br>Adolescent<br>Female<br>Male | 8–22 mg/kg<br>8–30 mg/kg<br>0.6–1.5 g/day<br>0.8–1.8 g/day | 71–195 μmol/kg<br>71–265 μmol/kg<br>5.3–13.3 mmol/day<br>7.1–15.9 mmol/day |
| pH | 4.5–8 | 4.5–8 |
| Phosphate[1] | 0.9–1.3 g/day | 29–42 mmol/day |
| Potassium[1] | 25–100 mEq/day | 25–100 mmol/day |
| Protein<br>Total<br>At rest | 1–14 mg/dL<br>50–80 mg/day | 10–140 mg/L<br>50–80 mg/day |
| Protein, quantitative | <150 mg/day | <0.15 g/day |
| Sodium[1] | 100–250 mEq/day | 100–250 mmol/day |
| Specific Gravity, random | 1.002–1.030 | 1.002–1.030 |
| Uric Acid, 24-hr | 250–750 mg | 1.48–4.43 mmol |

[1]Diet dependent

## Normal Laboratory Values—Drug Levels

| | | Drug Levels† | |
|---|---|---|---|
| | | **Reference Value** | |
| | **Drug Determination** | **Conventional Units** | **SI Units** |
| *Aminoglycosides* | Amikacin | | |
| | (trough) | 1–8 mcg/mL | 1.7–13.7 mcmol/L |
| | (peak) | 20–30 mcg/mL | 34–51 mcmol/L |
| | Gentamicin | | |
| | (trough) | 0.5–2 mcg/mL | 1–4.2 mcmol/L |
| | (peak) | 6–10 mcg/mL | 12.5–20.9 mcmol/L |
| | Kanamycin | | |
| | (trough) | 5–10 mcg/mL | nd |
| | (peak) | 20–25 mcg/mL | nd |
| | Netilmicin | | |
| | (trough) | 0.5–2 mcg/mL | nd |
| | (peak) | 6–10 mcg/mL | nd |
| | Streptomycin | | |
| | (trough) | <5 mcg/mL | nd |
| | (peak) | 5–20 mcg/mL | nd |
| | Tobramycin | | |
| | (trough) | 0.5–2 mcg/mL | 1.1–4.3 mcmol/L |
| | (peak) | 5–20 mcg/mL | 12.8–21.8 mcmol/L |
| *Antiarrhythmics* | Amiodarone | 0.5–2.5 mcg/mL | 1.5–4 mcmol/L |
| | Bretylium | 0.5–1.5 mcg/mL | nd |
| | Digitoxin | 9–25 mcg/L | 11.8–32.8 nmol/L |
| | Digoxin | 0.8–2 ng/mL | 0.9–2.5 nmol/L |
| | Disopyramide | 2–8 mcg/mL | 6–18 mcmol/L |
| | Flecainide | 0.2–1 mcg/mL | nd |
| | Lidocaine | 1.5–6 mcg/mL | 4.5–21.5 mcmol/L |
| | Mexiletine | 0.5–2 mcg/mL | nd |
| | Procainamide | 4–8 mcg/mL | 17–34 mcmol/mL |
| | Propranolol | 50–200 ng/mL | 190–770 nmol/L |
| | Quinidine | 2–6 mcg/mL | 4.6–9.2 mcmol/L |
| | Tocainide | 4–10 mcg/mL | nd |
| | Verapamil | 0.08–0.3 mcg/mL | nd |
| *Anti-convulsants* | Carbamazepine | 4–12 mcg/mL | 17–51 mcmol/L |
| | Phenobarbital | 10–40 mcg/mL | 43–172 mcmol/L |
| | Phenytoin | 10–20 mcg/mL | 40–80 mcmol/L |
| | Primidone | 4–12 mcg/mL | 18–55 mcmol/L |
| | Valproic acid | 40–100 mcg/mL | 280–700 mcmol/L |
| *Antidepressants* | Amitriptyline | 110–250 ng/mL[3] | 500–900 nmol/L |
| | Amoxapine | 200–500 ng/mL | nd |
| | Bupropion | 25–100 ng/mL | nd |
| | Clomipramine | 80–100 ng/mL | nd |
| | Desipramine | 115–300 ng/mL | nd |
| | Doxepin | 110–250 ng/mL[3] | nd |
| | Imipramine | 225–350 ng/mL[3] | nd |
| | Maprotiline | 200–300 ng/mL | nd |
| | Nortriptyline | 50–150 ng/mL | nd |
| | Protriptyline | 70–250 ng/mL | nd |
| | Trazodone | 800–1600 ng/mL | nd |
| *Antipsychotics* | Chlorpromazine | 50–300 ng/mL | 150–950 nmol/L |
| | Fluphenazine | 0.13–2.8 ng/mL | nd |
| | Haloperidol | 5–20 ng/mL | nd |
| | Perphenazine | 0.8–1.2 ng/mL | nd |
| | Thiothixene | 2–57 ng/mL | nd |

†The values given are generally accepted as desirable for treatment without toxicity for most patients. However, exceptions are not uncommon.
[3]Parent drug plus N-desmethy7l metabolite
nd — No data available

## Normal Laboratory Values (Cont.) Drug Levels

| Drug Levels† | | | |
|---|---|---|---|
| | | Reference Value | |
| | Drug Determination | Conventional Units | SI Units |
| *Miscellaneous* | Amantadine | 300 ng/mL | nd |
| | Amrinone | 3.7 mcg/mL | nd |
| | Chloramphenicol | 10–20 mcg/mL | 31–62 mcmol/L |
| | Cyclosporine[1] | 250–800 ng/mL (whole blood, RIA) | nd |
| | | 50–300 ng/mL (plasma, RIA) | nd |
| | Ethanol[2] | 0 mg/dl | 0 mmol/L |
| | Hydralazine | 100 ng/mL | nd |
| | Lithium | 0.6–1.2 mEq/L | 0.6–1.2 mmol/L |
| | Salicylate | 100–300 mg/L | 724–2172 mcmol/L |
| | Sulfonamide | 5–15 mg/dl | nd |
| | Terbutaline | 0.5–4.1 ng/mL | nd |
| | Theophylline | 10–20 mcg/mL | 55–110 mcmol/L |
| | Vancomycin | | |
| | (trough) | 5–15 ng/mL | nd |
| | (peak) | 20–40 mcg/mL | nd |

†The values given are generally accepted as desirable for treatment without toxicity for most patients. However, exceptions are not uncommon.
[1]24 hour trough values
[2]Toxic: 50–100 mg/dl (10.9–21.7 mmol/L)

# Reorder and Prices for the 11th Edition

Medical Abbreviations: 24,000 Conveniences at the
Expense of Communications and Safety
by Neil M Davis
(ISBN 0-931431-11-5)

| 1–24 copies | $24.95 each plus S&H |
|---|---|
| 25 or more copies | $17.50 each plus S&H |

Plus U.S. Shipping and Handling Charges

| Number of Books Ordered | U.S. S&H charges to be added to each **order** |
|---|---|
| 1 | $5.00 + price shown above |
| 2 | $7.00 + price shown above |
| 3–6 | $9.00 + price shown above |
| 7–11 | $12.00 + price shown above |
| 12–25 | $16.00 + price shown above |
| 26–50 | $28.00 + price shown above |
| 51 or more | $42.00 + price shown above |

Orders shipped to Pennsylvania must add 6% sales tax.
No sales tax for other states (subject to change).
Purchase orders are accepted.

**Payable by–**

| Visa | MasterCard | Discover |
|---|---|---|
| American Exp. | Check | Money Order |

**Order from and make check payable to–**

Neil M. Davis Associates
1143 Wright Drive
Huntingdon Valley PA 19006-2721

**Orders may be mailed to above address or**

**Phone**   215 947 1752 (9 AM–4:30 PM EST, MON–FRI)
**Fax**   215 938 1937
**Secure Web site**   www.medabbrev.com
**E-mail**   med@neilmdavis.com

Where applicable, please have ready credit card number and
expiration date, phone number, and mailing address. A PO
box address is not acceptable for orders as they are shipped
via UPS.

# Reorder and Price Information—continued

## Outside of the United States

- Pay by credit card (VISA, MasterCard, Discover, American Express), or in U.S. dollars through a corresponding U.S. bank, or an International Money Order in U.S. currency.
- Prices as shown on the previous page plus shipping costs.
- To obtain shipping cost, fax query to 1 215 938 1937 or E-mail to med@neilmdavis.com

### Information Needed on Order Form

PLEASE PRINT OR TYPE

Name _____

Address (PO Box addresses not acceptable) _____

_____

City _____ State _____ Zip Code _____

Phone ( ) _____

Attention (If Applicable) _____

Number of copies ordered _____ PO # (If Applicable) _____

Method of payment:

_____ Check or money order enclosed

_____ Visa          _____ MasterCard

_____ Discover     _____ American Express

Card Number _____

Exp. Date _____

Cardholder's Name _____

Signature _____

## Internet Access

Each book purchased includes, at no extra cost, a single-user access license for the website version of this 11th edition, which is updated monthly. This license is valid for 24 months from the date of the initial log-in. Multi-User Site Licenses are available. To obtain a copy of the Multi-User Site License, fax request to 1 215 938 1937 or E-mail to med@neilmdavis.com

## To Order the PDA Versions

Palm OS or Pocket PC PDA versions of "Medical Abbreviations: 24,000 Conveniences at the Expense of Communications and Safety," the 11th edition, 2003, by Neil M Davis, are available from Lexi-Comp Inc., at either:

| | |
|---|---|
| Their website | www.lexi.com |
| Phone | 1 800 837 5394 |
| Fax | 330 656 4308 |

The PDA versions are updated with 80-120 new entries per month. The Palm version is approximately 1.7MB. The Pocket PC version is approximately 2.2MB.

**Pricing:** If you list on the Lexi-Comp website order form or mention on the telephone or FAX order, the Promotion Code **"KT8BK"** you will be given a 10% discount, lowering the price to $31.50 for one year. The normal price is $35.00.

## Additions

Please forward additional meanings for these abbreviations, additional abbreviations and their meanings, or corrections to the author so that the web-version, PDA versions, and book can be updated. Thank you. Dr. Neil M Davis, 1143 Wright Drive, Huntingdon Valley, PA 19006. FAX (215) 938 1937. E-mail med@neilmdavis.com

_____

_____

_____

_____

_____

_____

_____

_____

_____

_____

_____

_____

_____

# Additions